AF344431

General Surgery/GI Words and Phrases

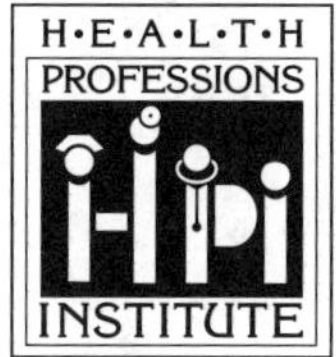

Health Professions Institute • Modesto, California • 2001

General Surgery/GI Words and Phrases

Developed by

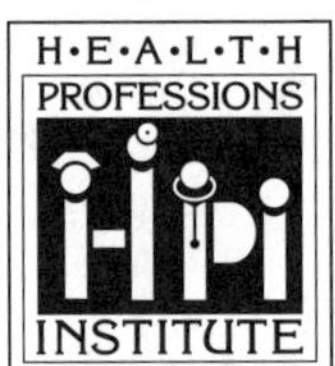

Sally C. Pitman
Editor & Publisher
Health Professions Institute
P. O. Box 801
Modesto, CA 95353-0801
Phone 209-551-2112
Fax 209-551-0404
Web site: http://www.hpisum.com
E-mail: hpi@hpisum.com

Printed by
Parks Printing & Lithograph
Modesto, California

ISBN 0-934385-36-X
Last digit is the print number: 9 8 7 6 5 4 3 2 1

In loving memory

of Rose Moore

Preface

In today's fast-paced, high-tech society, the quest to improve healthcare documentation is an ongoing challenge. Medical breakthroughs, new surgical techniques, and advances in pharmacology have given way to thousands of new medical terms. Every procedure must be documented in detail, each surgery described accurately, and every drug spelled correctly.

To stay abreast of the ever-changing world of healthcare documentation, it is vital to have direct access to the most accurate, comprehensive, up-to-date references. To this end we have produced *General Surgery/GI Words and Phrases,* truly a milestone in excellence and value.

General Surgery/GI Words and Phrases combines terminology from general surgery practice—a vast field in and of itself—with a multitude of terms from gastroenterology. Over 60,000 entries make word researching easier and more accurate for the production-oriented healthcare professional who needs help with general surgery instruments and devices; anatomic landmarks; dressings and bandages; wound management; gastroenterology practice (conditions, diseases, diagnosis, treatment); gastrointestinal surgery; hernia surgery; bariatric surgery; minimally invasive surgery; endoscopic and laparoscopic surgery; intra-abdominal transplantation; colorectal surgery; surgical oncology; trauma surgery; endocrinology practice (conditions, diseases, diagnosis, treatment); endocrine surgery; breast conditions and surgery; and breast devices.

A special feature in this edition is the Appendix with Tables of Arteries, Muscles, and Veins. Medical transcriptionists especially will appreciate listings of these common anatomic structures in both English and their Latin equivalents.

General Surgery/GI Words and Phrases is extensively cross-referenced to assure greater success in finding a desired word or phrase. Terms were gathered from thousands of actual surgical and gastrointestinal transcripts, from medical journals and textbooks, and through extensive research on the Internet.

Research for this second edition was done primarily by Linda C. Campbell, CMT; Georgia Green, CMT; and Diane S. Heath, CMT. Our warmest gratitude is also extended to those readers who called or wrote with comments and suggestions; this book is better because of their feedback.

Sally C. Pitman, M.A.
Editor & Publisher

How to Use This Book

The words and phrases in this book are alphabetized letter by letter of all words in the entry, ignoring punctuation marks and words or letters in parentheses. The possessive form ('s) is omitted from eponyms for ease in alphabetizing. Numbers are alphabetized as if written out, with the exception of subscripts and superscripts which are ignored.

Eponyms appear alphabetically as well as under the nouns they modify. For example, *Wise areola mastopexy breast augmentation (WAMBA)* is found alphabetically in the W's as well as under the main entries *mammoplasty* and *operation*. *Gastrografin* is found in the G's as well as under *imaging agent* and *medications*. The names of hundreds of medications used in general surgery and gastroenterology included in this book appear under the entry *medications*. Names of instruments appear under individual main entries like *catheter* and *forceps*, and in addition various kinds of technology are listed under the broad terms *device* and *system*.

In medical dictation physicians may arbitrarily refer to an operative procedure as an *approach*, *method*, *operation*, *procedure*, *repair*, or *technique*, or by the type of procedure, such as *gastrostomy* and *herniorrhaphy*. Thus, all procedures are listed alphabetically by the eponym, such as *Payne-DeWind jejunoileal bypass*, as well as under the type of procedure and under the main entry *operations*.

Many anatomical terms are found in the book, but no attempt was made to be comprehensive. The Appendix includes Tables of Arteries, Muscles, and Veins, with both English and Latin forms in tabular form for quick reference.

Main entries with a lengthy list of subentries include the following:

anesthesia	flap	operation
bandage	forceps	plate
biopsy	graft	retractor
blade	hernia	rongeur
cannula	hook	scissors
carcinoma	imaging	stent
catheter	incision	suture
clamp	knife	syndrome
device	laser	system
disease	lesion	test
dressing	medications	tube
elevator	nail	tumor
endoscope	needle	view

A, a

AA (acetabular anteversion)
AA (Alcoholics Anonymous)
AAA (aromatic amino acid)
AAA ("triple A") (abdominal aortic aneurysm)
Aagenaes syndrome (cholestasis-lymphedema syndrome)
AAI (axial acetabular index)
Aaron sign
Aarskog syndrome
AASLD (American Association for the Study of Liver Diseases)
Aastrom CPS (cell-production system)
abarelix
abate, abatement
Abbe operation
ABBI (advanced breast biopsy instrumentation) system
Abbokinase (urokinase)
Abbott esophagogastrostomy
Abbott gouge
Abbott-Miller tube
Abbott pump
Abbott-Rawson double-lumen gastrointestinal tube
Abbott tube
Abbreviated Injury Scale (AIS)
ABC (airway, breathing, circulation)

ABC (argon beam coagulator)
ABCD (amphotericin B colloid dispersion)
abdomen
    accordion
    acute
    acute surgical
    apertures of
    boardlike rigidity of
    boatlike
    boat-shaped
    concave
    diffusely tender
    distended
    doughy
    dull to percussion
    exquisitely tender
    fascia of
    flabby
    flat
    flat plate of
    free air in
    guarding of
    hyperdistended
    hyperresonant
    nondistended
    postlymphangiography
    postsurgical

abdomen *(cont.)*
  protuberant
  prune-belly
  resonant
  roof of
  rotund
  scaphoid
  silent
  soft
  splinting of
  surgical
  tight
  tympanitic
abdomen closed in anatomical layers
abdomen was deflated and laparoscope
  removed
abdominal abscess (see *abscess*)
abdominal angina
abdominal aorta
abdominal aortic aneurysm (AAA)
abdominal aortic artery
abdominal aortic plexus
abdominal aponeurosis
abdominal apron
abdominal bandage
abdominal binder
abdominal brace position
abdominal canal
abdominal cavity
abdominal colectomy
abdominal colic
abdominal compartment syndrome
  (ACS)
abdominal contents
abdominal cramp
abdominal distention
abdominal exploration
abdominal fat
abdominal fat pad
abdominal fissure
abdominal fistula
abdominal flap
abdominal fluid wave
abdominalgia, periodic

abdominal girth
abdominal impalement
abdominal incision dehiscence
abdominal iron deposition
abdominal kidney
abdominal lap (laparotomy) pad
abdominal lavage
abdominal lymph node
abdominal lymphatics
abdominal mass
abdominal migraine (cyclic vomiting
  syndrome)
abdominal muscle
abdominal muscle deficiency syndrome
  (prune-belly syndrome)
abdominal ostium
abdominal pad
abdominal panniculus
abdominal paracentesis
abdominal-perineal resection
abdominal peritoneum
abdominal pool
abdominal pregnancy
abdominal pull-through
abdominal pulse
abdominal raphe
abdominal rectopexy
abdominal reflex
abdominal region
abdominal retractor
abdominal rigidity
abdominal ring
abdominal sac
abdominal-sacral colpoperineopexy
abdominal scissors
abdominal scoop
abdominal section
abdominal situs inversus
abdominal stoma
abdominal stool
abdominal tap
Abdominal Trauma Index (ATI)
abdominal trocar
abdominal ultrasound

abdominal vascular accident
abdominal view
abdominal viscus (pl. viscera)
abdominal wall, elevation of
abdominal wall fistula
abdominal wall hernia
abdominal wall venous pattern
abdominal x-ray (AXR)
abdominal x-ray and computed
    tomography (AXR/CT)
abdominal zone
abdominis rectus muscle
abdominis transversus muscle
abdominocardiac reflex
abdominogenital
abdominojugular reflux
abdominopelvic abscess
abdominopelvic cavity
abdominopelvic mass
abdominopelvic viscera
abdominoperineal or abdominal-
    perineal resection (APR)
abdominoperineal proctectomy
abdominoscrotal
abdominothoracic arch
abdominovaginal
abdominovesical
ABD pad dressing
Abel scissors
Aberdeen knot suture
Abernethy sarcoma
aberrant goiter
aberrant pancreas
aberrant umbilical stomach
aberrant vessel
ABGs (arterial blood gases)
A bile
Ablatherm HIFU (high-intensity
    focused ultrasound) system
ablation
    celiac alcohol
    endoscopic
    endoscopic mucosal
    heater probe

ablation *(cont.)*
    laparoscopic uterine nerve
    laser
    laser uterosacral nerve (LUNA)
    Livewire TC
    percutaneous
    photothermal laser
    radioiodide
    radioiodine
    thermal
    thyroid
ablation catheter
ablation of tumor
ablative laser therapy
ablator
    Concept
    R.F. tissue
    Sonablate 200 tissue
ablepharon-macrostomia syndrome
    (AMS)
ABMTR (Autologous Bone Marrow
    Transplant Registry)
abnormal bleeding
abnormal clotting
abnormal feeding blood vessel
abnormality (pl. abnormalities)
    anatomic
    bleeding
    clotting
    DNA ploidy
    electrolyte
    mucosal
    persistent breast
    skeletal
    small-bowel congenital
abnormal mammographic findings
ABP (acute biliary pancreatitis)
abraded wound
Abrami disease
Abrams biopsy needle
Abrams needle
Abramson catheter
Abrikosov tumor

abscess (pl. abscesses)
   abdominal
   abdominopelvic
   actinomycotic brain
   acute
   amebic or amoebic
   amebic liver
   amoebic or amebic
   anal
   anorectal
   appendiceal
   arthrifluent
   Aspergillus cerebral
   atraumatic
   bacterial
   bone
   bowel
   brain
   breast
   Brodie metaphyseal
   cerebral
   chronic subareolar
   collar button
   colonic
   crypt
   cuff
   daughter
   debridement of
   deep
   deep interloop
   drainage of palate
   draining
   echinococcal
   encapsulated brain
   entamebic
   enteroperitoneal
   epidural
   epiploon
   extradural
   extraperitoneal
   fluctuant
   frontal
   fungal
   gallbladder wall

abscess *(cont.)*
   gas-forming liver
   growth plate
   hepatic
   Highmore
   horseshoe
   incision & drainage (I&D) of
   interloop
   intersphincteric
   intra-abdominal
   intractable
   intradural
   intrahepatic
   intramesenteric
   intramural
   intramuscular
   intraosseous
   intraperitoneal
   ischiorectal
   kidney
   liver
   local
   localized
   lumbar epidural
   mesenteric
   metaphyseal
   midpalmar
   missile track
   necrotic
   nonpuerperal breast
   omental
   Paget
   pancreatic
   paracolic
   pararectal
   parasitic
   parotid
   parumbilical
   pelvic
   pelvirectal
   perianal
   periappendiceal
   pericecal
   pericholecystic

access *(cont.)*
  transjugular
  transjugular liver
  transcervical tubal
  transcutaneous
  transperitoneal aortic
  vascular
  venous
  ventricular
accessible lesion
accessory breast
accessory gland
accessory nipple
accessory pancreas
accessory pancreatic duct
accessory spleen
accessory trocar
accommodation reflex
accordion abdomen
accordion sign
Accu-Chek Advantage blood glucose monitor
Accu-Chek Complete blood glucose monitor
Accu-Chek Compass glucose management software
Accu-Chek Easy blood glucose monitor
Accu-Chek Instant blood glucose monitor
Accu-Chek Instant Plus blood glucose monitor
Accu-Chek Simplicity blood glucose monitor
Accu-Chek II Freedom blood glucose monitor
Accu-Chek Voicemate blood glucose monitor
Accucore II core biopsy needle
accuDEXA bone mineral density assessment device
Accu-Flo dura film
Accu-Flo ventricular catheter
AccuGuide injection monitor
AccuLase excimer laser

Accu-Line guide
Acculink self-expanding (carotid) stent
Acculite Contour Tip endoprobe
AccuPort seal
Accuprep HPF powder
AccuProbe 600 cryotherapy probe
AccuSpan tissue expander
Accutom low-speed diamond saw
Accuzyme enzymatic debriding ointment
Ace adherent bandage
Acephen (acetaminophen) analgesic suppository
Aceta (acetaminophen)
Aceta with Codeine (codeine phosphate; acetaminophen)
acetabular cup detaching rod
acetabular cup push (pushing) rod
acetabular guide
acetabular knife
acetabular reamer
acetabular reconstruction plate
acetabuloplastic round chisel
acetaminophen overdose
acetaminophen poisoning
acetohexamide
achalasia
  classic
  cricopharyngeal
  esophageal
  pelvirectal
  sphincteral
  vigorous
Achard-Thiers syndrome
Achiever balloon dilatation catheter
achlorhydria
  gastric
  histamine-resistant
achlorhydric
acholangic biliary cirrhosis
acholic stool
acholuric jaundice
achondroplastic dwarfism
achylia gastrica

achylia pancreatica
acid
  arachidonic
  aromatic amino (AAA)
  bile
  branched chain amino (BCAA)
  carbonic
  caustic
  chenodeoxycholic
  choleic
  conjugated bile
  essential fatty (EFA)
  fecal bile (FBA)
  folinic
  gastric
  hepatoiminodiacetic (HIDA)
  hydrochloric
  intraesophageal
  intraluminal
  isovaleric
  medium chain fatty (MCFA)
  short chain fatty (SCFA)
  ursodeoxycholic
acid base imbalance
acid clearance test (ACT)
acid cell
acid dyspepsia
acidemia, isovaleric
acid-fast bacillus (AFB)
acid-fast bacteria
acid-fast organism
acid gland
acid hypersecretion
acidification of stool test
acidophilic adenoma
acidophilic body
acidophilus capsule
acidophilus milk
Acidose-Aqua
acidosis
  compensated
  diabetic
  hyperchloremic metabolic
  hypochloremic metabolic

acidosis *(cont.)*
  hypokalemic metabolic
  hypovolemia-induced metabolic
  ketoacidosis
  lactic
  metabolic
  normochloremic
  persistent
  pure respiratory
  renal tubular
  respiratory
  severe
  starvation
  uncompensated
acid-pepsin reflux esophagitis
acid peptic disease
acid peptic disorder
acid peptic juice
acid peptic ulcer
acid perfusion test
acid reflux disease
acid reflux test
acid regurgitation
acid-related disorder (ARD)
acid suppression
Acidulin (glutamic acid hydrochloride)
acid water, electrolyzed
Acier stainless steel suture
acinar cell
acinarization
acinar tissue
Acinetobacter calcoaceticus var. *lwoffi*
  (formerly *Mima polymorpha*)
acinous adenoma
acinous cell carcinoma
Aciphex (rabeprazole sodium) proton
  pump inhibitor
Ackland mouth gag
Acland-Banis arteriotomy set
Acland clamp-applying forceps
Acland microvascular clamp
ACL drill guide
ACL graft
ACMI Martin endoscopy forceps

ACMI monopolar electrode
ACMI rigid laparoscope
ACMI ulcer measuring device
AC137 analog of human amylin used with insulin
acorn-tipped bougie
acorn treatment
acoustic papilla
acoustic shadowing (in ultrasonography)
acoustic window
acquired benign adrenal androgenic overactivity
acquired disorder of coagulation
acquired esophagocele
acquired hemolytic jaundice
acquired hernia
acquired hypothyroidism
acquired immunodeficiency syndrome (AIDS)
acquired lactose deficiency
acquired lesion
acquired megacolon
acquired reflex
ACR (adenomatosis of colon and rectum)
Acra-Cut wire pass drill
acral lentiginous melanoma
Acremonium falciform
Acremonium kiliense
Acremonium recifei
acrodermatitis enteropathica (AE)
Acro-Lase Plus
AcroMed VSP plate
acromegaly
acroparesthesia
AcryDerm border island dressing
AcryDerm Sheet dressing
AcryDerm Strands dressing
ACS (abdominal compartment syndrome)
ACS Concorde catheter
ACS Endura coronary dilation catheter
ACS Hi-Torque Balance Middleweight guidewire

ACS Multi-Link OTW (over-the-wire) Duet stent
ACS:180 BR breast cancer screening test
ACS OTW (over-the-wire) Lifestream coronary dilatation catheter
ACS OTW (over-the-wire) Photon catheter
ACS RX Comet coronary dilatation catheter
ACS RX Multi-Link coronary stent
ACS SULP II balloon
ACS Tourguide II guiding catheter
ACT (acid clearance test)
ACT (activated clotting time)
Actalyke ACT (activating clotting test)
ACTH (adrenocorticotropic hormone) deficiency
Acticoat burn dressing
Acticoat foam dressing
Acticon neosphincter implantable prosthesis
ACTID (analgesic cell therapy implantable device)
Actidose Aqua (activated charcoal)
Actidose with Sorbital (activated charcoal; sorbital)
Actifoam collagen sponge
Actigall (ursodiol-ursodeoxycholic acid)
Actimmune (interferon gamma-1b)
actinomycotic brain abscess
Actiprep skin preparation
Actiq lozenge ("lollipop") oral transmucosal fentanyl citrate
activated attapulgite
activated charcoal
activated clotting time (ACT)
activated coagulation time
activated partial thromboplastin time (APTT)
activated thromboplastin time (ATT)
active bowel sounds
active duodenal ulcer
Active Life barrier
active source of bleeding

actively bleeding varices
activity tolerance
Actos (pioglitazone hydrochloride)
Actron (ketoprofen) pain reliever
Acucise retrograde procedure
ACU-derm wound dressing
ACU-dyne ointment
ACU-dyne wash
Acufex bioabsorbable Suretac suture
   and anchor
Acufex convex rasp
Acufex curved basket forceps
Acufex distractor pin
Acufex double-lumen cannula
Acufex gouge
Acufex mallet
Acufex nerve hook
Acufex probe
Acufex rasp
Acufex rotary biting basket forceps
Acufex rotary punch
Acufex scissors
Acufex TAG rod
Acufex T-fix suture anchor
Acufex tibial guide
Acumed suture anchor
AcuNav ultrasound catheter
acupuncture anesthesia
acupuncture laser
Acuson Aspen ultrasound system
acute abdomen
acute abdominal series
acute abdominal vascular disease
acute abscess
acute alcoholism
acute appendicitis
acute biliary pancreatitis (ABP)
acute cholangitis
acute cholecystitis
acute diverticulitis
acute erosive gastritis (AEG)
acute fatty liver of pregnancy
acute gallstone pancreatitis
acute gastritis

acute gastroenteritis (AGE)
acute hemorrhagic gastritis
acute hemorrhagic pancreatitis
acute hepatocellular degeneration
acute hypersensitivity reaction
acute idiopathic inflammatory bowel
   disease
acute infectious colitis
acute infectious diarrhea
acute infectious gastroenteritis
acute intermittent porphyria (AIP)
acute interstitial pancreatitis
acute juvenile cirrhosis
acute malaria
acute mononucleosis-like hepatitis
acute obstructive cholangitis
acute pancreatitis
acute parenchymatous hepatitis
acute peptic ulcer
acute porphyria
acute proctitis
acute prostatitis
acute sclerosing hyaline necrosis
   (ASHN)
acute self-limited colitis (ASLC)
acute septic splenitis
acute surgical abdomen
acute tubular necrosis
acute viral hepatitis (AVH)
Acutrainer for urinary incontinence
Acutrim
acyl-CoA dehydrogenase deficiency,
   long-chain
ad lib. (L. *ad libitum*, freely; at
   pleasure)
ADA (American Diabetes Association)
ADA (American Dietetic Association)
Adair-Allis forceps
Adair breast clamp
Adair clamp
Adair forceps
Adair tenaculum
Adams-DeWeese vena caval clip
Adams saw

adapter
  Carlens tube
  clip
  diamond Ohio
  DISS body
  dual irrigation
  Lamis
  open laparoscopy cannula
  VCS clip
Adaptic dressing
Adaptic packing
adaptive colitis
ADCC (antibody-dependent cell-mediated cytotoxicity)
Adcon-A
Adcon-C
Adcon-I
Adcon-L gel
Adcon-P adhesion control barrier
Adcon-P solution
Adcon-T/N gel
Addison disease
addisonian crisis
Addison point
AddOn-Bucky imaging device
adefovir dipivoxil
ADEKs multivitamin pediatric supplement
adelomorphous cell
adenitis, mesenteric
adenocarcinoma
  annular
  colloid
  esophageal
  exophytic
  gastric
  giant cell
  infiltrating
  malignant mucoid
  papillary
  prostate
  scirrhous
  tubular
  ulcerating

adenocystic carcinoma
adenoid cystic carcinoma
adenoid pattern
adenoid squamous cell carcinoma
adenoma
  acidophilic
  acinous
  ACTH-producing
  adnexal
  adrenocortical
  apocrine
  basal cell
  basophilic
  benign liver
  benign solitary
  bile duct (BDA)
  bronchial
  canalicular
  chromophil
  chromophobe
  colloid
  colonic
  embryonal
  eosinophil
  fibroid
  follicular
  Fuchs
  gallbladder
  gonadotropin-producing
  growth hormone-producing
  hepatic
  hepatocellular (HCA)
  Hürthle (Huerthle) cell
  islet cell
  lactating
  Leydig cell
  liver cell
  macrofollicular
  microfollicular
  moderately differentiated
  monomorphic
  mucinous
  nephrogenic
  nipple

adenoma *(cont.)*
  null cell
  ovarian tubular
  oxyphil
  pancreatic
  papillary cystic
  Pick tubular
  pituitary
  pleomorphic
  polypoid
  poorly differentiated
  prolactin-producing
  prostatic
  renal cortical
  sessile
  solitary benign
  testicular tubular
  thyroid
  thyrotropin-producing
  tubular
  tubulovillous
  undifferentiated
  villoglandular
  villous
  well-differentiated
adenoma prevention with celecoxib
  (APC) study
adenomatosis of colon and rectum
  (ACR)
adenomatous goiter
adenomatous hyperplasia (AH)
adenomatous polyp
adenomatous polyposis coli (APC)
adenomatous polyposis coli, familial
adenomatous polyposis coli gene
adenomyoma of gallbladder
adenomyomatosis
adenopapillomatosis, gastric
adenopathy
  axillary
  cervical
  inguinal
  lymph node

adenopathy *(cont.)*
  palpable
  paraductal
  splenic hilar
adenosquamous carcinoma
adenoviral p53 gene
adenovirus, enteric
adenovirus infection
adenovirus test kit
Adenovirus EIA test kit
Adept (icodextrin) antiadhesion solution
ADH (alcohol dehydrogenase)
ADH (antidiuretic hormone)
adhesion
  attic
  bandlike
  banjo-string
  bleb-like
  cell-cell
  dense
  fibrinous
  fibrous
  filmy
  freeing up of
  hard
  intra-abdominal
  intraperitoneal
  lysis of
  meningeal
  mesenteric
  omental
  pelvic
  pericholecystic
  peritoneal
  postop
  primary
  secondary
  takedown of
  taking down of
  thick
  thin
  tight
  violin-string

adhesive (see also *bandage*; *cement*;
    dressing; *glue*)
  APR cement fixation
  Aron Alpha
  autologous fibrin tissue (AFTA)
  BEMA (bioerodible mucoadhesive)
  benzoin
  Biobrane
  Bioerodible Mucoadhesive (BEMA)
  BioGlue surgical
  CicaCare topical gel sheeting
  Coe-pak paste
  Comfeel skin
  CoSeal resorbable synthetic sealant
  CoStasis
  Coverlet
  Cover-Roll gauze
  Colly-Seel
  cyanoacrylate (Superglue) tissue
  Dermabond topical skin
  Dynastat
  EMLA anesthetic disc
  Fibrijet
  fibrin glue
  fibrin sealant
  FloSeal matrix hemostatic sealant
  FocalSeal-S surgical sealant
  gelatin-resorcin-formalin tissue glue
  HemaMyst aerosol
  Hemaseel APR fibrin
  Hemaseel HMN biological tissue
    glue
  HemaSyst sealant
  Histoacryl Blue (HAB) tissue
    adhesive
  Histoacryl glue (cyanoacrylate)
    tissue
  hydroxyapatite (HA)
  Implast bone cement
  Indermil topical tissue
  isobutyl 2-cyanoacrylate (IBC) tissue
  ligand
  LPPS hydroxyapatite
  medical

adhesive *(cont.)*
  methyl methacrylate
  Palacos cement
  Proceed hemostatic surgical sealant
  ReliaSeal skin barrier
  Simplex
  Soothe-N-Seal
  Superglue (cyanoacrylate) tissue
  Surfit
  Tisseel "surgical glue"
  Vitex tissue
  Zimmer low viscosity
adhesive bandage
adhesive band
adhesive dressing
adhesive plastic drape
adhesive tape
ADICOL insulin delivery system
Adipex-P (phentermine HCl)
adipose fold
adipose graft
adipose tissue
adiposis dolorosa
adiposogenital dystrophy
adjacent organ invasion
adjunctive chemotherapy
adjunctive suppressive medical therapy
adjustable angle guide
adjustable nail
adjustable saline breast implant
adjustable silicone gastric banding
adjuvant chemotherapy
adjuvant radiotherapy
adjuvant systemic therapy
adjuvant therapy
Adler Eagle Vision laparoscope
Adler P.L.U.S. laparoscope
admitting diagnosis
adnexal carcinoma
ADOPT (diabetes outcome progres-
  sion) trial
adrenal cortex hyperfunction
adrenal cortex hypofunction
adrenal gland

adrenal medulla
adrenal medulla graft
adrenal medullary insufficiency
adrenal pseudocyst
adrenal pseudohermaphroditism
adrenal tumor
adrenalectomy
   bilateral total
   complete
   laparoscopic
   partial
adrenocortical carcinoma
adrenogenital syndrome
adrenoleukodystrophy (ALD)
Adriamycin (doxorubicin)
Adrucil (fluorouracil)
Adson-Anderson cerebellar retractor
Adson aneurysm needle
Adson baby forceps
Adson baby retractor
Adson bayonet dressing forceps
Adson bipolar forceps
Adson brain-exploring cannula
Adson brain suction tube
Adson-Brown clamp
Adson-Brown tissue forceps
Adson cerebellar retractor
Adson chisel
Adson clamp
Adson clip applier
Adson clip-introducing forceps
Adson cranial rongeur
Adson dissecting hook
Adson dressing forceps
Adson drill guide
Adson dura protecting forceps
Adson dural hook
Adson dural knife
Adson dural needle holder
Adson dural protector guide
Adson forceps
Adson ganglion scissors
Adson hemilaminectomy retractor
Adson hemostatic forceps

Adson hook
Adson hypophyseal forceps
Adson laminectomy chisel
Adson lightweight plain forceps
Adson lightweight toothed forceps
Adson micro tissue forceps
Adson-Mixter neurosurgical forceps
Adson nerve hook
Adson periosteal elevator
Adson retractor
Adson right-angle knife
Adson rongeur forceps
Adson saw guide
Adson scalp needle
Adson suction tube
Adson tissue forceps
Adson-Toennis scissors
Adson twist drill
Adson wire saw
adsorbent
adult chronic immune thrombo-
   cytopenic purpura
adult-onset (now type 2) diabetes
   mellitus
adult-onset obesity
adult polycystic disease
adult respiratory distress syndrome
   (ARDS)
adult sigmoidoscope
adult-to-adult living related donor liver
   transplant
advanced breast biopsy instrumentation
   (ABBI) system
Advance formula
advancement
   mucosal
   rectal sleeve
   transanal pouch
advancement flap graft
advancement of rectal flap
advance to regular diet
AdvaSeal
adventitial forceps
adverse event profile

adynamic ileus
adynamic intestinal obstruction
adynamic paralytic ileus
AE (acrodermatitis enteropathica)
AEG (acute erosive gastritis)
Aerobacter (old name for *Enterobacter*)
AER Plus (automatic endoscope reprocessor) infection
aerobic bacteria
aerobic culture
aerobilia
aerophagia
Aeroplast dressing
AeroView optical intubation system
AERx (morphine sulfate)
AERx diabetes management system
AERx electronic inhaler
AERx pain management system
Aesculap ABC cervical plate
Aesculap bipolar cautery forceps
Aesculap saw
AESOP (Automated Endoscopic System for Optimal Positioning)
AESOP 2000 surgical robot system
AESOP 3000 surgical robot system
Aestiva/5 MRI anesthesia machine
AFB (acid-fast bacillus) smear
afebrile
afferent
    spinal
    vagal
afferent jejunostomy
afferent limb
afferent loop
afferent loop syndrome
afferent vessels of kidney
Afipia felis
AFP (alpha-fetoprotein) globulin
AGA (American Gastroenterological Association)
agalsidase beta
agammaglobulinemia
aganglionic bowel
aganglionic segment of colon

aganglionosis, congenital
Agaricus (mushroom)
AGE (acute gastroenteritis)
AGE (advanced glycosylation end product)
agency, organ procurement
agenesis, congenital sacral
agent (see also *imaging agents*)
    5-ASA
    antitubulin
    immunosuppressive
    lymphocyte-depleting
    prokinetic
    wetting
ageusia
aggressive malignancy
agnogenic intestinal infarction
agonal clot
agonal infection
Agoral (mineral; phenolphthalein)
Agris-Dingman submammary dissector
AH (adenomatous hyperplasia)
AHD (arteriohepatic dysplasia)
Ahn thrombectomy catheter
AIDS (acquired immunodeficiency syndrome)
AIDS-related complex (ARC)
Ailee needle
Ailee suture
Ainsworth modification of Massie nail
AIOD (aortoiliac obstructive disease)
AIO (all-in-one) parenteral solution
AIP (acute intermittent porphyria)
air
    bowel loop
    colonic
    expired
    free
    Hampton
    inspired
    intramural colonic
    intraperitoneal
    Ohio
    Oxequip

air *(cont.)*
   room
   subcutaneous
   swallowed
airborne infection
air collection
air contrast barium enema
air cyst
air density
air-dried smear
air drill
air embolism
air enema
air exchange
air-filled loop
air-fluid level
Airis II open MRI system
airless lung
Airlift balloon retractor
air-powered cutting drill
air-powered saw
Air Pulse Sensory Stimulator
air sac
airsick
airsickness
airspace-filling pattern
airway
   Berman oropharyngeal
   COPA cuffed oropharyngeal
   disposable
   esophageal gastric tube (EGTA)
   esophageal obturator
   Guedel disposable
   Guedel plastic
   Guedel rubber
   Harrell Y
   LMA-Unique
   oropharyngeal
   pharyngeal
airway, breathing, circulation (ABC)
airway obstruction
airway pattern
AJ (ankle jerk)

Ajmalin liver injury
A-K diamond knife
akinesia, rectal
Akros extended-care mattress
ALA (alpha lipoic acid)
Alagille syndrome
Alamag (aluminum hydroxide;
   magnesium hydroxide)
Alamag Plus (aluminum hydroxide;
   magnesium hydroxide; simethicone)
alanine aminotransferase (ALT)
   (formerly SGPT) liver function test
Al-Anon
Alan-Parks rectal speculum
alar fold
alar plate
AlaSTAT latex allergy test
Alatest Latex-specific IgE allergen test
   kit
Albarran deflecting level
albatross syndrome
Albee bone graft
albendazole
Albenza Tiltab (albendazole)
Albert suture
Albright syndrome
albuminoid liver
albumin, serum
alcohol consumption
alcohol dehydrogenase (ADH)
alcoholic cirrhosis
alcoholic consumption
alcoholic fatty liver
alcoholic fibrosis
alcoholic gastritis
alcoholic hepatitis
alcoholic hyalin
alcoholic hypoglycemia
alcoholic ketoacidosis
alcoholic liver disease
alcoholic pancreatitis
Alcoholics Anonymous (AA)
alcoholic varices

alcoholism
　　acute
　　chronic
　　gamma
ALD (adrenoleukodystrophy)
ALD (alcoholic liver disease)
Aldactone (spironolactone)
Aldara cream 5%
Alden loop gastric bypass
Alderkreutz tissue forceps
aldesleukin
aldolase
aldosterone-producing carcinoma
aldosterone-secreting carcinoma
aldosteronism
Aldrete needle
Aldurazyme
Alenic Alka (aluminum hydroxide;
　　magnesium trisilicate)
Alenic Alka Extra Strength (aluminum
　　hydroxide; magnesium carbonate)
Alexa 1000 noninvasive breast
　　diagnostic system
Alexagram breast lesion diagnostic test
Alexander biopsy forceps
Alexander chisel
Alexander-Farabeuf rasp
Alexander gouge
Alexander rasp
alexandrite (solid-state) laser
AlexLazr or AlexLAZR laser
"alfa and new sling" configuration
　　of gracilis muscle
Alferon N (interferon alfa-n3)
Alfred M. Large clamp
algesimeter (pain monitor), Aly
Algicon
AlgiDERM alginate wound dressing
AlgiDERM calcium alginate gel
　　dressing
alginate wound dressing
AlgiSite alginate wound dressing
alglucerase
AlgoMed drug infusion system

Algosteril alginate wound dressing
Alibra (alprostadil/prazosin HCl)
alignment guide
alignment pin
alignment rod
alimentary canal
alimentary hypoglycemia
alimentary lipemia
alimentary mucosa
alimentary obesity
alimentary system
alimentary tract
alimentary tract smear
alimentation
　　enteral
　　forced
　　parenteral
　　peripheral intravenous
　　rectal
　　total parenteral
Aliminase
AlitraQ formula
alitretinoin
alkaline esophagitis
alkaline gastritis
alkaline phosphatase (ALP)
alkaline reflux gastritis
Alka-Mints (calcium carbonate)
Alka-Seltzer (sodium bicarbonate; citric
　　acid; aspirin; phenylalanine)
Alkets (calcium carbonate)
Alldress composite wound dressing
Allen anastomosis clamp
Allen-Brown vascular access shunt
Allen clip applier
Allen intestinal clamp
Allen intestinal forceps
Allen-Kocher clamp
Allen stirrups
allergic colitis
allergic gastritis
allergic granulomatous angiitis
allergic ileitis
allergic jejunitis

allergic sigmoiditis
allergy
  cow's milk protein
  food
  insulin
  latex
  wheat gliadin
Allevyn foam dressing
Allevyn nonadherent dressing
alligator forceps
alligator grasper
alligator grasping forceps
alligator jaws forceps
alligator scissors
Allis-Adair clamp
Allis atraumatic tissue forceps
Allis clamp
Allis forceps
Allison gastroesophageal reflux repair
Allison lung retractor
Allis-TC tissue forceps
Allis tissue forceps
Alliston GE reflux correction procedure
Allis-Willauer forceps
AlloDerm processed tissue graft
Allofix freeze-dried cortical bone pin
allogenic (also allogeneic)
allogenic bone graft
allogenic peripheral blood mono-
  nuclear cells
allogenous bone graft
allograft
  functioning
  hepatic
  intestinal
  pancreatic
AlloMatrix injectable putty bone graft
  substitute
Allon system
allostimulation
allotransplantation
  islet
  liver
Allovectin-7 (DNA/lipid complex)

Allport multiple clip applier
Allport retractor
Alm self-retaining retractor
Alm wound retractor
Almacone II (aluminum hydroxide;
  magnesium hydroxide; simethicone)
Aloe Vesta perineal dressings
Alogsteril (sterile alginate) dressing
Aloka 650 ultrasound system
Alond (zopolrestat)
alosetron HCl
ALP (alkaline phosphatase)
alpha$_1$ (also alpha-1)
alpha$_1$-antitrypsin deficiency disease
alpha$_1$-antitrypsin globulin
alpha$_2$ (also alpha-2)
alpha$_2$-antiplasmin functional assay
alpha chain disease
alpha chain syndrome
alpha-D-galactosidase enzyme
alpha-fetoprotein (AFP) globulin
alpha-Gal antibody
alpha-Gal epitope
alpha-galactosidase deficiency
alpha heavy chain disease
alpha lipoic acid (ALA)
AlphaNine
alpha sigmoid loop
alpha *Streptococcus viridans*
alprostadil
Alprox-TD (alprostadil)
ALPS (autologous leukapheresis,
  processing, and storage)
Alramucil (psyllium hydrophilic
  mucilloid)
ALRT1550 capsules
Alstrom syndrome
ALT (alanine aminotransferase)
  (formerly SGPT)
ALTE (apparent life-threatening event)
Altemeier repair of rectal prolapse
altered mucosal defenses
altered nutrition
altered thought processes due to
  advanced cirrhosis

altered tissue perfusion
ALternaGEL (aluminum hydroxide gel)
alternating blue and white mattress suture
alternating pressure mattress
Alteromonas putrefaciens
Altex polypropylene mesh
ALT (alanine aminotransferase) (formerly SGPT) liver function test
Altracin (bacitracin)
altumomab pentetate
Alu-Cap (aluminum hydroxide gel)
Aludrox (aluminum hydroxide; magnesium hydroxide; simethicone)
aluminum carbonate gel
aluminum hydroxide gel
aluminum sulfate
Alu-Tab (aluminum hydroxide gel)
alveolar cell carcinoma
alveolar mucosa
alveolar pattern
alveolar soft-part sarcoma (ASPS)
alvine calculus
Aly algesimeter
Alzate catheter
AMA (antimitochondrial antibody)
Amaryl (glimepiride) tablets
Amazr catheter
ambulant edema
ambulatory anesthesia
ambulatory surgery center
AMC needle
amebiasis, indigenous
amebic (also amoebic)
amebic abscess
amebic appendicitis
amebic colitis
amebic cyst
amebic granuloma
amebic hepatitis
amebic liver abscess
amebic ulcer
amelanotic melanoma
ameloblastic carcinoma

ameloblastic sarcoma
American ACMI flexible sigmoidoscope
American Association for the Study of Liver Diseases (AASLD)
American Association for the Surgery of Trauma Organ Injury Scale
American Cancer Society (ACS)
American College of Gastroenterology (ACG)
American Diabetes Association (ADA)
American Dietetic Association (ADA)
American Digestive Health Foundation (ADHF)
American Endoscopy mechanical lithotriptor
American Gastroenterological Association (AGA)
American Hernia Society (AHS)
American Liver Foundation (ALF) hepatitis screening
American Pancreatology Association (APA)
American Society for Gastrointestinal Endoscopy (ASGE)
American Society of Colon and Rectal Surgeons (ASCRS)
Amicus separator blood collection device
amifostine
Amin-Aid powdered feeding
amine precursor uptake and decarboxylation cell
Aminofusin L Forte amino acid solution
aminoglutethimide
Amino Mel Hepa
aminopyrine breath test
aminosalicylic acid
aminosidine
aminosterol
Aminosyn (multiple essential and nonessential amino acids)
Aminosyn M
Aminosyn II

Amitone (calcium carbonate)
AML (angiomyolipoma) solid renal
   tumor
ammonia
   blood
   serum
   urinary
ammonium molybdate tetrahydrate
ammonia N 13 test
amniotic fluid
amniotic fold
amoebic (see *amebic*)
amoebic cyst (also amebic)
Amoena breast prosthesis
amorphous material
Amphojel (aluminum hydroxide gel)
amphotericin B
ampicillin
Ampique
Amplatz dilator
Ampligen
ampulla of Vater
ampulla, rectal
ampullary carcinoma
ampullary stenosis
ampullary tumor
ampullectomy
ampulloma
amputating saw
amputation knife
amputation retractor
AMS (ablepharon-macrostomia
   syndrome) Endoview camera
Amset R-F rod
Amsterdam stent
Amussat operation
amylase
   ascitic
   pancreatic
   P-type (pancreatic)
   salivary
   serum
   S-type (salivary)
   urinary

amylase/creatinine clearance ratio
amyloglucosidase
amyloid degeneration of liver
amyloid kidney
amyloidosis, hepatic
amylo-1,6-glucosidase deficiency
   (Forbes disease)
amylopectinosis
amyotrophy, diabetic
ANA (antinuclear antibody)
Anaconda stent and delivery system
anaerobe, obligate
anaerobic bacteria
anaerobic culture
anakinra
anal abscess
anal anastomosis
anal atresia
anal bulging
anal canal
anal cellulitis
anal cleft
anal column
anal condyloma
anal crypt
anal dilatation
anal dilator
anal disk
anal endoscopy
anal epithelial neoplasia
analeptic enema
anal fascia
anal fissure
anal fistula
analgesia, patient-controlled
anal gland
anal ileostomy with preservation
   of sphincter
anal intermuscular septum
anal intersphincteric groove
anal manometry
anal mapping
anal membrane
analog, nucleoside

analogous tissue
anal orifice
anal papillae
anal pit
anal plate
anal pouch angle
Analpram-HC (hydrocortisone acetate; pramoxine)
anal procidentia
anal prolapse
anal protrusion
anal pruritus
anal reflex
anal region
anal retractor
anal sac
anal seton
anal sinus
anal spasm
anal speculum
anal sphincter
anal sphincteroplasty
anal sphincter squeeze pressure
anal sphincter tone
anal squamous dysplasia
anal squamous intraepithelial lesion
anal stenosis
anal stretch
anal stricture
anal triangle
anal valve
anal vein
anal verge
anal wink
analysis (pl. analyses)
   automated image
   fecal
   gastric
   Monte Carlo
   multivariate
analyzer
   automated blood cell
   BiliChek
   bilirubin

analyzer *(cont.)*
   Body Logic Pro body fat
   BVA-100 blood volume
   ChromaVision digital
   HemoCue
   Hitachi Model 737 multichannel
   LARA
   Piccolo blood
   Sequential Multiple (SMA)
   Sequential Multiple Analyzer C (SMAC)
anaphylactic shock
anaplastic carcinoma of thyroid gland
anaplastic tumor
anasarca
Anaspaz (hyoscyamine sulfate)
Anastaflo stent
anastamose
anastomosed
anastomosing fiber
anastomosing veins
anastomosis (pl. anastomoses)
   anal
   arteriolovenular
   arteriovenous
   Braun
   coloanal
   crucial
   end-to-end
   end-to-end invaginating
   end-to-side
   extracorporeal
   gastroduodenal
   gastrojejunal
   handsewn
   heel-toe
   ileoanal
   ileorectal
   intracorporeal
   LAMA (laser-assisted microvascular anastomosis)
   LAMA (laser-assisted microanastomosis)
   LeDuc

anastomosis *(cont.)*
   longitudinal
   low pelvic
   microvascular
   portacaval
   primary
   side-to-side
   supraoptic
   tension-free
   two-layer
anastomosis clamp
anastomosis of arteries
anastomotic area, portal systemic
anastomotic branch
anastomotic dehiscence
anastomotic fiber
anastomotic leakage
anastomotic stoma
anastomotic ulceration
anastomotic vein
anastrozole
anatomic abnormality
anatomical dead space
anatomical landmark
anatomical layer
anatomical root
anatomical snuffbox
anatomical sphincter
anatomical tooth
anatomical tubercle
anatomic diagnosis
anatomic landmark
anatomic nervous system
anatomic pathology
anatomy, anomalous
Anatrast (barium sulfate)
Ancef (cefazolin sodium)
ancestral organ
anchor (also suture anchor)
   Acufex bioabsorbable suture
   Acufex T-fix suture
   Acumed suture
   Anchorlok soft tissue
   Anspach suture

anchor *(cont.)*
   AxyaWeld bone anchor system
   Bio-Anchor suture
   Biologically Quiet mini-screw
     suture
   Bio-Phase suture
   BioROC
   Bio-Sphere suture
   Bio-Statak suture
   Catera suture
   ConTack
   ConvaTec Flextrak gastrostomy
   Cope suture
   Corkscrew suture
   fascia
   FASTak suture
   Fastin
   GLS suture
   GII EasyAnchor
   GII Snap-Pak
   Harpoon suture
   In-Tac bone-anchoring system
   intraosseous suture
   knotless suture
   Mainstay urologic soft tissue
   MicroMite suture
   Micro QuickAnchor
   Mini GLS
   Mini QuickAnchor
   Mini-Revo Screw suture
   Mitek bone
   Mitek GII suture
   Mitek knotless suture
   Mitek Superanchor
   Mitek suture
   Multitak SS suture
   OBL RC5 soft tissue
   Ogden
   Panalok RC absorbable soft tissue
   Parachute corkscrew suture
   PeBA suture
   Radial Osteo Compression (ROC)
     soft tissue
   ROC EZ

anchor *(cont.)*
   ROC XS
   Sherlock threaded suture
   SmartAnchor suture
   Statak suture
   StatLock Universal Plus
   Stryker wedge suture
   SuperAnchor suture
   suture
   T
   Tacit threaded
   TAG suture
   T-fix suture
   traction
   UltraFix MicroMite suture
anchoring suture
Anchorlok soft tissue anchor
anchor plate
Ancure system for minimally invasive
   repair of abdominal aortic aneurysm
ancylostomiasis (also ankylostomiasis)
Andersen disease
Anderson-Adson scalp retractor
Anderson clamp
Anderson forceps
Andractim (dihydrotestosterone gel)
André hook
Andrews gouge
Andrews Pynchon suction tube
Androderm testosterone transdermal
   patch
Androgel (testosterone)
androgen therapy
Androsorb
anemia
   autoimmune hemolytic
   congenital hemolytic
   iron-deficiency
   microcytic
   pernicious
   sickle cell
   splenic
anergy, clonal
aneroid manometry

anesthesia
   acupuncture
   ambulatory
   axillary
   balanced
   basal
   Bier block
   block
   bolus
   brachial
   caudal
   cervical
   circle absorption
   circuit
   closed
   closed circuit
   combined
   compression
   conduction
   continuous epidural
   continuous-flow catheter
   continuous spinal
   crossed
   diagnostic
   differential spinal
   dissociated
   dissociative
   dolorosa (painful)
   electric
   endotracheal
   epidural
   endotracheal
   extradural
   field block
   fractional epidural
   fractional spinal
   general
   general endotracheal
   general mask
   girdle
   glove
   gustatory
   high spinal
   hyperbaric

anesthesia *(cont.)*
  hyperbaric spinal
  hypnosis
  hypobaric spinal
  hypotensive
  hypothermic
  hysterical
  induced under
  induction
  infiltration
  inhalation
  inhalation mask
  insufflation
  intercostal
  intramedullary
  intranasal
  intraoral
  intraosseous
  intraspinous
  intravenous (IVA)
  intravenous regional
  intravenous sedation
  ischiorectal fossa block
  isobaric spinal
  I.V., IV (intravenous)
  local
  low spinal
  lumbar epidural
  MAC (monitored anesthesia care)
  mask
  nerve block
  Nerve Block Infusion Kit
  nonrebreathing
  ON-Q anesthesia delivery system
  open
  open drop
  oropharyngeal
  outpatient
  painful
  paracervical block
  paravertebral
  patient-controlled (PCA)
  peridural
  perineural

anesthesia *(cont.)*
  periodontal
  Ponka technique for local
  postoperative
  presacral
  pressure
  pudendal
  rapid-acting
  Raplon (rapacuronium bromide)
  rebreathing
  rectal
  refrigeration
  regional
  retrobulbar
  sacral
  saddle
  saddle block
  segmental
  semiclosed
  semiopen
  spinal
  splanchnic
  stocking
  stocking glove
  subarachnoid
  supraclavicular block
  surgical
  tactile
  therapeutic
  thermal
  to-and-fro
  topical
  topical oropharyngeal
  total intravenous (TOPA)
  total spinal
  Tracrium (atracurium besylate)
  transdermal
  traumatic
  unilateral
  variable-dose patient-controlled
  vecuronium bromide
  visceral
anesthesia adjunct
anesthetic hepatitis

aneuploid tumor
AneuRX graft
AneuRX stent
aneurysm, abdominal aortic (AAA)
aneurysmal dilatation
aneurysmal sac
aneurysm clip applier
aneurysm needle
Angelchik antireflux ring prosthesis
Angell James hypophysectomy forceps
Angell James reverse-action hypophy-
  sectomy forceps
angiitis, granuloma
angina
  abdominal
  intestinal
  mesenteric
  pseudomembranous
  Vincent
angina dyspeptica
angiocatheter
Angiocath PRN catheter
angiocentric immunoproliferative lesion
angiocholecystitis
Angiocidin
angiodysplasia
  intestinal
  jejunal
angioedema, hereditary
Angiografin contrast agent
angiogram, cystic duct
angiographic catheter
angiographic variceal embolization
AngioLaz Medi-Vu endoscope
angiolithic sarcoma
angioma (pl. angiomata)
  capillary
  cavernous
  cherry
  hemangioma
  lymphangioma
  petechial
  spider
  telangiectatic

AngioMark contrast agent
angiomatosis
angioneurotic edema
AngioOptic microcatheter
angioprokinetic effect
angiosarcoma, hepatic
AngioStent
Angiovist
Angiozyme
angle
  anal pouch
  anorectal
  cardiohepatic
  epigastric
  hepatic-renal
  hepatorenal
  splenic-renal
  splenorenal
angled awl
angled-down forceps
angled jaw rongeur
angled peripheral vascular clamp
angled pituitary rongeur
angled pleural tube
angled probe
angled rasp
angled retractor
angled-up forceps
angle of His
angle suture
angular bone rongeur
angular elevator
angular hinge clamp
angularis body
angular knife
angulated lesion
angulus of stomach
anhaustral colonic gas pattern
anhemolytic strep (streptococcus)
anhepatic jaundice
anhepatic stage of liver transplantation
anicteric hepatitis
anicteric sclerae
anicteric skin

aniline cancer
animal bite infection
anismus
anisotropine methylbromide
Ankeney sternal retractor
ankle jerk (AJ)
ankle region
anlage of pancreas
annamycin
annular adenocarcinoma
annular esophageal stricture
annular pancreas
anococcygeal raphe
anoderm-preserving hemorrhoidectomy
Anogesic (nitroglycerin ointment)
anomaly
    cloacal
    Cruveilhier-Baumgarten
    vascular
anomaly of Zahn
anoperineal fistula
anoplasty (see *operation)*
anorectal abscess
anorectal angle
anorectal fistula
anorectal impalement
anorectal junction
anorectal line
anorectal lymph node
anorectal malformation
anorectal manometry
anorectal melanoma
anorectal mucosal prolapse
anorectal myomectomy
anorectal ring
anorectal sphincter
anorectal wall
anorectic
anorectoplasty
anorectovaginoplasty
anorexia
anorexia-cachexia syndrome
anorexia nervosa
anorexic

anoscope (also *endoscope, proctoscope,*
    rectoscope, speculum)
    ACMI
    Alan-Parks
    Arakawa
    Bensaude
    Blond
    Brinkeroff
    disposable
    di-wing
    Enproct disposable
    Fansler-Ives
    front-lifting hood
    Gabriel
    Galencia disposable
    Heine
    Hirschman
    Ives
    Ives-Fansler
    Jasan
    Karl Storz
    Kelly
    KleenSpec disposable
    Medix
    Naunton Morgan
    Newman
    Pratt
    Romanoscope
    Sani-Scope
    Sapimed
    Sklar disposable
    slotted
    St. Mark's
    Storz
    Strauss
    tri-wing
    two-valved
    UniSpec disposable
    video
    Welch Allyn
anoscopy
anosigmoidoscopy
anovestibular fistula
Anspach power drill

Anspach reamer
Anspach suture anchor
antacid
  liquid
  pain relieved by
  phosphate-binding
  p.r.n. (as needed)
antagonism, drug
antagonist, histamine-2 (H_2) receptor
antecolic anastomosis
antecolic gastrojejunostomy
antegrade femoral nail
antegrade scrotal sclerotherapy
antelmycin (also anthelmycin)
antemesenteric corner
antemortem clot
antenatal diagnosis
antepartum constipation
anterior abdominal wall
anterior abdominal wall syndrome
anterior band of colon
anterior colon resection
anterior forceps
anterior iliac crest graft
anterior rectopexy
anterior rectus fascia
anterior rectus sheath
anterior resection clamp
anterior sliding tibial graft
anterior superior iliac spine
anterior surface of pancreas
anterior view
anterior wall antral ulcer
anterolateral thoracotomy incision
anteromedial incision
antero-oblique position
anthelmintic
anthelmycin (also antelmycin)
anthracene-type laxative
anthraquinone of cascara
anthrax colitis
Anthron heparinized catheter
anthropometry
antiangiogenesis

Antibacterial Personal Catheter
antibiotic
  broad-spectrum
  perioperative
  postoperative
  preoperative
  prophylactic
antibiotic-associated colitis (AAC)
antibiotic-induced diarrhea
antibody
  alpha-Gal
  anticolonic
  antidelta IgM
  anti-HA (anti-hepatitis A)
  anti-HAV (anti-hepatitis A virus)
  anti-HB (anti-hepatitis B)
  anti-HB_c (anti-hepatitis B core)
  anti-HB_c-IgM (anti-hepatitis B
    core-IgM)
  anti-HB_e (anti-hepatitis B "e")
  anti-HB_s (anti-hepatitis B surface)
  anti-HCV (anti-hepatitis C virus)
  anti-interleukin (IL)-2 receptor
  antimitochondrial (AMA)
  antinuclear (ANA)
  anti-pig
  anti-VEGF (vascular endothelial
    growth factor)
  cA2 monoclonal
  CEA-Cide (^{131}I-labeled humanized
    antibody against carcinoembry-
    onic antigen)
  cold-hemolytic
  C100-3 hepatitis C virus
  Cotara
  CytoTAb purified monoclonal
  detection
  HACA (human antichimeric
    antibody)
  HB_cAb (hepatitis B core antibody)
  HB_eAb (hepatitis B "e" antibody)
  HB_sAb (hepatitis B surface
    antibody)
  HCV (hepatitis C virus) (formerly
    non-A, non-B)

antibody *(cont.)*
 Herceptin (trastuzumab) monoclonal
 human antihepatitis B
 infliximab monoclonal
 islet cell
 LeuTech radiolabeled
 OST-577 human antihepatitis B
 serum HCV-specific
 transglutaminase
antibody-dependent cell-mediated cyto-
 toxicity (ADCC)
antibody-mediated attack (hyperacute
 rejection)
antibody-mediated immune reaction
 (type III)
antibody-mediated immunity
antibody to HCV (anti-HCV)
anticholinergic drug
anticholinergic therapy
anticoagulant-treated blood
anticolonic antibody
Anticort
antidelta IgM antibody
antidiarrheal
antiemetic drug
antiendomysial antibody test
antifibrin antibody imaging
antigastrin therapy
antigen
 Australian
 CA 19-9
 delta (delta-Ag)
 endogenous
 enterobacterial common (ECA)
 exogenous
 HbAg, HB Ag ("H-bag") (hepatitis
  B antigen)
 HB_eAg (soluble "e" antigen in
  hepatitis B antigen)
 HB_sAg (hepatitis B surface antigen)
 HDAg (hepatitis D antigen)
 hepatitis-associated
 hepatitis B antigen (HbAg)
 hepatitis B_e (anti-HBe)

antigen *(cont.)*
 histocompatibility
 Histoplasma capsulatum polysaccha-
  ride antigen (HPA)
 HLA (human lymphocyte antigen)
 HSP (heat shock protein)
 human lymphocyte antigen (HLA)
 PCNA (proliferating cell nuclear)
antigen-antibody complex
antigen-antibody ratio
antigenemia
antigen load
antigenic properties of blood
antigenic triggering of immune inflam-
 mation
antigen-presenting cell (APC)
anti-HA, anti-HAV antibody (antibody
 to hepatitis A virus)
anti-HB antibody
anti-HB_c antibody
anti-HB_e antibody
anti-HB_e antigen
anti-HB_s antibody
anti-HB_c-IgM antibody
anti-HB_e-positive chronic hepatitis
anti-HCV antibody
anti-interleukin (IL)-2 receptor antibody
antilymphocyte globulin
antilymphocyte induction therapy
antimesenteric border of distal ileum
antimesenteric fat pad
antimesocolic side of the cecum
antimicrobial prophylaxis
antimicrobial therapy
Antiminth (pyrantel pamoate)
antimitochondrial antibody (AMA)
antimotility drug
antinauseant
antineoplastic drug
antinuclear antibody (ANA)
antiperistaltic operation
anti-pig antibody
antiprostaglandin
Anti-Pr-3 ELISA autoimmune test

antireflux mechanism
antireflux operation
antireflux regimen
antireflux surgery for esophageal
  stricture
antireflux therapy
antireflux valve
antirejection medication
anti-Schiff stain
antischistosomal drug
antisecretory drug therapy
antisense technology
antiseptic dressing
Antispas (diclyclomine HCl)
antispasmodic drug
anti-Tamm-Horsfall protein
anti-TNF (anti-tumor necrosis factor)
  therapy
antitubulin agent
anti-VEGF (vascular endothelial growth
  factor) antibody
Antivert (meclizine)
antivibratory glove
antiviral therapy
antral edema
antral G cell hyperplasia
antral gastric cell
antral gastritis
antral mucosa
antral pouch
antral sphincter
antral stasis
antral stenosis
antral stricture
antral ulcer
antrectomy
Antrenyl (oxyphenonium bromide)
Antrocol (atropine sulfate; pheno-
  barbital)
antrotomy
antrum
  cardiac
  gastric
  prepyloric

antrum *(cont.)*
  pyloric
  retained
antrum of stomach
antrum of Willis
Anucort HC (hydrocortisone acetate)
Anumed (bismuth subgallate)
anus
  artificial
  ectopic
  high imperforate
  imperforate
  low imperforate
  patulous
  preternatural
Anusol (pramoxine HCl; zinc oxide)
Anusol-HC (hydrocortisone acetate)
anvil portion of EEA stapler
anvil-shaft assembly of stapling device
Anvirzel
anxiety-related diarrhea
Anzemet (dolasetron mesylate)
AO blade plate
AO condylar blade plate
AO contoured T plate
AODM (adult-onset diabetes mellitus)
  (now type 2)
AO hook plate
AOI blade plate
A-OK ShortCut knife
AO reconstruction plate
AO reduction forceps
AO semitubular
AO slotted medullary nail
AO small-fragment plate
aorta
  abdominal
  coarctation of
  dissecting
  esophageal artery of
  supraceliac
  thoracic
aortic aneurysm clamp
aortic arch

aortic bifurcation
aortic clamp
aortic hiatus
aortic occlusion clamp
aortic orifice
aortic root perfusion needle
aortic sac
aortic valve stenosis
aortoduodenal fistula
aortoenteric fistula
aortoesophageal fistula
aortofemoral bypass graft (AFBG)
aortohepatic arterial graft
aortosigmoid fistula
AP (anteroposterior)
APA (American Pancreatology
    Association)
APC (adenoma prevention with
    celecoxib) study
APC (adenomatous polyposis coli) gene
APC (argon plasma coagulation)
APECED syndrome
    APE (autoimmune polyendo-
        crinopathy)
    C (candidiasis)
    ED (ectodermal dysplasia)
aperient
aperistalsis, esophageal
aperitive
apertures of abdomen
apex (pl. apices)
    bladder
    duodenal bulb
    external ring
    fibrous
    fibula
    heart
    ischiorectal fossa
    lingual
    lung
    nose
    prostate
apex cordis
apex pulmonis

Apex Plus excimer laser
AP (anteroposterior) film
aphtha (pl. aphthae)
aphthoid ulcer
aphthous ulcer
apical duodenal ulcer
apical infection
apical lordotic view
apical segment
apical suture
apical view
apicoposterior segment
Apligraf (graftskin)
AP (anteroposterior) nail
apocrine carcinoma
apocrine gland
apocrine metaplasia
Apo-Domperidone (domperidone
    maleate)
Apollo3 triple-lumen papillotome
Apomate radiopharmaceutical imaging
    agent
apomorphine
aponeurosis of internal oblique muscle
aponeurosis of external oblique muscle
aponeurosis, transversus abdominis
aponeurotic layer
apophyseal pouch
apoplectic pancreatitis
apoptosis (programmed cell death)
apoptotic index
apoptotic potential
apparatus (see *device*)
apparent death
apparent life-threatening event (ALTE)
appearance
    bat-wing
    beads-on-a-string
    beefy
    cobblestone
    collar-button (in colon)
    corkscrew
    dewy
    granular

appearance *(cont.)*
 ground-glass
 hobnailed
 honeycomb(ed)
 lead pipe
 macroscopic
 meaty
 moth-eaten
 mottled
 nutmeg
 onion peel
 onionskin
 orange peel
 signet ring
 speckled
 steamy
 string-of-beads
 tigroid
 whorled
appearance infarct
appendage clamp
appendage, epiploic
appendectomy
 emergency
 emergent
 incidental
 inversion-ligation
 laparoscopic
 laser-assisted
 McBurney
 negative
 percutaneous
appendiceal abscess
appendiceal colic
appendiceal concretion
appendiceal constriction
appendiceal fecalith
appendiceal fistula
appendiceal hyperplasia
appendiceal intussusception
appendiceal lumen
appendiceal mass
appendiceal mucocele
appendiceal retractor

appendiceal stercolith
appendiceal stump
appendicitis
 acute
 amebic
 chronic
 complex
 early
 fulminating
 gangrenous
 helminthic
 inflamed
 lumbar
 nonperforated
 obstructive
 perforated
 perforated acute
 recurrent
 relapsing
 segmental
 stercoral
 subacute
 subperitoneal
 suppurative
 traumatic
appendicitis obliterans
appendicocele
appendicoenterostomy
appendicolith
appendicolithiasis
appendicolysis
appendicopathy
appendicovesicotomy
appendicular artery
appendicular colic
appendicular lymph node
appendicular muscle
appendicular skeleton
appendicular vein
appendix (pl. appendices)
 auricular
 cecal
 ensiform
 epiploic

appendix *(cont.)*
  gangrenous
  hot
  indurated
  inflamed
  inflammation
  mesentery of
  Morgagni
  nonperforated
  normal
  orifice of
  paracecal
  perforated
  preileal
  retrocecal
  retrocolic
  retroileal
  right auricular
  ruptured
  serpentine
  subcecal
  suppurative
  testis
  ventricle of larynx
  vermiform
  vesicular
  xiphoid
appendix fibrosa
appendix of epididymis
appendix of testis
appendolithiasis
apperceptive mass
appetite juice
apple-core configuration of mass
apple-core lesion
apple-peel bowel
apple-peel syndrome
appliance (see *barrier; device; pouch*)
  Bard colostomy
  closed-end ostomy
  ConvaTec colostomy
  Dansac DuoSoft pouch
  Dansac Nova ostomy
  Divine colostomy

appliance *(cont.)*
  Erlangen magnetic colostomy
  Gentle Touch colostomy
  Hollister
  Hollister Karaya
  Karaya ring ileostomy
  loop ostomy
  Nu-Comfort
  Nu-Flex
  Nu-Hope ostomy
  Nu-Self
  ostomy
  Remedy
applicator (see also *applier; forceps*)
  cotton
  cotton-tipped
  Eder cotton
  Endo Clip
  Farrell cotton
  Frankenfeldt cotton
  Olympus rotatable clip
applier (see also *applicator; forceps*)
  Absolok clip
  Adson clip
  Allen clip
  Allport multiple clip
  aneurysm
  Aslan clip
  Auto Suture Endo Clip
  bayonet clip
  clip
  Cyanamid clip
  double clip
  Duraclose clip
  Endo clip
  Endo Hernia
  endoscopic
  Ethicon clip
  Filshie clip
  Hulka clip
  Imagyn endoscopic clip
  laparoscopic clip
  Ligaclip ERCA endoscopic clip
  ligating clip

applier *(cont.)*
   Mayfield miniature clip
   Mayfield temporary aneurysm clip
   mini
   Mirage ostomy
   Multifire Endo Hernia clip
   MUR (Multiuse Reposable) clip
   multiple ligating clip
   Olympus clip
   Olympus rotatable clip
   One Shot vascular clip
   PermaClip endoscopic clip
   Reflex ELC clip
   reposable clip
   Richard Allen clip
   right-angle
   rotatable
   Sovereign Multifire clip
   Stahl clip
   Sur-Fit AutoLock
   Sur-Fit Natura ostomy
   Surgiclip
   USSC clip
   Vari-angle clip
   VCS clip
   VitaClip
   Weck clip
applying forceps
Appolito suture
Appraise blood glucose monitor
approach
   axillary
   cervical
   double seton modified surgical
   extraperitoneal
   inframammary
   Kugel
   laparoscopic
   preperitoneal
   retroperitoneal
   sacroperineal
   sternal split
   supraduodenal
   takedown abdominal

approach *(cont.)*
   transabdominal
   transabdominal preperitoneal
   transanal
   transcoccygeal
   transsacral
   transthoracic
   transumbilical
approximated
approximating forceps
approximation
   skin
   tissue
   wound
approximation suture
approximator clamp
"appy" (appendectomy) tape
APR (abdominoperineal or abdominal-perineal resection)
APR cement fixation adhesive
Apra (CT-2584 mesylate)
APRL (Army Prosthetics Research Laboratory)
apron (panniculus)
   abdominal
   fatty
   vascular
AP (anteroposterior) supine view
Aptosyn (exisulind)
APTT (activated partial thromboplastin time)
APUD (amine precursor uptake and decarboxylation) cell
APUDoma
AP (anteroposterior) view
Aquacel Hydrofiber wound dressing
Aquacel Hydrofiber wound packing
Aquaphor gauze dressing
Aquasorb transparent hydrogel dressing
Aquilion CT scanner
arachadonic acid
arachnoid fibrosis
arachnoid knife
arachnoid-shaped Beaver blade

Arakawa anoscope
arbaprostil
arborization of ducts
ARC (AIDS-related complex)
arcade, ileocolic
arch, aortic
arch cookie (pad)
archimedean hand drill
architectural atypia
architecture
    hepatic
    lobular
arcitumomab (CEA-Scan) imaging
    agent
arclofenin hepatic function test
Arco-Lase (amylase; protease; lipase;
    cellulase)
Arco-Lase Plus
arc reflex
arcuate artery of kidney
arcuate line
ARD (acid-related disorder)
ARDS (adult respiratory distress
    syndrome)
area gastrica (pl. areae gastricae)
area of mucosal irregularity
areola (pl. areolae)
areola of breast
areolar gland
areolar lesion
areolar tissue
ArF (argon fluorine) excimer laser
argentaffin cell
argentaffin reaction test
Arglaes antimicrobial barrier film
    dressing
argon beam coagulator (ABC)
argon/krypton laser
argon laser
argon plasma coagulation (APC)
Argyle chest tube
Argyle Medicut R catheter
Argyle-Salem sump tube
Argyle Sentinel Seal chest tube

argyrophil (or argyrophilic) cell
Aria coronary artery bypass graft
Arias syndrome
Aries-Pitanguy correction of mammary
    ptosis
Arimidex (anastrozole)
A ring, esophageal
A ring of esophagus
arm
    MINI 6600 C-arm
    PinPoint stereotactic
    robotic
arm abducted to 90 degrees
Armanni-Ebstein kidney
Armanni-Ebstein lesion
arm board
Armenian syndrome
Armstrong plate
Army bone gouge
Army-Navy retractor
Aromasin (exemestane)
aromatic amino acid (AAA)
aromatic cascara fluid extract
aromatic cascara sagrada
Aron Alpha adhesive
Aronson esophageal retractor
Aroplatin
Arrequi laparoscopic knot pusher
Arrestin (trimethobenzamide HCl)
arrhythmia mapping system catheter
Arrowgard Blue Line catheter
Arrow-Howes multilumen catheter
Arrow Twin Cath catheter
Arruga needle
Arruga-Nicetic forceps
arsenic, inorganic
arsenic trioxide (ATO)
ArtAssist compression dressing
arteria lusoria
arterial arcade of jejunum
arterial blood
arterial blood gases
arterial line
arterial missile embolism

arterial obstruction
arterial stenosis
arterial thrombosis
arteries were skeletonized
arteriogram
arteriography
arteriohepatic dysplasia (AHD)
arteriolar necrosis
arteriosclerotic kidney
arteriovenous (AV) fistula
arteriovenous malformation (AVM)
arteritis, necrotizing
artery (see Table of Arteries in
    Appendix)
artery forceps
Arthrex coring reamer
Arthrex femoral guide
Arthrex tibial guide
arthrifluent abscess
Arthrinium
arthritis panel
Arthrocare Wand probe
Arthroderma
arthropathy, neurogenic
arthroplasty gouge
arthropod-borne virus
ArthroProbe laser
arthroscopic blade
arthroscopic cannula
arthroscopic knife
arthroscopic probe
arthroscopic scissors
arthroscopy basket
arthroscopy grasping forceps
ArthroSew suture
Arthrotek RC needle
Arthrotek rigid laparoscope
ArthroWand
articular cartilage autograft
articular fluid
articulating dissector
artificial anus
artificial bezoar
artificial gut

artificial kidney
artificial sphincter
Artiflex bandage
aryepiglottic fold
aryepiglottis
arytenoid gland
Asacol (mesalamine)
ASAP antimicrobial solution
ascariasis, biliary
Ascaris lumbricoides
ascending cholangitis
ascending colon
Ascent guiding catheter
Asch forceps
ascites
    bile
    blood-tinged
    bloody
    chylous
    cloudy
    dialysis-related
    exudative
    fatty
    hemorrhagic
    hydremic
    milky
    myxedema
    nephrogenic
    pancreatic
    progressive
    pseudochylous
    refractory
    straw-colored
    tense
    transudative
ascites drainage tube
ascites trocar
ascitic amylase
ascitic fluid (see *fluid*)
Ascriptin A/D
ASCRS (American Society of Colon
    and Rectal Surgeons)
ASCUS (atypical squamous cells
    of uncertain significance)

ASE (axilla, shoulder, elbow) bandage
AS-800 artificial sphincter
Aselli pancreas
aseptic necrosis
aseptic technique
aseptic wound
Asepto irrigation syringe
ASGE (American Society of Gastro-
   intestinal Endoscopy)
Asherson syndrome
ASHN (acute sclerosing hyaline
   necrosis)
ASIF chisel
ASIF right-angle blade plate
Askin tumor
Ask-Upmark kidney
Aslan clip applier
ASLC (acute self-limited colitis)
aspartate transaminase (AST)
   (formerly SGOT) liver function test
A-Spas S/L (hyoscyamine sulfate)
Aspen laparoscopy electrode
Aspen ultrasound system
Aspergillus cerebral abscess
aspirate
   bilious
   bone marrow
   gastric
   NG (nasogastric)
aspirating needle
   large-bore slotted
   mediastinoscopy
aspiration
   cervical
   cyst
   fine-needle
   hematoma
   iliac crest bone
   needle
   percutaneous
   peritoneal
   puncture
aspiration associated with gastrostomy
   feeding

aspiration biopsy
aspiration biopsy cytology
aspiration needle
aspiration syringe
aspirator
   Cavitron ultrasonic
   Cavitron surgical
   Cooper Cavitron surgical
   CUSA (Cavitron ultrasonic surgical
     aspirator)
   CUSA EXcel surgical
   Dissectron ultrasonic
   Lysonix 2000 soft tissue
   Millennium ultrasonic
   PSI-TEC
   Selector ultrasonic
   ultrasonic surgical
   Vabra
aspirin-induced gastritis
asplenia syndrome
ASPS (alveolar soft-part sarcoma)
assay (see also *test*)
   alpha-2 antiplasmin functional
   Bioclot protein S
   bladder tumor (BTA)
   BTA stat bladder tumor
   BTA TRAK bladder tumor
   CA15-3 RIA
   CA27.29 antigen
   coagulation factor
   ELISA (enzyme linked immuno-
     sorbent assay)
   Emit 2000 cyclosporine specific
   EndoCab ELISA
   enzyme-linked immunosorbent
   ER-ICA (estrogen receptor immuno-
     chemical assay)
   Escherichia coli O157:H7
   FLU OIA
   Glycacor
   Heprofile ELISA
   Innofluor FPIA (fluorescence-
     polarization immunoassay)
   intact molecule

assay *(cont.)*
   intragraft polymerase chain reaction
     (PCR)
   IOS immunoassay system
   Limulus amoebocyte lysate (LAL)
     chromogenic endotoxin
   MATRIX
   N High Sensitivity CRP (C-reactive
     protein)
   OncoChek immunoassay
   OnCyte
   plasma assay coagulation panel
   PP-CAP IgA enzyme immunoassay
   PreVue *Borrelia burgdorferi*
     antibody detection
   PTH
   PyloriProbe
   recombinant immunoblot (RIBA)
   RIBA (recombinant immunoblot
     assay)
   RIBA HCV 3.0 SIA (strip
     immunoblot assay)
   sandwich radioimmunoassay
   SIA (strip immunoblot assay)
   steroid-binding
   strip immunoblot assay (SIA)
   thyrocalcitonin assay
   Truquant BR radioimmunoassay
   Velogene rapid VRE
assay of altered DNA exfoliated
   into stool
assessment of bowel function
assessment, preoperative
ASSI (Accurate Surgical and Scientific
   Instruments) device
ASSI No-scalpel vasectomy fixator ring
   clamp
Assure blood glucose monitoring
   system
AST (aspartate aminotransferase) liver
   function test (formerly SGOT)
asterixis
asteroid body

ASTRA profile
astrovirus gastroenteritis
Astwood-Coller staging system
   for carcinoma
asymmetric mural thickening
asymmetrical breast prosthesis
asymmetry, breast
asymptomatic appendicitis
asymptomatic cholelithiasis
asymptomatic gallstone
Atabrine
ataxia, late-onset
atelectasis, postoperative
atelectatic lung
Atgam (lymphocyte immune globulin;
   antithymocyte)
atherectomy catheter
AtheroCath Bantam coronary atherec-
   tomy catheter
AtheroCath catheter
atheromatous ulcer
atherosclerotic lesion
Athlete coronary guidewire
athyrotic cretinism
ATI (Abdominal Trauma Index)
Atkinson scoring system for dysphagia
Atkinson silicone rubber tube
Atlantic Ileostomy Catheter
Atlas 2.0 diagnostic ultrasound system
AtLast blood glucose monitor
ATL UM 9 HDI Colorflow ultrasound
   system
atmospheres of pressure in balloon
   catheter
ATO (arsenic trioxide; As2O$_3$)
atonic consti pation
atonic esophagus
atony
   colonic
   gastric
   intestinal
   sphincter
atorvastatin calcium
atovaquone/proguanil

ATPase (adenosine triphosphatase)
  inhibitors
atracurium besylate
Atraloc needle
Atrauclip hemostatic clamp
AtrauGrip forceps
atraumatic abscess
atraumatic forceps
atraumatic grasper
atraumatic suture
atraumatic vascular clamp
atresia
  anal
  biliary
  congenital
  congenital biliary
  duodenal
  esophageal
  extrahepatic biliary (EBA)
  intestinal
  intrahepatic (IHA)
  posterior choanal
  prepyloric
atrial retractor
atriocaval shunt
atrioventricular orifice
Atrisol aerosol
Atrocholin
atrophic cirrhosis
atrophic gastritis
atrophic-hyperplastic ulcer
atrophic kidney
atrophy
  crypt
  gastric
  healed yellow
  intestinal villous
  mammary
  mucosal
  muscular
  villous
  yellow
atropine sulfate
ATS (autotransfusion) catheter

attachment
  mesenteric
  peritoneal
  point of
Attain parenteral nutritional therapy
attapulgite
attenuated
attic adhesion
atypia, architectural
atypical gallbladder disease
atypical squamous cells of uncertain
    significance (ASCUS)
Auchincloss modified radical
    mastectomy
auditory mucosa
Auerbach mesenteric plexus
AU5 Harmonic ultrasound system
Aufranc awl
Aufranc cobra retractor
Aufranc cup
Aufranc gouge
Aufranc hook
Aufranc periosteal elevator
Aufranc psoas retractor
Aufranc reamer
Aufricht dissecting scissors
Aufricht glabellar rasp
augmentation, breast
augmentation mammoplasty
augmentation of anesthesia
Augustine boat nail
Aura desktop ENT laser
auricular appendix
auricular perichondritis
Aurora diode soft tissue laser
Aurora MR breast imaging system
auscultation of bowel sounds
Austin awl
Austin Moore chisel
Austin Moore extractor
Austin Moore hook
Austin Moore pin
Austin Moore rasp
Austin Moore reamer

Australian antigen
Auth atherectomy catheter
Autoblock safety syringe
autochthonous graft
autochthonous malaria
autoclavable
Autoclix fingerstick device
autocount sponge
autocrine mediator of bone metastasis
autodigestion
autoerotic rectal trauma
Autofuse Byron infiltration pump
autogenous bone graft
autogenous dermal graft
autogenous fascial heterograft
autogenous inlay graft
autogenous soft tissue graft
autograft harvesting
AutoGuard-P catheter
autoimmune attack
autoimmune disease
autoimmune disorder
   diabetes mellitus
   hypoadrenalism
   hypoparathyroidism
   pernicious anemia
   thyroiditis
autoimmune hemolytic anemia
autoimmune hepatitis
autoimmune hypoglycemia
autoimmune polyendocrinopathy (APE)
autoimmune process
autoimmune thyroiditis
autoinoculation
auto-Lancet
AuTolo Cure Process
autologous blood
autologous bone marrow transplant
   (AuBMT)
Autologous Bone Marrow Transplant
   Registry (ABMTR)
autologous clot
autologous crest bone graft
autologous fat graft

autologous leukapheresis, processing,
   and storage (ALPS)
autologous rectus abdominis fascia
autologous reverse graft
autologous transfusion
autologous tumor cells
autologous vein-covered stent
automated blood cell analyzer
Automated Cellular Imaging System
   (ACTS)
automated computerized axial
   tomography (ACAT)
Automated Endoscopic System for
   Optimal Positioning (AESOP)
automated image analysis
automated islet-cell shaking device
automatic knot-tying device
automatic skin retractor
automatic staple
autonomously hyperfunctioning nodule
autonomy, nutritional
autopepsia
autopsy knife
auto-reinforced polyglycolide rod
autosomal dominant disease
autosomal dominant genetic trait
autosomal dominant polycystic disease
autosomal recessive disorder
autosomal recessive genetic trait
AutoSonix system
autosplenectomize
autostapler, TA-55
autostapling device
Auto Suture ABBI system
Auto Suture Multifire Endo GIA 30
   stapler
Auto Suture One-Shot anastomotic
   device
Auto Suture Premium CEEA stapler
Auto Suture Premium TA-55 surgical
   stapler
Auto Suture Soft Thoracoport obturator
Auto Suture SurgiStitch
Auto Suture suture

autosuture technique
Auto Suture universal retractor base
autotransfusion system
autotransplantation, parathyroid, to
  forearm
autotransplant, islet
Autovac autotransfusion system
Autovac LF autotransfusion system
Auvard speculum
auxiliary transplant
AV (arteriovenous) fistula
Avakine (infliximab)
Avandia (rosiglitazone maleate)
avascular necrosis (AVN)
AVA 3Xi advanced venous access
  device
AVCO aortic balloon
Avelox (moxifloxacin)
AVH (acute viral hepatitis)
avian leukosis virus
avian malaria
Avicine therapeutic cancer vaccine
Avitene "flour" dressing
Avitene Hemostat
Avitene macrofibrillar collagen
  hemostatic material
Avitene Ultrafoam collagen hemostatic
  sponge
AVM (arteriovenous malformation)
avulsed wound
avulsion of appendiceal tip
awl
  angled
  Aufranc
  Austin
  bone
  curved
  DePuy
  Ender
  Küntscher (Kuentscher)
  Mark II Kodros radiolucent
  pointed
  reaming

awl *(cont.)*
  rectangular
  Rush
  square-shaped
  Swanson lunate
  Swanson scaphoid
  T-handled
  Zuelzer
axial hiatal hernia
axial plate
axial sesamoid view
axial wall
Axid (nizatidine)
Axid AR ("acid reducer")
axilla (pl. axillae)
axillary adenopathy
axillary anesthesia
axillary approach in surgery
axillary artery
axillary contents
axillary dissection
axillary envelope
axillary fat pad
axillary fold
axillary fossa
axillary line
axillary lymphadenectomy
axillary lymphadenopathy
axillary lymph node
axillary node dissection
axillary region
axillary tail
axillary vein
axillary view
axiom double sump tube
axis
  bowel
  celiac
  enteroinsular
  hypothalamic-pituitary
  hypothalamic-pituitary-adrenal
Axokine (ciliary neurotrophic factor
  [CNTF])

AXR (abdominal x-ray)
AXR/CT (abdominal x-ray and
    computed tomography)
AxyaWeld Bone Anchor System
Ayers needle holder
Aylett operation
Ayre brush
Ayre knife
Ayre spatula
Ayre tube

ayw1, ayw2, ayw3, ayw4, ayr (hepatitis
    B surface antigen subdeterminants)
AZA (azathioprine)
azathioprine
azotemia
aztreonam
Azulfidine (sulfasalazine)
Azulfidine EN-tabs
azygos vein
azygous system

B, b

Babcock atraumatic tissue forceps
Babcock clamp
Babcock grasping forceps, double-
　action
Babcock intestinal forceps
Babcock retractor
Babcock stainless steel suture wire
Babcock-TC tissue forceps
Babcock wire-cutting scissors
Babesia divergens
Babinski percussion hammer
baby Adson forceps
baby Allis tissue forceps
baby Babcock tissue forceps
baby Balfour abdominal retractor
baby Deaver retractor
baby Doyen intestinal forceps
baby Gelpi retractor
baby Harrington retractor
baby Jones towel clip
baby Metzenbaum dissecting scissors
baby Mollison retractor
baby Payr pylorus clamp
baby Poole suction tube
baby Reynolds dissecting scissors
baby Roux retractor
Babytherm IC gel mattress
baby Tischler biopsy forceps

baby Yankauer suction tube
Bacher flexible biopsy forceps
bacillary colitis
bacillary diarrhea
bacillary dysentery
bacillary necrosis
bacillus Calmette-Guérin (BCG)
Bacillus cereus
bacitracin ointment
Backhaus clamp
Backhaus dilator
Backhaus forceps
Backhaus knife
Backlund biopsy needle
back pain
backup of portal pressure
backward-cutting knife
backwash ileitis
Bacon bone rongeur
Bacon cranial rongeur
Bacon rasp
Bacon rongeur forceps
Bacon thoracic shears
BACTEC system
bacteremia
　community-acquired
　fulminant
　persistent

bacteremia *(cont.)*
  polymicrobial
  transient
bacteria (pl. of bacterium)
  acid-fast
  Acinetobacter
  aerobic
  anaerobic
  Calymmatobacterium
  Campylobacter
  Candida
  Chauveau
  coliform
  colonic
  corkscrew-shaped
  corynebacteria
  Cryptococcus
  defense against
  Enterobacter
  fibrillary
  fungus-like
  gas-forming
  gram-negative
  gram-positive
  Haemophilus
  helical
  intestinal
  intracellular
  Klebsiella
  Lactobacillus
  luminal
  mesophilic
  Nocardia
  pathogenic
  Proteus
  Pseudomonas
  pus-forming
  pyogenic
  Salmonella
  Serratia
  Shigella
  spiral-shaped
  toxigenic
  Toxoplasma

bacteria-impervious seal
bacteria in stool
bacteria in urine
bacterial abscess
bacterial cellular protein
bacterial cholangitis
bacterial cirrhosis
bacterial co-infection
bacterial colitis
bacterial colony
bacterial colonization
bacterial culture
bacterial culture media
bacterial dissociation
bacterial enterocolitis
bacterial esophagitis
bacterial flora
bacterial food poisoning
bacterial gastroenteritis
bacterial infection
bacterial lipopolysaccharide
bacterial meningitis
bacterial metabolism
bacterial myocarditis
bacterial nephritis
bacterial overgrowth
bacterial pericarditis
bacterial peritonitis
bacterial pneumonia
bacterial pneumonitis
bacterial protein
bacterial toxemia
bacterial toxin
bacterial vaginosis
bacterial virus
bactericidal antibiotic
bactericidal oxygen radical
bacteriocholia
bacteriologic smear, AFB (acid-fast
  bacillus)
bacteriostatic, mafenide acetate
bacteriostatic water
bacterium (see *bacteria*)
bacteriuria

Bacteroides bividius
Bacteroides capillosus
Bacteroides distasonis
Bacteroides fragilis
Bacteroides nodosus
Bacteroides praeacutus
Bacteroides putredinis
Bacteroides splanchnicus
Bacteroides thetaiotamicron
Bacteroides ureolyticus
Bacteroides vulgatus
Bactigen *Salmonella-Shigella* slide test
Bactrim (trimethoprim, sulfamethoxazole)
Baculovirus Expression Vector System (BEVS)
Badgley laminectomy retractor
Badglcy plate
BA-EDTA (bile acid-EDTA) solution
Baer bone-cutting forceps
Baer bone rongeur
Baermann stool filter
Baermann stool test
Baer rib shears
bag (see also *appliance*; *pouch*)
   bile
   bowel
   colostomy
   Endopouch Pro specimen
   Endosac specimen
   Hollister
   ileostomy
   intestinal
   Karaya seal stoma
   Lahey
   Lapides
   Marlen
   ostomy
   Perry
   Petersen
   pneumatic
   Ponsky Endo Sock retrieval
   Rutzen ileostomy
   stomal
   Whitmore

bag and mask
bag breathing
Bagby angled compression plate
BAGF (brachioaxillary bridge graft fistula)
bagged
Baggish biopsy forceps
Bahnson aortic clamp
Baho endoscope
Bailey aortic clamp
Bailey aortic valve-cutting forceps
Bailey-Dubow nail
Bailey-Gibbon rib contractor
Bailey-Gigli saw
Bailey-Gigli saw guide
Bailey rib contractor
Bailey wire saw
Bainbridge intestinal clamp
Bainbridge intestinal forceps
Baird forceps
Bakamjian flap
Baker intestinal decompression tube
Baker jejunostomy tube
Bakes common duct dilator
Bakes probe
Bak-Pac portable ultrasound scanner
BAL (bronchoalveolar lavage)
balanced anesthesia
balanced diet
balanced electrolyte solution (BES)
balanced salt solution (BSS)
balance, equal fluid
balantidial colitis
BalAsa (balsalazide disodium) (now Colazal)
bald gastric fundus
Baldy-Webster operation
Balfour abdominal retractor
Balfour center blade
Balfour retractor
Balfour self-retaining retractor
Ballance sign
ball-and-socket towel forceps
Ballantine clamp
Ballantine forceps

Ballantine hemilaminectomy retractor
Ballenger-Hajek chisel
Ballenger sponge-holding forceps
Ballenger swivel knife
ballerina-foot pattern
ball guide pin
ballistic wound
Ballobes gastric balloon
balloon
    ACS SULP II
    AVCO aortic
    Ballobes gastric
    banana-shaped
    bifoil
    BioEnterics gastric
    Blakemore
    Blue Max
    Brandt cytology
    DURAglide stone removal
    DURAglide 3 stone removal
    Duralon occlusion
    esophageal
    Extra View
    Extractor three-lumen retrieval
    Fogarty
    Garren-Edwards
    gastric
    Gau gastric
    Grüntzig (Gruentzig)
    Hartzler angioplasty
    Hartzler Micro II
    Hunter-Sessions
    hydrostatic
    Inoue
    intra-aortic (IAB)
    intragastric
    kissing
    Kontron intra-aortic
    low-compliance hydrostatic
    LPS
    Mansfield
    mercury-containing
    Microvasive endoscopic
    Microvasive Mini Button low-profile

balloon *(cont.)*
    Microvasive Rigiflex TTS
    Monorail
    Origin
    PDB laparoscopic
    PEG
    Percival gastric
    Percor DL-II (dual-lumen)
        intra-aortic
    Percor-Stat intra-aortic
    PET
    preperitoneal distention (PDB)
    pulsation
    Quantum
    rectal
    Rigiflex TTS
    Sci-Med Express Monorail
    scintigraphic
    self-positioning
    Sengstaken
    Sengstaken-Blakemore tamponade
    slave
    Soto USCI
    Stack autoperfusion
    Taylor gastric
    traction
    transendoscopic
    trefoil
    TTS (through-the-scope)
    Wilson-Cook gastric
balloon biliary catheter
balloon catheter
balloon catheter fenestration
balloon cholangiogram
balloon decompression
balloon dilating catheter
balloon dilation
balloon dissector
balloon-expandable flexible coil stent
balloon-expandable intravascular stent
balloon expulsion test
balloon extraction technique
balloon fenestration procedure
ballooning degeneration of hepatocytes

ballooning of hepatocytes
balloon occlusion
balloon pump
balloon reflex manometry
balloon sphincterotome
balloon tamponade of varices
balloon-tipped catheter
balloon-tipped end-hole catheter
Ball operation for treatment of pruritus
   ani
ballotable liver
ballottement, abdominal
ball-point guide pin
ball reamer
ball-tip electrode
ball-tip guide pin
ball-tipped Küntscher (Kuentscher)
   guide
ball-wedge catheter
balm of Gilead
Balneol
balsalazine
balsalazide disodium
Balser fatty necrosis
BAMBI (breast augmentation mammo-
   plasty by injection)
Banalg (methyl salicylate; camphor;
   menthol)
banana Beaver blade
banana knife
banana-shaped balloon
band
   anterior
   colon
   fascial
   free
   gastric
   Harris
   Ladd
   Lane
   Marlex
   mesocolic
   musculoaponeurotic
   omental

band *(cont.)*
   peritoneal
   ReliefBand NST
   silicone elastomer
bandage (see also *dressing*)
   Ace
   Ace adherent
   adhesive
   Artiflex
   ASE (axilla, shoulder, elbow)
   Band-Aid
   Barton
   butterfly
   capeline
   Cellona
   Champ elastic
   chip mat
   "chocolate bar"
   Clean Seals
   collodion
   Comperm
   Comperm PD
   Comperm tubular elastic
   compression
   Comprilan
   Conco Gauze
   cotton elastic
   Cover-Roll
   cravat
   crepe
   Daverbinde K
   Dema-Band
   Dema Pad
   demigauntlet
   Desault
   Dressinet netting
   Durelast
   E Cotton
   elastic
   elastic wrap
   Elastic Foam
   elastomer
   Elastomull
   Elastoplast

bandage *(cont.)*
   Esmarch
   Fabco gauze
   figure-of-8 interscapular
   Flex-Foam
   Flexilite conforming elastic
   Flex-Master
   FlexTube
   foam roll
   foam sheet
   Fractura Flex
   gauntlet
   Gibney
   Gibson
   gray foam
   gum rubber Martin
   Hamilton
   hand piece
   Heliodorus
   Hippocrates
   Hueter
   Hydron burn
   Idealbind
   immobilizing
   Isoband
   Kerlix
   Kling elastic
   K.T. Medical
   Komprex
   Komprex-Binde
   LiquiBand topical wound-closure
     glue
   Liquiderm liquid
   Luekosilk
   malleable metal finger splint
   Martin sheet rubber
   Mollelast
   "muff"
   nonadhesive
   Nu Gauze sterile gauze
   Ortho-Trac adhesive
   Ortho-Vent nonadhesive
   Pavlik
   POP (plaster of Paris)

bandage *(cont.)*
   pre-cut foam
   PRN
   Profore four-layer
   Redigrip pressure
   replantation
   restrictive
   Ribble
   Richet
   Rosidal
   Sayre
   scultetus
   self-adhering
   Silverlon wound packing strips
   sling and swathe
   Snugs
   spica
   spiral
   starch
   stockinette
   Tg
   Transelast
   Tricodur compression support
   Tricodur Epi (elbow) compression
   Tricodur Omos (shoulder)
     compression
   Tricodur Talus (ankle) compression
   Tricofix
   Tru-Support EW (elastic wrap)
   Tru-Support SA (self-adhering)
   Tubigrip
   tubular elastic
   tubular stockinette
   tumescent absorbent bandage (TAB)
   two-inch gauze
   Velpeau
   Webril
bandage and utility scissors
bandage scissors
Band-Aid
Band-Aid dressing
band and cut
band and snare
band circling needle

bandeau defect
Bandeau post-augmentation bra, The
banded bag
banding
    adjustable silicone gastric
    gastric
    hemorrhoidal
band ligation of esophageal varices
band-ligator device
bandlike adhesion
band sigmoidopexy
band slippage
band-snare technique
Bane mastoid rongeur
Bane rongeur forceps
Bane-Hartmann bone rongeur
Bangerter muscle forceps
banjo curet
banjo-string adhesion
Bankart lesion
Bankart shoulder retractor
Banks bone graft
Bantam coagulator
Bantam irrigation set
Bantam wire-cutting scissors
Banthine (methantheline bromide)
Banti disease
Banti syndrome
BAO:MAO (basal:maximal acid output
    ratio)
bar, cricopharyngeal
barbed staple
barber chair position
barber pole sign (on x-ray)
Barbidonna #2
Bard BTA test
Bard colostomy appliance
Bard Composix mesh graft material
Bard-Davol trumpet valve
Bardeleben bone-holding forceps
Bardeleben rasp
Bard Eliminator 1 balloon dilator
Bard endoscopic suturing system
Bard Extra Ileo B pouch

Bard flexible endoscopic injection
    system
Bard gastrostomy button
Bard gastrostomy catheter
Bard gastrostomy feeding tube
Bard Integrale pouch
Bard Memotherm colorectal stent
Bard-Parker blade
Bard-Parker knife
Bard Protective Barrier for ostomy skin
Bard Safety Excalibur catheter
    introducer
Bard Safety Excalibur PICC introducer
Bard Sperma-Tex preshaped mesh
Bard Visilex mesh graft
Bard XT bifurcated stent
bare area of liver
bare area of stomach
bariatric operation
bariatric surgery
Baricon contrast medium for GI
    imaging
barium
    residual
    retained
barium enema (BE)
barium enema with air contrast
barium esophagram
barium meal
barium sediment in urine
barium sulfate (BaSO$_4$)
barium sulfate-impregnated shunt
barium sulfate suspension
barium suspension, oral
barium swallow
Barnes-Neville forceps
Barnes perineorrhaphy scissors
Barnhill adenoid curette
Barobag contrast for GI imaging
Baro-cat contrast for GI imaging
Baroflave contrast medium
Baron suction tube
Baros adjunct for GI imaging
Barosperse contrast for GI imaging

barotrauma
Barouk microstaple
Barraquer cilia forceps
Barraquer Colibri forceps
Barraquer needle
Barraquer needle holder
Barraquer suture-removing forceps
Barr body analysis
Barr crypt hook
Barr D/E fistula probe
barrel guide
barrel reamer
barrel-shaped stone
Barr-Epstein virus
Barrett disease
Barrett epithelium
Barrett esophagus (BE)
Barrett intestinal forceps
Barrett mucosa
Barrett placenta forceps
Barrett syndrome
Barrett tenaculum forceps
Barrett ulcer
Barr fistula hook
Barr fistula probe
Barr hook
barrier (see also *appliance; dressing; mesh; ointment; pouch*)
   Active Life skin
   BioMesh surgical mesh
   CenterPointLock skin
   Coly-Seel ostomy
   ConvaTec skin
   CoStop surgical adhesion
   cut-to-fit skin
   Cymed colostomy
   gastric mucosal
   Gore-Tex surgical mesh
   Guidor surgical mesh
   Interceed surgical adhesion
   MicroSkin skin
   Nu-Hope skin
   Resolut surgical mesh
   SecureLife skin

barrier *(cont.)*
   SprayGel adhesion
   stockinette
barrier pack
Barr nail
Barron hemorrhoidal band
Barron hemorrhoidal ligator
Barron scalpel
Barr rectal probe
Barr rectal retractor
Barr rectal speculum
Barr-Shuford rectal speculum
Barsky skin hook
Barth curette
Barth hernia
Bartholin gland
Barton bandage
Bartonella bacilliformis
Barton obstetrical forceps
Bartter syndrome
basal acid secretion
basal anesthesia
basal cell
basal cell carcinoma
basal cell nevus syndrome
basal cell papilloma
basal granular cell
Basaljel (aluminum carbonate gel, basic)
basal:maximal acid output ratio (BAO:MAO)
basaloid carcinoma
basal plate
basal secretory flow rate (BSFR)
basal sphincter
bascule volvulus
baseball stitch
baseball suture
base deficit
Basedow disease
Basedow goiter
base excess
baseline, gastric
baseline mammogram

baseline tenting
baseline view
base material
basement membrane
base of appendix
base of tongue
base plate, bipod
base radical
basic fibroblast growth factor (bFGF)
basidiobolomycosis
basilar skull fracture
basilar suture
basiliximab
basket
    biliary stone
    CBD (common bile duct)
    Dormia stone
    four-wire
    gallstone
    intraductal biliary
    Pursuer CBD helical stone
    Pursuer CBD mini helical
    Segura CBD
    Segura stone
    six-wire
    sphincterotomy
basket extraction technique
basket forceps
basket impaction
basket retrieval
basket rongeur
basket sphincterotome
basket-type crushing forceps
basket weave pattern
$BaSO_4$ (barium sulfate)
basophil, basophile
basosquamous cell carcinoma
Bassen-Kornzweig syndrome (acantho-
    cytosis)
Bassini herniorrhaphy
Bassini inguinal hernia repair
    modified
    standard
basting suture

Batchelor plate
bathroom privileges (BRP)
bath, sitz
bathygastry
BAT (B-mode acquisition and targeting)
    system
batten graft
battery-driven hand drill
battledore (racquet-shaped) incision
Battle incision
Battle operation
Battle sign
bat-wing appearance
bat-wing catheter
Bauer and Black hernia belt
Bauer forceps
Bauhin gland
Bauhin, valve of
Baumgarten-Cruveilhier cirrhosis
Baumgartner needle holder
Baum wall unit
Baxter K-modified hose
Baxter mini-K thermia pump
Baylor sump tube
bayonet bipolar forceps
bayonet bone file
bayonet clip applier
bayonet forceps
bayonet fracture position
bayonet knife
bayonet rongeur
bayonet saw
bayonet-shaped forceps
bayonet-shaped hook
bayonet-shaped scissors
bayonet-type incision
B bile
B Braun/McGaw
BCAA (branched chain amino acids)
BCAA/AAA plasma ratio
B cell (fetal liver and bone marrow
    derived)
B-cell lymphoma
BCG (bacillus Calmette-Guérin)

BCT (breast-conserving therapy)
BDA (bile duct adenoma)
BDD (body dysmorphic disorder)
B-D Easy A1c test kit
BD Insyte Autoguard shielded I.V.
    catheter (also Autoguard-P)
BD Sensability breast self-examination
    aid
B-D Weiss epidural needle with fixed
    wings
BE (barium enema)
BE (Barrett esophagus)
Beacham amniotome
beach chair position
beach chair shoulder drape
Beacon Technology System (BTS)
beaded hepatic duct
beaded hip pin
beaded reamer guide pin
beading sign
beads
    PPMA (polymethyl-methacrylate-
        copolymer)
    Septopal
beads-on-a-string appearance
beaker cell
Beall circumflex artery scissors
Beamer injection stent system
Beamer Plus ABC unit
Beano (alpha-D-galactosidase enzyme)
bear-claw ulcer
Beardsley esophageal retractor
Bear-E-Bag Pediatric contrast medium
Bear-E-Yum GI contrast medium
Bearn-Kunkel-Slater syndrome
Beasley-Babcock forceps
Beath needle
Beath pin
Beath view
Beaver blade
    arachnoid shape
    banana
    cataract
    discission
    keratome

Beaver blade *(cont.)*
    retrograde
    rosette
    sickle shape
Beaver cataract blade
Beaver-DeBakey blade
Beaver-DeBakey knife
Beaver keratome blade
Beaver saw
BEB (blind esophageal brushing)
becaplermin
Beck aortic clamp
Becker breast implant
Becker external drain
Becker One-Piece cannula
Becker suture
Becker tissue expander/breast prosthesis
Becker Toomey syringe cannula
Beckman-Adson laminectomy blade
Beckman-Adson laminectomy retractor
Beckman-Eaton laminectomy blade
Beckman-Eaton laminectomy retractor
Beckman nasal speculum
Beckman pH probe
Beckman retractor
Beckman thyroid retractor
Beckman-Weitlaner laminectomy
    retractor
Beck miniature aortic clamp
Beck-Potts clamp
Beck triad
Beck vascular clamp
Beckwith syndrome
Beckwith-Wiedemann chromosome
    region
Beckwith-Wiedemann syndrome
Béclard hernia
Becton Dickinson introducer
Becton Dickinson Teflon-sheathed
    needle
Becton Dickinson Vacutainer
bed
    bladder
    capillary
    gallbladder

bed *(cont.)*
hepatic
liver
nail
pancreatic
portal vascular
stomach
ulcer
Bedel drape
Bedford syndrome
Bedge antireflux mattress
Beebe wire-cutting scissors
beef-lung heparin
beefy appearance
beefy texture
bee pollen
Beer cilia forceps
B.E. Glass abdominal retractor
Behçet disease
Behçet syndrome
Behrend cystic duct forceps
Bel-Phen-Ergot SR (belladonna
alkaloids; phenobarbital;
ergotamine tartrate)
belching
Bellacane elixir (atropine sulfate;
scopolamine hydrobromide;
hyoscyamine sulfate; phenobarbital)
Bellacane SR (sustained release)
(belladonna alkaloids; phenobarbi-
tal; ergotamine tartrate)
Belladenal
Bellafoline
Bell/ans tablets (sodium bicarbonate)
Bellatal (phenobarbital)
bell-clapper deformity
Belle-Amie breast prosthesis
Bellergal-S (belladonna extract; pheno-
barbital; ergotamine tartrate)
bellows, inflating sigmoidoscopic
Bell suture
Bellucci alligator forceps
Bellucci alligator scissors
"belly button" augmentation mammo-
plasty

Belsey antireflux operation
Belsey IV fundoplasty
Belsey Mark IV antireflux procedure
Belsey Mark IV 240° fundoplication
Belsey two-thirds wrap fundoplication
belt
Bauer and Black hernia
spigelian hernia
belt loop gastropexy
Belzer organ preservation unit
Belzer solution
BEMA (bioerodible mucoadhesive)
bendable metallic rod
Benedict-Talbot body surface area
method
BeneFix (coagulation factor IX
[recombinant])
Benelli mastopexy
Bengash-type needle
Bengolea artery forceps
benign adenomatous polyp
benign bile duct tumor
benign biliary stricture
benign breast condition
benign breast disease (BBD)
benign cyst
benign disease
benign epidermal tumor
benign fibrocystic disease of breast
benign gastric ulcer
benign hamartoma
benign hyperplastic gastropathy
benign in appearance
benign inflammatory thyroid
benign juvenile melanoma
benign liver adenoma
benign lymphoepithelial lesion
benign neoplasm
benign papillary stenosis
benign paroxysmal peritonitis
benign pigmented lesion
benign polyp
benign postoperative jaundice
benign primary tumor

benign prostatic hypertrophy or hyper-
  plasia (BPH)
benign recurrent intrahepatic cholestasis
benign solitary adenoma
benign squamous papilloma
benign subcutaneous cyst
benign tertian malaria
benign thyroid nodule
benign tumor
benign ulcer
benign uveal melanoma
benign vascular tumor of the liver
Benique catheter guide
Benjamin-Havas fiberoptic light clip
Bennett bone elevator
Bennett bone retractor
Bennett self-retaining retractor blade
Bennett tibia retractor
Bensaude proctoscope
Bensaude rectal speculum
Benson pylorus separator
Benson pylorus spreader
bent inner tube
bent malleable retractor
bent-tine, forklike retractor
bentiromide test
bentonite flocculation test
Bentyl (dicyclomine HCl)
benzalkonium chloride
benzidine
benzimidazoles, substituted
benzocaine
benzodiazepine
benzoin adhesive
benzquinamide
benztropine; benztropine mesylate
Beppu score
Berci-Shore choledochoscope
Berens clamp
Berens esophageal retractor
Berens muscle clamp
Berens muscle forceps
Berger disease
Berger magnifying loupe

Bergstrom cannula
Berkeley-Bonney self-retaining 3-blade
  abdominal retractor
Berkson-Gage calculation of breast
  cancer survival rates
Berliner percussion hammer
Berman airway
Berman aortic clamp
Berman oropharyngeal airway
Bernard-Sergent syndrome
Bernstein acid perfusion test
Bernstein esophageal acid infusion test
Berry sternal needle holder
Berry-TC wire-twisting forceps
Beset right-angle colon clamp
Bessauds-Hilmand-Augier syndrome
Bessey-Lowry unit for alkaline
  phosphatase
beStent Rival coronary stent system
Best gallstone forceps
Best intestinal clamp
Best right-angle colon clamp
beta-adrenergic blockade
beta blockade therapy
beta blocker
Beta-Cath system catheter
beta cell function
beta cell protective agent
beta cells of pancreatic islets
beta cell tumor of pancreas
Betadine (povidone-iodine)
Betadine dressing
Betadine gel
Betadine scrub
Betadine-soaked Owen gauze dressing
Betadine soap
Betadine solution
Betadine Surgi-Prep
beta hCG (human chorionic
  gonadotropin)
beta hemolytic strep (streptococcus)
Beta LT (beta-alethine)
beta-lactamase enzyme
beta 1 and beta 2 agonist

beta-naphthylamine
Betathine (beta-alethine)
betazole stimulation test
betel cancer
bethanechol
Bethea sheet holder
Bethune-Coryllos rib shears
Bethune periosteal elevator
Bethune rib shears
Bethune rongeur
Bevan abdominal incision
Bevan gallbladder forceps
beveled chisel
beveled knife
beveled speculum
beveled thin-walled needle
BEVS (Baculovirus Expression Vector
    System)
Bexxar (tositumomab, ^{131}I tositumomab)
Beyer paracentesis needle
Beyer forceps
Beyer rongeur
Beyer-Stille bone rongeur
bezoar formation
BFDR (bronchospasm, flushing,
    diarrhea, right-sided heart failure)
bFGF (basic fibroblast growth factor)
Biafine WDE (wound dressing
    emulsion)
biarticular bone shears
biarticular bone-cutting forceps
bias stockinette wrap
Biaxin XL (clarithromycin) extended-
    release tablets
BIB (biliointestinal bypass)
bicanalicular sphincter
BiCAP (Bipolar Circumactive Probe)
BiCAP bipolar diathermy
BiCAP cautery
BiCAP electrocoagulation probe
BiCAP endoscopic probe
BiCAP hemostatic system
Bicarbolyte
bicarbonate (HCO$_3^-$)

bicarbonate concentration
bicarbonate, sodium
biceps jerk (BJ)
bichloroacetic acid
Bickel intramedullary nail
Bickel intramedullary rod
BiCOAG bipolar forceps
bicortical iliac bone graft
bicortical ilial strip graft
bidomal shield template
Bier amputation saw
Bier block anesthesia
Bier lumbar puncture needle
Bierman needle
Biermer disease
Biesenberger technique of mastopexy
Biethium ostomy rod
bifid hook
Bifidobacterium bifidum
biflanged drill
bifoil balloon
bifoil balloon catheter
bifrontal incision
bifurcated cable
bifurcation
    aortic
    bile duct
    common bile duct
    hepatic
    iliac vessel
bifurcation lesion
bifurcation tumor
Big Bag 3000
Bigelo calvarium clamp
Bihrle dorsal clamp
bikini skin incision
BiLAP bipolar cautery
BiLAP bipolar cutting and coagulating
    probes
BiLAP bipolar needle electrode
bilateral adrenal hemorrhage
bilateral adrenalectomy
bilateral cortical necrosis
bilateral hernia

bilateral herniorrhaphy
bilateral hyperplasia
bilateral incarcerated scrotal hernia
bilateral inguinal hernia
bilateral inguinofemoral lymphadenec-
  tomies
bilateral mammogram
bilateral mastectomies
bilateral nodular dysplasia
bilateral pleural tube
bilateral recurrent laryngeal nerve
  damage
bilateral right-sidedness sequence
bilateral subcostal incision
bilateral total adrenalectomy
bilateral ureteral obstruction (BUO)
bilateral vagotomy
bilayer patch hernia repair
bilayer polypropylene mesh
bile
  A
  B
  C
  canaliculus
  clear
  cloudy
  conjugated
  extrahepatic
  gallbladder
  inspissated
  limy
  lithogenic
  liver
  stagnant
  supersaturated
  thick
  turbid
  viscid
  viscous
  white
bile acid
  conjugated
  fecal
  oxidized
  total

bile acid binder
bile acid breath test
bile acid-EDTA (BA-EDTA) solution
bile acid pool
bile acid sequestrant
bile acid tolerance test
bile antigen
bile ascites
bile bag
bile capillary
bile concretion
bile duct
  common (CBD)
  extrahepatic
  infundibulum of
  interlobular
  preampullary portion of
  sphincter of
bile duct abscess
bile duct adenoma (BDA)
bile duct calculus
bile duct carcinoma
bile duct colic
bile duct cystadenocarcinoma
bile duct dyskinesia
bile duct epithelium
bile duct gland
bile duct hamartoma
bile duct injury
bile duct lumen
bile duct obstruction
bile duct pressure
bile duct proliferation
bile duct stasis
bile duct stone
bile duct stricture
bile-induced gastritis
bile lake
bile leakage
bile papilla
bile peritonitis
bile pigment in basal ganglia
bile plug
bile reflux
bile reflux gastritis

bile salt-binding resin
bile salt diarrhea
bile salt-losing enteropathy
bile salts in the skin
bile sludge
bile solubility test
bile spillage, intraoperative
bile-stained fluid
bile-stained vomitus
bile stasis
bile supersaturated with cholesterol
bile-tinged fluid
Bilezyme
bilharzial carcinoma
"bili" (see *bilirubin*)
biliary atresia
   distal
   cxtrahepatic
biliary balloon catheter
biliary balloon probe
biliary calculus
biliary canal
biliary cirrhosis
biliary cirrhotic liver
biliary colic
biliary conduit
biliary-cutaneous fistula
biliary decompression
biliary dilation; dilatation
biliary duct
biliary ductule
biliary-duodenal fistula
biliary-duodenal pressure gradient
biliary dyskinesia
biliary dyspepsia
biliary endoprosthesis
biliary endoscopy
biliary-enteric anastomosis
biliary-enteric bypass
biliary-enteric fistula
biliary fistula
biliary gland
biliary manometry
biliary mud
biliary obstruction, malignant

biliary pancreatitis
biliary passage
biliary peritonitis
biliary piecemeal necrosis
biliary plexus
biliary radicle (*not* radical)
biliary reconstruction
biliary saturation index
biliary scintiscan
biliary sludge
biliary sphincter
biliary sphincterotomy and stent
   placement
biliary stasis
biliary stenosis
biliary stent
biliary stone disease
biliary stricture, long-segment intra-
   hepatic
biliary structure
biliary tract disease
biliary tract infection
biliary tract stone
biliary tree
BiliChek bilirubin analyzer
Biligrafin contrast medium
Bili mask
bilioenteric fistula
biliointestinal bypass (BIB)
biliopancreatic bypass (BPB)
biliopancreatic shunt
Biliopaque
bilious aspirate
bilious colic
bilious diarrhea
bilious emesis
biliousness
bilious pneumonia
bilious remittent malaria
bilious stool
bilious vomiting
bilirubin ("bili")
   conjugated
   direct
   elevated

biopsy *(cont.)*
    random needle
    scan-directed
    serial liver
    shave
    SiteSelect breast
    small bowel endoscopic
    snare loop
    Sonopsy 3-D ultrasound
    StereoGuide stereotactic needle core
    stereotactic aspiration
    stereotactic brain
    stereotactic breast
    stereotactic core needle (SCNB)
    stereotactic needle
    strip
    suction
    sural nerve
    synovial
    targeted brain
    temporal artery
    TNB (transthoracic needle)
    transfemoral liver
    transjugular liver
    transnasal
    transpapillary
    transvenous liver
    Tru-Cut needle (TCNB)
    ultrasonography-guided fine-needle
        aspiration
    ultrasound-guided anterior subcostal
        liver
    ultrasound-guided echo
    ultrasound-guided needle
    ultrasound-guided stereotactic
    vertebral body
    Vim-Silverman needle
    wedge
    wedge hepatic (or liver)
biopsy and brushings
biopsy cannula
biopsy excisors
biopsy cup forceps
biopsy needle

biopsy of breast, needle core
biopsy of cyst wall
biopsy of kidney
biopsy of pancreas
biopsy punches
biopsy specimen
biopsy suction curette
biopsy trephine
Biopty cut needle for breast biopsy
Biörck syndrome
BioROC absorbable suture anchor
Biosafe PSA4 test
BioSorb resorbable urology stent
BioSorb suture
Biostent stent
BioStinger
biosurgery
Biosyn synthetic monofilament suture
biotinylated IL-10 monoclonal
    antibody
Biotrack coagulation monitor
Bio-Tract proprietary strain of
    Lactobacillus salivarius
BioTwist
BioVue PICC catheter
BiPAP S/T-D 30 ventilatory support
BiPAP S/T-D ventilatory support
biparietal suture
biplanar aortography
biplane sector probe
bipod base plate
bipod suspension apparatus
bipolar cable
bipolar cautery (BiCAP)
bipolar cautery forceps
bipolar cautery probe
bipolar cautery scissors
bipolar coagulation
bipolar connecting cables
bipolar electrocoagulation
bipolar forceps
bipolar probe
bipolar urological loop
BiQ bipolar hand instrument

BI-RADS (Breast Imaging Reporting
    and Data System)
Bircher bone clamp
Bircher cartilage clamp
Bircher-Ganske cartilage forceps
Bircher meniscus knife
bird-beak configuration or narrowing
bird-breeder's lung
bird's nest lesion
biricodar dicitrate
BIS Sensor
BIS Sensor Plus
bisacodyl tannex
Bisco-Lax (bisacodyl)
Bishop chisel
Bishop clamp
Bishop gouge
Bishop-Harmon forceps
Bishop-Koop ileostomy
Bishop saw
Bismatrol (bismuth subsalicylate)
bismuth compounds
bismuth subcarbonate
bismuth subgallate
bismuth subsalicylate
Bismuth classification of benign bile
    duct stricture, types I-V
Bisound AP 3000 Colorflow ultrasound
    system
bisoxatin; bisoxatin acetate
BiSure laparoscopic forceps
bite down
bite of tissue
bite, surgical
bithionol
Bitin (bithionol)
bivalve (noun); bivalved (verb)
Bivona tracheostomy tube
BJ (biceps jerk)
BK DNA virus
Black and Decker drill
black blood clot
black death
Black-Draught syrup (casanthranol;
    senna extract)

Black-Draught tablets (senna
    concentrate)
black faceted stone
black liver disease
black lung
black pigment gallstone
Black rasp
black stone
black suture
black tarry stool
black widow spider bite
bladder bed
bladder carcinoma classification
bladder decompression
bladder fistula
bladder incontinence
bladder injury
bladder neck spreader
bladder neck support prosthesis
bladder pheochromocytoma
BladderScan
bladder scissors
bladder sound
bladder spatula
bladder stone
bladder tumor
bladder tumor assay (BTA)
blade (see also *knife*)
    arachnoid shape
    arthroscopic
    banana
    Bard-Parker
    Beaver cataract
    Beaver discission
    Beaver keratome
    Beaver-DeBakey
    Beckman-Adson laminectomy
    Beckman-Eaton laminectomy
    Bennett self-retaining
    carotid
    cartilage shaver
    Caspar
    cataract
    chisel
    chondroplasty

blade *(cont.)*
copper
craniotome
crescentic
Curdy
deep
Dennis
discission
double-edged razor
Doyen vaginal retractor
drill
Dyonics arthroscopic
Feild (not Field)
full curve
Gigli saw
Gomel
guillotine
Hebra
Hibbs
Incisor arthroscopic
K
keratome
knife
laminectomy
laryngoscope
LaserSonics EndoBlade
LaserSonics Nd:YAG LaserBlade
LaserSonics Surgiblade
malleable
McIntosh laryngoscope
meniscal trimmer
meniscectomy
Meyerding laminectomy
Meyerding-Scoville
MicroAire
mini meniscus
MVR
notchplasty
oscillating
partial curve
Paufique
PowerCut drill
RAD Airway laryngeal
razor

blade *(cont.)*
retractor
retrograde
ring-cutter
Rosenkranz deep retractor
rosette
saw
scalpel
Scoville
sickle-shaped
skin
spinal retractor
spoon
S/P surgical
Superblade
Surgiblade sterile scalpel
Swann-Morton surgical
Synovator arthroscopic
synovectomy
Taylor spinal retractor
Temperlite saw
3M Maxi Driver
tongue
tracheal
triradial resector
UltraCision ultrasonic knife
UltraClean electrosurgical
bladebreaker knife
blade handle
blade holder
blade plate
blade plate driver
blade-safe
Blair chisel
Blair elevator
Blair palate hook
Blair saw guide
Blair silicone drain
Blaivas classification of urinary incontinence
Blake drain
Blake gallstone forceps
Blakemore-Sengstaken tube
Blakemore tube

Blakesley suction flow forceps
Blake wound drain
Blalock-Niedner clamp
Blalock pulmonary clamp
Blalock-Taussig clamp
blanching of mucosa
blanching spider telangiectasias
bland diet
bland food
Blandin gland
bland thrombosis
blastic lesion
bleb-like adhesion
bleed (noun)
   GI
   herald
   slow
   variceal
BLEED (bleeding, low BP, elevated PT,
   erratic mental status, disease
   [comorbid]) classification
bleeder
bleeding
   abnormal
   active source of
   colorectal
   concomitant
   dysfunctional uterine (DUB)
   excessive
   external
   gastrointestinal tract
   GI (gastrointestinal)
   retroperitoneal
   intra-abdominal
   massive
   massive lower GI
   occult
   painless rectal
   pinpoint gastric mucosal defect
   portal hypertension-induced variceal
   postcoital
   postmenopausal
   purpuric
   rectal

bleeding *(cont.)*
   recurrent
   refractory
   variceal
   widespread
bleeding abnormality
bleeding controlled with direct pressure
bleeding controlled with electrocautery
bleeding diathesis
bleeding esophageal ulcer
bleeding esophageal varices
bleeding esophagogastric varices
bleeding from gastroduodenal artery
bleeding gastric varices
bleeding gums
bleeding into cyst
bleeding into joint
bleeding into parenchyma
bleeding into pericardial sac
bleeding lesion
bleeding per rectum
bleeding points were cauterized
bleeding polyp
bleeding time
   Duke
   Ivy
   Mielke
   Simplate
bleeding time coagulation panel
bleeding ulcer
bleeding vessel, embolization of
blenderized diet
BLEND waveform desiccation
Blickman Health Industries
blind clamping
blind enema
blind esophageal brushing (BEB)
blind gut
blindness
blind limb
blind loop syndrome
blind medullary nail
blind needle insufflation
blind percutaneous liver biopsy

blind pouch
blind stump
blind upper esophageal pouch
BlisterFilm transparent dressing
bloat; bloated
bloating, gas
Bloch-Paul-Mikulicz operation
block
 intercostal nerve
 ischiorectal fossa
 neuroplexus
blockade
block anesthesia
blocked shunt tube
blocked sweat gland
Blom-Singer tracheoesophageal fistula
Blond anoscope
blood
 anticoagulant-treated
 antigenic properties of
 arterial
 autologous
 bright red
 capillary
 gross
 Hemolink blood substitute
 hemolyzed
 Hextend blood substitute
 intraperitoneal
 iron-binding capacity of
 laky
 mass of congealed
 microscopic
 mixed venous
 nonoxygenated
 occult
 oozing
 oxygenated
 oxygen-carrying capacity of
 PentaLyte
 peripheral
 platelet-poor (PPB)
 PolyHeme blood substitute
 sludged

blood *(cont.)*
 spurting
 stagnation of
 transfusion of incompatible
 typed and crossmatched
 venous
 whole
blood admixed with stool
blood-borne organism
blood cell filtration, Hemasure r/LS
 circulating
blood clot (see *clot*)
blood coagulation
blood culture
 defibrinated
 degenerated
 dissecting (from the retroperitoneal)
 donor
 extravasated
 fecal occult
 frank
blood flow
 increased collateral
 reduced transhepatic
blood gas
 arterial
 base excess
 bicarbonate (bicarb)
 HCO_3^-(bicarbonate)
 $PaCO_2$
 PaO_2
 pCO_2
 pH
 pO_2
blood gas on oxygen (FiO_2—fractional
 percentage of inspired oxygen)
blood gas on room air
blood glucose, fasting
blood glucose monitor
 Accu-Chek Advantage
 Accu-Chek Complete
 Accu-Chek Easy
 Accu-Chek Freedom II
 Accu-Chek Instant

blood glucose monitor *(cont.)*
   Accu-Chek Instant Plus
   Accu-Chek Simplicity
   Accu-Chek Voicemate
   Appraise
   Assure
   AtLast
   Chemstrip MatchMaker
   Companion 2
   Diasensor 1000
   Digital Response
   Duet
   ExacTech
   ExpressView
   FastTake
   FreeStyle
   FreeStyle glucose
   Glucochek Pocketlab II blood
   Glucometer DEX system
   Glucometer Elite
   Glucometer Elite R
   Glucometer Elite XL
   Glucometer Encore
   Glucometer II
   Gluco-Protein OTC self-test
     glucose system
   GlucoWatch
   Glycosal
   In Charge
   Medisense Pen 2
   One Touch Basic
   One Touch FastTake
   One Touch Profile
   One Touch II
   One Touch Ultra
   Precision QID
   Precision Xtra
   Prestige Smart System (PSS)
   Select GT
   self (SBGM)
   Sof-Tact
   Supreme II
   SureStep
   SureStep Pro

blood glucose monitor *(cont.)*
   TD Glucose
   Tracer
   Visidex
   Visidex II
Bloodgood syndrome
blood in cyst aspirate
blood in stool
   gross
   microscopic
   occult
blood in toilet bowl
blood irradiator, portable
bloodless field
bloodless operation
bloodless zone of necrosis
blood mixed with stool
blood on surface of stool
blood on toilet paper
blood outflow line
blood passed with stool
blood pool
blood pressure, orthostatic
blood pressure titration
blood sludge
blood smear
blood-stained effusion
blood-streaked stool
blood substitute
   HemAssist (hemoglobin
     crosfumaril)
   Hemolink
   Hemopure
   Oxygent (emulsified perflubron)
   PolyHeme (human hemoglobin
     cross-linked with glutaral)
blood-sucking intestinal parasite
blood-tinged ascites
blood-tinged discharge
blood-tinged fluid
blood-tinged sputum
blood transfusion, mismatched
blood urea level
blood urea nitrogen (BUN)

blood vessel invasion
blood volume
blood volume expander
   Plasbumin-5
   Plasbumin-25 (human albumin)
   Plasmanate
   Plasma-Plex
   Plasmatein
   Protenate
blood volume expansion
blood vomitus
Bloodwell forceps
bloody ascites
bloody aspirate
bloody diarrhea
bloody discharge
bloody fluid
bloody nipple discharge
bloody peritoneal fluid
bloody spinal fluid
bloody stools
bloody vomitus
Bloom syndrome
Blount anvil retractor
Blount blade plate
Blount disease
Blount hip retractor
Blount knee retractor
Blount knife
Blount staple
blowhole ileostomy
blowing wound
blown pupil
blowout of suture ties
blue and white mattress suture
blue and white Tycron suture
Blue Cushion anesthesia face mask
blue diaper syndrome
blue dot sign
Blue FlexTip catheter
Blue Goo (Iamin hydrating gel) dressing
blue line Murphy tracheal tube
blue liver
Blue Max balloon

blue rubber-bleb nevus syndrome
blue rubber nevus syndrome
blue stone
bluish discoloration
Blumberg sign of peritonitis
Blumenthal bone rongeur
Blumenthal lesion
Blumenthal rongeur
Blumer rectal shelf
Blumgart technique for hepatico-
   jejunostomy
blunt abdominal trauma
blunt and sharp dissection
blunt caliper
blunt dissection
blunt elevator
blunt grasping forceps, double-action
blunt hook
blunting of valve
blunt injury
blunt nerve hook
blunt-nose grasper
blunt-point suture
Bluntport disposable laparoscopic trocar
blunt probe
blunt rupture of liver
blunt rupture of spleen
blunt tapered T-handled reamer
blunt-tip cannula
blunt-tipped scissors
blunt trauma
blunt trocar
blurred pericecal fat (on CT scan)
B lymphocyte (B cell)
BM (bone marrow)
BM (bowel movement)
BMI (body mass index) (pl. indices)
B-mode acquisition and targeting (BAT)
B-mode ultrasonography
BMP (bone morphogenic protein)
BMT (bone marrow transplant, bone
   marrow transplantation)
boardlike rigidity of abdomen
Boas point of gastric ulcer

Boas sign of gastric ulcer
Boas test of gastric ulcer
boatlike abdomen
boat nail
boat-shaped abdomen
Bobechko hook
Bochdalek, foramen of
Bochdalek hernia
Bodenhammer rectal speculum
Bodnar retractor
body
   acidophilic
   asteroid
   Barr
   Councilman
   esophageal
   foreign
   gallbladder
   Heinz
   Howell-Jolly
   inclusion
   Lafora
   Mallory
   malpighian
   Pappenheimer
   pancreas
   psamomma
   Schaumann
   stomach
   vermiform
body access instrumentation
body cell mass
body composition
body density
body dysmorphic disorder (BDD)
body fat calipers
body fluid
body habitus
body hair loss
body mass index (or indices) (BMI)
body of gallbladder
body of pancreas
body of stomach
body wall

Boeck, sarcoid of
Boehler (Böhler)
Boehler bone rongeur
Boehler calcaneal view
Boehler lumbosacral view
Boehler plaster cast breaker
Boehler plaster shears
Boehringer suction regulator
Boerema anterior gastropexy
Boerema hernia repair
Boerhaave syndrome (esophageal
   rupture)
Boettcher artery forceps
Bogros space
Böhler (Boehler)
Böhler clamp
Böhler pin
Bohlman pin
Boies forceps
Bolivian hemorrhagic fever virus
bolster
   cotton
   Dacron velour
bolster suture
bolus anesthesia
bolus challenge test
bolus dressing
bolus feeding
bolus of cotton
bombesin
Bondek absorbable suture
bone abscess
bone awl
bone biopsy
bone biopsy needle
bone-biting forceps
bone-breaking forceps
Bone Bridge suture passer
Bone Bullet suture anchor
bone chip graft
bone chisel
bone curette
bone-cutting instrument
bone drill

bone elevator
bone extension clamp
bone extractor
bone flap fixation plate
bone gouge
bone graft punch
bone graft substitute
bone-grasping forceps
bone-holding clamp
bone-holding forceps
bone hook
bone mallet
bone marrow (BM)
bone marrow aspirate
bone marrow augmentation,
    donor-specific
bone marrow biopsy
bone marrow dysfunction
bone marrow transplant, bone marrow
    transplantation (BMT)
bone metastasis
bone morphogenic protein (BMP)
bone-nibbling rongeur
bone peg graft
BonePlast
bone plate
bone plug extractor
bone punch
bone punch forceps
bone reamer
bone-retinaculum-bone autograft
bone retractor
bone round needle
bone saw
bone-splitting forceps
bone staple
bone-tendon-bone graft
bone tumor
bone wax
bone wire guide
Bonfiglio bone graft
Bonine (meclizine)
Bonner position
Bonney forceps

Bonney insufflator
Bonney needle
Bonney stress incontinence test
Bonn scissors
bony landmarks
bony plate
Bookler swivel-ball laparoscopic
    instrument holder
Bookwalter retractor
boomerang needle holder
BOOP (bronchiolitis obliterans
    with organizing pneumonia)
Boorman gastric cancer typing system
    (types 1–4)
boot
    O_2 Boot
    pneumatic compression
    Unna
borborygmus (pl. borgorygmi)
border, antimesenteric (*not* ante-)
border cell
borderline malignancy
bore needle
borescope
    ITI rigid
    KLI rigid
borescope endoscope
Borge clamp
boring pain
Bornholm disease
Borrelia burgdorferi
bosselated stone
Bosworth drill
Bosworth spine plate
Botox injection
Botox sphincter injection
botryoid sarcoma
bottle and specimen forceps
bottle, DISS suction
bottle-nose forceps
bottle-nose grasper
botulinum toxin
botulism
Bouchard disease

Bouge needle
bougie
  acorn-tipped
  Celestin dilator
  Clutton urethral
  EndoLumina
  esophageal
  filiform
  French
  Hegar
  Hurst mercury
  Jackson esophageal
  large-diameter
  Lister
  Maloney
  mercury-filled
  mercury-weighted
  Savary
  tapered rubber
  Trousseau esophageal
  Van Buren urethral
bougie and catheter
bougienage
  esophageal
  peroral
bougie à boule
Bouin fixative solution
Bouin fluid
Bouin solution
bound down with adhesions
Bourne test
Boutin thoracoscope
Bouveret syndrome
bovie; bovied (verb)
Bovie 2100 coagulating electrosurgical
  device
Bovie electrocautery
Bovie knife
bovine collagen graft
bovine heterograft
bovine immunoglobulin concentrate
bovine pericardium graft
bovine pericardium strip

bowel
  aganglionic
  apple-peel
  dead
  friable
  gangrenous
  infarcted
  intussuscepted
  ischemic
  knuckle of
  large
  necrotic
  nonviable
  small
  strangulated
bowel abscess
bowel adherent to omentum
bowel axis
bowel bag
bowel contents
bowel continuity
bowel dilatation
bowel disease with protein loss
bowel elimination disorder
bowel entrapment (internal hernia)
bowel evacuant (see *bowel prep; enema*)
bowel function, assessment of
bowel gas
bowel gas pattern
bowel grasper
bowel habits
bowel incontinence
bowel infarction
bowel intussusception
bowel loop
bowel loop air
bowel lumen
bowel mass, intramural
bowel mobilization
bowel movement (BM)
bowel necrosis
bowel obstruction
  functional
  mechanical

bowel packed out of the way
bowel perforation
bowel prep (see also *enema*)
   Ceo-Two suppository
   ChloraPrep One-Step
   Colonlite
   CoLyte
   Davol
   Dulcolax
   Emulsoil
   Evac-Q-Kit
   Fleet
   Go-Evac
   GoLYTELY
   inadequate
   ipepac syrup
   magnesium citrate
   magnesium sulfate
   NuLytely
   OCL
   syrup of ipecac
   Tridrate Bowel Evacuant Kit
   Visicol
   X-Prep
bowel preparation (bowel prep)
bowel pseudo-obstruction
bowel rest
bowel retractor
bowel scissors
bowel sounds
   absent
   active
   crescendoing
   decreased
   diminished
   gurgling
   high-pitched
   hyperactive
   hypoactive
   low-pitched
   musical
   negative
   normal
   normoactive (NABS)

bowel sounds *(cont.)*
   positive
   quiet
   return of
   rumbling
   tinkling
bowel stenosis
bowel stoma
bowel tones
bowel wall, compromised
bowel wall hematoma
bowel wall involvement
Bowen chisel
Bowen disease of anal canal
Bowen periosteal elevator
Bowen syndrome
Bowlby tracheal dilator
bowler hat sign
Bowles scope
Bowles stethoscope
Bowman probe
Bowman scissors
Bowman tube
bow-shaped spatula
bow-type saw
box chisel
boxer's punch or fracture (of fifth
   metacarpal)
boxwood mallet
Boyce modification of Sengstaken-
   Blakemore tube
Boyce sign
Boyd dual-onlay bone graft
Boyden sphincter
Boyden test meal
Boyes-Goodfellow hook
Boyes-Goodfellow retractor
Boyes muscle clamp
Boyle uterine elevator
Boynton needle
Boynton needle holder
Bozeman (knee-elbow) position
Bozeman sponge-holding forceps
Bozeman-Thomson Walker needle
   holder

Bozicevich test
BPB (biliopancreatic bypass)
BPB (bone-patellar ligament-bone)
    autologous graft
BPB (bone-patellar tendon-bone)
    autologous graft
BPI (bactericidal/permeability-
    increasing) protein
BPM (Laserflo blood perfusion
    monitor)
BPS spinal angiographic catheter
bra
    Caromed postaugmentation
    "Laser Bra" procedure (see *L.I.F.T.*)
    postaugmentation mammoplasty
    The Bandeau postaugmentation
BRACAnalysis test for detection of
    hereditary breast and ovarian cancer
brace drill
brace-type reamer
brachial anesthesia
brachial plexus
brachial plexus root retractor
brachioaxillary bridge graft fistula
    (BAGF)
brachiocephalic vein
brachiosubclavian bridge graft fistula
    (BSGF)
Brachmann-de Lange syndrome
Bracht-Wachter lesion
BrachySeed iodine [125]I
brachytherapy, gamma
Braden score
Bradley disease
bradyarrhythmia
braided Nurolon suture
braided silk suture
braided suture
braided tape
brain abscess
brain biopsy
brain clip forceps
brain death
brain-exploring cannula

brain forceps
brain metastasis
brain retractor
brain scissors
brain spatula forceps
brain suction tube
brain swelling
brain tumor forceps
Braithwaite knife
Bralon braided nylon suture
Bramber head mirror
branched chain amino acid (BCAA)
brancher deficiency glycogenosis
brancher enzyme deficiency
brancher glycogen storage disease
branches of superior mesenteric artery
branchial cleft cyst
branchial fistula
branchial pouch
branching pattern
branchiogenous cyst
branch of celiac axis
Brand tendon-holding forceps
Brand tendon-passing forceps
Brand tendon-tunneling forceps
Brandt cytology balloon
Brandt syndrome
Branhamella catarrhalis (formerly
    Neisseria catarrhalis)
Branham sign
brash
    sour
    water
BRAT (bananas, rice cereal, apple-
    sauce, toast) diet
BRATS (bananas, rice, apples, toast,
    saltines) diet
Braun anastomosis
Braun depressor
Braun episiotomy scissors
Braun hook
Braun-Jaboulay gastroenterostomy
Braun skin graft
Braun-Stadler scissors

Braun tenaculum forceps
BRBPR (bright red blood per rectum)
BRCA (breast cancer [gene]) mutation
BRCA1 (breast cancer one) gene
BRCA2 (breast cancer two) gene
breadlike material
BreakAway absorptive wound dressing
breakaway pin
breakdown product
breaker
   blade
   Boehler plaster cast
   Castroviejo blade
   Swiss-pattern blade
breakfast, Ewald
break-screw extractor
breast
   accessory
   fibroadenoma of
   fibrocystic
   proemial
   shotty
breast abscess
BreastAlert differential temperature
   sensor (DTS)
breast asymmetry
breast atrophy
breast augmentation (see *mammoplasty*)
breast binder, Expand-A-Band
breast biopsy system, Mammotest
breast bolster
breast bone (also, breastbone)
breast calcifications
breast cancer (carcinoma)
   cystosarcoma phyllodes
   in situ
   inflammatory
   intraductal
   invasive
   metastatic
   Paget disease
breast cancer genes
   BRCA1
   BRCA2

breast cancer metastasis
Breast Cancer Prevention Trial
breast carcinoma (see *breast cancer*)
BreastCheck device
breast-conserving surgery
   lumpectomy
   partial mastectomy
   quadrantectomy
   wide-excision
breast-conserving therapy (BCT)
   (lumpectomy, axillary dissection,
   and radiation therapy)
breast contour
breast cyst
breast degeneration
BreastExam device for breast cancer
   detection
breast examination, B-D Sensability
   Breast Self-Examination Aid
breast feeding
breast fibroadenoma
breast fibrocystic disease
breast form—see *breast implant; prosthesis*
Breast Imaging and Reporting System
   (BI-RADS) of the American College
   of Radiology
breast implant (also see *prosthesis*)
   adjustable saline
   Amoena
   asymmetrical
   Becker
   Belle-Amie
   Biocell RTV saline-filled
   filled
   BioDimensional
   calcified
   Contour Profile
   Cronin breast
   custom
   Discrene
   Dow Corning
   encapsulated
   explantation of

bronchial mucosa
bronchial polyp
bronchial sponge
bronchial stenosis
bronchioalveolar carcinoma
bronchiolar edema
bronchiolitis obliterans with organizing
   pneumonia (BOOP)
bronchioloalveolar carcinoma
Bronchitrac L catheter
bronchoalveolar lavage (BAL)
bronchobiliary fistula
Broncho-Cath endobronchial tube
Broncho-Cath endotracheal tube
Broncho-Cath with carinal hook
bronchocavitary fistula
bronchoesophageal fistula
bronchoesophageal forceps
bronchoesophageal scissors
bronchogenic carcinoma
bronchopleural fistula
bronchopulmonary segment
bronchoscopic smear
bronchospasm
bronchus forceps
bronze diabetes (iron storage disease)
bronze edema
bronze liver
Brooke-Bookwalter retractor
Brooke ileostomy
Brooker femoral nail
Brooker-Wills nail
Brook stitch scissors
Brophy periosteal elevator
Brophy scissors
Broviac catheter
brow-down skull view
Brown-Adson tissue forceps
Brown-Cushing forceps
Brown dietary method for colon
   preparation
Browne pneumatic impactor
Brown-McHardy pneumatic dilator
Brown needle holder

brown pigment gallstone
Brown rasp
brown stones
brown stool
Brown tissue forceps
brown tumor
brow-up skull view
Broxine (broxuridine) radiosensitizer
broxuridine radiosensitizer
BRP (bathroom privileges)
Brucella abortus
Brucella canis
Brucella melitensis
Brucella suis
brucellosis
Bruel-Kjaer 3535 ultrasound scanner
Bruening chisel
Bruening-Citelli rongeur
bruisability, easy
bruit, Cruveilhier-Baumgarten
Brunetti chisel with guard
Brun metacarpal saw
Brunner gland
Brunner gland adenoma
Brunner gland of duodenum
Brunner intestinal forceps
Brunner modified incision
Brunner palmar incision
Brunner rib shears
brunneroma
Bruns curette
Brunschwig artery forceps
Brunschwig operation
Bruns shears
Bruser skin (knee) incision
brush
   ERCP
   facial cannula
   Olympus cytology
brush and biopsy
brush biopsy
brush border of intestine
brush cytology
brushings and biopsy

brushings and washings
Bryan laparoscope
Bryan rigid laparoscope
BSA (body surface area)
BSD-2000 (*Lactobacillus salivarius*)
BSFR (basal secretory flow rate) test
BSGF (brachiosubclavian bridge graft fistula)
BSP (bromosulfophthalein) test
BTA stat bladder tumor assay
BTA TRAK bladder tumor assay
BTI-322 monoclonal antibody
bubble (see *balloon*)
   duodenal
   Garren-Edwards gastric (GEG)
   gastric
   intragastric
bubonocele
buccal frenulum
buccal gland
buccal mucosa
buccal region
buccal ulcer
Buck elevator
Buck-Gramcko gouge
Buck-Gramcko retractor
Buckley chisel
Buck neurological percussion hammer
Buck periosteal elevator
Buck scissors
Bucky imaging device
Bucky view
Bucladin-S
buclizine; buclizine HCl
bucrylate sclerosant
bucrylate (or bucrilate) tissue adhesive
Bucy chordotomy (or cordotomy) knife
Bucy-Frazier coagulating suction cannula
Bucy laminectomy rongeur
Budd-Chiari syndrome
Budd cirrhosis
Budd disease
Budde-Greenberg-Sugita retractor

Budd jaundice
Budd syndrome
budesonide
buffalo hump
buffer local instillation
buffer system
Buffets II (acetaminophen; aspirin; caffeine; aluminum hydroxide)
Buie fistula clamp
Buie fistula forceps
Buie fistula probe
Buie pile clamp
Buie position
Buie rectal forceps
Buie rectal probe
Buie rectal scissors
Buie rectal suction tip
Buie rectal suction tube
Buie-Smith retractor
Buie sigmoidoscope
Buie suction tube
Build Up enteral feeding
buildup of secretions
bulb and Air-Flo control valve
bulbar peptic ulcer
bulb, duodenal
bulbocavernous gland
bulbourethral gland
bulb suction
bulge
bulging of mucosa
bulimia nervosa
bulimorexia
bulk laxative
bulky dressing
bulky stools
bulky tumor
bulldog clamp
bulldog clamp-applying forceps
bulldog forceps
bullet driver
bullet-nose grasper
bullet-nose grasping, tissue well, double-action forceps

bullous appearance
bullous dermatitis
bullous-like edema
Bullseye guide
bull's-eye lesion
Bumex (bumetanide)
Bumm placenta curette
bumper (bolster)
BUN (blood urea nitrogen)
bunching suture
bundle suture
bunion retractor
Bunnell crisscross suture
Bunnell dissecting probe
Bunnell dressing
Bunnell forwarding probe
Bunnell hand drill
Bunnell probe
Bunnell tendon needle
Bunnell wire pullout suture
Bunyavirus infection
BUO (bilateral ureteral obstruction)
bupivacaine; bupivacaine HCl
Burch colposuspension
Burch iliopectineal ligament
   urethrovesical suspension
Burch laparoscopic procedure
burden, disease
Burdick paper
Burford-Finochietto retractor
Burford retractor
Burhenne biliary duct stone extraction
Burhenne steerable catheter
buried bumper syndrome
buried interrupted suture
buried-knot suture
buried penis
buried suture
buried vaginal island
Burke biopsy forceps
Burkitt lymphoma
burn
   chemical
   contact

burn (cont.)
   electrical
   first-degree
   flame
   scald
   second-degree
   third-degree
burn classification
burn debridement
burned-out mucosa (on x-ray)
burned-out pancreas
Burnett syndrome
burning pain
burning vulvar syndrome
burn scar carcinoma
burn wound
Burns plate
Buro-Sol (aluminum sulfate)
Burow solution (aluminum sulfate)
burp; burping
bursoscopy, supragastric
Burton headlight
Burton Nova exam light
Burton reflector light
Burton ultraviolet light
Busch suture scissors
Busch umbilical scissors
Buscopan
busulfan
Busulfex (busulfan)
butenafine
Butibel (belladonna extract; butabarbital
   sodium)
Butler bayonet forceps
butterflies in the stomach
butterfly bandage
butterfly needle
butterfly pattern
butterfly sponge
butter meal
buttocks
button
   Bard gastrostomy
   gastrostomy

button *(cont.)*
   Medicina percutaneous
   MIC-Key gastrostomy
   one-stage gastrostomy
   stoma
button electrode
buttonhole puncture technique for
   hemodialysis needle insertion
button hook
button of duodenum
button suture
Button gastrostomy feeding device
Button-One Step gastrostomy feeding
   device
buttonpexy fixation for stomal prolapse
buttress plate
buttress the sphincter
buttressed hook
butyrylcholinesterase
BVA-100 blood-volume analyzer
BVM (bag-valve-mask) device
BV-1 needle
BV130-5 needle
BV-175-6 needle
BV-175-8 needle
BV-2 needle
Bx Velocity coronary artery stent
Bx Velocity sirolimus-coated stent
Bx Velocity stent
Byler disease
bypass (see *operation*)
   Alden loop gastric
   aortofemoral
   Aria coronary
   biliary enteric
   biliointestinal (BIB)
   biliopancreatic (BPB)

bypass *(cont.)*
   cardiac
   cardiopulmonary
   carotid artery
   coronary artery
   duodenoileal (DIB)
   end-to-end jejunoileal
   end-to-side jejunoileal
   exclusion
   femoral-popliteal artery
   femoropopliteal artery
   gastric
   gastric loop
   Greenville gastric
   Griffen Roux-en-Y
   Hallberg biliointestinal
   hepatorenal
   jejunal
   jejunoileal (JIB)
   intestinal
   laparoscopic gastric
   laparoscopic Roux-en-Y gastric
   Litwak aortic
   long-limb gastric artery
   lymphaticovenous
   mini gastric
   operative biliary
   partial ileal
   Payne-DeWind jejunoileal
   Roux-en-Y biliary
   Roux-en-Y gastric
   Scopinaro pancreaticobiliary
   Scott jejunoileal
   transected vertical gastric
   venovenous
   vertical gastric

C, c

CAB (combined androgen blockade)
cabergoline
CABG (coronary artery bypass)
cable
   bifurcated
   bipolar
   bipolar connecting
   fiberoptic light
   monopolar
cable graft
Cabot CCD 3000 endoscopic camera
Cabot cystoscope
Cabot insufflator
Cabot laparoscope
Cabot rigid laparoscope
Cabot trumpet valve
cachectic-appearing
cachectic diarrhea
cachexia
   malignant
   pituitary
CAD (continuous analgesia delivery)
cadaveric donor
cadaveric liver
cadaveric organ
caddy (dark sandy mud) stool
CadPlan cancer planning therapy
cafe coronary syndrome

caffeinated beverage
caffeine gut
CA 15-3 RIA (radioimmunoassay) serum tumor marker
CAGEIN (catheter-guided endoscopic intubation)
CAH (chronic active hepatitis)
Cairns artery forceps
Cairns hemostatic forceps
Cairns-Oliver hook
Cairns ribbon retractor
cake kidney
"cake mix" kit for hematopoietic progenitor assay
Calandruccio side plate
calcaneal pin
calcaneal region
calcaneal stance position
calcareous material
calcareous pancreatitis
calcar reamer
calcifediol
calcification
   breast
   clustered
   focal
   linear
   multiple

calcification *(cont.)*
   questionable
   suspicious
calcified breast implant
calcified gallbladder
calcified lesion
calcified outline of cyst
calcified scar tissue in gallbladder wall
calciform cell
calcifying pancreatitis
Calcijex (calcitriol)
calcineurin inhibitor
Calcitite graft
calcitonin level
calcitonin, serum
calcitriol
calcium (Ca)
calcium alginate dressing
calcium bilirubinate stone
calcium carbonate
calcium gluconate
calcium lactate
calcium metabolism regulation
calcium polycarbophil
calcium supplementation
calculator, body mass index (BMI)
calculous cholecystitis
calculous gallbladder disease
calculus
   alvine
   bile duct
   biliary
   cholesterol
   common duct
   decubitus
   ductal
   gallbladder
   gastric
   hepatic
   hepatic duct
   impacted
   intestinal
   jackstone calculus
   mammary

calculus *(cont.)*
   metabolic
   mulberry
   nephritic
   nonopaque
   pancreatic
   pocketed
   prostatic
   radiopaque
   renal
   salivary
   staghorn
   stomach
   stonelike
calculus cirrhosis
Calcutript lithotriptor
Calderol (calcifediol)
caliber of stool
calibrate
calibrated pin
calibrated pin guide
calibration of the cardia
calibration tube
Caliciviridae
calicivirus gastroenteritis
calipers
   blunt
   body fat
   Castroviejo
   CV
   Harpenden
   Lange skin-fold
   Mitutoyo digital
   Thomas walking
   Townley femur
   vernier
   weight-relieving
Callaway formula for calorie intake
Calman carotid artery clamp
Calman ring clamp
Calmette-Guérin bacillus
Calm-X (dimenhydrinate)
Calogen LCT emulsion
caloric supplement

Calot node
Calot triangle
Caltagirone chisel
Caluso PEG (percutaneous endoscopic
    gastrostomy) tube
calvarial free bone graft
calvarium clamp
Calymmatobacterium granulomatis
    (formerly *Donovania granulomatis*)
Calypso Rely catheter
Camalox
cambendazole
camera
    AMS Endoview
    Concept 8160 IntraVision Lumi-Trac
        endoscopic
    Dyonics Vision 325z endoscope
    EndoMate
    Endoview endoscopy
    Enview
    Fujinon FG-135 endoscopic
    MedCam Pro Plus video
    Olympus OM-2N endoscopic
    Olympus OTV-S2 Hi-Resolution
        Soakable Surgical color
        endoscopic
    Olympus SCA-3 endoscopic
    Pentax endoscopic
    Polaroid endocamera EC-3
    StereoScope
    still
    Storz 9050B AutoexposureColor
        endoscopic
    Storz KSA-2S SuperCam
        endoscopic
    Storz laparoscopic video
    Stryker 590 color endoscopic
camera light source
camera trocar
Cameron-Haight periosteal elevator
Cameron-Miller electrocoagulation unit
Cameron-Miller electrode
Cameron-Miller monopolar probe
Cameron-Miller suction-coagulator

Camey ileocystoplasty
Camey reservoir
Camino ICP (intracranial pressure)
    catheter
Camino microventricular bolt catheter
Campbell gouge
Campbell nerve root retractor
Campbell onlay graft
Campbell periosteal elevator
Campbell reamer
Campbell rongeur
Camper fascia
Camptosar (irinotecan hydrochloride)
    injection
Campylobacter coli
Campylobacter concisus
Campylobacter fennelliae
Campylobacter fetus enteritis
Campylobacter hyointestinalis
    (Vibrio coli)
Campylobacter intestinalis
Campylobacter jejuni
Campylobacter lari
Campylobacter pylori (Helicobacter
    pylori)
Canada-Cronkhite syndrome
Canakis pin
canal
    abdominal
    alimentary
    anal
    biliary
    femoral
    Hering
    inguinal
    Nuck
    pleuroperitoneal
    stomach
canalicular cholestasis
canalicular sphincter
canaliculus, bile
Canasa (mesalamine)
cancelling A's (mental test for hepatic
    encephalopathy)

cancellous bone graft
cancellous chip bone graft
cancer (see *carcinoma*)
cancer embolism
cancer-inducing virus
cancerization
cancer of cervix
cancer of head of pancreas
cancer prophylaxis
Cancidas (caspofungin acetate)
Candela 405 nm pulsed-dye laser
Candela SPTL laser
Candida albicans esophagitis
candidal esophagitis
candidal infection
candida mucositis
candidiasis
   disseminated
   esophageal
   intestinal
Candistat-G
Candistroy
C&S (culture and sensitivity)
Candy Cane One-Piece cannula
Candy Cane superficial cannula
CA 19-9 (carbohydrate antigen) test
CA 19-9 tumor marker
canker sore
cannabinol
cannister, Guardian suction
cannula
   Acufex double-lumen
   Adson brain-exploring
   arthroscopic
   Becker One-Piece
   Becker Toomey syringe
   Bergstrom
   biopsy
   blunt-tip
   brain-exploring
   Bucy-Frazier coagulating suction
   Bucy-Frazier suction
   Candy Cane One-Piece
   Candy Cane superficial

cannula *(cont.)*
   Chieftan aspirating
   Clagett S
   coagulating
   coagulating suction
   Cohen
   Coleman infiltration
   Concorde
   cone biopsy
   Congreve
   cystic duct
   DeRoyal
   Dohrmann-Rubin
   Dorsey ventricular
   Duke
   Dyonics
   Elsberg brain
   Elsberg ventricular
   Endotrac
   Entree thoracoscopy
   ERCP
   Eriksson muscle biopsy
   exploring
   Fischer ventricular
   Ford Hospital ventricular
   Fournier One-Piece
   Fournier Toomey syringe
   Franklin-Silverman biopsy
   Frazier brain-exploring
   Frazier ventricular
   Gilliland etching
   Grinfeld cannula
   Hasson blunt-end cannula
   Hasson laparoscopy
   Hasson open laparoscopy
   Hasson SAC (stable access)
   Haynes brain
   high-flow
   inflow
   infusion
   intraventricular
   Iotec
   Jarcho self-retaining uterine
   J-hook

cannula *(cont.)*
    Kahn uterine trigger
    Kanavel brain-exploring
    Keel Cobra Toomey syringe
    Killian antrum
    LaparoSAC single-use
    large-bore inflow
    large egress
    Las Vegas One-Piece
    Leech Wilkinson
    Mayo-Ochsner suction
    Mayo subclavian
    McCain TMJ
    Mercedes
    Mercedes One Piece
    Mercedes tip
    Mercedes Toomey syringe
    microirrigating
    Mladick
    Mladick concave
    Mladick liposuction
    MultAport
    Neal fallopian
    Nelson
    Olympus monopolar
    One Piece
    outflow
    Pereyra improved ligature
    perfusion
    polyethylene
    portal
    Portnoy ventricular
    Provis
    Ray ventricular
    reusable
    Rumel tourniquet flex
    Scott attic
    Scott ventricular
    Sedan-Vallicioni
    Simple Suction Probe
    single-use
    slotted
    small egress
    soft tissue shaving (liposhaver)

cannula *(cont.)*
    SpaceSEAL cannula
    spatula One-Piece
    spatula-tip Toomey syringe
    standard One-Piece
    Stöckert
    suction
    suprapatellar
    Teflon ERCP
    thoracoscopy
    USCI
    ventricular
    Veress
cannula grommet
cannula reducer
cannula system
cannulated drill
cannulated Henderson reamer
cannulated nail
cannulated pin cutter
cannulation catheter
    common bile duct
    cystic duct
    retrograde
    selective
Canny Ryall retractor
canstatin
Cantil (mepenzolate bromide)
Cantlie line
Cantor tube
CA1-18 tumor marker
CA 72–4 gastric cancer antigen tumor
    marker
cap
    duodenal
    endoscopic suction
cap-and-anchor plate
Caparosa wire-crimping forceps
CAPD (continuous ambulatory
    peritoneal dialysis)
capecitabine, UFT (uracil plus tegafur),
    leucovorin (UFT/LV) chemotherapy
    regimen
capeline bandage

capillary angioma
capillary bed
capillary blood
capillary endothelial cell
capillary fill
capillary leak
capillary sludging
Capio CL transvaginal suture-capturing
    device
capitonnage
Capmul 8210 (glyceryl 1-mono-
    octanoate)
Capner gouge
capsaicin
Capset (calcium sulfate) bone graft
    barrier
capsular cirrhosis
capsular contracture following breast
    reconstruction
capsular incision
capsular invasion
capsular release forceps
capsule
    enteric-coated
    Glisson
    hepatic
    liver
    splenic
capsulectomy, periprosthetic
capsulitis, thyroid
Captopril test
caput medusae
Carafate (sucralfate)
CaraKlenz wound cleanser dressing
carbantel; carbantel lauryl sulfate
carbohydrate complex, refined
carbohydrate-deficient glycoprotein
    syndrome (CDGS), type 1a
carbohydrate polymer gel wound
    dressing
carbon dioxide (CO_2)
carbon dioxide content
carbon dioxide insufflator
carbon dioxide laser

carbon dioxide pneumoperitoneum
carbon fiber
carbon fiber graft
carbon fiber synthetic ligament
carbonic acid concentration
carbon steel surgical blade
carbon tetrachloride poisoning
carbon-tungsten rasp
carbonyl iron
carboplatin-coated plastic biliary stent
Carbo-Seal
carboxypeptidase
carboxypolypeptidase
carcinoembryonic antigen (CEA)
carcinogenicity
carcinoid syndrome
carcinoid tumor
carcinoma (also *cancer*; *sarcoma*; *tumor*)
    acinous cell
    adenocystic
    adenoid cystic
    adenoid squamous cell
    adenosquamous
    adnexal
    adrenocortical
    aldosterone-producing
    aldosterone-secreting
    alveolar cell
    ameloblastic
    ampullary
    aniline
    apocrine
    basal cell
    basaloid
    basosquamous cell
    betel
    bile duct
    bilharzial
    biologically active thyroid
    bladder
    breast
    bronchioalveolar
    bronchioloalveolar
    bronchogenic

carcinoma *(cont.)*
    burn scar
    cerebriform
    chimney-sweep's
    cholangiocarcinoma
    cholangiocellular
    cholangitis
    chorionic
    choroid plexus
    clear cell
    clear cell hepatocellular
    clay pipe
    colloid
    colon
    colorectal
    columnar cuff
    comedo
    contact
    corpus
    cortisol-producing
    cribriform
    cutaneous metastatic breast
    cylindrical
    cystic
    dendritic
    disseminated
    ductal
    duct cell
    Dukes (not Duke's)
    dye worker's
    eccrine
    embryonal
    embryonal cell
    encephaloid gastric
    endometrial
    epidermal
    epidermoid
    excavated gastric
    exophytic
    extrahepatic abdominal
    extrahepatic bile duct
    familial pancreatic
    fibrolamellar hepatocellular
        (FL-HCC)

carcinoma *(cont.)*
    follicular
    gallbladder
    gastric
    gastric stump
    gelatinous
    genital
    giant cell
    glandular
    glans
    granulosa cell
    hepatic
    hepatic cell
    hepatocellular (HCC)
    hepatocholangiolitic
    hereditary
    hereditary nonpolyposis colorectal
        (HNPCC)
    high-grade angioinvasive follicular
    hormone-sensitive breast
    Hürthle (Huerthle) cell
    hypernephroid
    infantile embryonal
    infiltrating ductal
    infiltrating lobular
    infiltrative
    inflammatory breast
    intraductal
    intraepidermal
    intraepithelial nonkeratizing
    invasive
    invasive breast
    invasive ductal
    invasive lobular
    juvenile embryonal
    kidney
    Kulchitsky cell
    large cell
    laryngeal
    latent
    lenticular
    leptomeningeal
    lobular
    Lucké

carcinoma *(cont.)*
  lung
  melanotic
  medullary
  melanotic
  meningeal
  Merkel cell
  metastatic
  metatypical
  microinvasive
  micropapillary
  microscopic multifocal medullary
  microtrabecular hepatocellular
  mixed hepatocholangiocellular
  moderately well-differentiated
  mucinous
  mucoepidermal
  mucoepidermoid
  mucous
  mule-spinner's
  nasopharyngeal
  neuroendocrine skin
  noninfiltrating lobular
  non-small cell lung
  oat cell
  occult
  oral
  oropharyngeal
  osteoid
  ovarian
  Paget
  pancreatic
  pancreatic ductal
  papillary gastric
  paraffin
  parathyroid
  perforated
  periampullary
  pitch worker's
  polypoid
  poorly differentiated
  preinvasive
  prickle cell
  primary

carcinoma *(cont.)*
  primary bile duct
  primary hepatic
  primary intraosseous
  protruded gastric
  rectosigmoid
  renal cell
  residual
  retinoblastoma hereditary human
  scar
  schistosomal bladder
  schneiderian
  scirrhous
  sclerosing hepatic (SHC)
  sclerosing well-differentiated
  sebaceous
  sessile nodular
  sigmoid
  signet ring
  small cell
  small cell anaplastic
  small cell lung
  small round cell
  spindle cell
  squamous cell (SCC)
  staging of cervical
  string cell
  submucosal
  superficial gastric
  swamp
  systemic effects
  tar
  T cell
  terminal duct
  thyroid
  transitional cell
  tubular
  undifferentiated squamous cell
  uterine cervix
  uterine corpus
  verrucous
  villous
  well-differentiated
  yolk sac

carcinoma arising from epidermal cells
carcinoma de novo
carcinoma en cuirasse
carcinoma ex mixed tumor
carcinoma ex pleomorphic adenoma
carcinoma in situ
    ductal (DCIS)
    lobular (LCIS)
carcinomatosis
    diffuse
    disseminated
carcinomatous implant
carcinomatous pericarditis
carcinosarcoma
cardia
    gastric
    patulous
cardiac allograft vascular disease
    (CAVD)
cardiac antrum
cardiac arrhythmias
cardiac catheter
cardiac cirrhosis
cardiac edema
cardiac function, compromised
cardiac impression on liver
cardiac lung
cardiac mucosa of stomach
cardiac obstruction
cardiac of stomach
cardiac orifice
cardiac polyp
cardiac reflex
cardiac retraction clip
cardiac segment
cardiac sphincter (stomach)
cardiac stomach
cardiac tamponade
cardiac valvular lesion
cardiac valvular stenosis
Cardiac Assist intra-aortic balloon
    catheter
Cardima Pathfinder microcatheter
cardinal suture

Cardiocap 5 patient monitor
cardiochalasia
cardioesophageal (CE) junction
cardioesophageal mucosal junction
cardioesophageal sphincter
cardiograms, serial
Cardio-Green (CG) (indocyanine green)
cardiohepatic angle
cardiohepatic triangle
Cardiomed Bodysoft epidural catheter
Cardiomed endotracheal ventilation
    catheter
Cardiomed thermodilution catheter
cardiomyotomy
    Heller
    laparoscopic
    stomach
    videolaparoscopic
cardioplegic needle
cardiopulmonary bypass
cardiospasm
Cardio Tactilaze peripheral angioplasty
    laser catheter
cardiovascular silk suture
CARDS O.S. mono test
CaREpair endoscope repair
Cariel gel dressing
carina
Carlens tube adapter
Carmalt (Walter) splinter forceps
Carmalt artery forceps
Carmalt clamp
Carmalt forceps
Carmalt hemostat
C-arm fluoroscope
carminative
CARN 750 (now CarraVex injectable)
Carnett sign
carnitine deficiency
    myopathic
    primary
    secondary
carnitine deficiency secondary
    to MCAD deficiency

Caroid (bisacodyl)
Caroli disease
Caroli syndrome
Caromed postaugmentation bra
carotene
carotid artery clamp
carotid artery injury
carotid blade
carotid bruit
carotid fork
carotid retractor
carotid sheath
carotid wall
carpal tunnel glove
carpal tunnel stretch
carpal tunnel view
Carpenter syndrome
CarraFilm transparent film dressing
CarraGauze wound strips dressing
CarraSmart foam dressing
CarraSmart self-adhesive foam dressing
Carra Sorb H wound dressing
Carra Sorb M freeze-dried gel dressing
Carrasyn hydrogel wound dressing
Carrasyn V dressing
Carrasyn wound gel dressing
Carrasyn wound gel spray dressing
CarraVex injectable
Carrel patch
carrier, hepatitis
Carr-Locke snare
Carr-Locke stent remover
Carroll-Bennett retractor
Carroll bone-holding forceps
Carroll dressing forceps
Carroll hand retractor
Carroll-Legg periosteal elevator
Carroll skin hook
Carroll tendon retriever
Carroll tendon-pulling forceps
Carroll tissue forceps
carsick
carsickness
Carson Zero Tip balloon dilator

Carter-Horsley-Hughes syndrome
Carter pillow for immobilization and elevation in replantation procedures
Carter-Rowe view
Carter-Thomason suture passer
Carticel autologous cultured chondrocytes
Cartilade (shark cartilage)
cartilage
    cricoid
    shark
cartilage clamp
cartilage-derived inhibitor (CDI)
cartilage forceps
cartilage graft
cartilage knife
cartilage scissors
cartilage shaver blade
cartilaginous growth plate
cartwheel pattern
casanthronol
cascade, metastatic
cascade stomach
caseation
Casec calcium supplement
caseous necrosis
CASH (classic abdominal Semm hysterectomy)
Casoni skin test
CASP (contoured anterior spinal) plate
Caspar alligator forceps
Caspar blade
Caspar cervical plate
Caspari suture punch
caspofungin acetate
Castanares facelift scissors
Castaneda anastomosis clamp
Castaneda vascular clamp
cast breaker
Casten classification of groin hernias (stage 1–3)
Casten hernia staging
castlike tube
castor oil

Castroviejo blade breaker
Castroviejo caliper
Castroviejo-Colibri forceps
Castroviejo marker
Castroviejo-Mayo needle
Castroviejo-Mayo needle holder
Castroviejo needle
Castroviejo needle holder
Castroviejo scissors
Castroviejo-TC needle holder
cast saw
cast spreader
cast syndrome
catabolic activity
catabolism, tissue
cataract blade
cataract knife
cataract needle
Catarex surgical device for cataract
   removal
catarrhal colitis
catarrhal gastritis
catch in chest on inspiration
cat's eye calculi
cat-eye syndrome
catecholamine crisis
catecholamine-induced vasoconstriction
catecholamine production
catechol
Catera suture anchor
catgut suture
cathartic
cathartic abuse
cathartic colon
cathartic (see also *bowel prep*)
   magnesium citrate
   magnesium sulfate
   syrup of ipecac
catheter
   ablation
   Abramson
   Abscession fluid drainage
   Accu-Flo ventricular
   ACE

catheter *(cont.)*
   Achiever balloon dilatation
   ACS (Advanced Catheter or Cardiac
     Systems)
   ACS angioplasty
   ACS balloon
   ACS Concorde
   ACS Endura coronary dilation
   ACS JL4 (Judkins left 4 French)
   ACS mini
   ACS OTW (over-the-wire)
     Lifestream coronary dilatation
   ACS OTW (over-the-wire) Photon
   ACS RX Comet coronary dilatation
   ACS RX coronary dilatation
   ACS Tourguide II guiding
   AcuNav ultrasound
   Ahn thrombectomy
   AL-1
   AL II guiding
   Alzate
   Amazr
   Amplatz cardiac
   Amplatz femoral
   Amplatz right coronary
   Angiocath
   Angiocath PRN
   Angiocath PRN flexible
   angiographic
   angiographic balloon occlusion
   Angio-Kit
   Angiomedics
   AngioOptic microcatheter
   angiopigtail
   angioplasty balloon
   angled balloon
   angulated
   Anthron heparinized antithrombo-
     genic
   Antibacterial Personal
   aortogram
   Arani double-loop guiding
   Argyle Medicut R
   arrhythmia mapping system

catheter *(cont.)*
    Arrow pulmonary artery
    Arrow Twin Cath
    Arrow Twin Cath multilumen
      peripheral
    Arrow-Berman balloon
    ARROWgard Blue
    ARROWgard central venous
    Arrow-Howes multilumen
    arterial embolectomy
    AR-2 diagnostic guiding
    Ascent guiding
    atherectomy
    atherectomy, peripheral
    AtheroCath
    AtheroCath Bantam coronary
      atherectomy
    Atlantic ileostomy
    Atlas LP PTCA balloon dilatation
    Atlas ULP balloon dilatation
    Atri-Pace I bipolar-flared pacing
    Auth atherectomy
    AutoGuard-P
    AV-Paceport thermodilution
    Axiom DG balloon angioplasty
    bail-out
    Baim pacing
    Baim-Turi monitor/pacing
    ball-wedge
    balloon
    balloon biliary
    balloon dilatation
    balloon dilating
    balloon embolectomy
    balloon flotation
    balloon septostomy
    balloon-flotation pacing
    balloon-tipped angiographic
    balloon-tipped end-hole
    balloon-tipped flow-directed
      pulmonary artery
    Bard guiding
    Bardic cutdown
    bat-wing

catheter *(cont.)*
    Baxter
    BD Insyte Autoguard-P shielded I.V.
    Benique
    Berman angiographic
    Bernstein
    Beta-Cath system
    bicoudate
    bifoil balloon
    biliary balloon
    BioEnterics gastric balloon suction
    BioVue PICC
    bipolar pacing electrode
    bipolar temporary pacemaker
    Block right coronary guiding
    Blue FlexTip
    Blue Max triple-lumen
    BPS spinal angiographic
    Brevi-Kath epidural
    Brockenbrough mapping
    Brockenbrough modified bipolar
    Brockenbrough transseptal
    bronchial
    Bronchitrac L
    bronchospirometric
    Broviac
    Broviac atrial
    Buchbinder Omniflex
    Buchbinder Thruflex
    Burhenne steerable
    Calypso Rely
    Camino ICP (intracranial pressure)
    Camino microventricular bolt
    cannulation
    cardiac
    Cardiac Assist intra-aortic balloon
    Cardima Pathfinder microcatheter
    Cardio Tactilaze peripheral
      angioplasty laser
    Cardiomarker
    Cardiomed Bodysoft epidural
    Cardiomed endotracheal ventilation
    Cardiomed thermodilution
    Castillo

catheter *(cont.)*
    Cath-Finder
    Cathlon I.V.
    Caud-A-Kath epidural
    CCOmbo
    central venous (CVC)
    Cheetah angioplasty
    Chemo-Port
    Chilli cooled ablation
    cholangiography
    ChronoFlex
    CliniCath peripherally inserted
    Closure System by VNUS
    Cloverleaf
    coaxial
    Cobra
    Cobra over-the-wire balloon
    cobra-shaped
    coil-tipped
    Comfort Cath I or II
    Conceptus Soft Seal cervical
    Conceptus Soft Torque uterine
    Conceptus VS (variable softness)
    Concord Portex epidural
    conductance
    constantly perfused side-hole
    Constellation mapping
    Cook arterial
    Cook pigtail
    Cook TPN
    Cool Tip
    Cordis Brite Tip guiding
    Cordis Ducor I (or II, III) coronary
    Cordis Ducor pigtail
    Cordis high-flow pigtail
    Cordis Predator PTCA balloon
    Cordis Son-II
    Cordis Trakstar PTCA balloon
    coronary dilatation
    coronary guiding
    coronary sinus thermodilution
    corset balloon
    coudé
    Cournand cardiac

catheter *(cont.)*
    Cragg-McNamara valved infusion
    CR Bard
    Critikon
    CrossSail coronary dilatation
    cryoablation
    cutdown
    Cutting Balloon microsurgical
        dilatation
    CVP (central venous pressure)
    Dacron
    Dale Foley
    Datascope
    Datascope DL-II percutaneous
        translucent balloon
    decapolar
    deflectable quadripolar
    diagnostic
    Diasonics
    dilatation balloon
    dilating
    DLP cardioplegic
    Doppler coronary
    Dormia stone basket
    Dorros brachial internal mammary
        guiding
    Dorros infusion/probing
    Dotter
    Dotter caged balloon
    Dotter coaxial
    Double J indwelling
    Double J ureteral
    double-lumen
    double-lumen femoral vein
    double-lumen subclavian vein
    Dow Corning ileal pouch
    drainage
    Ducor balloon
    Duette
    dummy seed
    Du Pen long-term epidural
    DURAglide stone removal
    DVI Simpson atherocath
    DynamicDeca steerable

catheter *(cont.)*
    EAC (expandable access catheter)
    EchoMark
    EchoMark angiographic
    Edwards diagnostic
    eight-lumen esophageal manometry
    El Gamal coronary bypass
    Elecath thermodilution
    electrode
    electrophysiologic (EP)
    11 French JCL 3.5 guiding
    Elite
    embolectomy
    Encapslon
    end-hole
    EndoCPB (endovascular cardiopul-
        monary bypass)
    Endosound endoscopic ultrasound
    Endotak C lead
    enhanced torque 8F (8 French)
        guiding
    EnSite cardiac
    EP (electrophysiologic)
    epidural
    Eppendorf
    ERCP (endoscopic retrograde
        cholangiopancreatography)
    Erythroflex
    Erythroflex hydromer-coated central
        venous
    esophageal balloon
    e-TRAIN 110 AngioJet
    Evert-O-Cath
    eXamine cholangiography
    expandable access (EAC)
    Express
    Express PTCA
    extraction
    ExtreSafe
    extrusion balloon
    FACT (Focal Angioplasty
        CatheterTechnology)
    Falcon coronary
    FAST (flow-assisted, short-term)
        balloon

catheter *(cont.)*
    Fast-Cath introducer
    FasTracker
    female
    femoral guiding
    Feth-R-Kath epidural
    Finesse large-lumen guiding
    Flexguard Tip
    Flexxicon Blue dialysis
    flotation
    flow-directed
    flow-oximetry
    fluid-filled
    Fogarty adherent clot
    Fogarty arterial embolectomy
    Fogarty balloon
    Fogarty balloon biliary
    Fogarty-Chin extrusion balloon
    Fogarty embolectomy
    Fogarty graft thrombectomy
    Fogarty irrigation
    Fogarty occlusion
    Fogarty venous thrombectomy
    Foley
    Foltz
    Force balloon dilatation
    FR4 guiding
    Freezor cryocatheter
    French
    French 5 (5 French) angiographic
    French MBIH
    French mushroom-tip
    Ganz-Edwards coronary infusion
    Gensini coronary
    Gentle-Flo suction
    Gold Probe bipolar hemostasis
    Goodale-Lubin cardiac
    Gorlin pacing
    Gould PentaCath 5-lumen thermo-
        dilution
    graft-seeking
    Greenwich
    Grollman
    Grollman pigtail

catheter *(cont.)*
    Groshong
    Groshong double-lumen
    Groshong PICC
    Grüntzig (Gruentzig)
    Grüntzig arterial balloon
    Grüntzig Dilaca
    guide
    guiding
    Halo
    Hanafee
    Hartzler ACX-II or RX-014 balloon
    Hartzler LPS dilatation
    Hartzler Micro II
    Hartzler Micro XT dilatation
    headhunter visceral angiography
    HealthShield
    HealthShield antimicrobial media-
        stinal wound drainage catheter
    HealthShield wound drainage
    helical-tip Halo
    helium-filled balloon
    hep lock
    hexapolar
    Hickman
    Hickman indwelling right atrial
    Hidalgo
    Hieshima coaxial
    high-fidelity
    high-fidelity microtipped
    high-flow
    high-pressure
    high-speed rotation dynamic
        angioplasty
    HNB angiographic
    Hohn central venous
    hot-tip
    Hurwitz dialysis
    HydraCross TLC PTCA
    Hydrolyser microcatheter
    hydrostatic balloon
    hyperthermia
    IAB (intra-aortic balloon)
    ICP (intracranial pressure)

catheter *(cont.)*
    Illumen-8 guiding
    ILUS (intraluminal ultrasound)
    indwelling
    Infiniti
    InfusaSleeve II
    Inoue balloon
    Insyte AutoGuard
    interstitial
    intra-aortic balloon
    intra-aortic balloon double-lumen
    intra-arterial chemotherapy
    Intracath
    intracoronary guiding
    intracoronary perfusion
    Intran disposable pressure measure-
        ment
    intratumoral
    intravascular ultrasound (IVUS)
    intravenous pacing
    intraventricular
    Intrepid PTCA angioplasty
    ITC balloon
    ITC radiopaque balloon
    IVUS (intravascular ultrasound)
    Jackman orthogonal
    Jackson-Pratt
    jejunostomy
    Jelco I.V.
    Jelco intravenous
    Jelco winged I.V.
    JL4 (Judkins left 4 cm curve)
    JL5 (Judkins left 5 cm curve)
    JR4 (Judkins right 4 cm curve)
    Judkins 4 diagnostic
    Judkins left 4 cm (JL4)
    Judkins left coronary
    Judkins right 4 cm (JR4)
    Judkins right coronary
    Judkins USCI
    Kaye tamponade balloon
    KDF-2.3
    Kensey
    Kensey atherectomy

catheter *(cont.)*
    Kidney Internal Splint/Stent (KISS)
    Kifa
    King multipurpose coronary graft
    kinking of CNS
    Kinsey atherectomy
    Kish urethral illuminated
    KISS (Kidney Internal Splint/Stent)
    Koala pressure
    Konton
    Kontron balloon
    large-bore
    large-lumen
    laser
    Lawrence Add-A-Cath
    L-Cath peripherally inserted
      neonatal
    left coronary
    left heart
    left Judkins
    left ventricular sump
    Lehman
    Lehman ventriculography
    LeMaitre biliary
    Leonard
    LeVeen
    Lifestream coronary dilatation
    Livewire duo-decapolar steerable
    Livewire TC ablation
    Longdwel Teflon
    Lo-Profile balloon
    Lo-Profile II balloon
    Lo-Profile steerable dilatation
    low-pressure
    low-speed rotation angioplasty
    LPS
    Lumaguide
    Malecot
    Malinckrodt
    Mallinckrodt angiographic
    MammoSite RTS (radiation therapy
      system)
    manometer-tipped cardiac
    Mansfield

catheter *(cont.)*
    Mansfield Atri-Pace 1
    Mansfield orthogonal electrode
    Mansfield Scientific dilatation
      balloon
    Marathon guiding
    Mark IV Moss decompression-
      feeding
    Max Force
    McGoon coronary perfusion
    McIntosh double-lumen
    Medi-Tech
    Medi-Tech balloon
    Medicut
    Medina ileostomy
    medium-pressure
    Medtronic balloon
    Mercator atrial high-density array
    Mewi-5 sidehole infusion
    Micro-Guide
    micromanometer-tip
    MicroMewi multi-sidehole infusion
    midstream aortogram
    Mikro-tip micromanometer-tipped
    Millar micromanometer
    Millar MPC-500
    Millar pigtail angiographic
    Millenia balloon
    Miller septostomy
    Mini-Profile dilatation
    Mirage over-the-wire balloon
    Mitsubishi angioscopic
    Molina needle
    Mon-a-therm Foley
    Monorail angioplasty
    Monorail balloon
    Moss decompression feeding
    MPF
    MS Classique balloon dilatation
    Mullins transseptal
    multi-electrode impedance
    Multi-Med triple-lumen infusion
    multifiber
    multiflanged Portnoy (for hydro-
      cephalus shunts)

catheter *(cont.)*
  multilumen
  multipolar impedance
  multipurpose
  Multipurpose-SM
  mushroom
  MVP
  Mylar
  nasobiliary
  Navi-Star
  Naviport
  Naviport deflectable tip guiding
  NBIH
  Nelaton solid-tip red latex
  Neo-Sert umbilical vessel
  nephrostomy-type
  NeuroVasx (Sub-Microinfusion)
  Nexus 2 linear ablation
  NIH (National Institutes of Health)
  NIH cardiomarker
  NIH left ventriculography
  9 Fr JL 4 guiding (9 French Judkins
     left 4 guiding)
  nontraumatizing
  NoProfile balloon
  NovaCath multi-lumen infusion
  Nutricath
  Nycore
  octapolar
  Oligon
  OmniCath atherectomy
  Omniflex balloon
  On-Command (male and female)
  one-hole angiographic
  OptiQue sensing
  Optiscope
  Optiva I.V.
  Oracle Focus
  Oracle Megasonics
  Oracle Micro
  Oracle Micro Plus
  Oreopoulos-Zellerman
  over-the-wire balloon
  oximetric

catheter *(cont.)*
  Pace bipolar pacing
  Paceport
  Pacewedge dual-pressure bipolar
     pacing
  pacing
  P.A.S. (peripheral access system)
     Port catheter
  P.A.S. Port Fluoro-Free
  Passage catheter
  Pathfinder
  Pathfinder microcatheter system
  Pathfinder mini microcatheter
  PA Watch position-monitoring
  PBN
  PEG
  PE Plus II balloon dilatation
  Percor DL balloon
  Percor DL-II balloon
  Percor-Stat-DL
  percutaneous
  percutaneous transhepatic biliary
     drainage (PTBD)
  percutaneous transhepatic pigtail
  perfusion
  Periflow peripheral balloon
  peripherally inserted central (PICC)
  peritoneal
  peritoneal dialysis (PDC)
  PermCath double-lumen ventricular
     access
  pervenous
  Pezzer
  Phantom 5 Plus balloon
  Phoenix ventriculostomy
  PIBC (percutaneous intra-aortic
     balloon counterpulsation)
  PIC (peripherally inserted)
  PICC (peripherally inserted central)
  Pico-ST II
  pigtail
  Pipelle endometrial suction
  Polaris RF
  polyethylene

catheter *(cont.)*
- PolyFlo peripherally inserted central (PICC)
- Polystan
- Polystan venous return
- Port-A-Cath
- portal
- Portnoy ventricular
- Positrol II
- preformed
- preshaped
- probing
- ProCross Rely over-the-wire balloon
- Profile Plus dilatation
- Proflex 5 dilatation
- Pro-Flo
- Pro-Flo XT
- PRO infusion
- Pruitt-Inahara balloon-tipped perfusion
- PTBD (percutaneous transhepatic biliary drainage)
- PTCA (percutaneous transluminal coronary angioplasty)
- Pudenz peritoneal
- pulmonary artery
- pulmonary flotation
- pulmonary triple-lumen
- pusher
- quadripolar electrode
- quadripolar steerable electrode
- Quanticor
- Quinton
- Quinton Mahurkar dual-lumen peritoneal
- Raaf Cath vascular
- radial artery
- radiopaque Teflon biliary dilating
- Raimondi peritoneal
- Raimondi spring
- Raimondi ventricular
- Ranfac cholangiographic
- Rashkind balloon
- Rashkind septostomy balloon

catheter *(cont.)*
- Rebar microcatheter
- recessed balloon septostomy
- red Robinson
- red rubber
- Reddick cystic duct cholangiogram
- Reddick-Saye screw
- Redifurl TaperSeal IAB
- Release-NF
- Reliance urinary control insert
- remote access perfusion (RAP)
- Rentrop infusion
- Response electrophysiology
- retroperfusion
- RF (radiofrequency-generated thermal) balloon
- right coronary
- right heart
- right Judkins
- Rigiflex TTS balloon
- Ring
- Rivas vascular
- Robinson
- Rodriguez
- Rodriguez-Alvarez
- Rosch-Uchida transjugular liver access needle-catheter
- Royal Flush angiographic flush
- Rumel
- Sable
- Sarns wire-reinforced
- SCA-EX ShortCutter
- Schneider
- Schneider-Shiley
- Schoonmaker femoral
- Schoonmaker multipurpose
- Schwarten balloon
- Schwarten balloon dilatation
- Sci-Med SSC Skinny
- SCOOP 1
- SCOOP 2
- Scott silicone ventricular
- Seletz nonrigid ventricular
- sensing

catheter *(cont.)*
    Seroma-Cath wound drainage
    serrated
    SET three-lumen thrombectomy
    Shaldon
    shaver
    Shaw
    Sheldon
    Sherpa guiding
    Shiley guiding
    Shiley-Ionescu
    SHJR4s (side-hole Judkins right,
       curve 4, short)
    side-hole
    sidewinder
    Silastic
    silicone
    silicone rubber Dacron-cuffed
    Silicore
    Simmons-type (sidewinder)
    Simplus PE/t dilatation
    Simpson
    Simpson atherectomy
    Simpson peripheral AtheroCath
    Simpson-Robert
    Simpson Ultra Lo-Profile II balloon
    single-stage
    Skinny
    Skinny dilatation
    sliding rail
    Slinky
    Smec balloon
    snare
    Soaker
    Softip arteriography
    Softip diagnostic
    Soft Torque uterine
    Softouch guiding
    Soft-Vu Omni flush
    solid-state esophageal manometry
    Solo catheter with Pro/Pel coating
    SoloPass
    Sones cardiac
    Sones Cardio-Marker

catheter *(cont.)*
    Sones catheter
    Sones Hi-Flow
    Sones Positrol
    Sones woven Dacron
    Speedy balloon
    SPI-Argent II peritoneal dialysis
    SpineCATH intradiscal
    split sheath
    Spyglass angiography
    Stack perfusion coronary dilatation
    Stamey-Malecot
    standard Lehman
    steerable electrode
    Steerocath
    Stertzer brachial guiding
    Stertzer guiding
    stimulating
    St. Jude 4F Supreme electro-
       physiology
    straight flush percutaneous
    subarachnoid
    subclavian
    subcutaneous ventricular reservoir
    subdural drainage
    Sub-Microinfusion
    Suction Buster
    SULP II
    sump
    Supreme electrophysiology
    SureCuff
    Sure-Flex dilatation
    surgically implanted hemodialysis
       (SIHC)
    Swan-Ganz
    Swan-Ganz balloon-flotation
       pulmonary artery
    Swan-Ganz flow-directed
    Swan-Ganz Guidewire TD
    Swan-Ganz Pacing TD
    Swan-Ganz pulmonary artery
    Swan-Ganz thermodilution
    swan-neck
    Swartz SL Series Fast-Cath
       introducer

catheter *(cont.)*
    Syntel latex-free embolectomy
    TAC atherectomy
    Tactilaze angioplasty laser
    Targis microwave
    Taut cystic duct
    Teflon
    temporary pacing
    Tenckhoff peritoneal dialysis
    Tennis Racquet
    tetrapolar esophageal
    thermistor
    thermodilution
    thermodilution balloon
    thermodilution pacing
    thermodilution Swan-Ganz
    thoracic
    thrombectomy
    Thruflex PTCA balloon
    Tiemann
    Tis-U-Trap endometrial suction
    toposcopic
    Torcon NB selective angiographic
    Tourguide guiding
    Tracker
    Tracker-10
    Tracker-18 Soft Stream
    TrakBack ultrasound
    transcutaneous extraction
    transducer-tipped
    transjugular access
    transluminal extraction (TEC)
    transseptal
    transtracheal oxygen
    transvenous pacemaker
    trefoil balloon
    Triguide
    triple-lumen central venous
    triple-lumen manometric
    triple thermistor coronary sinus
    tripolar
    tripolar electrode
    T-TAC (transcervical tubal access)
    TTS (through the scope)

catheter *(cont.)*
    twist drill
    Tygon
    Uldall (not Udall) subclavian
        hemodialysis
    ULP (ultra-low profile)
    Ultra 8 balloon
    UltraLite flow-directed micro-
        catheter
    ultra low-profile fixed-wire balloon
        dilatation
    umbilical artery (UAC)
    UMI
    Ureflex
    UroMax II
    USCI Bard
    USCI guiding
    USCI Mini-Profile balloon dilatation
    valvuloplasty balloon
    Van Andel
    Van Tassel pigtail
    vanSonnenberg-Wittich
    Vantex central venous
    Variflex
    Vas-Cath
    Vector and VectorX large-lumen
        guiding
    venous
    venous thrombectomy
    venting
    Ventra
    ventricular
    ventriculography
    Ventureyra ventricular
    Verbatim balloon
    Veripath peripheral guiding
    vessel-sizing
    VIPER PTA
    Visa II PTCA
    Vision PTCA
    Vitalcor venous
    Vitesse Cos laser
    Vitesse E-II
    VNUS Restore

catheter *(cont.)*
  Voda
  Von Andel
  Vygon Nutricath S
  Was-Cath
  washing
  water-infusion esophageal
    manometry
  Webster coronary sinus
  Webster orthogonal electrode
  Wexler
  whistle-tip ureteral
  Williams L-R guiding
  Wilton-Webster coronary sinus
  Witzel enterostomy
  Workhorse percutaneous trans-
    luminal angioplasty balloon
  Wurd
  X-trode electrode
  XL-11
  Xpeedior
  Xpeedior 60
  Z-Med
  Zucker
  Zuma guiding
catheter balloon valvuloplasty
catheter-directed thrombolysis and
  endovascular stent placement
catheter entrapment
catheter-guided endoscopic intubation
  (CAGEIN)
catheter introducer, Bard Safety
  Excalibur
catheter-introducing forceps
catheterization (see also *catheter*)
  bile duct
  cardiac
  coronary artery
  cystic duct
  double-lumen
  endoscopic
  endoscopic transpapillary
  hepatic vein

catheterization *(cont.)*
  indwelling
  percutaneous
  percutaneous transhepatic
  portal vein
  Seldinger cystic duct
  selective
  transhepatic
  transnasal bile duct
  transpapillary
  two-lumen
  urinary
  venous
catheter sepsis
catheter tip placement
catheter vitrector
Cath-Finder catheter tracking system
Cath-Secure hypoallergenic tape
CathLink implantable vascular access
  device
Cathlon I.V. catheter
CathTrack catheter locator system
cation
Catlin amputating knife
CAT (computerized axial tomography)
  scan
cA2 monoclonal antibody
caudad
Caud-A-Kath epidural catheter
caudal anesthesia
caudal dysplasia sequence
caudal hook
caudal pancreatic artery
caudal regression syndrome
caudate lobe of liver (also quadrate)
caudocephalad projection
cause-and-effect relationship
caustic acid (poison)
caustic alkali (poison)
caustic digestive enzymes
caustic ingestion
cauterization
cauterize

cautery (electrocautery)
   Aesculap bipolar
   BiCAP
   BiLAP
   BiLAP bipolar
   bipolar
   Bovie
   ClearCut 2 electrosurgical handpiece
   Cloward
   Concept handheld
   Electroloop
   Endocut
   endoscopic laser
   hook
   Hotsy
   insulated
   looped
   Malis
   Mira
   insulated
   NeoKnife
   Neo-Med
   Olympus BiQ bipolar
   Op-Temp
   RollerLOOP
   Scheie ophthalmic
   snare
   wet field
cautery bend
cautery hook
cautery knife
cautery pencil
caval fold
CAVD (cardiac allograft vascular disease)
CaverMap surgical device
cavernous angioma
cavernous hemangioma
CAVH (chronic active viral hepatitis)
CAVH (continuous arteriovenous hemofiltration)
CAVH-B (chronic active viral hepatitis, type B)
CAVH-NAB (chronic active viral hepatitis, non-A, non-B)

caviar lesion
Cavilon barrier ointment
cavitary fluid
Cavitron ultrasonic surgical aspirator (CUSA)
cavity
   abdominal
   peritoneal
   retroperitoneal
   thoracic
   wound
cavity wall
CAVU (continuous arteriovenous ultrafiltration)
cavum conchal cartilage graft
C-bar web-spacer
C-bloc continuous nerve block system
CBC (complete blood count):
   hematocrit
   hemoglobin
   MCH (mean corpuscular hemoglobin)
   MCHC (mean corpuscular hemoglobin concentration)
   MCV (mean corpuscular volume)
   red blood cell count (RBC)
   white blood cell count (WBC)
CBC with a left shift
CBC with diff (differential)
CBD (common bile duct) stone
CBDE (common bile duct exploration)
CBG (corticosteroid-binding globulin)
CB erbium/2.94 laser
C bile
CBP (chronic bacterial prostatitis)
CBP (copper-binding protein)
C cell
CCD Apex autoclavable camera head
CCFA (Crohn's and Colitis Foundation of America)
CCK (cholecystokinin)
CCK-PZ (cholecystokinin-pancreozymin)
C-cholyl-glycine breath excretion test
C clamp

CCOmbo catheter
CCP (colitis cystica profunda)
CCS (colitis cystica superficialis)
CCS (Composite Cultured Skin)
CD (celiac disease)
CD (Crohn disease)
CDA (chenodeoxycholic acid)
CDAD (*Clostridium difficile*-associated diarrhea)
CDAI (Crohn disease activity index)
CDC (Centers for Disease Control and Prevention)
CDC (Crohn disease of colon)
CDCA (chenodeoxycholic acid)
CDE (common duct exploration)
CD-45RB monoclonal antibody
CDGS (carbohydrate-deficient glycoprotein syndrome), type 1a
CDI (cartilage-derived inhibitor)
CDIS (controlled distention irrigation system)
CDI 2000 blood gas monitoring system
CDS (choledochoduodenostomy)
Cd-texaphyrin photosensitizing agent
CdTOX A OIA kit
CDUS (color-flow Doppler ultrasound)
CE (cardioesophageal) junction
CEA (carcinoembryonic antigen) test
CEA and CA 19-9 (pancreatic tumor markers)
CEA-Cide (^{131}I-labeled humanized antibody against carcinoembryonic antigen)
CEAP (clinical manifestations, etiologic factors, anatomic involvement, and pathophysiologic features) classification
CEA-Scan (arcitumomab) imaging agent
CEA-[99mTc] carcinoembryonic antigen
Cebotome drill
cecal appendix
cecal bascule
cecal diverticulitis

cecal fold
cecal hernia
cecal serosa
cecal volvulus
 mesenterico-axial (cecal bascule)
 organo-axial (true volvulus)
cecitis
cecopexy
cecorrhaphy
cecostomy
 percutaneous catheter
 tube
CECT (contrast enhancement of computed tomographic) head and body imaging
cecum, coned
cecum twisted in a clockwise direction (cecal volvulus)
Cedax (ceftibuten)
Cedecea davisae
Cedecea lapagei
Cedecea neteri
cedelizumab monoclonal antibody
CEEA (curved end-to-end anastomotic)
CEEA 21, 25, 28, 31 stapling device
cefadroxil
cefazolin
cefdinir
cefotetan
cefoxitin
ceftibuten
Ceftin (cefuroxime)
cefuroxime
Celebra (celecoxib) (now Celebrex)
Celebrex (celecoxib)
celecoxib
Celestin dilator bougie
Celestin esophageal tube
Celestin graduated dilator
Celestin intraluminal tube
Celestin latex rubber tube
Celestin procedure
celiac alcohol ablation
celiac artery aneurysm

celiac artery compression syndrome
celiac axis
celiac clamp
celiac crisis
celiac dimple
celiac disease (CD)
celiac gland
celiac infantilism
celiac lymph node
celiac node
celiac rickets
celiac sprue disease
celiac trunk
celiacography
celiotomy
   exploratory
   staging
celiotomy and resection of pancreatic
   tumor
celiotomy incision
cell
   acid
   acinar
   adelomorphous
   antral gastric
   APUD (amine precursor uptake
     and decarboxylation)
   argentaffin
   argyrophil
   B
   basal granular
   beaker
   border
   Cajal, interstitial
   calciform
   capillary endothelial
   central
   centroacinar
   chalice
   chief
   Davidoff
   delomorphous
   dendritic reticular
   ECL (enterochromaffin-like)

cell *(cont.)*
   enterochromaffin
   fat
   fat-storing liver
   foam
   G
   gastric pacemaker
   gastrin-secreting
   Gaucher
   gelbe
   giant
   goblet
   ground-glass
   Heidenhain
   helle
   helper T
   interstitial
   Ito
   killer T
   Kulchitsky
   Kupffer
   L
   mucous neck
   mucus-secreting
   Namalwa
   natural killer (NK)
   non-alpha, non-beta pancreatic islet
   nuclear-tagged
   oxyntic
   pacemaker (gastric)
   pale
   pancreatic islet
   Paneth
   parietal
   peptic
   phagocytic stellate
   Pick
   plasma
   PP
   ptyocrinous
   pulpar
   S
   signet-ring
   silver

cell *(cont.)*
 small granule
 specialized columnar
 spindle
 stellate
 suppressor T
 T
 target
 undifferentiated
 von Kupffer
 xanthoma
 zymogenic
cell atypia
cell-cell adhesion
CellCept (mycophenolate mofetil
 [MMF])
cell death
cell growth regulation program
cell-mediated delayed immune reaction
 (type IV)
cell-mediated immune inflammation
cell-mediated immune reaction
cell-mediated immunity
Cellolite patty material
Cellona bandage
Cell Recovery System (CRS)
Cell Saver
Cell Saver 5
Cell Saver Haemolite autotransfusion
 system
celltrifuge
cell turgidity
cellular debris
cellular immunity
cellular polyp
cellular xenograft rejection
cellular xenotransplantation
cellulitis
 anal
 perirectal
 rectal
 wound
cell wall
celomic pouch

celosomia
Celsior organ preservation solution
Cement Eater drill
cement, Implast bone cement
cement tube
Cenflex central monitoring system
Centara (priliximab)
Centauri Er:YAG laser system
centering balloon light guide
centering drill
CenterPointLock skin barrier
Centers for Disease Control and
 Prevention (CDC)
central cell
central cirrhosis
central cone technique reduction
central hyaline sclerosis
central hyperalimentation
central lesion
central line infection
central lymph node
central necrosis
central nervous system (CNS)
central scar
central venous catheter (CVC)
central venous pressure line
centrilobar pancreatitis
centrilobular necrosis
centrilobular pancreatitis
centrilobular region of liver
centroacinar cell
centrum retractor
Ceo-Two suppository (sodium bicar-
 bonate; potassium bitartrate)
cephalad
cephalic phase of acid secretion
cephalin-cholesterol flocculation test
cephalosporin
Cephulac
ceramic insulated coating
cerclage suture
cerebellar retractor
cerebral abscess
cerebral death

cerebral edema
cerebral malaria
cerebral radiation (CRN) necrosis
cerebriform carcinoma
cerebrohepatorenal syndrome
cerebroside lipidosis (Gaucher disease)
cerebrospinal fluid
cerebrotendinous xanthomastosis
Ceredase (alglucerase)
ceremidetrihexosidase
Cerezyme (imiglucerase)
ceroid-laden macrophage
ceroid-like histiocytic granuloma
Certican (everolimus)
Certiva vaccine
ceruloplasmin, serum
cervical adenopathy
cervical anesthesia
cervical aortic arch
cervical aspiration
cervical disk retractor
cervical drill
cervical esophagogastrostomy
cervical esophagotomy
cervical incision
cervical laminectomy punch
cervical laminectomy rongeur
cervical locking plate
cervical mallet
cervical motion tenderness
cervical node dissection
cervical polyp
cervical punch forceps
cervical roll
cervical stenosis
cervical stump
cervical support pillow
cervical ulcer
CESD (cholesterol ester storage disease)
Cestoda (genus, tapeworm)
cestode (pl. cestodes) (tapeworm)
Cetacaine (benzocaine; tetracaine; butamben)

cetraxate HCl
cetuximab
CFC BioScanner System
CF-HM colonoscope
CF-HM endoscope
CFIDS (chronic fatigue and immune dysfunction syndrome)
CF-LB3R colonoscope
CF-200Z Olympus colonoscope
CF-UM3 echocolonoscope
CG (Cardio-Green)
C-glycolic acid breath test
CGM (coffee-grounds material)
C graft
Chaffin-Pratt drain
CHAG (coralline hydroxyapatite Goniopora)
Chagas disease
chain suture
chain-of-lakes deformity
chain-of-lakes filling defect
chain-of-lakes sign
chalice cell
chalk stone
chamfer reamer
Champ elastic bandage
champagne shield template
Champion (nitinol coronary) stent
Champion Trauma Score (CTS)
Championnière bone drill
Chandler bone elevator
Chandler knee retractor
Chandler spinal perforating forceps
change in bowel habits
channel and core biopsy
channel, pyloric
char (following laser treatment)
CharcoAid (activated charcoal)
CharcoAid 2000
charcoal, activated
Charcoal Plus (activated charcoal)
CharcoCaps (charcoal)
Charcodote (activated charcoal)
Charcot cirrhosis

Charcot triad of symptoms (fever/chills, right upper quadrant pain, jaundice)
Charcot triangle
Chardonna-2 (belladonna extract; phenobarbital)
CHARGE (coloboma, heart, atresia of the choanae, retardation of growth and development, genital and urinary anomalies, and ear anomalies [also tracheoesophageal fistula])
CHARGE association
CHARGE syndrome
Charnley centering drill
Charnley compression clamp
Charnley deepening reamer
Charnley expanding reamer
Charnley femoral condyle drill
Charnley femoral prosthesis neck punch
Charnley horizontal retractor
Charnley incision
Charnley knee retractor
Charnley pin
Charnley pin retractor
Charnley rasp
Charnley reamer
Charnley retractor
Charnley self-retaining retractor
Charnley suction drain
Charnley suture forceps
Charnley taper reamer
Charnley tissue forceps
Charnley trochanter reamer
Charnley vertical retractor
Charnley wire-holding forceps
Charriere amputating saw
Charriere bone saw
Chaufford point
Chauveau bacterium
Cheatle-Henry hernia
Cheatle slit for takedown of colostomy
Cheatle sterilizing forceps
Check-Flo introducer
cheese handler's lung

cheesy necrosis
Cheetah angioplasty catheter
cheilosis
Chelsea-Eaton anal speculum
chem air
chem panel (chemistry)
Chem-7
Chem-10
chemical denaturing in vivo
chemical esophagitis
chemical exposure
chemical gastritis
chemical paralysis
chemical peritonitis
chemistries
chemistry panel
Chemo-Port catheter
chemoprevention
chemoprotective agent
chemoradiation
chemoradiotherapy, external beam radiotherapy and 5-FU
chemosis
chemotactic effects
chemotherapy (see also *medication*)
    adjunctive
    adjuvant
    combination
    intraperitoneal hyperthermic IPHC)
    multi-drug
    palliable
    primary
    systemic
chemotherapy-induced vomiting
chemotherapy protocol
chemotherapy regimen
Chemstrip MatchMaker blood glucose monitor
Chenix (chenodiol)
chenodeoxycholic acid (CDCA)
chenodiol
Chenofalk
Cherchevski disease
Cherney incision

Cherney lower transverse abdominal
   incision
Cheron dressing forceps
cherry (small dissecting sponge)
cherry angioma
Cherry-Austin drill
Cherry brain retractor
Cherry-Crandall method for testing
   serum lipase
cherry dissector sponge
cherry endosponge
Cherry extractor
Cherry-Kerrison laminectomy forceps
Cherry-Kerrison laminectomy rongeur
Cherry laminectomy retractor
cherry-pit sponge
cherry-red endobronchial lesions
   of Kaposi sarcoma
cherry sponge
CHESS (comprehensive health
   enhancement support system)
chest drainage unit
chest tube
chest wall fixation
chest wall invasion
chevron incision
chew-and-spit test
Cheyne periosteal elevator
CHF (congenital hepatic fibrosis)
CHF (congestive heart failure)
Chiari-Budd syndrome
Chiari disease
Chiba aspiration biopsy needle
Chiba cholangiography needle
Chiba percutaneous cholangiogram
chicken fat clot
Chick nail
chiclero ulcer
chief cell
chief-cell hyperplasia
chief (primary) complaint
Chieftan aspirating cannula
Chilaiditi sign
Chilaiditi syndrome

Child classification of cirrhosis
Child classification (A–C) of
   esophageal varices
Child classification (A–C) of hepatic
   reserve
Child classification of hepatic risk
   criteria
Child classification of liver disease
Childe approximating forceps
Childe hernia director
Child hepatic risk criteria
childhood thyroid irradiation
Child pancreaticoduodenostomy
Child-Pugh bleeding esophageal varices
   grading scale
Child-Pugh class A–C (used in hepatic
   disease)
Children's Hospital hand drill
Children's Hospital intestinal forceps
Child-Turcotte classification (used in
   hepatic surgery)
Childs-Phillips bowel plication
Chilli cooled ablation catheter
chills and fever
chills, shaking
chimney-sweep's cancer
CHIMPANZEES (calcium, hyper-
   parathyroidism/hyperthyroidism/
   hypocalciuric/hypercalcemia,
   immobility/iatrogenic, metastasis/
   milk alkali syndrome, Paget disease,
   Addison disease/acromegaly,
   neoplasm, Zollinger-Ellison
   syndrome, excessive vitamin D,
   excessive vitamin A, sarcoid)
chin lift
Chin-Up Strip
chip graft
chip mat bandage
Chirocaine (levobupivacaine)
chiropractic film
chisel (see also *gouge*)
   acetabuloplastic round
   Adson

chisel *(cont.)*
    Adson laminectomy
    Alexander
    ASIF
    Austin Moore
    Ballenger-Hajek
    beveled
    Bishop
    Blair
    bone
    Bowen
    box
    Brittain
    Bruening
    Brunetti
    Buckley
    Caltagirone
    Cinelli-McIndoe
    Cloward cervical
    Cloward spinal fusion
    cold
    Converse
    Cottle
    Dautrey
    Derlacki
    D'Errico lamina
    Farrior-Dworacek
    Fomon
    Freer
    gouge
    Hajek
    Hibbs
    hollow
    Lambert-Lowman
    laminectomy
    Lexer
    Lowman-Hoglund
    Lucas
    Martin cartilage
    meniscotomy
    Metzenbaum
    Meyerding
    Miles bone
    mortising

chisel *(cont.)*
    neurosurgical
    Partsch
    Passow
    Pick
    Puka
    Schwartze
    seating
    Sheehan
    Simmons
    Smillie cartilage
    Smillie meniscotomy
    Smith-Petersen
    square hollow
    Stille bone
    straight
    swan-neck
    Trautmann
    U.S. Army bone
    USA pattern
    West bone
chisel blade
chisel edge elevator
chisel elevator
chisel-tip wire
chitosan
Chlamydia pneumoniae
Chlamydia psittaci
Chlamydia trachomatis
Chloraprep preoperative skin
    preparation
ChloraPrep One-Step
Chloresium (chlorophyllin copper
    complex)
chloride (Cl⁻)
chloride ion
chloride, vinyl
chlormethazine
chloroform poisoning
chlorophyllin
Chloroplast membrane sulfolipids
    (blue-green algae) nutritional
    supplement
chloroprocaine

cholecystectomy *(cont.)*
  micro laparoscopic
  open
  prophylactic
  three-trocar technique
  transcylindrical
cholecystectomy and wedge resection of
  overlying liver
cholecystectomy clamp
cholecystectomy with incidental appen-
  dectomy
cholecystenteric fistula
cholecystitis
  acalculous
  acute
  asymptomatic
  calculous
  chronic
  emphysematous
  erythromycin-induced
  follicular
  gangrenous
  gaseous
  perforated
  suppurative
  typhoidal
  uncomplicated acute
  xanthogranulomatous
cholecystitis with cholelithiasis
cholecystobiliary fistulization
cholecystocholangiography
cholecystocholedochal fistula
cholecystocholedocholithiasis
cholecystocolonic fistula
cholecystoduodenal fistula
cholecystoduodenal ligament
cholecystoduodenocolic fistula
cholecystoduodenocolic fold
cholecystoduodenostomy, Jenckel
cholecystoenteric fistula
cholecystoenterostomy, direct
cholecystogram, oral (OCG)
cholecystojejunostomy
cholecystokinetic food

cholecystokinin (CCK)
cholecystokinin-pancreozymin
  (CCK-PZ)
cholecystokinin stimulation test
cholecystolithiasis
cholecystoscopy, percutaneous
  transhepatic
choledochal basal pressure
choledochal-colonic fistula
choledochal cyst
choledochal region
choledochal sphincter
choledochal stent
choledochitis, suppurative
choledochocele
choledochocholedochostomy,
  side-to-side anastomosis
choledochoduodenal area
choledochoduodenal fistula
choledochoduodenal junction
choledochoduodenal junctional stenosis
choledochoduodenostomy (CDS)
choledochofiberscope (see *endoscope)*
choledochojejunostomy
  end-to-side
  loop
  retrocolic end-to-side
  Roux-en-Y
choledocholith
choledocholithiasis
choledocholithotripsy
choledochopancreatic ductal junction
choledochoscope
  Berci-Shore
  flexible fiberoptic
  Jasan JFE
  Machida
  Olympus CHF-CB30
  Olympus CHF-P20
  Olympus CHF-P20Q
  Pentax ECN-1530 choledocho-
    nephroscope
  Pentax FCN-15H flexible

choledochoscopy
  Berci-Shore
  T-tube tract
choledochostomy
choledochotomy, longitudinal
choledochous cyst
choledochous duct
choledochus (noun)
choleic acid
cholelithiasis
  asymptomatic
  chronic
  weight loss-induced
cholelithic dyspepsia
cholelithiasis, cholesterol
cholelitholysis
cholelithotomy
cholelithotripsy
cholemia
  familial
  Gilbert
cholemesis
choleperitoneum
choleperitonitis
cholera morbus
cholera, pancreatic
choleric jaundice
cholescintigram
cholescintigraphy
Cholestagel (now Welchol)
cholestasis
  benign recurrent intrahepatic
    (of pregnancy)
  canalicular
  chlorpromazine-induced
  drug-induced
  extrahepatic
  familial
  familial intrahepatic
  hepatocellular
  intrahepatic
  intrahepatic in pregnancy (ICP)
  methyltestosterone-induced
  tolbutamide-induced

cholestasis-lymphedema syndrome
  (Aagenaes syndrome)
cholestasis with peripheral pulmonary
  stenosis
cholestatic cirrhosis
cholestatic jaundice
cholestatic liver disease
cholestatic syndrome
cholestatic viral hepatitis
Cholestech L.D.X. test
cholesterol
  blood
  dietary
  HDL
  LDL
  serum
  total
  VLDL
cholesterol calculus
cholesterol ester storage disease
  (CESD)
cholesterol gallstone
cholesterol precipitate
cholesterol stone
cholesterolosis of gallbladder
cholesterolosis of mucosal surface
CholesTrak test
Cholestron PRO test
Cholestron test
cholestyramine resin
Choletec (^{99m}Tc mebrofenin) imaging
  agent
choline chloride
Cholografin contrast medium
Cholografin Meglumine (iodipamide
  meglumine)
chondroplasty blade
chondroplasty knife
Chooz (calcium carbonate)
CHOP chemotherapy
chordotomy (cordotomy) knife
chorionic carcinoma
choristoma
choroid plexus carcinoma

choroid plexus papilloma
choroidal hemangioma
choroidal layer of the eye
Christensen interlocking nail
Christie gallbladder retractor
Christmas tree appearance of pancreas
   (on x-ray)
Christmas tree reamer
Christmas tree sign
Christopher-Williams overtube
Christoudias fascial closure device
chromatin pattern
ChromaVision digital analyzer
chromic catgut suture
chromic gut suture
chromic interrupted suture
chromium (Cr)
chromium picolinate supplementation
   (in diabetes)
chromium polynicotinate
chromium-51 (^{51}Cr)-tagged red blood
   cells
Chromobacterium violaceum
chromoscopy
chromosome 14$_q$ tumor marker
chromosome 23
   inverted duplication
   partial tetrasomy
   partial trisomy
chronic acholuric jaundice
chronic active hepatitis (CAH)
chronic active viral hepatitis (CAVH)
chronic active viral hepatitis B
   (CAVH-B)
chronic active viral hepatitis C
   (CAVH-C)
chronic active viral hepatitis non-A,
   non-B (CAVH-NAB) (now
   CAVH-C)
chronic aggressive hepatitis
chronic alcoholic cirrhosis
chronic alcoholic hepatic cirrhosis
chronic alcoholic liver disease
chronic alcoholic pancreatitis

chronic alcoholism
chronic appendicitis
chronic atrophic duodenitis
chronic atrophic gastritis
chronic bacillary diarrhea
chronic bacterial prostatitis (CBP)
chronic calcific pancreatitis
chronic calcifying pancreatitis
chronic cholecystitis
chronic congestive splenomegaly
chronic constipation
chronic cystic gastritis
chronic cystic mastitis
chronic dermatitis
chronic diarrhea
chronic diverticulitis
chronic Epstein-Barr virus infection
chronic erosive gastritis
chronic familial jaundice
chronic fatigue and immune dysfunction
   syndrome (CFIDS)
chronic fibrosing hepatitis
chronic fibrous thyroiditis
chronic fissure refractory to conserva-
   tive treatment
chronic follicular gastritis
chronic gastritis type B
chronic granulomatous disease
chronic hemolysis
chronic hepatitis
chronic hyperparathyroid state
chronic idiopathic intestinal pseudo-
   obstruction (CIIP)
chronic idiopathic jaundice
chronic infection
chronic inflammation of pancreas
chronic inflammatory process
chronic intermittent colitis
chronic interstitial hepatitis
chronic intestinal pseudo-obstruction
   (CIP)
chronic ischemic colitis
chronic ischemic enteritis
chronic ischemic enterocolitis

chronic laxative abuse
chronic lobular hepatitis (CLH)
chronic lymphocytic leukemia (CLL)
chronic lymphocytic thyroiditis
chronic mononucleosis
chronic myelogenous leukemia
chronic nonsuppurative destructive
  cholangitis
chronic obstructive pancreatitis
chronic pancreatitis
chronic peptic esophagitis
chronic peptic ulcer
chronic persistent hepatitis (CPH)
chronic progressive hepatitis
chronic proliferative peritonitis
chronic prostatitis
chronic regurgitation
chronic relapsing pancreatitis
chronic renal disease
chronic scab
chronic sclerosing hyaline fibrosis
chronic stool retention
chronic stricture of the small bowel
chronic subareolar abscess
chronic thyroiditis
chronic ulcer
chronic ulcerative colitis (CUC)
chronically inflamed gallbladder
Chronicle implantable hemodynamic
  monitor
ChronoFlex catheter
chrontropy
Chronulac (lactulose)
CHRYS CO_2 laser
Chrysalin
Chrysosporium parvum
chuck drill
Chuinard autogenous bone graft
CHUK (conserved helix-loop-helix
  ubiquitous kinase) protein
Church scissors
Chvostek sign
chyle cyst
chyliferous vessel

chylomicron retention disease
chylopoietic disease
chylous ascites
chylous ascitic fluid
chylous fluid
chylous hydrotherapy
chyme
Chymex (bentiromide)
chymosin
chymotrypsin
CI (cardiac index)
Ciaglia Blue Rhino tracheostomy set
Ciaglia percutaneous tracheostomy
  introducer
CicaCare topical gel sheeting
cicatricial kidney
cicatricial stricture
cicatricial tissue
cicatrix (cicatrices)
cicatrization
Cicherelli bone rongeur
Cidecin (daptomycin for injection)
Cidex OPA disinfectant solution
cidofovir gel dressing
cigarette drain
CIIP (chronic idiopathic intestinal
  pseudo-obstruction)
cilansetron
ciliary fold
ciliary neurotrophic factor (CNTF)
cimetidine HCl
Cincinnati incision
Cincinnati subzero unit
cinedefecogram
cinefluorography
cinefluoroscopy
cine-esophagogram
cine-esophagoscope
cine-esophagoscopy
cine-esophagram
cinegastroscopy
Cinelli-McIndoe chisel
cineradiography
cine view

Cintor bone rongeur
CIP (chronic intestinal pseudo-
	obstruction)
Cipro (ciprofloxacin)
ciprofloxacin
circle
circle absorption anesthesia
circle straight cutting
circomyotomy
Circon-ACMI electrohydraulic
	lithotriptor probe
Circon bipolar instrument
Circon continuous-flow resectoscope
Circon Corporation video camera
	system
Circon rigid laparoscope
Circon videohydrothoracoscope
CircPlus compression dressing
circuit anesthesia
circuit without filter
circular cherry-red lesion
circular fold
circular myotomy
circular saw
circular self-retaining retractor
circular stapler
circular suture
circular tape
circular wire suture
circulating antibody
circulating blood
circulating blood volume
circulating endotoxin
circulating T_3 and T_4
circulation
	bile acid
	collateral
	cutaneous collateral
	enterohepatic
	hyperkinetic
	portal
	portal-systemic; portosystemic
	systemic
circulator fold

circulatory decompensation
circulatory overload
Circulon dressing
Circulon System Step 1 (and Step 2)
	venous ulcer kit dressing
circumanal gland
circumareolar incision
circumcostal gastropexy
circumference
circumferential incision
circumferentially
circumferential suture
circumferential suture ligation
circumferentially sutured onlay patch
circumflex scissors
circumoral numbness and tingling
circumscribing incision
circumumbilical incision
circumvallate papilla
cirrhosis
	acholangic biliary
	acute juvenile
	alcoholic
	atrophic
	bacterial
	Baumgarten-Cruveilhier
	biliary
	Budd
	calculus
	capsular
	cardiac
	central
	Charcot
	cholangitic biliary
	cholestatic
	chronic alcoholic
	coarsely nodular
	congenital
	congestive
	congestive liver
	Cruveilhier-Baumgarten
	cryptogenic
	decompensated
	decompensated alcoholic

cirrhosis *(cont.)*
  dietary
  diffuse septal
  end-stage
  extrahepatic
  fatty
  fatty micromedionodular
  florid
  focal biliary
  frank
  glabrous
  Glisson
  Hanot
  hemochromatotic
  hepatic
  hepatolienal
  hobnail
  hypertrophic
  Indian childhood
  insular
  intrahepatic
  juvenile
  Laënnec
  liver
  lung
  macrolobular
  macronodular
  malarial
  medionodular
  metabolic
  microlobular
  micronodular
  monolobular
  multilobular
  nodular
  nonalcoholic
  nutritional
  obstructive biliary
  passive congestive
  pericholangiolitic biliary
  periportal
  pigment
  pigmentary
  pipestem

cirrhosis *(cont.)*
  portal
  posthepatic
  posthepatitic
  postnecrotic
  primary biliary (PBC)
  progressive familial
  pulmonary
  secondary biliary
  scptal
  splenomegalic
  stasis
  stomach
  syphilitic
  Todd
  toxic
  trabecular
  unilobular
  vascular
  xanthomatous biliary
cirrhosis of liver
cirrhosis of lung
cirrhosis of stomach
cirrhotic
cirrhotic gastritis
cirrhotic inflammation
cirrhotic liver
CIS (Colon Injury Score)
cisplatin/epinephrine gel
cisterna chyli
Citelli punch forceps
Citra pH (sodium citrate)
Citralax (magnesium citrate;
  magnesium sulfate)
citrate
citrate of magnesia
citrate test
Citrobacter amalonaticus
Citrobacter diversus
Citrobacter freundii
Citrocarbonate (sodium bicarbonate;
  sodium citrate)
Citrotein liquid feeding
Citrucel (methylcellulose)

Citrucel Sugar Free (methylcellulose;
  phenylalanine)
CK (conductive keratoplasty)
CKC (cold knife cone) biopsy
CKPT (combined kidney-pancreatic
  transplant)
Cl⁻ (chloride)
CLA (conjugated linoleic acid)
C lactose test
Cladosporium
Clagett Barrett esophagogastrostomy
Clagett S cannula
clammy
clamp (see also *clip*)
  Acland
  Adair
  Adair breast
  Adams-DeWeese vena caval
  Alfred M. Large
  Allen anastomosis
  Allen intestinal
  Allen-Kocher
  Allis
  Allis-Adair
  anastomosis
  Anderson
  angled peripheral vascular
  angular hinge
  anterior resection
  aortic
  aortic aneurysm
  aortic occlusion
  appendage
  approximator
  ASSI No-scalpel vasectomy fixator
    ring clamp
  Atrauclip hemostatic
  atraumatic vascular
  Atraumax
  Babcock
  baby Payr pylorus
  Backhaus towel
  Bahnson
  Bailey aortic

clamp *(cont.)*
  Bainbridge intestinal
  Ballantine
  Beck
  Beck-Potts
  Benjamin-Havas fiberoptic light
  Berens muscle
  Berman aortic
  Best right-angle colon
  Bigelo calvarium
  Bihrle dorsal
  Bircher bone/cartilage
  Bishop
  Blalock-Niedner
  Blalock pulmonary
  Blalock-Taussig
  Böhler (Boehler)
  bone extension
  bone-holding
  Borge
  Boyes muscle
  Brock
  Buie pile
  bulldog
  C
  Calman carotid artery
  Calman ring
  calvarium
  cardiac retraction clip
  Carmalt
  carotid artery
  cartilage
  Castaneda anastomosis
  Castaneda vascular
  celiac
  Charnley compression
  cholecystectomy
  Clark clamp
  coarctation
  colon resection
  Cooley anastomosis
  Cooley aortic
  Cooley-Beck
  Cooley bulldog

clamp *(cont.)*
    Cooley coarctation
    Cooley cross-action bulldog
    Cooley-Derra anastomosis
    Cooley iliac
    Cooley partial occlusion
    Cooley patent ductus
    Cooley pediatric
    Cooley renal
    Cooley-Satinsky
    Cooley vascular
    Cooley vena cava catheter
    Cope crushing
    Cope modification of Martel
      intestinal
    Cosgrove Flex
    Crafoord aortic
    Crafoord coarctation
    Crile appendix
    Crile-type
    Crutchfield carotid artery
    Cunningham
    curved
    curved Cooley
    curved Mayo
    Dandy
    Daniel colostomy
    Dardik
    Davidson vessel
    Davis aneurysm
    DeBakey aortic aneurysm
    DeBakey arterial
    DeBakey atraumatic bulldog
    DeBakey-Bahnson vascular
    DeBakey-Bainbridge
    DeBakey-Beck
    DeBakey bulldog
    DeBakey coarctation
    DeBakey colon resection
    DeBakey cross-action bulldog
    DeBakey-Derra anastomosis
    DeBakey-Harken
    DeBakey-Howard
    DeBakey-Kay

clamp *(cont.)*
    DeBakey patent ductus
    DeBakey pediatric
    DeBakey peripheral vascular bulldog
    DeBakey-Reynolds anastomosis
    DeBakey ring-handled bulldog
    DeBakey-Semb
    DeBakey sigmoid anastomosis
    DeBakey tangential occlusion
    DeBakey vascular
    DeMartel vascular
    DeMartel-Wolfson anastomosis
    Demos tibial artery
    Dennis
    Derra vena cava
    Derra vestibular
    DeWeese vena cava
    Dieffenbach bulldog
    Diethrich bulldog
    Diethrich micro bulldog
    Dingman bone and cartilage
    Dingman cartilage
    Dixon-Thomas-Smith
    double
    double-occluding
    Doyen intestinal
    Duval lung-grasping
    Earle hemorrhoid
    Edna towel
    Endo Babcock
    exclusion
    Fehland colon resection
    Fergusson
    Filshie female sterilization
    Fogarty
    Fogarty-Chin
    Fogarty Hydrogrip
    Foss intestinal
    Fukushima C-
    Furniss anastomosis
    Furniss-Clute
    Gant
    Garcia aorta
    Gardner neurosurgical skull

clamp *(cont.)*

 Gerbode patent ductus
 Glassman atraumatic bowel
 Glover bulldog
 Glover coarctation
 Glover patent ductus
 Glover vascular
 Goldblatt
 Goldstein Microspike approximator
 Grant aneurysm
 Greenberg
 Gregory baby profunda
 Gregory carotid bulldog
 Gregory DeBakey bulldog
 Gregory external
 Gross coarctation occlusion
 Grover
 Gusberg hysterectomy
 Gutgemann
 Guyonn-Pean kidney
 Gwilliam
 Haberer intestinal
 Halifax interlaminar
 Harken auricle
 Harrington hook
 Harrington rod
 Harvey Stone
 Hayes anterior resection
 Heaney
 Heifitz
 Hemoclip
 Hem-o-lok
 hemorrhoidal
 hemostatic
 Hendrin ductus
 Henley vascular
 Herrick kidney
 Hirschman pile
 Hoen
 hook
 Hopkins aortic
 Hufnagel aortic
 Humphries aortic
 Hurwitz esophageal

clamp *(cont.)*

 hyperinsulinemic-euglycemic
  glucose
 infant skull
 interlaminar
 intestinal
 intestinal crushing
 intracranial
 Jackson bone extension
 Jacobson bulldog
 Jacobson-Potts vascular
 Jahnke anastomosis
 Jarvis pile
 Javid carotid artery
 Johns Hopkins bulldog
 Johns Hopkins coarctation
 Jones thoracic
 Kantrowitz thoracic
 Kapp-Beck
 Kapp-Beck-Thomson
 Kartchner carotid artery
 Kay aorta
 Kay-Lambert
 Kelly
 Kelsey pile
 Kern bone-holding
 Kindt carotid artery
 Kinsella-Buie lung
 Kleinschmidt appendectomy
 Klintmalm
 Koala vascular
 Kocher
 Lahey
 Lambert aortic
 Lambert-Kay aorta
 Lambert-Kay vascular
 Lambert-Lowman bone
 Lamis patella
 Lane bone
 Lane bone-holding
 Lane intestinal
 Lane twin stomach
 Lang Stevenson intestinal
 Lee microvascular

clamp *(cont.)*
    Leland-Jones vascular
    Lewin bone-holding
    Liddle aorta
    Ligaclip
    Linnartz intestinal
    Locke
    long Péan
    Lowman bone
    Lowman bone-holding
    Lowman-Gerster bone
    Lowman-Hoglund bone-holding
    Maingot
    Martel
    Martin cartilage
    Martin meniscus
    Martin muscle
    Mason vascular
    Masters intestinal
    Masters-Schwartz liver
    Mastin muscle
    Matthew cross-leg
    Mattox aorta
    Mayfield neurosurgical skull
    Mayfield three-pin skull
    Mayo
    Mayo-Guyon kidney pedicle
    Mayo-Robson intestinal
    McCleery-Miller intestinal
    McDougal prostatectomy
    McLean pile
    M.D. Anderson
    Meeker gallbladder
    meniscus
    metal
    metallic
    Michel aortic
    micro cross-action bulldog
    Microspike approximator
    microvascular
    Mikulicz
    Mixter
    Mixter right-angle
    Mogen circumcision

clamp *(cont.)*
    Morris aorta
    mosquito
    Moynihan towel
    Muller pediatric
    Multiclip
    muscle biopsy
    Neuromeet nerve approximator
    Niedner anastomosis
    noncrushing bowel
    noncrushing vascular
    Noon AV fistula
    Nussbaum intestinal
    occluding
    occlusion
    Olsen cholangiogram
    Omed bulldog vascular
    O'Hanlon intestinal
    O'Neill
    Parham-Martin fracture
    Parker-Kerr intestinal
    partial occluding
    partial occlusion
    partially occluding vascular
    patch-clamp
    patellar
    patent ductus
    Payr gastrointestinal
    Payr pyloric
    Pean
    pediatric bulldog
    pediatric vascular
    pedicle
    Pemberton sigmoid
    Pemberton spur-crushing
    Pennington
    Perneczky aneurysm clamp
    Petz
    pin
    Poppen-Blalock carotid
    Poppen-Blalock-Salibi
    Potts aortic
    Potts coarctation
    Potts patent ductus

clamp *(cont.)*
    Potts-Niedner
    Potts-Satinsky
    Potts-Smith aortic occlusion
    Presbyterian Hospital tubing
    Presbyterian tube-occluding
    Price muscle biopsy
    Quick Bend flex
    Raney
    Rankin
    Rayport muscle biopsy
    rectal occlusion
    Redo intestinal
    Reinhoff
    Reynolds vascular
    Right Clip
    right-angle
    rod
    Roosevelt
    Rosenkranz universal
    rubber-shod
    Rumel myocardial
    Rumel thoracic
    saddle
    Salibi carotid artery
    Sarot bronchus
    Satinsky aortic
    Satinsky vascular
    Satinsky vena cava
    Schlein
    Schnidt (not Schmidt)
    Schumaker aortic
    Schwartz temporary intracranial
       artery
    Scudder intestinal
    Secu
    Sehrt
    self-retaining
    Selman
    Selverstone carotid
    Selverstone carotid artery
    Senning bulldog
    serrefine
    Sevrain cranial

clamp *(cont.)*
    Shoemaker intestinal
    side-biting
    sigmoid anastomosis
    single
    skull
    sliding
    Slocum meniscal
    Smith bone
    sponge
    spoon
    spur-crushing
    stainless steel
    Steinhauser bone
    Stetten intestinal
    Stille-Crawford
    Stille vessel
    Stockmann
    Stone-Holcombe intestinal
    Stone intestinal
    straight
    Strelinger colon
    St. Vincent tube occluding
    Subramanian
    Sugita right-angle aneurysm
    supraceliac aortic cross-
    suprarenal aortic cross-
    Swan aortic
    "sweetheart" (Harrington)
    swivel
    Thompson carotid artery
    Thomson Walker
    three-point skull
    tissue occlusion
    towel
    trochanter-holding
    tubing
    tube-occluding
    twin stomach
    Ulrich bone-holding
    vascular
    Verbrugge bone
    Veridien
    V. Mueller bulldog

clamp *(cont.)*
    Vorse-Webster
    VSF (Vermont spinal fixator)
    Walton cartilage
    Wangensteen anastomosis
    Wangensteen patent ductus
    Weber aortic
    Weck
    Wertheim
    Wertheim-Cullen
    Winston
    Winston-Acland
    wire fixation
    Wirthlin splenorenal
    Wister vascular
    Wolfson intestinal
    Wylie carotid artery
    Wylie hypogastric
    Yasargil carotid
    Z
    Zachary Cope-DeMartel
    Zeppelin
    Zinnanti Z
clamp-and-sew technique
clamp-applying forceps
clamped, cut, and ligated
clamshell incision
Clark clamp
Clark classification I–V
Clarke-Hadefield syndrome
Classen-Demling papillotome
classic abdominal Semm hysterectomy
    (CASH)
classic achalasia
classic coffee bean sign
classic hyperthyroidism
classic triad of palpitations, headache,
    episodic diaphoresis (PHE)
classic triad of Rigler
classification (also *grade; stage*)
    Abbreviated Injury Scale (AIS)
    American Association for the
        Surgery of Trauma Organ Injury
        Scale

classification *(cont.)*
    Bismuth bile duct stricture,
        types I-V
    bladder carcinoma classification
    Blaivas classification of urinary
        incontinence
    BLEED (bleeding, low BP, elevated
        PT, erratic mental status, disease
        [comorbid])
    Boorman gastric cancer typing
        system (types 1-4)
    Breast Imaging and Reporting Data
        System of the American College
        of Radiology (BI-RADS)
    Breslow
    Broders index of malignant tumors
    burn
    carcinoma of bladder
    Casten
    CEAP (clinical manifestations, etio-
        logic factors, anatomic involve-
        ment, pathophysiologic features)
    Child classification of cirrhosis
    Child esophageal varices (A–C)
    Child hepatic dysfunction
    Child hepatic reserve (A–C)
    Child hepatic risk criteria
    Child liver disease
    Child-Pugh class A–C used
        in hepatic disease
    Child-Turcotte hepatic surgery
    Couinaud liver anatomy
    cytoprotective agent
    Dagradi esophageal variceal
    diabetes mellitus
    Dubin and Amelar varicocele
    Dukes Astler-Coller, modified
    Dukes carcinoma
    ECOG (Eastern Cooperative Oncol-
        ogy Group) performance status
    Edmondson Grading System
    Edmondson-Steiner histologic
        grading of hepatocellular
        carcinoma

cleanser *(cont.)*
   DiabKlenz wound
   Hibiclens (chlorhexidine gluconate; alcohol)
   MicroKlenz wound
   Operand (povidone; iodine)
   Puri-Clens wound
   Sea-Clens wound
   Shur-Clens wound
   Skinvisible hypoallergenic hand lotion
   Surgi-Kleen skin
   Techni-Care surgical scrub
   UltraKlenz wound
   Zepiran
cleansing, intestinal
clearance, ineffective airway
clear bile
clear cell carcinoma
clear cell hepatocellular carcinoma
ClearCut 2 electrosurgical handpiece
clear effluent
clear fluid
clear-liquid diet
clear margins of tumor
clear otorrhea
clear rhinorrhea
ClearSite absorbent hydrogel wound dressing
ClearSite border dressing
ClearSite borderless dressing
ClearSite Hydro Gauze dressing
clear tap
ClearVac smoke evacuation system
ClearView CO_2 laser
"cleavoplasty" augmentation mammoplasty
cleft lip
clenched fist view
clenoliximab
Cleveland bone-cutting forceps
Cleveland bone rongeur
CLH (chronic lobular hepatitis)
clidinium bromide

Clik-Tite connector
clindamycin
clinical diagnosis
clinical parameters
clinical pathologic classification
clinical pathology
clinical picture
CliniCath peripherally inserted catheter
Clinifeed Iso enteral feeding
Clinimix E (amino acid with electrolytes in dextrose with calcium)
Clinipad Corporation
Clinistix reagent strips
Clinitest-negative stool
Clinitest-positive stool
Clinitest stool test
Clinoril (sulindac)
clip (see also *clamp*)
   Absolok locking PDS
   Absolok Plus
   Acland
   Adson scalp
   aneurysm
   aneurysm window
   Atrauclip
   baby Jones towel
   Biemer-Clip aneurysm
   brain
   Braun-Yasargil right-angle
   Children's Hospital scalp
   cobalt alloy aneurysm
   Codman aneurysm
   Cologne
   Cologne pattern scalp
   Drake aneurysm
   fenestrated Drake
   Filshie
   Heifitz
   Hem-o-lok ligating
   Hemoclip
   hemostasis
   hemostatic
   Horizon
   Housepan aneurysm

clip *(cont.)*
 Ingraham-Fowler tantalum
 Jones towel
 Khodadad
 Lapra-Ty absorbable suture
 Lapro-Clip
 Lapro-Clip ligating
 LeRoy-Raney scalp
 Liga
 Ligaclip
 Ligaclip hemostatic
 ligating
 M.A.R.C.
 Mayfield aneurysm
 MCAS (modular clip application
  system)
 McFadden temporary aneurysm
 McKenzie brain
 McKenzie hemostasis
 McKenzie silver
 Michel wound
 microclip
 MicroMark
 modular clip application system
  (MCAS)
 Multiclip
 Olivecrona aneurysm
 pin
 Raney hemostasis (hemostatic)
 Raney scalp
 ring angled
 scalp
 Schwartz aneurysm
 Schwartz micro
 Secu ("C-Q")
 Shardle towel
 silver
 skin
 sponge stopper
 Sugita aneurysm
 Sundt encircling
 Sundt-Kees aneurysm window
 supracondylar medial
 surgical

clip *(cont.)*
 surgical steel skin
 Sutured-Clip
 temporary vessel
 titanium aneurysm
 towel
 vari-angle aneurysm
 VCS
 vessel
 Weck
 Yasargil vessel
clip applier (see *applier; applicator*)
clip-applying forceps
clip-bending forceps
clip-cutting forceps
clip-inserting forceps
clip-introducing forceps
clipped, doubly
clipping of aneurysm
clipping of cystic artery
clip-removing forceps
cloacal anomaly
cloacogenic zone
cloagenic carcinoma
clockwise direction
Clomycin (polymyxin B sulfate;
 bacitracin; neomycin sulfate;
 lidocaine)
clonal anergy of T cells
clonal deletion
clonidine gel
clonidine hydrochloride injection
clonorchiasis
Clonorchis sinensis
C-loop of duodenum
Cloquet gland
Cloquet hernia
clorsulon
clortermine
clortermine HCl
closantel
closed anesthesia
closed circuit anesthesia
closed drainage system

closed-end ostomy pouch
closed hemorrhoidectomy
closed Küntscher (Kuentscher) nail
closed loop
closed loop bowel obstruction
closed loop intestinal obstruction
closed loop strangulation of bowel
closed nail
closed neck dissector
closed pin
closed suction
closed-system irrigation
closed unlocked nail
closed wound
Closer suture
Closer, The
CloseSure procedure kit
close-up view
Clostridium bifermentans
Clostridium botulinum
Clostridium botulinum toxin
Clostridium butyricum
Clostridium cadaveris
Clostridium difficile
Clostridium difficile-associated diarrhea
  (CDAD)
Clostridium histolyticum
Clostridium innocuum
Clostridium novyi
Clostridium paraputrificum
Clostridium perfringens
Clostridium putrificum
Clostridium ramosum
Clostridium septicum
Clostridium sordellii
Clostridium sphenoides
Clostridium subterminale
Clostridium tertium
Clostridium tetani
Clostridium tertium
Clostridium welchii
closure
  crural
  fascial

closure *(cont.)*
  Graham
  ileostomy
  latex
  marlex
  primary
  secondary
  single-layer continuous
  Smead-Jones
  transmural
  two-layer latex
  V-to-Y
  water-tight
  wound
Closure catheter/radiofrequency
  generator
Closure endovascular coagulation
  system
closure of colostomy
closure of fistula
closure of perforation
Closure System by VNUS catheter
clot
  agonal
  antemortem
  black blood
  blood
  chicken
  chicken fat
  currant jelly
  distal
  evacuating
  external
  fresh blood
  friable
  heart
  internal
  laminated
  marantic
  organized
  passive
  plastic
  postmortem
  proximal

clot *(cont.)*
   retraction of
   sentinel blood
   spider-web
   stratified
   washed
CLOtest (*Campylobacter*-like
   organism)
cloth shears
clothespin spinal fusion graft
clot lysis test
clot retraction coagulation panel
clot retraction test
clotting, abnormal
clotting abnormality
clotting factors
clotting parameters
clotting time (also, coagulation)
   activated
   Lee-White
   plasma
clotting time coagulation panel
clot tube
cloudy ascites
cloudy bile
cloudy fluid
clove-hitch suture
cloverleaf deformity
cloverleaf intramedullary nail
cloverleaf Küntscher (Kuentscher) nail
cloverleaf pin extractor
cloverleaf plate
Cloward blade retractor
Cloward brain retractor
Cloward hook
Cloward cervical chisel
Cloward cervical retractor
Cloward-Cushing vein retractor
Cloward drill
Cloward drill guide
Cloward dural hook
Cloward dural retractor
Cloward-English laminectomy rongeur
Cloward hammer

Cloward-Harper laminectomy rongeur
Cloward-Hoen hemilaminectomy
   retractor
Cloward-Hoen laminectomy retractor
Cloward intervertebral disk rongeur
Cloward large cervical rongeur
Cloward lumbar lamina retractor
Cloward nerve root retractor
Cloward osteophyte elevator
Cloward periosteal elevator
Cloward pituitary rongeur
Cloward punch forceps
Cloward rongeur forceps
Cloward skin retractor
Cloward small cervical retractor
Cloward spinal fusion chisel
Cloward tissue retractor
club-shaped bacillus
clustered calcifications
Clutton bladder sound
Clutton urethral bougie
clysma
Clysodrast (bisacodyl tannex)
CMBC (cutaneous metastatic breast
   cancer)
C-mount
CMV (cytomegalovirus) enteritis
CMV inclusion
CMV prophylaxis
CMV-IGIV (cytomegalovirus immune
   globulin, intravenous)
CMV-positive donor
CNS (central nervous system) tumor
CNS depression
CNTF (ciliary neurotrophic factor)
CO (cardiac output)
CO$_2$ (carbon dioxide)
CO$_2$ embolus
CO$_2$ gas filter
CO$_2$ Guard gas filter for laparoscopy
CO$_2$ insufflation
CO$_2$ laser
CO$_2$ laser vaporization
CO$_2$ medium

coagulopathy, consumption
COAG waveform desiccation
Coakley antrum trocar and wash tube
coalesce
coalescence
coalition view
coal-miner's lung
coaptation bioplar forceps
coaptation plate
coapting suture
coarctation clamp
coarctation of the aorta
coarse nodularity
coarsely nodular cirrhosis
coated suture
coated Vicryl Rapide (polyglactin 910) suture
Cobactin E (*Lactobacillus acidophilus*)
Coballoy twist drill
Cobalt Knife
cobalt-60 gamma knife
Coban dressing
Cobb periosteal elevator
Cobb spinal elevator
Cobb spinal gouge
Cobbett knife
cobblestone appearance of mucosa
cobblestone mucosa
cobblestone pattern of hepatocytes
cobblestoning of colon
cobblestoning of mucosa
cobblestoning on endoscopic exam
cobblestoning sign
Cobelli gland
Cobe stapler
Coblation-Channeling operation
Coblation technology
cobra grasping forceps, double-action
cobra retractor
Cobra rat-tooth grasping forceps
cobra-head plate
CO/BSA (cardiac output/body surface area = cardiac index)
coccidial colitis

Coccidioides immitis
coccidioidomycosis
coccidiosis
cockscomb papilloma
cocktail, immunosuppressant
codeine
Codivilla bone graft
Codman-Harper laminectomy rongeur
Codman-Kerrison laminectomy rongeur
Codman-Leksell laminectomy rongeur
Codman-Schlesinger cervical laminectomy rongeur
Codman wire pass drill
Coe-pak paste adhesive
coffee bean sign of cecal volvulus
coffee-grounds emesis
coffee-grounds vomitus
Coffey ureterointestinal anastomosis
Cohen cannula
Cohen periosteal elevator
Cohen rongeur
Cohen syndrome
Coherent CO_2 surgical
Coherent UltraPulse 5000C laser
CO/HR (cardiac output/heart rate = stroke volume)
coil
   Gianturco wool-tufted wire
   Stylet internal esophageal MRI
coil gland
coil of intestine
coil of jejunum
coinfection with hepatitis B
coin lesion of lung
Colace (docusate sodium)
Colanis maneuver
Colapinto transjugular liver biopsy needle
Colaris test
Co-Lav (polyethylene glycol electrolyte solution; electrolytes)
Colax (phenolphthalein; docusate sodium)
Colazal (balsalazide disodium)

Colazide (balsalazide disodium)
Colclough-Scheicher laminectomy
  rongeur
cold abscess
cold agglutinin pneumonia
cold agglutinins
cold biopsy
cold chisel
cold compressive dressing
cold cone biopsy
cold cup biopsy
cold defect
cold erythema
cold-hemolytic antibody
cold laser
cold light source
cold nodule
cold spot
colectomy
  abdominal
  hand-assisted laparoscopic
  laparoscopic
  left
  partial
  prophylactic
  subtotal
  total abdominal (TAC)
  transverse
Coleman infiltration cannula
colesevelam HCl
Cole sign
Colestid (colestipol)
colestipol
Cole tube
coli (see *Escherichia coli*)
colibacillemia
colibacillosis, enteric
Colibri forceps
colic
  abdominal
  appendiceal
  appendicular
  bile duct
  biliary

colic *(cont.)*
  bilious
  common duct
  Devonshire
  episodic
  esophageal
  flatulent
  gallbladder
  gallstone
  gastric
  hepatic
  hysterical
  infantile
  intestinal
  kidney
  lead
  liver
  mucous
  nephritic
  Painter
  pancreatic
  psychogenic
  saturnine
  spasmodic
  vermicular
colic artery
colic flexure
colic impression on the liver
colicky abdominal pain
colicky pain
colic omentum
colic patch
colic plexus
colic sphincter
colic surface
colic vein
coliform bacillus (pl. bacilli)
coliform bacteria
colipase
colistimethate
colistin
colitis (see also *enterocolitis*)
  acute infectious
  acute self-limited (ASLC)

colitis *(cont.)*
   adaptive
   allergic
   amebic
   anthrax
   antibiotic-associated
   bacillary
   bacterial
   balantidial
   Campylobacter
   catarrhal
   chronic intermittent
   chronic ischemic
   chronic ulcerative (CUC)
   coccidial
   collagenous
   Crohn
   croupous
   dietetic
   enterocolitis
   exudative
   familial ulcerative
   focal
   fulminant
   fulminating ulcerative
   functional
   gangrenous
   giardial
   granulomatous
   granulomatous transmural
   hemorrhagic
   idiopathic
   infectious
   infective
   intractable ulcerative
   ischemic
   left-sided
   left-sided ulcerative
   lymphocytic
   membranous
   microscopic
   mucous
   nondysenteric
   noninfectious

colitis *(cont.)*
   phlegmonous
   progesterone-associated
   pseudomembranous (PMC)
   psychogenic
   radiation
   radiation-induced
   regional
   Salmonella
   Shigella
   single-stripe (SSC)
   staphylococcus
   thromboulcerative
   toxic
   transmural
   trichomonal
   tuberculous
   ulcerative (UC)
   universal
   universal ulcerative
   Yersinia enterocolitica
colitis cystica profunda (CCP)
colitis cystica superficialis (CCS)
collagen accumulation
collagen-alginate wound dressing
collagen arranged in swirls
collagen deposition
collagen hemostat
collagen hemostatic material
collagenolysis
collagenous colitis
collagenous sprue
collagen suture
collagen synthesis inhibitor
collagen vascular disease
CollagENT wand
Collagraft bone graft matrix
collapsible pin
collar-button abscess
collar-button appearance in colon
collar-button-like ulcer
Collastat hemostatic sponge
CollaTape
collateral circulation

colon bacillus
colon cancer
colon conduit
colon cutoff sign
Colon Injury Score (CIS)
colon interposition
colonic abscess
colonic adenoma
colonic air
colonic atony
colonic bacteria
colonic balloon volume
colonic crypt region
colonic distention
colonic diverticulitis
colonic diverticulum
colonic fistula
colonic flora
colonic hypersecretion
colonic inertia
colonic lavage
colonic loop
colonic mesenteric plexus
colonic motility
colonic myenteric plexus
colonic necrosis
colonic obstruction
colonic patch
colonic perforation
colonic pit
colonic polyp
colonic pseudo-obstruction (Ogilvie
   syndrome)
colonic solitary ulcer syndrome
colonic transit study
colonic transit test
colonic tube
colonic tuberculosis
colonic varices
colonic volvulus
colonization infection
Colonlite bowel prep
colon mass

colonoscope (see also *endoscope*)
   ACMI
   CF-HM
   CF-LB3R
   CF-MB-M
   Fujinon EVC-M video
   MIS Source
   Olympus CF
   Olympus CF-140I video
   Olympus CF-140L video
   Olympus CF-140S video
   Olympus CF-1T10L flexible
      therapeutic
   Olympus CF-1T20L flexible
      therapeutic
   Olympus CF-20L flexible
   Olympus CF-30L flexible
   Olympus CF-ITS2 fiberoptic
   Olympus CF-MB/LB
   Olympus CF-P
   Olympus CF-Q160AL/I innoflex
      video
   Olympus CF-UHM
   Olympus CF-VL
   Olympus DF-HM magnifying
   Olympus PCF pediatric
   Olympus PCF-10 flexible pediatric
   Olympus PCF-140I pediatric video
   Olympus PCF-140L pediatric video
   Olympus PCF-160AL/I video
   Olympus SIF-M
   Pentax EC-3430F video
   Pentax EC-3430L video
   Pentax EC-3440F video
   Pentax EC-3440L video
   Pentax EC-3830 video
   Pentax EC-3830L video
   Pentax EC-3830TL video
   Pentax EC-3840L video
   Pentax EC-3840T video
   Pentax FC-38LV fiberoptic
   Pentax FC-38MV fiberoptic
   variable-stiffness

colonoscopic polypectomy
colonoscopy
  complete
  incomplete
  real-time
  stomal
  virtual
colonoscopy per rectum
colonoscopy per stoma
colon polyp
colon resection clamp
colon syndrome
colon tumor
Colopath test
colopexy
Coloplast Flange Mini Caps
Coloplast Flange pouch
Coloplast Mini pouch
Coloplast ostomy irrigation set
Coloplast skin barrier
coloplasty pouch
coloplasty procedure
coloproctitis
coloproctostomy
color and caliber of stool
Colorado microdissection needle
Colorado tick fever virus
colorectal bleeding
colorectal cancer (CRC)
colorectal cancer screening
colorectal carcinoma
colorectal disease
colorectal malignancy
colorectal mucosa
colorectal polyp
colorectal segment
Colormate TLc BiliTest System
colorrhaphy
Col-R-Sponge sponge
ColoScreen occult blood test
ColoScreen Self Test
ColoScreen Slide Test
Coloshield
colosigmoid resection

colostomy (see also *appliance; bag; barrier; mesh; pouch*)
  blow hole decompressing
  da Silva
  decompression
  descending loop
  Devine
  diverting
  diverting proximal
  divided-stoma
  double-barrel (or barreled)
  dry
  end
  end-loop
  end-sigmoid
  exteriorization
  Hartmann
  ileoascending
  ileosigmoid
  ileotransverse
  Lazaro da Silva technique
  loop
  Mikulicz
  permanent
  permanent end
  resective
  sigmoid-end
  sigmoid-loop rod
  temporary end
  terminal
  transverse
  transverse-loop rod
  Turnbull
  wet
colostomy bag
colostomy bridge
colostomy closure
colostomy rod
Colovage (polyethylene glycol-electrolyte solution)
colovaginal fistula
COLO-Vax
colovesical fistula
colpohysteroscope

colpoperineopexy, abdominosacral
colpopexy
colporrhaphy, posterior
colposcope
colposcopic diagnosis
colposcopically directed punch biopsy
colposuspension needle
colposuspension suture
column, anal
columnar cell lined
columnar cuff cancer
columnar epithelium
columnar-lined esophagus
columnar metaplasia
column of Morgagni
Colver tonsil-seizing forceps
Coly-Mycin M
Coly-Mycin S
Coly-Seel ostomy barrier
Colyte (polyethylene glycol-electrolyte
    solution)
coma
    diabetic
    hepatic
    hyperosmolar
    hyperosmolar nonketotic
    insulin
    myxedema
    nondiabetic insulin
    nonketotic
    nonketotic hyperglycemic-
        hyperosmolar (NKHHC)
Comamonas terrigena
CombiDerm absorbent cover dressing
Combidex imaging agent
combination chemotherapy
combined androgen blockade (CAB)
combined anesthesia
combined Collis gastroplasty-
    fundoplication operation for
    scleroderma reflux esophagitis
combined defect
combined hemorrhoids
combined hernia

combined liver and intestinal
    transplantation
combined modality therapy
comblike redness sign
combretastatin
comedo carcinoma
Comeg rigid laparoscope
Comfeel Plus dressing
Comfeel Purilon dressing
Comfeel Ulcus occlusive dressing
Comfort Cath I or II catheter
Commando procedure (glossectomy)
commensally (without harm)
commode, bedside
common bile duct (CBD)
common bile duct exploration (CBDE)
common bile duct obstruction
common bile duct stone
common cavity phenomenon
common cold virus
common duct
common duct calculus
common duct cholangiogram
common duct colic
common duct dilator
common duct exploration
common duct obstruction
common duct scoop
common duct sound
common duct stone
common gall duct
common hepatic artery
common hepatic duct
common iliac artery
common iliac node
common variable hypogamma-
    globulinemia
communicable infectious disease
communicating pseudocyst
community-acquired bacteremia
community-acquired infection
community-acquired pneumonia
comorbidity
Compaction pliers

comparison film
compartment, preperitoneal
compartment syndrome
Compazine suppositories (prochlor-
  perazine)
compensated acidosis
compensated dysphagia (for solid foods)
Compere threaded pin
Comperm bandage
Comperm PD bandage
Comperm tubular elastic bandage
competency of repair
competent ileocecal valve
competent valve
Compleat-B liquid feeding
Compleat modified formula
complete adrenalectomy
complete bowel obstruction
complete hemostasis
complete hernia
complete mastectomy
complete obstruction
complete rupture
complete thymectomy
complete thyroidectomy
complete wrap (Nissen operation)
complex
  esophagogastric
  gastroduodenal artery
  Meyenburg
  nipple-areola
  von Meyenburg
complex anorectal fistula
complex appendicitis
complex IV deficiency
complex lesion
complex regional pain syndrome
  (CRPS)
compliance
complicated residual hepatolithiasis
  with biliary stricture
complication
  concomitant obesity
  postsplenectomy
complication *(cont.)*
  surgery
  trocar wound site
Comply
composite graft
composite procedure
composition, body
Composix mesh
compound cyst
compound gland
compound volvulus
comprehensive health enhancement
    support system (CHESS)
compressed carbon dioxide gas
compressed malignant cells
compression
  extrinsic
  mechanical variceal
  vena cava
compression anesthesia
compression bandage
compression hook
compression of the hepatoduodenal
    ligament
compression plate
compression rod
compression stay suture
compression tape
compression wrap dressing
compressive dressing
compressive symptoms
Comprilan bandage
comprimeter
Compro (prochlorperazine)
compromise of blood supply
compromised bowel wall
compromised breathing
compromised cardiac function
Compton clavicle pin
computed tomography (CT) scan
computed tomography laser mammog-
    raphy (CTLM)
computer-assisted microsurgery
computerized axial tomography (CAT)

computerized lithotriptor
computerized peristaltic pump
computerized phonoenterography
Computerized Thermal Imaging system
computerized treatment planning
Comvax (*Haemophilus* purified
    capsular polysaccharide; *Neisseria*
    meningitidis OMPC; hepatitis B
    virus vaccine)
concave abdomen
concave obturator
concave sheath
concave wound
concealed hemorrhage
concealed vomiting
concentration, extracellular
concentration of lipopolysaccharide-
    binding protein
concentric hiatal hernia
concentric layers of epithelial cells
concentric lesion
concentric needle electrode
concentrically laminated mass
Concept 8160 IntraVision Lumi-Trac
    endoscopic camera
Concept ablator
Concept endoscope
Concept handheld cautery
Concept/Linvatec laparoscope
Concept rigid laparoscope
Conceptus Soft Seal cervical catheter
Conceptus Soft Torque uterine catheter
Conceptus VS (variable softness)
    catheter
Conco elastic bandage
Conco gauze bandage
concomitant acute alcoholic hepatitis
concomitant bleeding
concomitant complications of obesity
concomitant health problems
concomitant injury
concomitant spinal cord injury
Concorde cannula
Concord Portex epidural catheter

concretion
    appendiceal
    bile
    calculus
    fecal
    gallbladder
    intestinal
    preputial
    prostatic
    salivary
    tophic
concurrent chemotherapy and radiation
    therapy
conditioning
    interceptive
    semantic
condition, pathological hypersecretory
conduction anesthesia
conductive keratoplasty (CK)
conduit
    aortic
    arterial
    artificial
    autologous
    biliary
    Bricker
    bypass
    circumferential
    colon
    colonic
    continent
    flow
    free jejunal
    homograft
    jejunal
    ileal
    intestinal
    Kock
    mucosa-lined
    obstructed
    peristaltic
    prosthetic
    radial
    sigmoid

conduit *(cont.)*
  silicone
  substitute
  surgical
  synthetic
  thoracic
  transdermal
  T-shaped
  ureteroileal
  urinary
  valve
condylar plate
condylocephalic nail
condyloma (pl. condylomata)
  anal
  flat
  genital
  penile
  perianal
  vaginal
  venereal
condyloma acuminatum
condyloma latum
cone biopsy
cone biopsy cannula
cone biopsy needle
coned-down appearance of colon
coned-down view
cone laminectomy retractor
cone-nose forceps
cone retractor
cone scalp retractor
cone skull punch
cone skull punch forceps
cone suction tube
cone ventricular needle
cone view
cone wire-twisting forceps
confined to mucosa
confined to muscularis
confined to serosa
confirmatory needle biopsy
confluent
Conform dressing

Conforma 3000 photon beam therapy
  system
Conformant contact-layer wound
  dressing
ConforMAX MMLC (mini-multileaf
  collimator)
confusion, mental
congenital adrenal hyperplasia
congenital anomaly
congenital atresia
congenital biliary atresia
congenital cardiac malformation
congenital cavernous malformation
  of the splenic vein
congenital choledochal cyst
congenital choledochal dilatation
congenital cirrhosis
congenital cystic liver disease
congenital dilatation of intrahepatic bile
  duct
congenital disorder of coagulation
congenital diverticulum
congenital erythropoietic porphyria
congenital esophageal stenosis
congenital familial nonhemolytic
  jaundice
congenital goiter
congenital hemangioma
congenital hemolytic anemia
congenital hemolytic jaundice
congenital hepatic fibrosis (CHF)
congenital hernia
congenital hourglass stomach
congenital hypertrophic pyloric stenosis
congenital hypothyroidism
congenital lactose malabsorption
congenital lesion
congenital lipomatosis of pancreas
congenital malaria
congenital malrotation of the gut
congenital megacolon
congenital pulmonary arteriovenous
  fistula
congenital pyloric stenosis

congenital sacral agenesis
congenital splenomegaly
congenital sucrose intolerance
congenital sucrose-isomaltose
   deficiency (CSID)
congenital sucrose-isomaltose
   malabsorption
congenital thyroid deficiency
congenital virilizing adrenal hyperplasia
congenital zinc deficiency
congested kidney
congestive cirrhosis
congestive heart failure (CHF)
congestive hepatomegaly
congestive liver cirrhosis
congestive splenomegaly
Congo red dye
Congreve cannula
congruous cup-shaped reamer
conical cecum
conical mass
conical papilla
conical reamer
conical tectal plate
conical trocar
conization knife
conjoined tendon (also conjoint)
conjoining of the aponeurosis
   to the internal oblique
conjoint tendon (also conjoined)
conjugate forward gaze position
conjugated bile acid
conjugated bilirubin
conjugated hyperbilirubinemia
conjugated linoleic acid (CLA)
conjunctival icterus
Conley pin
Conmed Corporation
Conn syndrome
connecting plate
Conn pneumatic tourniquet
connective tissue disease (overlap
   syndrome)

connector
   banana plug
   Olympus
   tubing
Connell suture
Conray contrast medium
conscious sedation
Conseal ostomy irrigation set
consented
conservative measures
conservative therapy
conservative treatment with close
   observation
considerable fibrosis
consistency of stool
consolidated graft
constantly perfused side-hole catheter
Constellation mapping catheter
Constilac (lactulose)
constipated
constipation
   antepartum
   atonic
   chronic
   drug-induced
   functional
   gastrojejunal
   geriatric
   intermittent
   lifelong
   new-onset
   normal transit (NTC)
   outlet
   postpartum
   proctogenous
   refractory
   spastic
constipation and diarrhea, alternating
constipation due to ganglioneuromatosis
constipation-predominant irritable
   bowel syndrome
constricting pain
constriction, appendiceal
constrictive lesion

Constulose (lactulose)
consumption
    alcoholic
    dietary
    ethanol (EtOH)
consumption coagulopathy
ConTack suture anchor
contact cancer
contact laser hemorrhoidectomy
contact-layer wound dressing
contagious infectious disease
contaminated wound
contamination
    fecal
    peritoneal
ConTE-Pak-4 (multiple trace elements)
contents
    abdominal
    bowel
    digestive tract
    enteric
    gastric
    intestinal
    intraluminal
    refluxed gastric
contents of axilla
contiguous loop
contiguous spread
contiguous structures
continence, fecal
continent ileal pouch
continent ileal reservoir
continent ileostomy
continent of stool
continent supravesical bowel urinary
    diversion
continued blood per NG tube
continued clinical exploration
continuous ambulatory peritoneal
    dialysis (CAPD)
continuous analgesia delivery (CAD)
continuous compression
continuous drainage
continuous drip feeding

continuous electrocardiogram
    monitoring
continuous epidural anesthesia
continuous-flow catheter anesthesia
continuously perfused probe
continuous NG suction
continuous pull-through technique
continuous running suture
continuous spinal anesthesia
continuous suture
continuous thoracic epidural analgesia
Continuum total knee base plate
contour, breast
contoured tilting compression
    mammography
contoured T-plate
Contour Profile breast implant
Contour scalp retractor
contracted kidney
contractile capacity of esophageal body
contractile stricture
contractility
contraction (pl. contractions)
    esophageal
    gallbladder
    hypotensive esophageal
    intestinal muscle
    longitudinal muscle
    peristaltic
    phasic
    primary
    secondary
    tertiary
    tonic
contraction alkalosis
contraction band necrosis
contraction of gallbladder, decreased
contraction-relaxation cycles
contractive ring dysphagia
contractor
    Bailey rib
    Bailey-Gibbon rib
    Lemmon rib
    rib
    Sellors rib

Converse periosteal elevator
Converse-TC needle holder
conversion of T_4 to T_3
conversion to ileostomy
conversion to laparotomy
Converspaz
convert from laparoscopic to open
 procedure
convertible slipknot suture
Convertor drape
Convertor setup
Converzyame
convex border of
convex rasp
ConXn (recombinant human relaxin,
 H_2)
Cook aspiration biopsy needle
cookie (pad)
 arch
 Gelfoam
 navicular shoe
 scaphoid shoe
cookie cutter
Cook introducer
Cook Oasis biliary stent
Cook rectal speculum
Cook TPN catheter
Cook-Wilson gastric balloon
Cooley anastomosis clamp
Cooley aortic clamp
Cooley atrial retractor
Cooley-Baumgarten aortic forceps
Cooley-Baumgarten wire twisters
Cooley-Beck clamp
Cooley bulldog clamp
Cooley coarctation clamp
Cooley cross-action bulldog clamp
Cooley-Derra anastomosis clamp
Cooley graft suction tube
Cooley iliac clamp
Cooley intracardiac suction tube
Cooley partial occlusion clamp
Cooley patent ductus clamp
Cooley pediatric clamp

Cooley renal clamp
Cooley rib retractor
Cooley rib shears
Cooley-Satinsky clamp
Cooley vascular clamp
Cooley vascular forceps
Cooley vena cava catheter clamp
Cool Tip catheter
Coombs test, direct
Cooper Cavitron surgical aspirator
Cooper hernia
Cooper ligament
Cooper ligament repair
Cooper Surgical cystoscope
Cooper Surgical Marro Nu-Tip
Cooper Surgical trocar
COPA cuffed oropharyngeal airway
Cope (aspirin; caffeine; magnesium
 hydroxide; aluminum hydroxide)
Cope biopsy needle
Cope crushing clamp
Cope modification of Martel intestinal
 clamp
Cope needle
Cope suture anchor
copious amounts of saline
copious irrigation
copious peritoneal lavage
copious rice-water diarrhea
copious watery diarrhea
copper-binding protein (CBP) test
copper blade
copper mallet
copper-vapor pulsed laser
Corbett bone rongeur
cord
 hepatic
 spermatic
Cordis-Hakim shunt
Cordis Predator PTCA balloon catheter
Cordis Trakstar PTCA balloon catheter
cord lipoma
Cordonnier ureteroileal loop
cordotomy (chordotomy) knife

cordotomy hook
Cordox
cord structure
core biopsy
core needle biopsy
core of tumor
core probe
Core aspiration/injection needle
Core audible trocar
Core cannula system
Core CO$_2$ insufflation needle
Core Entree Plus laparoscopic trocar and cannula system
Core Entree II laparoscopic trocar system
Core laparoscopic aspiration/injection needle
Core laparoscopic dilator
Core laparoscopic Kittner dissector
Core laparoscopic smoke eliminator
Core reposable trumpet
Core shielded laparoscopic trocar
Core suction/irrigation probe
Core trocar
Corey forceps
Cori disease
corkscrew appearance
corkscrew dural hook
corkscrew esophagus
corkscrew femoral head extractor
corkscrew-shaped bacteria
corkscrew suture anchor
corneal shield sponge
corneal ulcer
CorneaSparing LTK system laser
Cornelia de Lange syndrome
corner, antemesenteric
corner mouth lift
cornflake esophageal motility test
corona mortis
coronal incision
coronal scalp incision
coronal suture
coronary arteriole vasodilation

coronary artery lesion
coronary artery of stomach
coronary artery scissors
coronary artery vasoconstriction
coronary ligament
coronary stent
coronary vein
coronavirus gastroenteritis
Corpak feeding tube
corpus carcinoma
correction of electrolytes
corrective soft dressing
Correctol (bisacodyl)
Correctol Extra Gentle (docusate sodium)
corrosive esophagitis
corrosive gastritis
corrugated reamer
corrugated tubing
corset effect
Corson needle electrode
CorTek laparoscope
CorTek semirigid microlaparoscope
Cortenema (hydrocortisone)
Cortenema retention enema
cortex drill
Corticaine
cortical bone graft
cortical drill
cortical plate
cortical strut graft
corticoadrenal insufficiency
corticocancellous bone graft
corticocancellous chip graft
corticorelin ovine triflutate
corticosteroid
corticosteroid-based immuno-suppression
corticosteroid-binding globulin (CBG)
corticotropin-releasing factor (CRF)
Cortifoam (hydrocortisone acetate)
cortisol analog
cortisol-binding globulin
cortisol-producing carcinoma

cortisol-secreting tumor
cortisol secretion
Coryllos-Doyen periosteal elevator
Coryllos rasp
Coryllos retractor
Coryllos rib shears
Corynebacterium genitalium
CoSeal resorbable synthetic vascular
  sealant
CoSeal surgical sealant
Cosgrove Flex clamp
Cosman coagulator
cosmetic conventional cutting suture
cosmetic reverse cutting suture
costal margin
costal rasp
CoStasis enterocolic hemostatic sealant
CoStasis surgical hemostat
costocolic fold
CoStop surgical adhesion barrier
costopleural reflection
costovertebral angle (CVA) tenderness
costovertebral angle tenderness (CVAT)
cot death
Cotara
Cotazym-S (lipase; protease; amylase)
Cotrel-Dubousset hook
Cottle chisel
Cottle-Kazanjiann rongeur
Cottle-MacKenty elevator
Cottle-MacKenty rasp
Cottle mallet
Cottle retractor
Cottle saw
Cottle style
Cottle suction tube
cotton, absorbable cellulose
cotton applicator
cotton carrier
cotton dressing
cotton elastic bandage
cotton suture
Cotton cartilage graft
coudé catheter

Couinaud liver disease grading
  classification
Coumadin (warfarin sodium)
coumarin green tunable dye laser
  lithotripsy
coumarin pulsed-dye laser
Councilman body (in viral hepatitis)
Councilman lesion
Count EZ sponge counter bag
counterirritant
counter rotating saw
count, sponge and needle
coupled suture
Cournand arteriogram needle
Cournand-Grino arteriogram needle
Cournand needle
Courvoisier gallbladder
Courvoisier gastroenterostomy
Courvoisier law
Courvoisier sign
Courvoisier-Terrier syndrome
couvade syndrome
Covaderm composite wound dressing
Covaderm Plus adhesive barrier
  dressing
Coventry staple
Coverlet adhesive surgical dressing
Cover-Roll adhesive gauze dressing
CoverTip safety syringe
Cowden disease
cow kidney
COX (cytochrome C oxidase) deficiency
  French-Canadian type
  infantile mitochondrial myopathy
  Leigh disease
  subacute necrotizing encephalo-
    myopathy
COX-1-sparing agent
COX-2 (cyclo-oxygenase-2) inhibitor
Cox-Uphoff International tissue
  expander (CUI)
Coxiella burnetii
coxsackievirus
CPAP (continuous positive airway
  pressure)

CPAP valve
CPAS-free (caffeine, alcohol, pepper, spicy foods) diet
CPC connector
C-peptide (protein)
CPH (chronic persistent hepatitis)
CPK (creatine phosphokinase)
C-plasty
Cr (chromium)
Crabtree dissector
cracked nipple
Crafoord aortic clamp
Crafoord coarctation clamp
Crafoord forceps
Crafoord thoracic scissors
Cragg endoluminal
Cragg Endopro System I stent
Cragg-McNamara valved infusion catheter
Craig biopsy needle
Craig scissors
Craig vertebral body biopsy instrument set
cramping
crampy abdominal pain
Crane mallet
cranial angled view
cranial bone fixation plate
cranial bone graft
cranial drill
cranial rongeur
cranial rongeur forceps
cranial suture
craniocaudad view
craniocaudal view
craniocerebral penetrating wound
craniopharyngioma
craniotome blade
craniotomy saw
craterlike (with jagged edges) ulcer
crater, ulcer
cravat bandage
Crawford aortic retractor
Crawford dural elevator

Crawford needle
CRC (colorectal cancer)
CRD canister
crease
   inframammary
   midline abdominal
   palmar
   skin
   torso
   wound
crease wound
creatinine
creatinine clearance
creatorrhea
Credé maneuver
creeping of mesenteric fat
Crego elevator
Crego-McCarroll pin
Crego retractor
cremasteric fascia
cremasteric fascial fibers
cremasteric fiber
cremasteric reflex
cremasteric sheath
cremasteric vessel
Creon
crepe bandage
crepitus
crescendoing bowel sounds
crescent knife
crescent of the cardia
crescentic blade
CREST syndrome
Crestor (rosuvastatin)
cretinism
   athyrotic
   endemic
   goitrous
CRF (corticotropin-releasing factor)
CRH (corticotropin-releasing hormone)
crib death
cribriform fascia
cribriform carcinoma
cribriform pattern

cribriform plate
Cricket stapler
cricoid cartilage
cricoid myotomy
cricopharyngeal achalasia
cricopharyngeal bar
cricopharyngeal dilation
cricopharyngeal diverticulum
cricopharyngeal myotomy
cricopharyngeal sphincter
cricopharyngeus muscle
cricopharyngeus myotomy
cricothyroid membrane
cricothyroid muscle
cricothyroidotomy
Crigler-Najjar syndrome
Crile appendix clamp
Crile artery forceps
Crile bile duct forceps
Crile clamp
Crile forceps, curved
Crile gasserian ganglion knife
Crile hemostat
Crile hemostatic forceps
Crile hook and dissector
Crile nerve hook
Crile-Rankin forceps
Crile retractor
Crile stone hook
Crile thyroid retractor
Crile-type clamp
Crile-Wood needle
Crile-Wood needle holder with
   tungsten carbide inlay
crisis
   addisonian
   celiac
   thyroid
   thyrotoxic
crisscross suture
criteria (see *classification*)
critical lesion
Criticare HN (high nitrogen) elemental
   liquid feeding

Cro-Man-Zin (chromium; manganese;
   zinc)
Crohn's and Colitis Foundation
   of America, Inc. (CCFA)
Crohn colitis
Crohn disease (CD)
Crohn disease (regional ileitis)
Crohn disease activity index (CDAI)
Crohn ileitis
Crohn ileocolitis
Crohn regional enteritis
Cronkhite-Canada disease
Cronkhite-Canada syndrome
Crosby-Kugler capsule for biopsy
crossbar
   inner
   outer
crossbridge cycle
cross-circulation
cross-clamp
cross-clamping
crosscut saw
crossed anesthesia
crossed embolism
crossed reflex
crossed-swords technique suture
CrossFlex LC coronary stent
CrossFlexTMLC coronary stent
cross-infection
crossing over (also, crossover)
cross-irrigation of wound
cross-linking
cross-lip pedicle flap
crossmatch
   HLA (human lymphocyte antigen)
   major
   minor
   pretransplant
   type and
crossmatching
crossover (also, crossing over)
cross pin
cross-reacting agglutinin
cross-reacting antibody

cross-reacting material (CRM)
cross-reactivation
cross-reactivity
cross-reference
cross-resistance
CrossSail coronary dilatation catheter
cross-section (noun, verb)
cross-sectional (adj.)
cross-sectional imaging technique
cross-sensitization
cross-table lateral film
cross-table view
"cross-the-heart" augmentation
    mammoplasty
cross-tunneling incision
Crotti-Kocher thyroid retractor
Crotti thyroid retractor
croup-associated virus (CA v.)
croupous colitis
Crowe-Davis mouth gag
Crowe pilot point on Steinmann pin
crown and collar scissors
crowns the liver
CRP (C reactive protein)
CRPS (complex regional pain
    syndrome)
CRS (Cell Recovery System)
Cr,TM,Ho:YAG crystal laser
cruciate four-strand suture
cruciate incision
crural closure
crural repair
crural ring
crura of the external oblique
crus (pl. crura) of diaphragm
crush kidney
crutch-and-belt femoral closed nail
crutched stick-type biliary duct stent
Crutchfield carotid artery clamp
Crutchfield hand drill
Cruveilhier-Baumgarten bruit
Cruveilhier-Baumgarten cirrhosis
Cruveilhier-Baumgarten syndrome
Cruveilhier sign

Cruveilhier ulcer
cryoablation, NeoCure
CRYOcare system
Cryo/Cuff ankle dressing
cryoglobulinemia, essential mixed
CRYOguide
CryoHit
cryoprecipitate
cryosurgery
cryosurgical lesion
cryotherapy
    endoscopic
    flexible gastrointestinal
cryotherapy for hemorrhoids
crypectomy
crypt
    anal
    enamel
    epithelium
    ileal
    Lieberkühn (Lieberkuehn)
    Morgagni
    tonsillar
crypt abscess
crypt and surface epithelium (from
    colonic biopsy specimens)
crypt atrophy
crypt epithelium
crypt hook
crypt hyperplasia
cryptitis
cryptogenic cirrhosis
cryptogenic infection
cryptogenic septicopyemia
cryptosporidiosis
Cryptosporidium parvum
Cryptosporidium parvum bovine
    colostrum IgG concentrate
crystal, cholesterol monohydrate
crystal tracheostomy tube
crystallized trypsin
crystalloid fluid
crystalloid infusion

crystalloid solution
CSF (cerebrospinal fluid)
CSF glucose
CSF glutamine test
CSF protein
CSF shunt
C-shaped incision
C-shaped microplate
C-shaped plate
CSID (congenital sucrose-isomaltose deficiency)
CSM Stretta system
C-spine traction
CT (computed or computerized tomography)
CT cholangiography
CT-directed hook-wire localization
CT-directed needle biopsy
CTE:YAG (CrTmEr:YAG) laser
CT-guided needle aspiration biopsy
CTLA4-Ig monoclonal antibody
CTLM (CT laser mammography)
CTLV (cross-table lateral view)
CTP-37 theraccine
CT PEG (CT-guided percutaneous endoscopic gastrostomy)
CT-scan-directed needle biopsy
CT scan, dual-energy
CT scan with I.V. contrast
CTS (Champion Trauma Score)
CTS Harvester bipolar scissors
CT-2584 mesylate
Cubbins incision
CUC (chronic ulcerative colitis)
Cuda endoscope
Cuda laparoscope
Cuda retractor
Cuda 0° 10 mm rigid laparoscope
cuff
   gastric
   musculotendinous
   one-tube
   rectal muscle
   rotator

cuff *(cont.)*
   suprahepatic caval
   vaginal
cuff abscess
cuffed endotracheal tube
cuffed fenestrated tube
cuff measurement
CUI (Cox-Uphoff International)
CUI gel breast prosthesis
CUI saline breast prosthesis
CUI tissue expander
Culbertson canal knife
cul-de-sac of Douglas
cul-de-sac smear
culdolaparoscopy
culdoscope
Cullen sign
Culler hook
culprit lesion
culture and sensitivity (C&S)
culture, blood
cultured epithelial autograft
cultured organism
Cunningham clamp
cup
   acetabular
   graduated metal
   Malmstrom
   stone
cup-and-spill stomach
cup forceps
cupped jaw
cup reamer
Curaderm hydrocolloid dressing material
Curafil hydrogel dressing
Curafoam foam wound dressing
Curagel hydrogel dressing
Curasol gel wound dressing
Curasorb calcium alginate dressing
curative operation
curative restorative resection
curative therapy
Curdy blade

¹⁴C urea (PYtest)
curettage
  blunt
  sharp
curette
  banjo
  Barnhill adenoid
  biopsy suction
  Bone
  Bruns
  Bumm placenta
  Derlacki
  dermal
  double-ended
  Fox
  Fukushima-Giannotta
  Guilford-Wright micro bone
  Heaney biopsy
  Hibbs-Spratt
  House-Paparella stapes
  House stapes
  Jansen
  Kevorkian-Townsend biopsy
  Kevorkian-Younge
  large sharp
  Lempert fine
  Milan
  Novak suction
  Paparella angled ring
  Paparella mastoid
  Randall suction
  Recamier
  Rheinstadter
  Semm biopsy suction
  serrated
  Sims
  Spratt
  Volkmann
  Williger
  Yankauer
Curity disposable sponge
Curity economy shave prep tray
Curity Oil emulsion dressing
Curity saline dressing

Curity sterile gauze pads
Curlin 2000 Plus infusion pump
Curling duodenal ulcer
Curling esophagus
Curling gastric ulcer
currant jelly clot
currant jelly stools
current
  coagulating
  cutting
Curry hip nail
Curtin incision
curvature of stomach
  greater
  lesser
curve
  duodenum
  Frank-Starling
  sigmoid
curved awl
curved bone rongeur
curved circular stapler
curved clamp
curved Cooley clamp
curved Crile forceps
curved dissecting scissors
curved double-action Metzenbaum
  scissors
curved end-to-end (CEEA) stapler
curved excavator
curved forceps, Crile
curved gouge
curved incision
curved Kelly forceps
curved Maryland dissector
curved Mayo clamp
curved Mayo scissors
curved micro-grasper
curved mosquito forceps
curved periosteal elevator
curved retractor
curved scissors
curved-tip Metzenbaum
curve of duodenum

curvilinear incision
CUSA (Cavitron ultrasonic surgical
    aspirator) dissector
CUSA EXcel surgical aspirator
Cusco Swiss pattern vaginal speculum
Cushing angular hook
Cushing bayonet forceps
Cushing bipolar forceps
Cushing brain retractor
Cushing-Brown forceps
Cushing-Cairns forceps
Cushing cranial rongeur
Cushing decompression retractor
Cushing delicate forceps
Cushing disease
Cushing dressing forceps
Cushing dural hook
Cushing dural hook knife
Cushing flat drill
Cushing forceps
Cushing gasserian ganglion hook
Cushing-Gigli saw guide
Cushing-Hopkins periosteal elevator
Cushing hook
Cushing intervertebral disk rongeur
Cushing Little Joker elevator
Cushing monopolar forceps
Cushing nerve hook
Cushing nerve retractor
cushingoid facies
cushingoid state
Cushing perforator drill
Cushing periosteal elevator
Cushing pituitary elevator
Cushing pituitary rongeur
Cushing reflex
Cushing retractor
Cushing rongeur
Cushing rongeur forceps
Cushing saw
Cushing saw guide
Cushing staphylorrhaphy elevator
Cushing suture
Cushing syndrome

Cushing tissue forceps
Cushing ulcer
Cushing vein retractor
Cushing ventricular needle
custocolic fold
custom breast implant
Cutalon nylon polyamide surgical
    suture
cutaneous enterostomy
cutaneous graft
cutaneous hyperesthesia
cutaneous metastatic breast cancer
    (CMBC)
cutaneous papilloma
cutaneous punch
cutaneous stoma
cutaneous tumor
cutaneous ulcer
cutaneous wound
cut-back procedure
cut, clamp, and tie
cutdown catheter
cuticle scissors
Cutinova Cavity wound filling material
Cutinova Hydro dressing
cutter (also see *dissector*)
    Circon continuous flow resectoscope
    ClearCut 2 electrosurgical handpiece
    Endopath ETS-FLEX endoscopic
      articulating linear
    Endopath linear
    Endo Mini Shears
    Endo Shears
    Evershears
    EZ45 thoracic linear
    finger ring
    Lempert malleus
    Modulap
    Neoknife
    Proximate linear
    Quadripolar
    Questus Leading Edge
    Ruskin-Liston bone
    Stille-Liston bone

cutting biopsy needle
cutting Bovie
cutting current
cutting forceps
cutting jig
Cutting Balloon microsurgical dilatation
    catheter
Cutting LOOP coagulator
cutting needle
CUT waveform desiccation
CVA (costovertebral angle) tenderness
CVAT (costovertebral angle tenderness)
CVC (central venous catheter)
CV caliper
CV forceps
CVI (common variable immuno-
    deficiency)
CVP (central venous pressure) line
CVP right atrium
CXR (chest x-ray)
CY-1899
Cyanamid clip applier
cyanoacrylate tissue adhesive
cyanoacrylate glue
cyanocobalamin radioactive agent
cyanosis
cyanotic kidney
cyclic changes of hyperplasia and
    colloid formation
cyclic pain
cyclic tenderness
cyclic vomiting
cyclic vomiting syndrome (abdominal
    migraine)
cyclizine
cyclooxygenase
cyclophilin
cyclophosphamide rescue
cycloserine (L-cycloserine)
cyclosporin A
cyclosporine steroid therapy
CycloTech cyclosporine delivery system
cylindrical carcinoma
cylindrical sponge

cymba conchal cartilage
Cymed colostomy barrier
Cymed Micro Skin one-piece drainage
    pouch
Cymetra tissue replacement material
CyPat
cyproheptadine
cyst
    air
    amebic, amoebic
    Baker
    benign liver
    benign subcutaneous
    blue dome breast
    branchial cleft
    branchiogenous
    breast
    chocolate
    choledochal
    choledochus
    chyle
    compound
    congenital choledochal
    corpus luteum
    daughter
    duplication
    echinococcal
    echinococcus liver
    enteric
    enterogenous
    epidermal inclusion
    epidermoid
    follicular
    ganglion
    gastric duplication
    granddaughter
    hepatic parasitic
    hydatic liver
    hydatid
    intraluminal
    mesenteric
    milk-filled
    mother
    multilocular

cyst *(cont.)*
    mytoid
    nabothian
    omental
    pancreatic
    parasitic
    pilonidal
    primordial
    Rathke pouch
    retention
    Sampson
    sebaceous
    splenic
    theca-lutein
    thymic
    thyroglossal
    thyroglossal duct
    Tornwaldt
    unilocular
    vitellointestinal
    wolffian
cystadenocarcinoma
    bile duct
    mucinous
    papillary
    pseudomucinous
    serous
cystadenoma
    ductal
    hyperplastic mucinous
    thyroid
cyst aspiration
cyst aspiration needle
cystectomy
cystica polyposa gastritis
cystic artery
cystic cancer
cystic carcinoma
cystic changes
cystic-choledochal junction
cystic degeneration
cystic duct cannula
cystic duct catheterization

cystic duct cholangiogram
cystic duct forceps
cystic duct leak
cystic duct lumen
cystic duct obstruction
cystic duct rupture
cystic duct stone
cysticercosis
cysticercus disease
Cysticercus dellulosae
cystic fibrosis
cystic fistula
cystic fluid
cystic goiter
cystic kidney
cystic lesion
cystic mass
cystic mastitis
cystic medial necrosis
cystic plexus
cystic polyp
cystic structure
cystine stone
cystitis
    acute
    allergic
    bacterial
    honeymoon
    interstitial
    radiation
cystoatrial shunt
cystoduodenostomy
cystogastrostomy, endoscopic
cystohepatic triangle
cystojejunostomy
cystopericystectomy
cystoperitoneal shunt
cystosarcoma phyllodes
cystoscope (see *endoscope*)
Cytadren (aminoglutethimide)
cytarabine liposomal
Cytobrush Plus
cytochrome C oxidase (COX)
    deficiency

CytoGam (cytomegalovirus immune
  globulin, solvent/detergent treated)
CytoImplant
cytokine induction
cytokine interleukin-10 (IL-10)
cytokine interleukin-8 (IL-8)
Cytolex (pexiganan acetate) (now
  Locilex)
Cytolex cream (pexiganan acetate)
cytologic diagnosis
cytologic examination
cytologic smear
cytology
  abnormal
  aspiration biopsy (ABC)
  brush
  equivocal pancreatic
  EUS-guided
  fine-needle aspiration (FNAC)
  gastric
  guided-needle aspiration
  peritoneal
  salvage
CytoLyt solution
cytomegalic inclusion virus disease
cytomegalovirus (CMV)

cytomegalovirus hepatitis
cytomegalovirus immune globulin,
  human
cytomegalovirus mucositis
Cytomel (liothyronine sodium)
cytopathologic examination
cytopathologic preparation
cytopathologist
cytoplasmic granules
cytoplasmic material
cytoprotective agent
cytoreductive surgery
CytoTAb antibody
Cytotec (misoprostol)
cytotoxic antibodies
cytotoxic lymphocyte
cytotoxic lymphocytic proliferation
cytotoxic T cell
Cytovene (oral ganciclovir)
Cytoxan (cyclophosphamide)
Czaja-McCaffrey endoscope
Czaja-McCaffrey rigid stent introducer
Czerny-Lembert suture
Czerny rectal speculum
Czerny retractor
Czerny suture

D, d

dacarbazine
dacliximab monoclonal antibody
Dacron-bolstered suture
Dacron-impregnated silicone rod
Dacron interposition graft
Dacron mesh
Dacron patch
Dacron suture
Dacron synthetic ligament material
Dacron tape
Dacron velour bolster
Dagradi classification of esophageal
  varices
Dagrofil suture
Dahedi 25 insulin delivery pump
Dahl-Iverson mastitis
Dahlgren cranial rongeur
daily weights
DairyCare
Dairy Ease (lactase enzyme)
Dakin solution
Dale abdominal binder
Dale first rib rongeur
Dale Foley catheter
Dale forceps
DALM (dysplasia with associated
  lesion or mass)
dalteparin sodium

dam, rubber
damage, macroscopic
danaparoid sodium
danazol
Danbolt-Closs syndrome
Dance sign
Dandy clamp
Dandy forceps
Dandy nerve hook
Dandy neurosurgical scissors
Dandy probe
Dandy hemostatic forceps
Dandy scalp hemostats
Dandy scissors
Dandy trigeminal nerve scissors
Dandy ventricular needle
Dane particle
Daniel colostomy clamp
Daniel iliac bone graft
Dansac DuoSoft pouch
Dansac DuoSoft wafer
Dansac Karaya Seal one-piece drainage
  pouch
Dansac Nova ostomy appliance
Dansac ostomy irrigation set
Dansac Skin Barrier for ostomy
Dansac Standard Ileo pouch
danthron

daptomycin for injection
Darbid
Dardik Biograft
Dardik clamp
Daricon PB
darifenacin
darkfield microscope
darkfield microscopy
dark green stools
dark stools
dark urine
Darrach elevator
dartos fascia
Darvocet-N 100
da Silva colostomy
Datascope catheter
daughter abscess
daughter cyst
Dautrey chisel
Daverbinde K
David Baker bleph retractor
Davidoff cell
David rectal speculum
Davidson pulmonary vessel clamp
Davidson retractor
Davidson-Sauerbruch-Doyen periosteal
   elevator
Davidson scapula retractor
Davidson thoracic trocar
da Vinci surgical laparoscopic system
Davis blade
Davis brain retractor
Davis clamp
Davis coagulating forceps
Davis forceps
Davis guide for Gigli saw
Davis monopolar forceps
Davis mouth gag
Davis muscle-pedicle graft
Davis percussion hammer
Davis pin
Davis retractor
Davis ribbon retractor
Davis saw

Davis saw guide
Davis scalp retractor
Davis spatula
Davol prep
Davol sump drain
dawn phenomenon
Dawson-Yuhl gouge
Dawson-Yuhl-Kerrison rongeur forceps
Dawson-Yuhl-Key elevator
Dawson-Yuhl-Leksell rongeur forceps
Dawson-Yuhl periosteal elevator
Dawson-Yuhl suction tube
Daxor quantitative injection syringe kit
Day pin
Day staple
dazopride, dazopride fumarate
DBx diagnostic system
DC softgels (docusate calcium)
DCBE (double-contrast barium enema)
DCC (deleted in colorectal carcinoma)
   gene
DCIS (ductal carcinoma in situ)
DCP (dynamic compression) plate
DDAVP (desmopressin acetate)
DDS-Acidophilus
dead bowel
deadly agaric (*Amanita phallodes*)
dead pancreatic tissue
dead space
Dean bone rongeur
Dean dissecting scissors
death
   apparent
   black
   brain
   cell
   cerebral
   cot
   crib
   fetal (early, intermediate, late)
   functional
   genetic
   liver
   local

death *(cont.)*
  molecular
  natural
  programmed cell
  SIDS (sudden infant death syndrome)
  somatic
  sudden cardiac
  unsuspected cause of
  voodoo
Deaver incision
Deaver retractor
Deaver scissors
DeBakey-Adson tissue forceps
DeBakey aortic aneurysm clamp
DeBakey arterial clamp
DeBakey arterial forceps
DeBakey AtrauGrip forceps
DeBakey atraumatic bulldog clamp
DeBakey atraumatic colon resection
  clamp
DeBakey atraumatic tissue forceps
DeBakey-Bahnson vascular clamp
DeBakey-Bainbridge atraumatic
  intestinal forceps
DeBakey-Bainbridge clamp
DeBakey-Beck clamp
DeBakey bulldog clamp
DeBakey coarctation clamp
DeBakey colon resection clamp
DeBakey-Cooley dissecting forceps
DeBakey-Cooley retractor
DeBakey cross-action bulldog clamp
DeBakey-Derra anastomosis clamp
DeBakey-Diethrich atraumatic tissue
  forceps
DeBakey-Diethrich vascular forceps
DeBakey dissecting forceps
DeBakey dissecting scissors
DeBakey double-action grasping
  forceps
DeBakey endarterectomy scissors
DeBakey forceps
DeBakey-Harken clamp
DeBakey-Howard clamp

DeBakey-Kay clamp
DeBakey-Mixter artery forceps
DeBakey needle
DeBakey needle holder with tungsten
  carbide inlay
DeBakey patent ductus clamp
DeBakey pediatric clamp
DeBakey peripheral vascular bulldog
  clamp
DeBakey pickups
DeBakey-Reynolds anastomosis clamp
DeBakey ring-handled bulldog clamp
DeBakey scissors
DeBakey-Semb clamp
DeBakey-Semb forceps
DeBakey sigmoid anastomosis clamp
DeBakey tangential occlusion clamp
DeBakey-TC needle holder
DeBakey tissue forceps
DeBakey vascular clamp
DeBakey vascular forceps
debrancher deficiency
debrancher enzyme
debrancher enzyme deficiency
debrancher glycogen storage disease
debrided
debridement of abscess
debridement tissue
debris
  amorphous
  cellular
Debrisan (dextranomer)
debulking of tumor
debulking surgery
decannulation plug
decanting device
decarboxylase
D cell tumor
Decholin (dehydrocholic acid)
DecisionMaker software
decitabine
deck plate
Decker alligator forceps
Decker micro scissors

Decker microsurgical forceps
Decker microsurgical rongeur
Decker microsurgical scissors
Decker pituitary rongeur
declamping
decompensated alcoholic cirrhosis
decompensated cirrhosis
decompensation
   circulatory
   metabolic
decompression
   balloon
   bladder
   duodenal
   endoscopic
   endoscopic biliary
   gastric
   gastrointestinal
   hydrostatic
   intestinal
   percutaneous
   transhepatic (PTD)
   portal
   tube
   variceal
decompression colostomy
decompression jejunostomy
decompression procedure
decompression retractor
decompression therapy, transduodenal
   endoscopic
decompression tube
decompressive surgery
decompression of varices
deconjugation, bilirubin glucuronide
Decon Mini-Plus kit
decreased afterload
decreased alveolar ventilation
decreased blood flow
decreased blood pressure
decreased bowel sounds
decreased breath sounds
decreased cardiac output
decreased colonic motility

decreased contraction of gallbladder
decreased cytoprotection
decreased gastric acid secretion
decreased gastric emptying
decreased gastric reservoir
decreased GI calcium absorption
decreased GI motility
decreased hematocrit
decreased ileus
decreased libido
decreased lower esophageal sphincter
   (LES) tone
decreased perfusion of the juxta-
   glomerular apparatus
decreased peristalsis
decreased pH
decreased pituitary production
decreased preload
decreased shunt fraction
decreased skin turgor
decreased testosterone
decreased uptake with patchy
   distribution
decreased urinary 17-OCHS
decreased venous return
decreased xylose absorption
decrease in systemic vascular resistance
decrease p.o. protein intake
decubitus calculus
decubitus film
decubitus position
decubitus ulcer
decubitus view
Deddish-Potts intestinal forceps
deep abscess
deep blade
deep blade knife
deep epigastric vessel
deep interloop abscess
deep perineal pouch
deep-purple spleen
deep retention suture
deep section
deep suture

deep tendon reflexes (DTRs)
deep to pectoral minor muscle
deep vein thrombophlebitis (DVT)
deep vein thrombosis (DVT)
deepening reamer
defatting of panniculus
defecate
defecation, painful
defecatory urgency
defecogram
defecography
defect
 bandeau
 cold
 combined
 diaphragmatic
 direct
 fascial
 filling
 frondlike filling
 hernia
 hot
 indirect
 large hernia
 pinpoint gastric mucosal
 postinjury immunologic
 skin
 slitlike
 small hernia
 thoracoscopic repair of diaphrag-
  matic
 ventricular septal wound
defective hemoglobin synthesis
defect of pyrrole metabolism
defense against bacteria
defenses, altered mucosal
deferoxamine mesylate infusion test
defervesce
defervescence of fever
defibrinated blood
deficiency
 acquired lactose
 ACTH
 alpha-galactosidase

deficiency *(cont.)*
 amylo-1,6-glucosidase
 bilirubin glucuronosyltransferase
 brancher
 brancher enzyme
 complex IV
 congenital thyroid
 congenital zinc
 COX (cytochrome C oxidase)
 debrancher
 debrancher enzyme
 essential fatty acid (EFAD)
 glucose-6-phosphorylase
 hepatic phosphorylase
 immune
 isolated thyroid-stimulating hormone
 isovaleric acid CoA dehydrogenase
 isovaleryl CoA carboxylase
 long chain acyl-CoA dehydrogenase
 low density beta lipoprotein
 medium chain acyl-CoA
  dehydrogenase (MCAD)
 muscle carnitine
 myopathic carnitine
 nutritional
 PEPCK (phosphoenolpyruvate
  carboxykinase)
 PiZZ alpha$_1$ antitrypsin
 prolactin
 sucrose-isomaltose (SI)
 systemic carnitine
 thyroid
 uridine diphosphate glucuronosyl-
  transferase
 vasopressin
deficit (see also *deficiency*)
 endocrine
 fluid volume
 focal neurologic
 neurologic
 nutritional
defined parenteral exposure
definitive care
definitive diagnosis

definitive surgery
Definity ultrasound contrast agent
deflecting mechanism
defocused (laser) beam
defogging of laparoscopic telescope
    immersion in warm saline
    intra-abdominal irrigation
    intra-abdominal wiping
    use of defogging agent
deformity
    Akerlund duodenal
    bell-clapper
    cloverleaf
    crossbar stomach
    duodenal bulb
    hourglass (on x-ray)
    phrygian cap
    splenic vein
    trefoil
    Whitehead
Defourmentel bone rongeur
defunctionalization
Degas (simethicone)
degenerated blood
degeneration
    acute hepatocellular
    amyloid
    feathery
    fibroid
    hepatolenticular
    lardaceous
    parenchymous
    sarcomatoid
degeneration of pancreas
degenerative liver
deglutition disorder
deglutition mechanism
deglutition reflex
deglutitive pharyngeal chamber
deglutitive tongue biomechanics
deglutitive tongue force modulation
Degos disease
degradable polyglycolide rod
degraded liver

degree of accuracy
degree of encephalopathy
degree of penetrance
degree of specificity
degrees centrigrade
dehisced (verb)
dehiscence
    abdominal incision
    anastomotic
    staple line
    suture line
    wound
DEHOP (diethylhomospermine)
DEHSPM (diethylhomospermine)
dehydration
dehydrocholic acid
dehydroemetine
dehydroepiandrosterone (DHEA)
DEI (diffraction-enhanced imaging)
Dejerine-Davis percussion hammer
Dejerine percussion hammer
Dejerine-Sottas syndrome
Deklene and Deklene II suture
Deknatel suture
Delafield fluid
Delaginiere abdominal retractor
Delasco electrocoagulator device
delayed closure of suture
delayed gastric emptying
delayed hypersensitivity reaction
delayed insertion of breast prosthesis
delayed primary intention healing
delayed splenic rupture
delayed umbilical ring closure
delayed whole gut transit
delayed xenograft rejection (DXR)
DeLee forceps
DeLee-Hillis stethoscope
DeLee suction trap
deletion
    chromosomal
    clonal
Delicot sponge
Deliver 2.0 formula

delomorphous cell
Delorme rectal prolapse repair
delphian lymph node group
delta-Ag (delta antigen)
delta agent hepatitis
delta antigen (HDAg, hepatitis D virus)
delta hepatitis
delta hepatitis superinfection
delta virus
deltoid region
deltoid-splitting incision
deltopectoral fascia
deltopectoral flap
deluxe lightweight quad cane
Dema-Band bandage
Dema Pad bandage
demarcator
DeMarneffe meniscotomy knife
DeMartel appendix forceps
DeMartel clamp
DeMartel dissecting scissors
DeMartel neurosurgical scissors
DeMartel scalp flap forceps
DeMartel vascular clamp
DeMartel vascular scissors
DeMartel wire saw
DeMartel-Wolfson anastomosis clamp
DeMeester score
Demel wire-tightening forceps
Demel wire-twisting forceps
dementia
Demerol
demigauntlet bandage
demineralized bone graft
Demir rigid laparoscope
demise
Demling-Classen sphincterotome
DeMorgan spot
Demos tibial artery clamp
denatured homograft
dendritic cancer
dendritic reticular cell
dengue fever
dengue virus

Denham pin
Denhardt mouth gag
Denis Browne abdominal retractor
Denis Browne intestinal holding forceps
Denis Browne pouch
Dennis blade
Dennis-Brooke ileostomy
Dennis forceps
Dennis intestinal clamp
Dennis intestinal tube
Dennis-Varco pancreaticoduodenostomy
Denonvillier fascia
de novo lesion
de novo presentation
dens (cervical spine) view
dense adhesions
dense breast tissue
density
   body
   radiopaque
DENSPM (diethylnorspermine)
Dent sleeve
dental drill
dental malocclusion
dental polyp
dentate line
dentate margin
dentate suture
dentinal fluid
dentinal papilla
dentoalveolar structures
denuded mucosa
denutrition
Denver hydrocephalus shunt
Denver peritoneal venous shunt
deoxyribonuclease
deoxyspergualin
Depage-Janeway gastrostomy
DePalma stapler
dependent drainage
dependent edema
dePezer gastrostomy tube
depigmented lesion
depilatory forceps

DepoCyt (cytarabine liposomal)
DepoMorphine (morphine sulfate)
deposition of porphyrins
depressed cell-mediated immunity
depression of left mainstem bronchus
depressor
 bone
 Braun
 blood pressure
 lifter-
 pin
 scleral
 tongue
depth of invasion
depth of wound
DePuy awl
DePuy femoral acetabular overlay guide
DePuy nerve hook
DePuy pin
DePuy plate
DePuy rasp
DePuy reamer
de Quervain thyroiditis
deranged electrolyte balance
derangement, metabolic
Derby nail
Dercum disease
Derf needle
Derf needle holder with tungsten
 carbide inlay
Derf-TC needle holder
Derifil (chlorophyllin)
Derlacki capsule knife
Derlacki chisel
Derlacki curette
Derlacki hook
Derlacki mobilizer
Dermabond dressing
Dermabond topical skin adhesive
Dermabond wound adhesive
DermaFreeze
Dermagraft human-based dermal
 replacement
Dermagraft-TC (transitional covering)

Dermagran hydrophilic wound dressing
Derma K laser
DermaLase ErCr:YSGG laser system
dermal collagen homograft
Dermalene suture
Dermalon suture
dermal papilla
dermal-subdermal plexus
dermal suture
DermaMend foam wound dressing
DermaMend hydrogel dressing
DermaMend moisture barrier cream
 dressing
DermaMend polyurethane foam
 dressing
DermaNet contact-layer wound
 dressing
DermaScan system
DermaSeptic iontophoresis device
DermaSorb dressing
DermAssist hydrocolloid dressing
DermAssist wound filling material
Dermatell hydrocolloid dressing
dermatitis herpetiformis
dermatitis of the nipple
dermatome pain
dermatomyositis
dermatophytic fungi
Derma 20 laser
Dermol HC (hydrocortisone)
Dermoplast (benzocaine; menthol)
dermotropic virus
Dermuspray (trypsin; Peruvian balsam)
DeRoyal surgical cannula
Derra vena cava clamp
Derra vestibular clamp
D'Errico-Adson retractor
D'Errico bayonet pituitary forceps
D'Errico hypophyseal forceps
D'Errico lamina chisel
D'Errico nerve root retractor
D'Errico perforating drill
D'Errico periosteal elevator
D'Errico pituitary forceps

device *(cont.)*
  BiPAP S/T-D 30 ventilatory support
  bipod suspension apparatus
  bipolar urological loop
  BiQ bipolar hand instrument
  BIS Sensor
  BIS Sensor Plus
  Bovie electrocoagulation unit
  Bovie 2100 coagulating electro-
    surgical
  BreastAlert differential temperature
    sensor (DTS)
  breast bolster
  BreastCheck
  BreastExam
  Bremer AirFlo Vest
  broach
  Bucky imaging
  Button and Button-One Step
    gastrostomy feeding
  BVA-100 (blood-volume analyzer)
  BVM (bag-valve-mask)
  Cameron-Miller electrocoagulation
    unit
  Capio CL transvaginal suture-
    capturing
  Carr-Locke stent remover
  Carroll tendon retriever
  Carter pillow
  Carter-Thomason suture passer
  Catarex
  catheter vitrector
  CathLink implantable vascular
    access
  CaverMap surgical aid
  C-bar web-spacer
  Cell Saver
  Cellolite patty material
  Cholestron PRO
  Christoudias fascial closure
  Cincinnati subzero unit
  CLC 2000 swabable intravenous
    connector
  ClearCut 2 electrosurgical handpiece

device *(cont.)*
  Closure catheter/radiofrequency
    generator
  Closure endovascular coagulation
  Conforma 3000 photon beam
    therapy
  decanting
  DermaSeptic iontophoresis
  Devine colostomy
  DeWitt-Stetten colostomy
    spur-crushing
  DiaScreen
  digital x-ray detector
  Digitizer Director
  DirectRay imaging
  Disetronic insulin pen
  Dissectron aspirator
  Diva laparoscopic morcellator
  Dix foreign body
  Dormia noose
  Draffin bipod suspension apparatus
  duodenal decompression
  Dynamic PACSPlus
  DynaWell
  8-lumen silicone recording assembly
  ELAD (extracorporeal liver assist)
  Elmor tissue morcellator
  Endo Babcock surgical grasping
  Endo Catch
  Endocut cautery
  Endo Lumenal Gastroplication
  EndoLumina II transillumination
  EndoMate Grab Bag
  Endopath EZ-RF linear cutter and
    coagulation
  Endopath laparoscopic trocar
  Endopath Optiview optical surgical
    obturator
  Endopath TriStar trocar
  Endo-P-Probe
  endoscopic "sewing machine"
  endoscopic suction cap
  Endo Mini Shears
  Endo Shears

device *(cont.)*

Enterra gastric stimulation
Erbotom F2 electrocoagulation unit
Erlangen magnetic colostomy
esophageal decompression
EU-M30S endoscopic ultra-
    sonography receiver
Favaloro-Morse rib spreader
First Warning breast cancer
    screening
Flexiflo Lap G laparoscopic
    gastrostomy kit
Flexiflo Lap J laparoscopic
    jejunostomy kit
Fuller shield
Gauderer Genie gastrostomy feeding
Glassman stone extractor
Gottschalk Nasostat
Gould polygraph
G-suit external counterpressure
Haemonetics Cell Saver 5
Hancke/Vilmann biopsy handle
    instrument
HandPort hand-assist
Harrison-Nicolle polypropylene
    pegs
Health Buddy health monitoring
Hemasure r/LS red blood cell
    filtration system
Hemi Sling
HemoCue photometer
hemodialyzer
hemofiltration
HemoSleeve
Hemotherapies Liver Dialysis Unit
HepatAssist bioartificial liver
Hercules 7000 mobile x-ray unit
HERMES Control Center for
    medical robotics
HERMES surgery monitoring unit
HumatroPen
Hummingbird wand
IMED infusion device
Import vascular-access port with
    BioGlide

device *(cont.)*

Innervasc
InstaTrak
InstaTrak 3000
IrrigaTORR
Irrijet DS
IsoMed implantable drug pump
IVAC Vital·Check
joker (slang for instrument)
Kao Lectrolyte
Karl Storz N2O Endoflator
Kelly sphincterotome
leading bar
Leonard Arm pneumatic action
    support
Licox monitoring
Lightstic 180 and 360 fiberoptic
    medical laser diffuser
LIMA-Lift
LIMA-Loop
Linvatec micro debrider
liposhaver
lithotrite
Littleford/Spector introducer
Liver Dialysis Unit
Lunderquist-Ring torque guide
M2A Swallowable Imaging Capsule
Maddacrawler
malleus nipper
Mammotome breast biopsy
Mandibular Excursiometer
Marlow Primus instrument
    collection
Masimo SET (signal extraction
    technology) pulse oximeter
Maxima Forté blood oxygenator
Medi-Jector Choice needle-free
    insulin injection
MedPulser
MegaDyne all-in-one hand control
MetraTie knot pusher
MicroAire power-assisted lipoplasty
    device
Microblater ArthroWand

device *(cont.)*
    Micro Diamond-Point microsurgery
      instruments
    Micro-Probe micro dissection tip
    MINI 6600 C-arm
    Mobetron electron accelerator
    morcellator
    MultApplier
    MultAvalue laparoscopic
    Navigator
    NeedleAid
    Neo-Med cautery
    Nerve Block Infusion Kit
    NeuroSector ultrasound
    Neurotone multipurpose
    Nibblit laparoscopic
    nitinol mesh-covered frame
    Nottingham Key-Med introducing
    One-Shot anastomotic
    On-Q postoperative pain
      management system
    Opal R.F. tissue ablation
    Origin Tacker
    OsmoCyte pillow
    PC Polygraf HR
    Pelosi Illuminator
    permanent lead introducer
    Phillips ultrasound
    Pilot suturing guide
    Pneumo-Needle reusable
    Pneumo Sleeve laparoscopic airlock
    PocketDop ultrasound
    Ponsky "Pull" gastrostomy feeding
    portable blood irradiator
    PROloop electrosurgical
    Prostar percutaneous closure
    Prostar Plus percutaneous closure
    Prostar XL percutaneous closure
    prosthetic
    Protect-a-Pass suture passer
    Protocult stool sampling device
    Quadripolar electrosurgical unit
    Quinton suction biopsy

device *(cont.)*
    R.F. tissue ablation
    roentgen knife stereotaxic
      radiosurgical
    Roho air-filled mattress
    Rolyan Firm D-Ring wrist support
    Rotablator
    Roth retrieval net
    roticulating endograsper
    rubber-band loader
    Sensability lubricated plastic sheet
      for breast self-examination
    Sepacell RZ-2000 leukoreduction
    Skin Skribe skin marker
    smoke evacuation unit
    Soehendra stent retriever
    Sofpulse pulsed magnetic energy
    Somogyi (amylase)
    Sonotron radiofrequency
    Spacemaker
    stapling
    Step minimally invasive surgical
      access
    Storz cholangiograsper
    Storz LaproFlator
    Stretta
    Surg-I-Loop
    SurgiScope robotic surgery
    Suture Assistant endoscopic suturing
    Suture Assistant knot-tying
    suture-welding
    SYBIOL (synthetic bio-liver)
    Tapertome sphincterotome
    targeted cryoablation
    Thora-Port
    Tissomat application
    tissue expander
    TissueLink Monopolar Floating Ball
    TQa (transcutaneous access flow)
    Trachlight
    TransScan TS 2000 electrical
      impedance breast scanning
    TransScan 2000 breast mapping

device *(cont.)*
   TraumaJet wound debridement
   Tru-Area Determination wound-
      measuring
   TULIP (transurethral laser-induced
      prostatectomy)
   20/30 Indeflator Inflation
   Ultramark 4 ultrasound
   USSC (United States Surgical
      Corp.)
   Valleylab laparoscopic and electro-
      surgical unit
   Valleylab SSE-2 cautery unit
   Vasotrax blood pressure/heart rate
      sensor
   VerreScope micro laparoscopic entry
   Vibra-Surge ultrasonic
   Volkmann spoon
   Wilson-Cook (modified) wire-
      guided sphincterotome
   XPS Straightshot
DeVilbiss cranial rongeur
DeVilbiss rongeur forceps
Devine procedure
devitalized bone graft
Devonshire colic
Devrom (bismuth subgallate)
DeWeese vena cava clamp
Dewey obstetric forceps
dewy appearance
dexamethasone sodium phosphate
dexamethasone suppression test
dexanabinol
Dexatrim
dexfenfluramine
dexmedetomidine
Dexon Plus suture
Dexon polyglycolic acid mesh
Dexon suture
Dexon II suture
dexpanthenol
dextran 40 plasma volume expander
dextranomer
dextrinizing time

dextrinosis, limit
dextrorotation
Dextrostix
Dey-Wash skin wound cleanser
Deyerle II pin
Deyerle pin
Deyerle plate
DFDR diamond fraise
DF-2 bacillus
DGHAL (Doppler-guided hemor-
   rhoidal artery ligation)
DG Softgut suture
DGR (duodenogastric reflux)
DHEA (dehydroepiandrosterone)
DHEA sulfate (DHEAS)
DHEAS (DHEA sulfate)
DiaBeta (glyburide)
diabetes induced by beta-cell toxins
diabetes insipidus
   acquired
   central
   idiopathic
   primary
   secondary
   vasopressin-sensitive
diabetes mellitus
   adult-onset
   brittle
   bronze
   gestational
   IDDM (insulin-dependent diabetes
      mellitus)
   insulin-dependent, associated with
      acanthosis nigricans
   juvenile-onset (now classified as
      type 1)
   lipoatrophic
   maturity-onset diabetes of the young
      (MODY)
   neonatal
   NIDDM (non-insulin-dependent
      diabetes mellitus)
   non-insulin-dependent
   nonclinical

diabetes *(cont.)*
    post-transplant diabetes mellitus
    type 1 (formerly classified as
        juvenile or juvenile-onset)
    type 2 (formerly classified as
        adult-onset)
    uncontrolled maternal
diabetes secondary to pancreatic disease
diabetic acidosis
diabetic amyotrophy
diabetic colitis
diabetic diet
diabetic enteropathy
diabetic gangrene
diabetic gastroparesis
diabetic gastropathy
diabetic hyperglycemia
diabetic hyperosmolar nonketotic coma
diabetic ketoacidosis (DKA)
diabetic mononeuropathy
diabetic neuropathy
diabetic polyneuropathy
DiabetiSweet sugar substitute
diabetologist
DiabGel hydrogel dressing
DiabKlenz wound cleanser
Diacol
Diagnex Blue gastric acid test
diagnosis (pl. diagnoses)
    admitting
    antenatal
    clinical
    colposcopic
    cytologic
    definitive
    differential
    discharge
    empirical
    fetal
    final
    frozen section
    genetic
    gross
    histologic

diagnosis *(cont.)*
    histopathologic
    initial
    microscopic
    neonatal
    operative
    pathologic
    physical
    postoperative
    preliminary
    prenatal
    prenatal genetic
    preoperative
    presumptive
    principal
    provisional anatomic
    tentative
    ultrasound
    working
diagnosis by exclusion
diagnostic and therapeutic administra-
    tion
diagnostic anesthesia
diagnostic cascade
diagnostic findings
diagnostic laparoscopy
diagnostic pancreatography
diagnostic peritoneal lavage (DPL)
diagnostic radiology procedures
    (see *operation*)
Diagnostix sphygmomanometer
Dialock hemodialysis access system
Dialose (docusate sodium)
Dialose Plus (yellow phenolphthalein;
    docusate sodium)
Dialume (aluminum hydroxide gel)
Dialyflex dialysis fluid
dialysis
    BioLogic-DT (now Liver Dialysis
        Unit)
    continuous ambulatory peritoneal
        (CAPD)
    kidney
    liver
    peritoneal

dialysis-related ascites
diamond fraise
diamond inlay graft
diamond knife sponge
diamond Ohio adapter
Diamond pin cutter
diamond rasp
diamond-shaped incision
diamond-shaped medullary nail
diaper rash
diaphoresis
diaphragm veins
diaphragmatic defect
diaphragmatic hernia
diaphragmatic hiatus
diaphragmatic hump
diaphragmatic injury
diaphragmatic irritation
diaphragmatic rupture
diaphragmatic surface of liver
Diapid (lypressin)
Diar-Aid (loperamide)
diarrhea
   acute infectious
   antibiotic-induced
   anxiety-related
   bacillary
   bile salt
   bilious
   bloody
   cachectic
   chronic
   chronic bacillary
   Clostridium difficile-associated
   colliquative
   copious rice-water
   copious watery
   Dientamoeba
   dysenteric
   enteral
   enterotoxin
   explosive
   familial chloride
   flagellate

diarrhea *(cont.)*
   functional
   gastrogenous
   hemorrhagic
   ileostomy
   infectious
   inflammatory
   intermittent
   intractable
   irritative
   lactose-associated
   lienteric
   liquid
   malabsorptive
   maldigestive
   mechanical
   mucous
   osmotic
   pancreatogenous
   postvagotomy
   rotavirus
   secretory
   serous
   stercoral
   toxic
   traveler's
   unexplained
   unrelenting
   viral
   virulent
   watery
diarrheal disease
diarrhea-predominant irritable bowel
   syndrome
diarrhea stools
Diascan reagent strips
DiaScreen reagent strips
Diasensor 1000 glucose monitor
Diasorb (activated attapulgite)
diastasis of suture
diastasis recti abdominis
Diastat vascular access graft
diastatic serosal tear
diastolic blood pressure

diastolic cardiac arrest
diastolic hypertension
diathermic loop
diathermic loop biopsy
diathermy dissection of the esophagus
diathermy-excision hemorrhoidectomy
diathermy forceps
diathermy rectal snare
diathermy scissors
diathermy suction tube
diathesis (pl. diatheses), bleeding
diatrizoate meglumine
diazepam
DIB (duodenoileal bypass)
Dibent (dicyclomine)
dibucaine
DIC (diffuse intravascular coagulation)
DIC (disseminated intravascular coagu-
  lopathy)
DIC (drip infusion cholangiography)
DIC parameters
dicarboxylicaciduria
dicyclomine HCl
DIDMOAD (diabetes insipidus,
  diabetes mellitus, optic atrophy,
  and deafness)
Dieffenbach bulldog clamp
Dieffenbach serrefine
diencephalic syndrome
Dientamoeba diarrhea
Dientamoeba fragilis
diet
  absolute
  ADA (American Diabetes Associa-
    tion or American Dietetic
    Association)
  balanced
  bland
  blenderized
  BRAT (bananas, rice cereal,
    applesauce, toast)
  BRATS (bananas, rice, apples, toast,
    saltines)
  CAPS-free (caffeine, alcohol,
    pepper, spicy foods)

diet *(cont.)*
  clear liquid
  diabetic
  elemental
  elimination
  exclusion
  fasting
  fluid-restricted
  fractionated
  full liquid
  gastric
  Glutasorb
  gluten-free
  grapefruit
  high-bulk, low-fat
  high-carbohydrate
  high-fiber
  high-protein
  high-residue
  hypercaloric
  hyperprotidic
  lactose-free
  liquid
  liver
  low-calorie
  low-fat
  low-fiber
  low-protein
  low-residue
  low-roughage
  low-sodium
  Meulengracht
  milk
  mixed elemental-fat
  mixed protein-fat
  Moro-Heisler
  ovolactovegetarian
  Portagen
  progressive
  ProSol 20%
  reduced lactose
  regular
  rice-fruit
  Schmidt

diet *(cont.)*
    semielemental
    Sippy
    smooth
    soft bland
    vegetarian
    very low calorie (VLCD)
    Weight Watchers
    Western
    yo-yo
diet ad lib.
dietary cholesterol
dietary cirrhosis
dietary fat
dietary fiber
dietary habits
dietary history
dietary protein
dietary protein restriction
dietary supplementation
dietetic colitis
dietetic ileitis
dietetic jejunitis
dietetic regimen
dietetic sigmoiditis
Diethrich bulldog clamp
Diethrich bulldog clip
Diethrich coronary scissors
Diethrich-Hegemann scissors
Diethrich micro bulldog clamp
Diethrich-TC needle holder
Diethrich valve scissors
Diethrich vascular scissors
diethylcarbamazine
diethylcarbamazine citrate
diethylhomospermine (DEHOP;
    DEHSPM)
diethylnorspermine (DENSPM)
diethylpropion
dieting plateau
dieting, yo-yo
diet therapy
Dieulafoy disease
Dieulafoy gastric lesion

Dieulafoy lesion of anal canal
Dieulafoy triad
Dieulafoy ulcer
Dieulafoy vascular malformation
difenoximide HCl
difenoxin HCl
differential diagnosis
differential spinal anesthesia
DiffGAM
difficulty breathing
Diffistat-G
diffraction-enhanced (breast) imaging
    (DEI)
diffuse abdominal pain
diffuse abdominal tenderness
diffuse abscess
diffuse breast involvement
diffuse carcinomatosis
diffuse colloid goiter
diffuse esophageal spasm (DES)
diffuse GI hamartoma polyps
diffuse goiter
diffuse intravascular coagulation (DIC)
diffuse lesion
diffuse lobular fibrosis
diffusely tender abdomen
diffuse microcalcifications
diffuse microvascular thrombosis
diffuse mucosal polyposis
diffuse multinodular goiter
diffuse necrosis
diffuse pain
diffuse pancreatitis
diffuse peritonitis
diffuser
    Lightstic 180 fiberoptic medical
        laser
    Lightstic 360 fiberoptic medical
        laser
diffuse septal cirrhosis
diffuse thyroid enlargement
diffuse toxic goiter
diffuse toxic non-nodular goiter
diffuse transmural ganglioneuromatosis

diffuse transmural intestinal ganglio-
neuromatosis
diffuse varioliform gastritis
diffusion problem
digastric impression
digastric triangle
Di-Gel (aluminum hydroxide; magne-
sium hydroxide; simethicone)
Di-Gel Advanced Formula (magnesium
hydroxide calcium carbonate;
simethicone)
DiGeorge syndrome
Digepepsin (pancreatin; pepsin;
bile salts)
digestant
digestive enzyme
Hi-Vegi-Lip (pancreatase; lipase;
protease; amylase)
lipase
Ku-Zyme HP (amylase; protease;
lipase; cellulase)
Kutrase
Pancrease MT 20 (lipase; protease;
amylase)
pancreatin
Pancreatin 8X (pancreatin; lipase;
protease; amylase)
Pancrecarb MS-8 (lipase; protease;
amylase)
pancrelipase
Pancrezyme 4X (pancreatin; lipase;
protease; amylase)
Papaya Enzyme (papain; amylase)
Trizyme
Ultralase MT 12, Ultralase MT 20
Vita-PMS, Vita-PMS Plus
digestive fluid
digestive tract
digestive tract contents
digestive tract sensorimotor physiology
and pathophysiology
Digestozyme (pancreatin; pepsin;
dehydrocholic acid)
Digibar 190 (barium sulfate for
suspension)

digital examination
digital rectal examination
digital subtraction angiography
digital subtraction film
digital subtraction imaging technique
digital wrist blood pressure monitor
digital x-ray detector
Digital Response (DRx) glucose
monitor
digitalization
Digitizer Director
Digitrapper MKIII device
dilatation (see also *dilation*)
anal
aneurysmal
bowel
ductal
esophageal
gastric
percutaneous transfemoral
periportal sinusoidal
pneumatic bag esophageal
urethral
dilatation of stenotic hepatico-
jejunostomy
dilatation of the pouch
dilated bowel
dilated gallbladder
dilated loop of bowel
dilating catheter
dilating forceps
dilating tip trocar
dilating window
dilation (see also *dilatation*)
balloon
biliary
cricopharyngeal
ductal
Eder-Puestow
endoscopic
endoscopic retrograde balloon
esophageal
extrahepatic biliary cystic
hepatic web

dilation *(cont.)*
    intrahepatic biliary cystic
    percutaneous balloon
    pneumatic balloon catheter
    postoperative ductal
dilation instrument
dilation of gastric outlet
dilation of stomach
dilation of subareolar duct
dilator
    American Dilation System
    Amplatz
    anal
    Bakes common duct
    Bard Eliminator balloon
    Bowlby tracheal
    Brown-McHardy pneumatic
    Carlson Zero Tip balloon
    Celestin graduated
    common duct
    Core laparoscopic
    CRE wireguided controlled radial
        expansion
    Eder-Puestow metal olive-tipped
    Einhorn
    Endo-Flex balloon
    esophageal
    Ferris biliary duct
    Flex-EZ balloon
    French
    Garrett
    Hegar
    Hegar rectal
    Hobbs
    Hurst bullet-tip
    Hurst mercury-filled
    Hurst-Tucker pneumatic
    Kollman urethral
    Kron bile duct
    Laborde
    Laborde tracheal
    Maloney esophageal
    Maloney mercury-filled

dilator *(cont.)*
    Maloney tapered-tip
    Med-Tech Teflon
    mercury-filled
    mercury-weighted
    Murphy common duct
    Plummer esophageal
    pneumatic balloon
    probe
    rectal
    Rigiflex balloon
    Savary-Gilliard
    Savary tapered thermoplastic
    Sippy esophageal
    Soehendra dilator
    Starck
    Stucker bile duct
    through-the-scope (TTS)
    Trousseau trachea
    Tucker spindle-shaped
    Wilson-Cook esophageal balloon
dilator system
diloxanide furoate
dimenhydrinate
dimercaptosuccinic acid scan
dimethyl iminodiacetic acid scan
dimethyl sulfoxide
diminished bowel sounds
DIMOAD syndrome (diabetes
    insipidus, diabetes mellitus,
    optic atrophy, and deafness)
dimple, celiac
dimpling of skin
Dinate (dimenhydrinate)
Dingman bone and cartilage clamp
Dingman bone-holding forceps
Dingman cartilage clamp
Dingman mouth gag
Dingman oral retractor
Dingman osteotome
Diocto-C (casanthranol; docusate
    sodium)
Diocto-K (docusate potassium)

Diocto-K Plus (casanthronol; docusate
potassium)
Dioctolose Plus (casanthronol; docusate
potassium)
diode laser
Dioeze (docusate sodium)
DiPAS-positive granule
Dipentum (olsalazine sodium)
diphenoxylate HCl
Diphtheria
diphtheria bacillus
Diphyllobothrium latum
Diplococcus pneumoniae
Diprivan (propofol)
Diquinol (iodoquinol)
Dirame (propiram)
direct and indirect component
direct antagonist
direct bilirubin
DirectBite disposable biopsy forceps
direct cholecystoenterostomy
direct contrast ductography
direct Coombs test
directed biopsy
direct extension
direct extension of tumor
direct hernia
direct hernia defect
direct inguinal hernia
direction
   clockwise
   counterclockwise
directional endotracheal tube
direct laryngoscopy
direct ligation of esophageal varices
director
   Childe hernia
   grooved
   Key hernia
   Kocher
   Koenig small
   Larry probe
   Lockhart Mummary fistula
   Payr
   St. Mark's fistula

Director biliary guidewire
direct pressure
direct tissue destruction
direct virtual control of biopsy
direct vision
direct-vision liver biopsy
direct visualization
DirectRay imaging device
disaccharidase deficiency
disaccharide intolerance I
disaccharide tripeptic glycerol
   dipalmitoyl
disaccharide tripeptide glycerol
   tripalmitoyl (ImmTher)
Disanthrol (casanthranol)
DISC (disabled infectious single cycle)
   vaccine
discharge
   blood-tinged
   bloody
   bloody nipple
   milky nipple
   mucopurulent
   mucosanguineous
   mucus
   spontaneous nipple
   suppurative
discharge diagnosis
discission blade
discission knife
discoloration of the flank
discolored mucosa
discomfort
   postprandial
   referred epigastric
discordant cellular xenograft
discordant organ xenograft
Discrene breast prosthesis
discrete bleeding source
discrete lesion
discrete mass (*not* discreet)
discrete stenosis
discrete tumor
discussion needle

disease
- Abrami
- acalculous gallbladder
- acid peptic
- acid reflux
- acute abdominal vascular
- acute idiopathic inflammatory bowel
- Addison
- adenomatous polyposis coli
- adiposis dolorosa
- adult polycystic
- AIOD (aortoiliac obstructive)
- alcoholic liver (ALD)
- alpha chain
- $alpha_1$-antitrypsin deficiency
- anal epithelial neoplasia
- Andersen
- anorectal melanoma
- atypical gallbladder
- autoimmune
- autoimmune thyroid
- autosomal dominant polycystic
- autosomal recessive
- Banti
- Barrett
- Basedow
- Behçet
- benign breast (BBD)
- Biermer
- biliary stone
- biliary tract
- black liver
- Bouchard
- Bowen
- Bradley
- brancher glycogen storage
- bronchiolitis obliterans
- bronze (Addison)
- Budd
- Byler
- calculous gallbladder
- Caroli (acute cholangitis)
- celiac (CD)
- celiac sprue

disease *(cont.)*
- Chagus
- Cherchevski
- Chiari
- cholestatic liver
- cholesterol ester storage (CESD)
- chronic granulomatous
- chronic renal
- chylopoietic
- classic triad of Rigler
- collagen vascular
- colonic mucosubmucosal elongated polyp
- colorectal
- congenital cystic liver
- connective tissue
- Cori
- Cowden
- coxsackie virus
- Crohn (CD)
- Cronkhite-Canada
- cryptosporidiosis
- cytomegalic inclusion virus
- Cushing
- cysticercus
- de Quervain thyroiditis
- debrancher glycogen storage
- Degos
- Dercum
- desmoid
- Dieulafoy
- diverticular (of the colon)
- diverticulitis
- Dubin-Sprinz
- Duncan
- duodenal ulcer
- echinococcal cyst
- end-stage liver
- erosive gastroesophageal reflux (GERD)
- esophageal reflux
- essential mixed cryoglobulinemia
- estrogen-induced liver
- extraluminal retrorectal tumor

disease *(cont.)*

    extramammary Paget
    Fabry
    familial adenomatous polyposis (FAP)
    familial visceral neuropathy
    fatty liver
    Fenwick
    fibrocystic breast
    Fiedler
    fistulizing Crohn
    Forbes
    fulminant Wilson
    functional bowel
    Gamna
    gastrocolic fistula
    gastroesophageal reflux (GERD)
    Gaucher
    Gee-Herter
    Gee-Herter-Heubner
    Gee-Thaysen
    GERD (gastroesophageal reflux)
    Gierke
    Gilbert
    glycogen storage
    gonococcal perihepatis pelvic inflammatory
    Gordon
    graft-versus-host (GVHD)
    Graves
    Grey Turner
    Gross
    Hartnup
    Hashimoto thyroiditis
    hepatic encephalopathy
    hepatic Hodgkin
    hepatic veno-occlusive
    hepatic venous web
    hepatobiliary
    hepatocellular
    hepatolenticular
    Hers
    Herter-Heubner
    Hirschsprung

disease *(cont.)*

    Huebner-Herter
    human ehrlichial infection, Sennetsu type
    Huntington
    Hutinel
    hydatid cyst
    hyperplastic mucinous cystadenoma
    IBD (inflammatory bowel)
    idiopathic inflammatory bowel
    ileocolic
    immunologically mediated
    immunoproliferative small intestinal (IPSID)
    immunoproliferative small intestine
    infectious
    inflammatory bowel (IBD)
    intercapillary glomerulosclerosis
    intrahepatic
    iron storage
    ischemic bowel
    ischemic heart
    ischemic mesenteric
    jejunal angiodysplasia
    kinky hair
    Kinnier Wilson
    Klemperer
    Lane
    leather-bottle stomach
    Leigh
    Leiner
    Leyden
    lithiumogenic goiter
    littoral cell angioma
    locoregional residual
    Lyme
    Mediterranean lymphoma
    Menetrier
    Meniere
    Menkes
    metastatic
    micrometastatic
    mixed cell Hodgkin
    Mondor

disease *(cont.)*
    necrotizing enterocolitis (NEC)
    necrotizing fasciitis
    neoplastic
    NERD (nonerosive reflux)
    Niemann-Pick
    nodular sclerosing Hodgkin
    nodular thyroid
    nonerosive reflux (NERD)
    nonobstructive hepatic parenchymal
    Ormond
    Osler-Weber-Rendu (OWR)
    osteitis fibrosa cystica generalisata
    Paget perianal
    parasitic
    paroxysmal motor
    Patella (pyloric stenosis)
    pathologic nipple
    pelvic inflammatory (PID)
    peptic ulcer (PUD)
    perianal Bowen
    pilonidal
    pneumatosis coli
    polycystic liver
    porphyria cutanea tarda
    primary biliary cirrhosis (PBC)
    primary sclerosing cholangitis (PSC)
    pseudomembranous colitis (PMC)
    Recklinghausen
    Rendu-Osler-Weber
    Riedel struma
    Rokitansky
    Ruysch
    Saunders
    Schaumann
    schistosomal liver
    scleroderma bowel
    sclerosing encapsulating peritonitis
    Sennetsu fever
    Siewerling-Creutzfeldt
    Simmonds
    small intestinal malignant lymphoma
    space-occupying
    Spencer

disease *(cont.)*
    stress-related mucosal (SMRD)
    struma lymphomatosis
    systemic mast cell
    systemic scleroderma
    Tangier
    terminal ileal
    triad of Rigler
    tuberculous Addison
    ulcerative colitis
    unilateral renal parenchymal
    Van Bogaert
    vancomycin-resistant *Enterococcus faecium* (VREF) infection
    veno-occlusive liver
    venous outflow obstructive
    von Hippel-Lindau
    von Recklinghausen
    von Rokitansky
    Von Gierke
    Waldmann
    Weber-Christian
    Weil
    Westphal-Strümpell
    Whipple
    Wilson
    winter vomiting
    Wolman
disease burden
disease flare
disease-free interval
disease-free survival
Disetronic diabetes management tools and instruments
Disetronic insulin pen
Disetronic insulin pump
DISH (diffuse idiopathic skeletal hyperostosis)
DISIDA scan
disinfectant
disinsertion of the papilla
disk, anal
disk forceps
disk kidney

disk punch
disk rongeur
dismal prognosis
disodium cromoglycate (DSC; DSCG)
Disolan (phenolphthalein; docusate
    sodium)
Disolan Forte (casanthranol;
    carboxymethylcellulose sodium;
    docusate sodium)
Disonate (docusate sodium)
Disoplex (carboxymethylcellulose
    sodium; docusate sodium)
disorder
    acid-peptic
    acid-related (ARD)
    bowel elimination
    deglutition
    esophageal motility
    evacuation
    exocrine pancreas
    extrapyramidal movement
    fat storage
    functional
    functional gastrointestinal (FGID)
    gastric motor
    gastric NK-like T cell lympho-
        proliferative
    helminthic
    iatrogenic pituitary
    immunologic deficiency
    infiltrative
    lymphoproliferative
    malignant gastrointestinal
    myeloproliferative
    neoplastic
    nonspecific esophageal motility
        (NEMD)
    peripheral neurologic
    post-transplant lymphoproliferative
    rectal evacuatory
    smooth-muscle motility
    underlying hematologic
disordered preoperative peristalsis
disordered vasculature

disorders of intestinal motility
Di-Spaz (dicyclomine)
dispersive electrodes
disposable airway
disposable biopsy punch
disposable proctoscope
Dispos-a-Ject plunger
disrupt impacted stone
disruption of blood supply
disruption of diaphragm
DISS air
DISS body adapter
Disse space
dissecting abdominal aneurysm
dissecting and grasping forceps
dissecting aorta
dissecting aortic aneurysm
dissecting blood from the retro-
    peritoneal cavity
dissecting forceps
dissecting hook
dissecting probe
dissecting scissors
dissecting sponge
dissection
    axillary
    blunt
    cervical node
    diathermy (of the esophagus)
    elective lymph node
    en bloc
    extensive lymph node
    finger
    finger fracture
    fingertip
    Freer
    groin
    laparoscopic
    lateral cervical node
    lymph node
    modified neck
    node
    radical mediastinal
    radical neck

dissection *(cont.)*
  scissor
  scissors
  sharp
  sharp and blunt
  sponge
  submucosal
  VasoView balloon dissection system
dissection injury
dissection of esophagus, diathermy
dissection of gallbladder from the liver
  bed
dissection of peritoneum overlying
  the cystic duct
dissection of terminal esophagus
  and fundus of stomach
dissector (also see *cutter, scissors,*
   shears)
  Agris-Dingman submammary
  articulating
  Circon continuous flow resectoscope
  ClearCut 2 electrosurgical handpiece
  Core laparoscopic Kittner
  CPC
  Crabtree
  Crile
  curved Maryland
  CUSA (Cavitron ultrasonic Surgical
   aspirator)
  dolphin-nose dissector
  Durham
  Endo Dissect
  Endopath ETS-FLEX endoscopic
   articulating linear cutter
  Endopath EZ45 endoscopic linear
   cutter
  Endo Shears cutter
  EZ45 thoracic linear cutter
  FD-43 micro dissector
  Freer
  Fukushima-Giannotta
  grooved
  GSI balloon dissector
  hernia

dissector *(cont.)*
  Howarth
  Hurd tonsil
  Jimmy
  Kittner blunt
  Kittner dissecting scissors
  Kocher thyroid
  Maryland
  McCabe flap knife
  McCormick
  McDonald
  micro
  monopolar
  Olivecrona
  orbital rim
  oval
  Penfield
  Pivotal
  right angle
  SaphFinder surgical balloon
  SAPHtrak balloon
  short right-angle
  Spacemaker balloon
  Spacemaker VBD-300
  sponge
  spud dissector
  straight
  Swedish pattern
  tapered Maryland
  tapered right-angle
  ultrasonic
  VaporTrode
  Watson-Cheyne
Dissectron ultrasonic aspirator
disseminated gonococcal infection
disseminated intravascular coagulation
  (DIC)
disseminated intravascular coagulopathy
  (DIC)
disseminated pheochromocytoma
dissociated anesthesia
dissociative anesthesia
dissolution of gallstone
dissolution, percutaneous stone

DISS suction bottle
Distaflo bypass graft
distal bile duct
distal bile duct obstruction
distal biliary atresia
distal blind stomach
distal clot
distal colon
distal cremasteric stump
distal duodenum
distal end of transected colon
distal esophageal ring
distal esophagus
distal flow
distal gastrectomy with excision of ulcer
distal ileitis
distal lymph node metastasis
distal near-total pancreatectomy
distal nephron
distal pancreatectomy (body/tail fistula)
distal pancreatic resection
distal pulses
distal resection
distal Roux-en-Y gastric procedure
distal spatula
distal splenorenal shunt (DSR)
distal stump of artery
distal subtotal pancreatectomy
distal transection of pancreas
distance from the anal verge
distant metastasis
distant skin recurrence
distend
distended abdomen
distended afferent loop
distended gallbladder
distended loop of sigmoid colon
distended loop of small bowel
distensibility
distention
   abdominal
   bladder
   colonic
   gallbladder

distention *(cont.)*
   gaseous
   gastric
   liver
   postprandial
   progressive abdominal
   rectal
distortion of normal parenchyma
distraction hook
distraction rod
distractor pin
disturbance of self-esteem
diuresis
diuretic therapy
Diva laparoscopic morcellator
diversion, biliopancreatic
diversion proctitis
diversionary ileostomy
diverticula (see *diverticulum*)
diverticular disease of the colon
diverticulectomy
   Harrington esophageal
   Meckel
   open
diverticulectomy of hypopharynx
diverticulitis
   acute
   cecal
   chronic
   recurrent episodes of
   sigmoid
diverticulization of duodenum
diverticuloscope
diverticulosis
diverticulum (pl. diverticula)
   colonic
   congenital
   cricopharyngeal
   end-stage
   epiphrenic
   esophageal
   false
   Ganser
   Graser

diverticulum *(cont.)*
  hepatic
  hyperplastic mucosal
  hypopharyngeal
  intestinal
  intraluminal duodenal (IDD)
  intramural
  juxtapapillary
  Kirchner
  large pharyngeal
  lateral
  Meckel
  midesophageal
  perforated
  perforation of
  periampullary
  pharyngoesophageal
  pulsion
  Rokitansky
  subdiaphragmatic
  traction
  true
  volvulated Meckel diverticulum
  wide-mouthed mucosal
  Zenker
diverticulum of Nuck
diverting colostomy
diverting ileostomy
diverting loop ileostomy
diverting proximal colostomy
diverting stoma
divided-stoma colostomy
Divine colostomy appliance
diving goiter
division of cystic duct between clips
division of short gastric vessels
division of stricture
di-wing anoscope
Dix foreign body device
Dixon-Thomas-Smith clamp
Dizmiss (meclizine HCl)
DJJ (duodenojejunal junction)
DKA (diabetic ketoacidosis)
DLP cardioplegic needle

DME (drug metabolizing enzyme)
D-Modem and insulin pump therapy
DMP 504
DMSO (dimethyl sulphoxide)
DNA flow cytometry
DNA ploidy abnormality
DNA repair gene
DNA tumor virus
Doane knee retractor
Dobbhoff biliary stent
Dobbhoff feeding tube
Dobbhoff gastrectomy feeding tube
DOBI (Dynamic Optical Breast
  Imaging System)
dobutamine
docetaxel
Docucal-P (phenolphthalein; docusate
  calcium)
documented loss of blood elements
docusate calcium
docusate potassium
docusate sodium
Döderlein (Doederlein) bacillus
dog-bite infection
Dohn-Carton brain retractor
Dohrmann-Rubin cannula
DOK (docusate sodium)
DoLi S extracorporeal shock-wave
dolichocolon
dolorosa (painful) anesthesia
dolphin-nose dissector
dolphin-nose grasper
dolphin-nose grasping forceps, tissue
  well, double-action
Domeboro powder, tablets (aluminum
  sulfate; calcium acetate)
dome of diaphragm
dome of liver
Dome-Paste (zinc oxide; calamine;
  gelatin)
dominant breast mass
domperidone
domperidone maleate
Donaghy angled suture needle holder

donation, organ
Donati suture
Don Congreve trocar set
Don Duralap scissors
Donnagel (attapulgite)
Donnagel-PG
Donnamar (hyoscyamine sulfate)
Donna-Sed (atropine sulfate; scopolamine hydrobromide; hyoscyamine hydrobromide; phenobarbital)
Donnatal (atropine sulfate; scopolamine hydrobromide; hyoscyamine sulfate; phenobarbital)
Donnazyme (pancreatic lipase; protease; amylase)
donor
  cadaveric
  CMV-positive
  living related
  non-heart-beating
  organ
donor blood
donor kidney
donor hepatectomy
donor pancreatectomy
donor-specific bone marrow augmentation
donor-specific transfusion (DST)
Don peritoneal scissors
Donphen
donut mastopexy
Dooley nail
dopa agonist
dopamine
dopamine agonist
Doppler-guided hemorrhoid artery ligation (DGHAL)
Doppler, Nicolet Elite obstetrical
Doppler sonography
Doppler ultrasonography
Doppler ultrasound intestinal blood flow measurement
Dorbane (danthron)
Dorbantyl Forte (danthron)

Dor fundoplasty
Dormia basket catheter
Dormia noose
Dornier gallstone lithotriptor
Dornier HM3 waterbath lithotriptor
Dorros infusion/probing catheter
dorsal linear incision
dorsal lithotomy (*not* dorsolithotomy) position
dorsal mesogastrium
dorsal pancreas
dorsal pancreatic artery
dorsal plate
dorsal point
dorsal position
dorsal recumbent position
dorsal supine position
dorsal surface of the thyroid gland
dorsal vein complex
Dorsey ventricular cannula
dorsiflexion view
dorsomedial incision
dorsoplantar view
dorsosacral position
dorsosupine position
Dosalax (senna concentrate; alcohol)
Dos Santos needle
DOS Softgels (docusate sodium)
Dostinex (cabergoline)
Dott retractor
Doubilet sphincterotomy
double-action jaws
double-action parallel pliers and wire cutter
double-action rongeur
double-action wire cutter
double-action wire extraction pliers
double-armed (DAS) suture
double barrel colostomy
double barrel ileostomy
double barrel reservoir
double binocular operating microscope
double-bladed knife
double bubble duodenal sign

double buttress laparoscopic hernio-
plasty
double channel
double channel endoscope
double clamp
double clamping
double contrast barium enema (DCBE)
double contrast barium meal
double drape
doubled semitendinosus and gracilis
autograft (DST&G)
double duct sign
double-edged razor blade
double-ended curette
double-ended nail
double-ended right-angle retractor
double gallbladder
double-head ceiling mount reflector
double-headed P190 stapler
double hernia
double hook
double hollow nail
double hook Lovejoy retractor
double-H plate
double incision
Double J indwelling catheter
double J-shaped reservoir
Double J ureteral catheter
double lumen endobronchial tube
double lumen endoprosthesis
double lumen papillotome
double lumen tube
double mesh graft
double-occluding clamp
double pedicle flap
double pedicle TRAM flap
double pigtail endoprosthesis
double pigtail stent
double-pointed needle
double-post Mayo stand
double prong fork
double puncture laparoscope
double pyloroplasty
double reverse alpha sigmoid loop

double seton modified surgical
approach to transsphincteric anal
fistula repair
double-spoon forceps
double S-shaped curvature
DoubleStent biliary endoprosthesis
double tertian malaria
double tracking of barium
double-wrap graciloplasty
doubly ligated
doubly ligated and divided
doubly ligated suture
doughnut kidney
doughy abdomen
Douglas cannula
Douglas, cul-de-sac of
Douglas fold
Douglas forceps
Douglas pouch
Douglas procedure (suture of tongue for
micrognathia)
Douglas rectal snare
Douglas rectouterine pouch
Douglas skin graft
Dow Corning breast prosthesis
Dow Corning ileal pouch catheter
dowel graft
Dowen forceps
downbiting rongeur
Down epiphyseal knife
Downey hemilaminectomy retractor
downhill esophageal varices
Downing cartilage knife
Downing retractor
Downing staple
Down syndrome
Doxidan (phenolphthalein; docusate
calcium)
Doxil (doxorubicin hydrochloride
liposome injection)
Doxinate
doxorubicin hydrochloride liposome
injection
Doyen abdominal retractor

drainage *(cont.)*
  green-brown
  internal biliary
  J-Vac closed wound
  mucopurulent
  nasobiliary
  nasogastric
  nasopancreatic
  needle
  percutaneous abscess and fluid
    drainage (PAFD)
  percutaneous antegrade biliary
  percutaneous transhepatic (PTD)
  perianal
  preoperative endoscopic
  presacral
  regional lymphatic
  retroperitoneal
  sanguineous
  Seroma-Cath wound drainage system
  serosanguineous
  suction
  surgical
  transduodenal
  transgastric
  transpapillary
  transrectal
  Tru-Close wound drainage system
  T-tube
  wound
drainage gastrostomy
drainage of palate abscess
drainage of pancreatic exocrine
  secretions
drainage of pus
drainage procedure
drainage tube
draining abscess
drain site evisceration
Drake-Willock peritoneal dialysis
  system
Dramamine (dimenhydrinate)
Dramamine II (meclizine HCl)

Dramanate (dimenhydrinate)
Dramilin (dimenhydrinate)
Drapanas shunt
drape
  adhesive
  adhesive plastic
  beach chair shoulder
  Bedel
  Convertor
  double
  Emerald
  fenestrated
  foot
  head
  impervious
  Incise
  Ioban antimicrobial incise
  Ioban Vi-Drape
  isolation
  Iso-Seal
  Kaycel towel
  lint-free
  Microban
  NeuroDrape surgical
  Opmi microscope
  Opraflex incise
  paper
  plastic
  povidone-iodine impregnated
  Sensability lubricated plastic sheet
    for breast self-examination
  shoulder
  Steri-Drape plastic incise
  sterile
  sterile paper
  3M skin
  U-drape
  Vi-Drape
draped out
drawing pin
drawtape
Dreiling tube
drenching sweat

Dressinet netting bandage
dressing (see also *bandage*; *packing*)
 ABD
 ABD pad
 absorbent gauze
 Accuzyme
 AcryDerm absorbent wound
 AcryDerm advanced wound
 AcryDerm border island
 AcryDerm hydrogel sheet
 AcryDerm Sheet
 AcryDerm Strands
 Acticoat burn
 ACU-derm wound
 Adaptic
 Adaptic X Xeroform gauze
  nonadhering
 Adcon-L
 Adcon-P
 adhesive
 adhesive tape
 Aeroplast
 AlgiDERM calcium alginate gel
 AlgiDERM alginate wound
 alginate wound
 AlgiSite alginate wound
 Algosteril alginate wound
 Alldress composite wound
 Allevyn hydrocellular foam
 Allevyn nonadherent
 Aloe Vesta protective ointment
 Alogsteril
 antiseptic
 Aquacel Hydrofiber
 Aquaphor
 Aquasorb hydrogel
 Aquasorb transparent hydrogel
 Arglaes antimicrobial barrier film
 ArtAssist compression
 Avitene "flour"
 Band-Aid
 Betadine
 Betadine-soaked Owen
 Bioclusive

dressing *(cont.)*
 Bioclusive transparent
 Biolex wound gel
 Biopatch foam wound
 BioPatch antimicrobial
 BlisterFilm transparent
 Blue Goo
 bolus
 BreakAway absorptive wound
 breast support
 bulky
 Bunnell
 Buro-Sol
 calcium alginate
 CaraKlenz
 carbohydrate polymer gel
 Cariel
 CarraFilm transparent film
 CarraGauze wound strips
 CarraSmart foam
 CarraSmart self-adhesive foam
 Carra Sorb H wound
 Carra Sorb M freeze-dried gel
 Carrasyn hydrogel wound
 Carrasyn V
 CicaCare topical gel sheeting
 cidofovir gel
 CircPlus compression
 Circulon
 Clean Seals
 ClearSite absorbent hydrogel wound
 ClearSite borderless
 ClearSite Hydro Gauze
 Coban
 cold compressive
 collagen-alginate wound
 collodion
 CombiDerm absorbent cover
 CombiDerm ACD
 Comfeel Plus
 Comfeel Purilon
 Comfeel Ulcus occlusive
 compression wrap
 compressive

dressing *(cont.)*
    Conform
    Conformant contact-layer wound
    corrective soft
    cotton
    Covaderm composite wound
    Covaderm Plus adhesive barrier
    Coverlet adhesive surgical
    Cover-Roll adhesive gauze
    Cryo/Cuff ankle
    Curaderm hydrocolloid
    Curafil hydrogel
    Curafoam foam wound
    Curagel hydrogel
    Curasol
    Curasorb calcium alginate
    Curity Oil emulsion
    Curity saline
    Dermabond
    Dermagran wound
    DermaMend foam wound
    DermaMend hydrogel
    DermaNet contact-layer wound
    DermaSorb
    DermAssist hydrocolloid
    DermAssist wound filling
    Dermatell hydrocolloid
    DiabGel hydrogel
    Domeboro powder
    Dome-Paste
    dry
    dry sterile
    DuoDerm CGF
    DuoDerm hydroactive gel
    DuoDerm SCB
    Dyna-Flex compression
    elastic salve
    elasticized gauze
    Elastikon
    Elastomull double-woven stretch
    Elastoplast
    Elta Dermal hydrogel
    ENTaxis nasal
    Epigard compositive wound

dressing *(cont.)*
    Epi-Lock wound
    epistaxis
    Esmarch
    Excilon sponge
    ExuDerm hydrocolloid
    Exu-Dry absorptive
    Fabco gauze bandage
    Fellonet ointment gauze
    felt
    Fibracol collagen-alginate
    Fibracol Plus collagen
    figure-of-8 (or figure-8)
    First Aid
    Flexinet
    Flexzan foam wound
    fluff
    foam gauze
    Forvade
    4 x 4 gauze
    4 x 8 gauze
    Fuller shield
    Furacin gauze
    FyBron alginate wound
    gauze
    Gentell alginate wound
    Gentell foam wound
    GeriMend
    Glasscock ear
    Greer goo
    Handages
    Hepafix
    hyCURE collagen hemostatic wound
    hyCURE G hydrogel
    HydraGran absorbent
    Hydrasorb foam wound
    Hydrofiber
    hydrogel
    hydrophilic powder
    hydrophilic semipermeable
        absorbent polyurethane foam
    HyFil hydrogel
    Hypafix
    Hypergel hydrogel

dressing *(cont.)*
Iamin
Iamin gel wound
iLEX skin
Inerpan flexible burn
Intelligent dressing
Interceed
Interceed TC7
IntraSite (graft T starch copolymer)
IntraSite gel
Iodoflex absorptive
iodoform gauze
Iodosorb absorptive
Irrijet DS
island
Jelonet (paraffin-soaked tulle)
Jobst breast support
Jones
Kalginate alginate wound
Kalginate calcium alginate
Kaltostat Fortex
Kaltostat wound packing material
Kerlix
Kling adhesive
Koch-Mason
LYOfoam A
LYOfoam C
LYOfoam T
LYOfoam tracheostomy
Maxorb alginate wound
Medifil collagen hemostatic wound
Medipore Dress-it surgical
Mepilex self-adherent foam
Mepitel contact-layer wound
Mepore absorptive
Merogel
Mesalt ribbon
Microfoam
Mills
Mitraflex
Mitraflex Plus
modified Robert Jones
moleskin strips
Montgomery strap

dressing *(cont.)*
Mother Jones (modified Robert Jones)
MPM hydrogel
Multidex hydrophilic powder
Multidex wound-filling material
No Sting Barrier Film
nonadherent gauze
nonadhesive
nonocclusive
Normigel hydrogel
Nu-Brede
NuDerm hydrocolloid
Nu Gauze sponge
Nu-Gel clear hydrogel wound
NUVO barrier film
Oasis wound
occlusive
O'Donoghue
Omiderm mesh
Omiderm plain
Omiderm transparent adhesive film
OpSite
OpSite Flexigrid transparent adhesive film
Optipore sponge
OsmoCyte PCA pillow wound
Owen gauze
palm-to-axilla
PanoPlex hydrogel
patch
Pedi-Boro Soak Packs
Peri-Strips Dry
Piliel hair
Pillo Pro
pledget
Polyderm foam wound
Polyderm hydrophilic polyurethane foam
Poly Mem
Polyskin II
pressure
Primaderm semipermeable foam
Primapore absorptive wound

dressing *(cont.)*
    Primer compression
    Pro-Clude transparent film wound
    ProCyte transparent adhesive film
    Proderm Topical
    Profore wound
    PSD Gel
    RepliCare hydrocolloid
    Repliderm collagen-based
    Repliderm wound
    Reston foam wound
    Reston hydrocolloid
    Restore
    rigid
    Robert Jones
    Robert Jones bulky soft
    Royl-Derm nonadherent wound
    SAF-Clens
    Saf-Gel hydrogel
    Scar Care
    Scarlet Red ointment
    SCB
    Schanz
    SeaSorb alginate wound
    2nd Skin wound
    Seprafilm bioresorbable membrane
    Shur-Clens
    SignaDress hydrocolloid
    Silastic
    silk mesh gauze
    Silon wound
    Silvadene (silver sulfadiazine)
    Silverlon wound packing strips
    SIS wound
    SiteGuard MVP transparent
        adhesive film
    SkinTegrity hydrogel
    Snugs
    Sof-Band bulky bandage
    Sof-Kling
    Sof-Rol
    SofSorb absorptive
    soft bulky
    SoftCloth absorptive

dressing *(cont.)*
    Sof-Wick sponge
    Solosite
    SoloSite wound gel
    SorbaView composite wound
    Sorbsan topical wound
    Spand-Gel
    Spyrogel hydrogel wound
    stent
    Stericare
    Steri-Strips
    sterile
    Stimson
    StrataSorb composite wound
    SurePress compression
    SureSite transparent adhesive film
    Surgicel
    Suture-Self
    Sween Prep skin
    Synthaderm occlusive wound
    SyringeAvitene
    TAB (tumescent absorbent bandage)
        wound
    Tegaderm
    Tegaderm HP
    Tegaderm transparent
    Tegagel hydrogel dressing and sheet
    Tegagen HG alginate wound
    Tegagen HI alginate wound
    Tegapore contact-layer wound
    Tegasorb
    Telfa
    Telfa gauze
    Telfa Plus
    Thera-Boot compression dressing
        or wrap
    THINSite with BioFilm hydrogel
        topical wound
    Tielle Plus absorbent adhesive
        dressing with multilayer structure
    tie-over
    toe-to-groin modified Jones
    Transeal transparent adhesive
    Transorbent multilayer

dressing *(cont.)*
   transparent
   transparent adhesive film
   transparent polyethylene
   Tubegauz
   Tubex gauze
   Tubigrip
   tumescent absorbent bandage (TAB)
   Ultec hydrocolloid
   UltraKlenz
   Ultrafera wound
   Ultrex
   Uniflex polyurethane adhesive
     surgical
   Uni-Site
   Unna-Flex compression
   Unna-Pak compression
   Vari/Moist wound
   Vaseline gauze
   Vaseline petrolatum
   Veingard transparent
   Velpeau
   Veni-Gard I.V. Stabilization
   Ventex wound
   Versalon
   Viasorb wound
   Vigilon occlusive
   Vitacuff
   Webril
   wet-to-dry
   wide-mesh petroleum gauze
   Wound Stick
   WoundSpan Bridge II
   Woun'Dres hydrogel
   Xeroflo
   Xeroflogauze
   Xeroform gauze
   Zipzoc stocking compression
dressing forceps
dressing scissors
DRG Sherlock threaded suture anchor
dried-out material
Driessen hinged plate
drifting spleen

Drilac dressing
drill
   Acra-Cut wire pass
   Adson twist
   air
   air-powered cutting
   Anspach power
   archimedean hand
   battery-driven hand
   biflanged
   Black and Decker
   bone
   Bosworth
   brace
   Bunnell hand
   cannulated
   Cebotome
   Cement Eater
   centering
   cervical
   Championnière bone
   Charnley centering
   Charnley femoral condyle
   Cherry-Austin
   Children's Hospital hand
   chuck
   Cloward
   Coballoy twist
   Codman wire pass
   Collison
   cortex
   cortical
   cranial
   Crutchfield hand
   Cushing flat
   Cushing perforator
   dental
   D'Errico perforating
   Elan-E power
   femoral condyle
   fingernail
   flat
   flex
   Gray bone

drill *(cont.)*
    Hall air
    Hall large-bore
    Hall Micro E
    Hall Surgairtome
    Hall Versipower
    hand
    hand-operated
    high-speed twist
    hip fracture compaction
    Hudson brace
    Hudson cranial
    Kirschner hand
    Kirschner wire
    Küntscher (Kuentscher)
    Mam
    Mathews hand
    McKenzie perforating twist
    MicroAire
    microsurgery
    Mira Mark III cranial
    Moore hand
    Osteone air
    otologic
    patellar
    Pease bone
    penetrating
    Penn fingernail
    perforating twist
    Phoenix cranial
    Pilot
    pneumatic
    Ralk hand
    Raney cranial
    Raney perforator
    right-angle dental
    Shea
    Smedberg hand
    Smedberg twist
    Smith automatic perforator
    Smith cranial
    spiral
    step
    Stille bone
    Stille cranial

drill *(cont.)*
    Stille hand
    Stille-Sherman bone
    Stryker microsurgery
    subchondral
    Synthes
    Toti trephine
    Treace
    trephine
    Trinkle
    twist
    wire
    wire pass
    Xomed
    Zimmer hand
drill bit
    cannulated
    hip fracture compaction
    Howmedica Microfixation System
    Leibinger Micro System
    Luhr Microfixation System
    Storz Microsystems
    Synthes Microsystems
drill blade
drill bushing
drill flat
drill guide
    ACL (anterior cruciate ligament)
    Adson
    neutral and load
drill hole
drill pin
drill point
    cannulated
    carbon steel
    Crutchfield
    Raney-Crutchfield
    Stille
drill/reamer, MicroAire
drill set, Hudson cranial
drill trephine
drinker
    binge
    social
    weekend

drinking habits
drip infusion cholangiography (DIC)
Drisite brand fabric reinforcement
driver
    blade plate
    bullet
    Flatt
    Hall
    Harrington hook
    Jewett
    Küntscher (Kuentscher) nail
    K-wire
    Linvatec
    Lloyd nail
    Massie
    Micro Series wire
    nail
    Orthoairtome wire
    Paramax angled
    plate
    power
    prosthesis
    staple
    supine position
    Sven-Johansson
    Teflon-coated
driver-bender-extractor, Rush
driver-extractor
    Hansen-Street
    Ken
    McReynolds
    Sage
    Schneider
    Zimmer
driving the camera
droloxifene
dromedary kidney
dronabinol
drop test
droperidol
droplet infection
drotaverine
drowned lung
drug antagonism

drug cessation
drug class
    aminosterol
    antacid
    anthelmintic
    anticholinergic
    antiemetic
    antihyperglycemic
    antihypertensive
    antinauseant
    antineoplastic
    antisecretory
    antispasmodic
    aperient
    aperitive
    ATPase (adenosine triphosphatase)
        inhibitors
    bacteriostatic
    benzodiazepine
    bile acid sequestrant
    bowel evacuant
    carminative
    cathartic
    cholagogue
    counterirritant
    COX-2 inhibitor
    digestant
    digestive enzyme
    discutient
    emetic
    5-hydroxytryptamine (5-HT)
        receptor antagonist
    fluoropyrimidine
    general anesthetic
    H_2 blocker
    hemorroidal agent
    hemostatic
    hepatics
    hydragogue
    hydrocholeretic
    immunizing agent
    immunosuppressant
    laxative
    local anesthetic

drug class *(cont.)*
  plasma expander
  proliferation signal inhibitor
  proton pump inhibitor
  purgative
  SSRI (selective serotonin reuptake
    inhibitor)
  substituted benzimidazole
  sulfonylurea
  taeniacide
  taxane, taxoid
  theraccine
  thiazolidinedione
  vaccine
  vermicide; vermifuge
  vulnerary
drug fever
drug-induced cholestasis
drug-induced constipation
drug-induced gastritis
drug-induced hepatitis
drug-induced steatosis
drug metabolism
drug-metabolizing enzyme (DME)
drug toxicity
Drummond hook
Drummond, marginal artery of
Drummond syndrome
DRx (Digital Response)
dry colostomy
dry dressing
dry heaves (retching)
dry necrosis
dry sterile dressing
dry swallow on esophageal manometry
dry vomiting
DSC; DSCG (disodium cromoglycate)
DSMC Plus (casanthranol; docusate
  potassium)
DSRS (distal splenorenal shunt)
D-S-S (docusate sodium)
DST (donor-specific transfusion)
DST&G (doubled semitendinosus and
  gracilis) autograft

DTAFA (descending thoracic aorta-
  to-femoral artery) bypass graft
D-thyroxine
D-TRON insulin delivery pump
DTRs (deep tendon reflexes)
DTT (dynamic transverse traction) hook
dual-cup grasping forceps, double-
  action
dual irrigation adapter
DualMesh biomaterial graft
dual onlay bone graft
dual phase spiral CT scan
dual plate
dual tracer imaging
Dubecq-Princeteau angulating needle
  holder
Dubin and Amelar classification
  of varicoceles
Dubin-Johnson syndrome
Dubin-Sprinz disease
Dubin-Sprinz syndrome
Dubois scissors
duckbill forceps
duckbill elevator
duckbill forceps
duckbill rongeur
duck nose micrograsper
duct
  accessory pancreatic
  beaded hepatic
  common bile (CBD)
  common hepatic
  cystic
  distal bile
  ductal
  extrahepatic bile
  extrahepatic biliary
  fusiform widening of
  gall
  hepatic (right and left)
  Hering
  interlobular bile
  intrahepatic
  intrahepatic bile

duct *(cont.)*
   intrahepatic biliary
   lactiferous
   main pancreatic (MPD)
   middle extrahepatic bile
   normal caliber
   omphalomesenteric
   pancreatic
   perilobular
   preampullary portion of bile
   prepapillary bile
   subvesical
   terminal bile
   thyroglossal
   vitelline
   vitellointestinal
ductal calculus
ductal carcinoma
ductal carcinoma in situ (DCIS)
ductal carcinoma of prostate
ductal dilatation
ductal dilation
ductal duct
ductal ectasia of breast
ductal epithelium
ductal irregularities with dilation and
   stenosis
ductal obstruction
ductal proliferation
duct cell carcinoma
duct ectasia
duct lesion
ductless gland
duct lumen
duct of Luschka
duct of Santorini
duct of Wirsung
ductogram, mammary
ductography, direct contrast
duct papilloma
duct-to-duct anastomosis
ductus arteriosum
Duecollement hemicolectomy
Duecollement maneuver

Duet glucose monitor
Duette catheter
Duffield scissors
Duhamel colon operation
Duhamel laparoscopic pull-through
   procedure
Duke bleeding time (BT)
Duke cannula
Dukes Astler-Coller modified staging
   system
Duke trocar
Dulcagen (bisacodyl)
Dulcolax (bisacodyl)
Dulcolax Bowel Prep Kit (bisacodyl)
dullness
   hepatic
   liver
   shifting
   splenic
   tympanitic
dullness to percussion
dull pain
dull purple lung
dull right upper quadrant pain
dumbbell-shaped shadow
dummy seed catheter
Dumon-Gilliard prosthesis introducer
Dumon-Gilliard prosthesis pushing tube
Dumont dissecting forceps
Dumont microdissecting forceps
dumping stomach
dumping syndrome
Duncan disease
Dunhill artery forceps
Dunlop-Shands view
Dunn biopsy
duodenal aspirate
duodenal atresia
duodenal bubble
duodenal bulb
duodenal bulb apex
duodenal bulb deformity
duodenal cap
duodenal C-loop

duodenal contents examination
duodenal decompression
duodenal diversion
duodenal end of dorsal pancreatic duct
duodenal end of main pancreatic duct
duodenal erosion
duodenal fistula
duodenal fold
duodenal fossa
duodenal gland
duodenal ileus
duodenal impression on liver
duodenal ligament
duodenal loop
duodenal lumen
duodenal mucosal cells
duodenal papilla
duodenal perforation
duodenal polyp
duodenal recess
duodenal rupture
duodenal scarring
duodenal seromyectomy
duodenal sphincter
duodenal string test
duodenal stump
duodenal sweep
duodenal switch
duodenal terminus
duodenal ulcer
duodenal ulcer disease
duodenal ulcer perforation (DUP)
duodenal ulceration
duodenal vein
duodenal villi
duodenal wall hamartoma
duodenal web
duodenitis
   chronic atrophic
   erosive
duodenobiliary pressure gradient
duodenobiliary reflux
duodenocolic fistula
duodenoenterostomy

duodenogastric reflux (DGR)
duodenogastroscopy, retrograde (RDG)
duodenoileal bypass
duodenoileitis
duodenojejunal angle
duodenojejunal flexure
duodenojejunal fold
duodenojejunal fossa
duodenojejunal junction (DJJ)
duodenojejunal recess
duodenojejunal sphincter
duodenojejunostomy
duodenomesocolic fold
duodenopancreatic reflux
duodenorenal ligament
duodenoscope (see also *endoscope*)
   Fujinon EVD-XL video
   master
   MIS Source
   Olympus
   Olympus JF-1T20 flexible
     therapeutic
   Olympus JF-1T30 flexible
     therapeutic
   Olympus JF-V10 video
   Olympus JTI-T10
   Olympus PJF-7.5 pediatric duodeno-
     fiberscope
   Olympus TJF-160F video
   Olympus TJF-V10
   Pentax ED-3430T video
   Pentax ED-3440T video
   Pentax FD-34V fiberoptic
   two-channel
   transverse
duodenum
   C-loop of
   curve of
   descending
   distal
   scarified
   supravaterian
   suspensory muscle of
duodenum deformed by scarring

DuoDerm CGF (control gel formula)
  dressing
DuoDerm dressing
DuoDerm SCB (sustained compression
  bandage) dressing
Duopress guide
Duopress plate
DUP (duodenal ulcer perforation)
Du Pen epidural catheter
Du Pen long-term epidural catheter
Duphalac (lactulose)
duplex kidney
duplication cyst
DuPont Cronex x-ray film
Duraclon (clonidine hydrochloride
  injection)
Duraclose clip applier
DuraGen graft
Duragesic-25 (fentanyl) transdermal
  patches
DURAglide stone removal balloon
DURAglide3 stone removal balloon
Duralap J-hook
Duralap Metzenbaum scissors
dural elevator
dural graft
dural hook
dural knife
dural needle
Duralone-40 (methylprednisolone
  acetate)
Duralon occlusion balloon
dural punch
dural retractor
dural scissors
dural tack-up suture
dural tenting suture
dural traction suture
Duramorph (morphine sulfate)
Duranest MPF (etidocaine; epinephrine)
Durapatite graft
Duraprep kit
dura-protecting forceps
duration of loop formation

Duray-Read gouge
Durelast bandage
Duret lesion
Durham dissector
Durham retractor
Durmarker
Durmont-style dissecting forceps
Duros implant
duskiness, stomal
dusky cyanosis
dusky medulla
dusky stoma
dust-borne infection
duToit staple
Duval clamp
Duval distal (caudal) pancreatico-
  jejunostomy
Duval elevator
Duval-Scheie hemorrhoidal forceps
Duval tissue-grasping forceps
Duverney gland
DuVries incision
DVP flush shunt
DVT (deep vein [venous] thrombosis)
dwarfism
    achondroplastic
    cretin
    diastrophic
    Lorain-Levi
    pituitary
Dwyer-Hall plate
D-xylose absorption test
Dyclone (dyclonine HCl)
dyclonine HCl (Dyclone)
dye (see also *stain*)
    Congo red
    Evans blue
    indigo carmine
    Lymphazurin
    methylene blue
    radiopaque
    rapid emptying of
dye laser
dye spraying

dye worker's cancer
dymanthine HCl
dimantine HCl
Dymelor (acetohexamide)
Dymenate (dimenhydrinate)
Dyna-Flex compression dressing
Dyna-Flex compression wrap
Dynalink self-expanding biliary stent
   system
   lipolytic
   liver
   liver phosphorylase
   medium chain acyl-CoA
     dehydrogenase
   pancreatic
   protease digestive
   proteinase
   proteolytic
   serum liver
dynamic compression (DCP) plate
DynamicDeca steerable catheter
dynamic graciloplasty
dynamic ileus
dynamic locking nail
Dynamic Optical Breast Imaging
   System (DOBI)
Dynamic PACSPlus
dynamic pharyngeal radiography
dynamic/spastic ileus
dynamic stress x-ray view
dynamometer, Collin
Dynarex
DynaStat surgical hemostatic
DynaWell
dynograph
Dyonics arthroscopic blade
Dyonics cannula
Dyonics cystoscope
Dyonics laparoscope system
Dyonics rod-lens endoscope
Dyonics Vision 325z endoscope camera
Dyonics 0° 10 mm rigid laparoscope
Dyonics 7208130 rigid laparoscope
Dyonics 8007 rigid laparoscope

DyoVac suction punch
dysarthria
dyschezia
dysenteric algid malaria
dysenteric diarrhea
dysentery, bacillary
dysentery bacillus
dysfunction
   bone marrow
   endocrine
   gastrointestinal
   hepatocyte
   multiorgan
   neuroimmune
   peristaltic
   polyglandular
   sphincter of Oddi
   stress-induced organ
dysfunctional uterine bleeding (DUB)
dysgenesis, anorectal
dysimmunity
dyskinesia
   bile duct
   biliary
   esophageal
dysmotility
   esophageal
   generalized gut
   gut
   small intestinal
dyspepsia
   acid
   biliary cholelithic
   flatulent
   functional
   gastric
   nonorganic
   nonulcer
   postcholecystectomy flatulent
   ulcer-like
dyspeptic symptoms
dysphagia
   contractile ring
   esophageal

dysphagia *(cont.)*
  intermittent
  liquid food
  oropharyngeal
  postfundoplication
  postoperative
  postvagotomy
  pre-esophageal
  progressive
  sideropenic
  soft food
  solid food
  vallecular
dysphagia lusoria
dysphagia nervosa
dysphagic
dyspituitarism

dysplasia
  anal squamous
  arteriohepatic
  bilateral nodular
  caudal
  epithelial
  focus of hepatocyte
  high-grade
  mammary
  polypoid
dysplasia with associated lesion or mass
  (DALM)
dysplastic lesion
dysproteinemia, familial
dysrrhythmia, gastric
dyssynergia
dyssynergic esophagus
dystrophy, adiposogenital

E, e

EAC (expandable access catheter)
EAEC (enteroadherent *E. coli*)
Eagle-Barrett syndrome (prune-belly syndrome)
eagle's beak bone-cutting forceps
ear and endaural instruments
ear blade
ear forceps
Earle hemorrhoid clamp
Earle rectal probe
ear loop
early appendicitis
early gastric cancer (EGC)
early ligation of venous drainage
early menarche
early menopause
early postoperative complication
early recurrence
early satiety
Early Treatment Diabetic Retinopathy Study
early zoster
ear packing sponge
ear wick sponge
Easi-Lav
easily reducible hernia
EASL (European Association for the Study of the Liver)

Eastern Cooperative Oncology Group (ECOG)
East-West retractor
Easy A1$_c$ test
easy bruisability
easy fatigability
EasySafe disposable syringe
Eating Attitudes Test
eating habits
Eaton agent
EBA (extrahepatic biliary atresia)
EBCT (electron-beam computed tomography)
Ebner gland
EBL (endoscopic band ligation)
EBL (estimated blood loss)
Ebstein lesion
EBV (Epstein-Barr virus) infection
EBVS (EBV susceptibility)
ECA (enterobacterial common antigen)
E-CABG (endoscopic coronary artery bypass graft)
E-cadherin expression test for classification of breast carcinoma
E.CAM+ coincidence-imaging
E.CAM dual-head emission imaging system
eccentric drill guide

eccentric dynamic compression
   (EDCP) plate
eccentric lesion
eccentric restenosis lesion
eccentrically
ecchymosis (pl. ecchymoses)
ecchymosis of inguinal ligament
ecchymosis, perineal
ecchymotic
eccrine carcinoma
echinococcal cyst
echinococcal cyst disease
echinococciasis
Echinococcus granulosus
Echinococcus multilocularis
Echinococcus liver cyst
Echlin bone rongeur
Echlin duckbill rongeur
Echlin laminectomy rongeur
Echlin-Luer rongeur
Echlin rongeur forceps
ECHO (enterocytopathogenic human
   orphan) virus infection
echocolonoscope (see *colonoscope*)
echoendoscope (see *endoscope*)
echogastroscope (see *gastroscope*)
EchoGen (perflenapent)
echogenic liver
Echols retractor
EchoMark catheter
Eck fistula
Eckhoff mapping pen
Eckhout vertical gastroplasty
ECL (enterochromaffin-like) cell
Eclipse TMR laser
ECOG (Eastern Cooperative Oncology
   Group) performance status
E. coli 0157:H7 pathogen
E. coli serotype O157:H7
E Cotton bandage
Ecotrin
ectasia
   duct
   ductal (of breast)

ectasia *(cont.)*
   mammary ductal
   vascular
ectatic aneurysm
ecthyma, contagious
ecthyma gangrenosum
ectodermal cells of neural crest origin
ectopic ACTH syndrome
ectopic antidiuretic hormone secretion
ectopic anus
ectopic cortisol-producing tumor
ectopic gastric mucosa
ectopic hormone production
ectopic hyperinsulinism
ectopic hyperparathyroidism
ectopic midline thyroid tissue
ectopic pancreatic tissue
ectopic placement of thyroid tissue
   in the tongue
ectopic pregnancy
ectopic spleen
ectopic testis
ectopic thyroid nodule
edema
   ambulant
   angioneurotic
   antral
   bronchiolar
   bronze
   bullous-like
   cardiac
   cerebral
   dependent
   epithelial
   focal
   generalized (anasarca)
   gestational
   heat
   hereditary angioneurotic
   ileocecal
   inflammatory
   laryngeal
   local
   lymphatic

eflornithine
Egan mammography
EGC (early gastric cancer)
EGD (esophagogastroduodenoscopy)
EGF (epidermal growth factor)
EGG (electrogastrogram)
Eggers bone plate
EG (esophagogastric) junction
EGS Model 100 electrogalvanic
    stimulator
EGTA (esophageal gastric tube airways)
Egyptian splenomegaly
EHEC (enterohemorrhagic *E. coli*)
EHL (electrohydraulic lithotripsy)
Ehlers-Danlos syndrome
EHM (extrahepatic metastasis)
ehrlichial infection, human, Sennetsu
    type
EHT (electrohydrothermo) electrode
EIA-2 (enzyme-linked immunoassay)
EIC (extensive intraductal carcinoma)
eicosapentaenoic acid
EIEC (enteroinvasive *E. coli*)
eight-lumen esophageal manometry
    catheter
Eikenella corrodens (formerly
    Bacteroides corrodens, HB-1)
Einhorn dilator
Einhorn string test
EIT (endoscopic injection therapy)
ELAD (extracorporeal liver assist
    device)
Elan-E power drill
Elase (fibrinolysin; desoxyribonuclease)
Elastase
elastic band ligation
elastic bandage
elastic ligature
elastic salve dressing
elastic stable intramedullary nail (ESIN)
elastic wrap bandage
Elastic Foam bandage
elasticized gauze dressing
Elastikon dressing
Elastikon elastic tape

elastomer bandage
Elastomull bandage
Elastomull double-woven stretch
    dressing
Elastoplast bandage
Elastoplast dressing
ELCA laser
Elder Helio cystoscope
Eldisine (vindesine sulfate)
elective herniorrhaphy
elective lymph node dissection
elective shunt procedure
elective sigmoid resection
elective surgical procedure
electrical impedance breast scanning
    system
electrical neutrality
electrical shock
electric anesthesia
electric cast saw
electrocautery
    bipolar
    Bovie
    Bugbee
    EndoClip
    Fine
    hook
    low-current
    monopolar
    multipolar
    needle-tip
    needlepoint
    Neoflex bendable
    Ultrashear
    Valleylab
electrocautery knife
electrocautery pencil
electrochemical glucose-monitoring
    test strip
electrocoagulating biopsy forceps
electrocoagulation
    bipolar
    monopolar
    transendoscopic
electrocoagulator (see *coagulator*)

electrode
    ACMI monopolar
    Aspen laparoscopy
    ball-tip
    BiLAP bipolar needle
    Bugfee
    button
    Cameron-Miller
    coagulation
    Coaguloop resection
    concentric-needle
    Corson needle
    EHT (electrohydrothermo)
    glass pH
    J-hook
    L-diamond
    L-wedge
    Mitek VAPR™ T thermal
    Salinetrode
    short spatula
    SingleBAR
    SilverBullet
    single-fiber EMG
    spatula
    spoon
    square-L
    StarBAR
    suction irrigation (SIE)
    surface
electrode and probe
electrode introducer
electrode pad
electrodesiccation of tumor
electrogalvanic stimulator
electrogastrogram (EGG)
electrogastrography
electrohydraulic lithotripsy (EHL)
electrohydraulic probe
Electrolase
electrolyte abnormality
electrolyte balance
electrolyte concentration
electrolyte disturbance
electrolyte imbalance

electrolyte losses
electrolyte management
electrolyte panel
    bicarbonate (bicarb) (HCO_3^-)
    calcium (Ca)
    chloride (Cl^-)
    CO_2
    potassium (K)
    sodium (Na)
electrolyte solution, polyethylene glycol
electrolyte, stool
electrolyte therapy
    Multilyte-40
    Normosol-M and 5% Dextrose
    Normosol-R and 5% Dextrose
    Normosol-R, Normosol-R pH 7.4
    Nutrilyte II
    Plasma-Lyte A pH 7.4
    Plasma-Lyte R
    Plasma-Lyte 56
    Plasma-Lyte 148
    Rehydralyte
    Resol
    Ringer injection
    Ringer injection, lactated
electrolyte-polyethylene glycol lavage
    solution
electrolyzed acid water
electromagnetic focusing field (EFF)
    probe
electromechanical coupling
electromechanical dissociation and
    gastroparesis
electromyogram, electromyography
    (EMG)
    colonic
    conventional concentric
    pelvic floor
    single-fiber
    ureteral
electron accelerator, Mobetron
electron-beam computed tomography
    (EBCT)
electronic microscopy

electrophoresis
  hemoglobin
  pulsed-field gel
  serum protein
ElectroProbe
Electroscope disposable laparoscopic
  scissors
Electrosurgery Insulation Test Set
electrosurgical cutting knife
electrosurgical desiccation
electrosurgical pencil
electrosurgical snare polypectomy
electrosurgical therapy
electrosurgical unit (see *cautery; cutter;*
  dissector; knife)
elemental diet
elevated alkaline phosphatase
elevated alpha-fetoprotein
elevated bilirubin
elevated BUN
elevated ESR
elevated LFTs
elevated pancreatic tumor markers
elevated plasma basal calcitonin level
elevated plasma stimulated calcitonin
  level
elevated portal pressure
elevated reticulocyte count
elevated serum calcitonin
elevated total serum T_4
elevated WBC
elevating spoon
elevation of anterior abdominal wall
elevation of head of the bed
elevation of right hemidiaphragm
elevator
  Adson periosteal
  angular
  Aufranc periosteal
  Bennett bone
  Bethune periosteal
  Blair
  blunt
  bone

elevator *(cont.)*
  Bowen periosteal
  Boyle uterine
  Bristow periosteal
  Brophy periosteal
  Buck
  Buck periosteal
  Cameron-Haight periosteal
  Campbell periosteal
  Carroll-Legg periosteal
  Chandler bone
  Cheyne periosteal
  chisel edge
  Cloward osteophyte
  Cloward periosteal
  Cobb periosteal
  Cobb spinal
  Cohen periosteal
  Converse periosteal
  Coryllos-Doyen periosteal
  Cottle-MacKenty
  Crawford dural
  Crego
  curved periosteal
  Cushing-Hopkins periosteal
  Cushing Little Joker
  Cushing periosteal
  Cushing pituitary
  Cushing staphylorrhaphy
  Darrach
  Davidson-Sauerbruch-Doyen
    periosteal
  Dawson-Yuhl-Key
  Dawson-Yuhl periosteal
  D'Errico periosteal
  Doyen costal
  Doyen rib
  duckbill
  dural
  Duval
  Endotrac
  Farabeuf periosteal
  flat narrow
  Fomon periosteal

elevator *(cont.)*
    Forman nasal
    fracture-reducing
    Frazier dural
    Freer periosteal
    Freer septal
    Freer septum
    Gardner
    Guilford-Wright duckbill
    Hajek-Ballenger septal
    hand
    Harrington spinal
    Henahan
    Herczel rib
    Hibbs chisel
    Hoen periosteal
    House endaural
    House stapes
    Iowa University periosteal
    Jannetta duckbill
    joker periosteal
    Joseph periosteal
    J periosteal
    Kahre-Williger periosteal
    Kennerdell-Maroon
    Key periosteal
    Kirmission periosteal
    Kleinert-Kutz periosteal
    Kocher
    Lambotte
    lamina
    Lane
    Lane periosteal
    Langenbeck
    Langenbeck periosteal
    Lempert narrow
    Lempert periosteal
    Lewis periosteal
    liberator
    Locke
    Love-Adson periosteal
    lumbosacral fusion
    M.H.G.
    MacKenty periosteal

elevator *(cont.)*
    Malis
    Matson-Alexander
    Matson rib
    McGlamry
    Mead periosteal
    Molt periosteal
    Moore bone
    nasal
    OSI Extremity
    osteophyte
    Paparella duckbill
    Penfield
    periosteal
    Phemister
    Presbyterian Hospital staphylor-
        rhaphy
    Ray-Parsons-Sunday staphylor-
        rhaphy
    Rhoton
    rib
    Rish periosteal
    Roberts-Gill periosteal
    Rochester lamina
    Rochester spinal
    Rosen
    round-tapped periosteal
    Sauerbruch rib
    Sayre
    Sayre periosteal
    Scott-McCracken periosteal
    Sebileau periosteal
    Sedillot periosteal
    septal
    Shambaugh-Derlacki duckbill
    Shambaugh narrow
    Sheffield hand
    Sisson fracture reducing
    spinal
    staphylorrhaphy
    Stille
    straight periosteal
    Sunday staphylorrhaphy
    Swanson

elevator *(cont.)*
  Tabb
  Take-Apart
  Tegtmeier
  Tenzel
  T handle
  Tronzo
  von Langenbeck periosteal
  Ward periosteal
  Wiberg periosteal
  wide periosteal
  Willauer-Gibbon periosteal
  Williger periosteal
  Woodson
  Yankauer periosteal
  Yasargil
elevator dissector
elimination diet
elimination of stool
ELISA (enzyme-linked immunosorbent assay)
ELISA buffer
ELISA IgG
ELISA titer; ELISA-3 titer
Elite Farley retractor
Ellence (epirubicin hydrochloride)
Elliot forceps
Elliott B solution
Elliott femoral condyle blade plate
Elliott gallbladder forceps
elliptical incision
ElMed rigid laparoscope
Elmor tissue morcellator
Elmore radiofrequency tissue morcellator
elongated colon
elongated mass
elongate pattern
elongated PR interval
Eloxatin (oxaliplatin)
Elsberg brain cannula
Elsberg ventricular cannula
Elta Dermal hydrogel dressing
Elta gauze dressing

Elta wound cleanser
Eltroxin (levothyroxine sodium)
Elucigene test
embalming fluid
embarrassment, circulatory
embolic mesenteric infarction
embolic necrosis
embolism
  air
  amniotic fluid
  arterial missile
  bile pulmonary
  gas
  mesenteric
  multiple
  pulmonary
  shotgun pellet
  tumor
embolization
  angiographic variceal
  transcatheter variceal
  transhepatic (THE)
embolization of bleeding vessel
embolize bleeding vessel
embolus, massive pulmonary
embryological line
embryological remnant of the third pharyngeal pouch
embryonal cell carcinoma
embryonal tumor of neural crest origin
embryonic cell transplantation
embryonic chromaffin cells
embryotomy scissors
Emdogain enamel matrix protein
Emerald drape
Emerald fabric
emergency appendectomy
emergency intubation
emergency laparotomy
emergency operation
emergency tracheostomy
emergent appendectomy
emergent endoscopic sclerotherapy
emergent herniorrhaphy

emergent operation
emergent surgery
emesis (see *vomiting*)
   coffee-grounds
   gagging without
   induction of
   retching of
   retching without
Emete-con
emetic reflex
Emetrol (fructose, dextrose, and
   phosphoric acid)
EMG (electromyogram) needle
Emit 2000 cyclosporine specific assay
Emitasol (metoclopramide) nasal spray
emitefur
Emmett cotton swab forceps
Emmett fistula hook
Emmett tenaculum hook
emollient laxative
emphysema, subcutaneous
emphysematous cholecystitis
emphysematous gastritis
emphysematous lung
empiric antibiotic regimen
empirical diagnosis
empirical therapy
emptying
   delayed gastric
   gallbladder
   gastric
empyema of gallbladder
EMR (endoscopic mucosal resection)
   suction cap method
EMT emergency medicine tube
emulsification
emulsified perflubron blood substitute
emulsion
   intravenous fat
   lipid
Emulsoil
EN (enteral nutrition)
enamel crypt
enamel matrix protein for wound
   healing

ENANB (enterically transmitted non-A,
   non-B) hepatitis (former name)
en bloc augmentation mammoplasty
en bloc axillary node dissection
en bloc distal pancreatectomy
en bloc resection
en bloc splenectomy
en bloc vein resection
Encapslon catheter
encapsulated brain abscess
encapsulated breast implant
encapsulated fluid collection
encapsulated mass
encapsulated neoplasm
encapsulated nodule
encasement of splenic vein
encephaloid gastric carcinoma
encephalomyocarditis virus
encephalomyopathy, subacute necro-
   tizing
encephalopathy
   bilirubin
   hepatic (HE)
   portal-systemic (PSE)
   portosystemic (PSE)
   post-shunt
   Wernicke
encircled
encircling
encopresis
encroachment of tumor
endamebic abscess
endarterectomy scissors
endarterectomy shunt
endaural instrument
endaural retractor
end-biting forceps
end colostomy
end-cutting reciprocating saw
end-diastolic volume
endemic (colloid) goiter
endemic cretinism
endemic goiter
endemic nonbacterial gastroenteritis

Ender awl
Ender flexible medullary nail
Ender pin
Ender rod
end-expiratory pressure
end expiration
End-Flo laparoscopic irrigating system
end ileostomy
Endius endoscope
Endius spinal endoscopic camera
    endoscope
end-loop colostomy
end-loop ileocolostomy
end-loop ileostomy
Endo-AID suction irrigation
EndoALPHA integrated endosurgical
    system
endoanal coil
endoanal ultrasound
Endo Avitene hemostatic agent
Endo Babcock clamp
Endo Babcock surgical grasper
Endobag laparoscopic specimen
    retrieval system
endobiliary stent
endobiliary stenting
endobrachyesophagus
endobronchial fistula
endobronchial lesion
EndoCab ELISA
EndoCab enzyme linked immuno-
    sorbent assay (ELISA)
endocardial tumor
ENDOcare nitinol stent (urinary)
Endo Catch specimen retrieval bag
endocervical mucosa
Endocet (oxycodone/acetaminophen)
Endo Cinch laparoscopic grasper
Endo Cinch suturing system
endoclip, absorbable
Endo Clip laparoscopic clip applicator
Endo Close surgical stapler
Endocodone (oxycodone hydrochloride)
EndoCoil biliary stent

EndoCoil esophageal stent
EndoCPB (endovascular cardio-
    pulmonary bypass) catheter
endocrine dysfunction
endocrine function
endocrine gland
endocrine pancreas hormone
endocrine pathology
endocrine therapy
endocrine tumor of the pancreas
endocrinopathy
Endocut cautery device
Endodan (oxycodone/oxycodone
    terephthalate/aspirin)
endodermal
Endo Dissect laparoscopic instruments
endoesophageal probe
endoesophageal tube
Endo-Flex balloon dilator
Endo-Flo irrigation system
Endo-Flo probe
end-of-treatment response
Endo-Gauge
endogenous bacteria
endogenous infection
endogenous inflammatory mediator
    production
endogenous insulin
endogenous obesity
endogenous parathyroid hormone
endogenous TSH stimulation
Endo GIA suture stapler
Endo GIA II stapler
Endo Grasp laparoscopic forceps
Endo Grasp roticulator
Endo Hernia clip applier
Endo Hernia surgical stapler
Endo Hernia Universal stapler
Endoknot suture needle
Endolap laparoscope
Endolap rigid laparoscope
Endolase laparoscope
Endolase rigid laparoscope
Endolav lavage pump

Endoloop disposable chromic ligature
   suture instrument
Endoloop ligature
Endoloop suture
Endo Lumenal gastroplication device
EndoLumina bougie
EndoLumina II transillumination
   system
endoluminal ultrasound (EUS)
Endo Lung device
endolymphatic sac
endolymphatic shunt
EndoMate camera
EndoMate Grab Bag endoscopic
   specimen retrieval bag
EndoMed laparoscopic systems
EndoMed LSS laparoscopic system
endometrial carcinoma
endometrial polyp
endometrial resection and ablation
   (ERA) resectoscope sheath
endometrial stromal sarcoma
endometriosis
endometritis
Endopath circular stapler
Endopath curved intraluminal stapler
Endopath EMS hernia stapler
Endopath ES reusable endoscopic
   stapler
Endopath ETS-FLEX endoscopic
   articulating linear cutter
Endopath EZ-RF linear cutter
   and coagulation device
Endopath EZ45 endoscopic linear
   cutter
Endopath EZ45 No Knife endoscopic
   linear stapler
Endopath EZ46 No Knife endoscopic
   linear stapler
Endopath laparoscopic trocar
Endopath linear cutter
Endopath multifeed stapler
Endopath no-knife stapler
Endopath Optiview optical surgical
   obturator

Endopath TriStar trocar
Endopath trocar
Endopath Ultra Veress needle
endopelvic fascia
endophlebitis hepatica obliterans
Endopouch Pro specimen bag
Endo-P-Probe for endorectal ultra-
   sonography
endoprosthesis (see also *prosthesis*)
   biliary
   double-lumen
   double-pigtail
   IntraStent Double Strut biliary
   IntraStent Double Strut XS
   IntraStent LP biliary
   large-bore bile duct
   Medoc-Celestin
   Procter-Livingstone
   Wallstent enteral
   Wilson-Cook
endorectal ileal pouch
endorectal ileal pull-through
endorectal pull-through procedure
Endo Retract
end-organ response
Endosac specimen bag
endoscope (see also *endoscopy*)
   ACMI rigid laparoscope
   ACMI S3565 flexible sigmoidoscope
   Adler Eagle Vision laparoscope
   Adler P.L.U.S. laparoscope
   adult endoscope
   AESOP (Automated Endoscopic
      System for Optimal Positioning)
   AESOP 2000; 3000
   AngioLaz Medi-Vu endoscope
   anoscope (proctoscope)
   Arthrotek rigid laparoscope
   Baho endoscope
   Bard flexible endoscope
   borescope
   Boutin thoracoscope
   bronchoscope
   Bryan rigid laparoscope

endoscope *(cont.)*
   Buie sigmoidoscope
   Cabot cystoscope
   Cabot rigid laparoscope
   CF-200Z Olympus colonoscope
   CF-UM3 echocolonoscope
   Cho/Dyonics two-portal endoscopic system
   choledochofiberscope
   Circon rigid laparoscope
   Circon videohydrothoracoscope
   colonoscope
   Comeg rigid laparoscope
   Concept/Linvatec hysteroscope
   Concept/Linvatec laparoscope
   Concept rigid laparoscope
   Cooper Surgical cystoscope
   Cor/Tek laparoscope
   Cuda 0° 10 mm rigid laparoscope
   cystoscope
   Czaja-McCaffrey rigid laparoscope
   Demir rigid laparoscope
   Desormaux endoscope
   double-channel endoscope
   double-puncture laparoscope
   duodenoscope
   Dyonics cystoscope
   Dyonics laparoscope
   Dyonics rod-lens endoscope
   Dyonics 3625 laparoscope
   Dyonics 7208130 rigid laparoscope
   Dyonics 8007 rigid laparoscope
   Dyonics 8017 laparoscope
   Dyonics 0° 10 mm rigid laparoscope
   echocolonoscope
   echogastroscope
   Eder 180° 10 mm rigid laparoscope
   Effner/Arthrotek laparoscope
   Effner rigid laparoscope
   Elder Helio cystoscope
   ElMed rigid laparoscope
   Endius spinal endoscopic camera
   EndoALPHA integrated end surgical system

endoscope *(cont.)*
   Endolap rigid laparoscope
   Endolase rigid laparoscope
   endometrial resection and ablation (ERA) resectoscope sheath
   enteroscope
   esophagoscope
   EVII endoscopic video system
   Fansler-Ives anoscope
   FCS-ML gastroscope
   fiberoptic choledochoscope
   fiberoptic gastroscope
   fiberoptic laryngoscope
   fiberoptic sigmoidoscope
   fiberscope
   flexible sigmoidoscope
   flexible, steerable nasolaryngopharyngoscope
   Fujinon EVS-E flexible sigmoidoscope
   Fujinon FG-100FP flexible gastroscope
   Fujinon FG-100PE flexible gastroscope
   Fujinon PRO-PC flexible sigmoidoscope
   Fujinon SIG-E2 flexible sigmoidoscope
   Fujinon SIG-EK flexible sigmoidoscope
   Fujinon SIG-ET flexible sigmoidoscope
   Fujinon SIG-PC flexible sigmoidoscope
   Fujinon UGI-PE flexible gastroscope
   gastroscope
   Heine sigmoidoscope
   Henke-Sass rigid laparoscope
   Henke-Sass Wolf laparoscope
   Hirschman anoscope
   Hopkins rigid glass lens
   Iglesias fiberoptic resectoscope
   InjecTx customized cystoscope
   Inspex rigid laparoscope

endoscope *(cont.)*
  InstrumentMakar laparoscope
  intubating laryngoscope
  InVISION to endoscope
  ITI (Instrument Technology Inc.)
    0.5 mm rigid borescope
  Jacobscope-Palmer laparoscope
  Jarit cystoscope
  Jarit 0° 10 mm rigid laparoscope
  Jarit 0° 5 mm rigid laparoscope
  Jasan flexible fiberoptic sigmoido-
    scope
  Jasan JFE choledochoscope
  Jasan rigid proctoscope
  Kantor-Berci videolaryngoscope
  Karl Storz rigid laparoscope
  Kelly anoscope
  Kendall esophageal sonascope
  Killian-Lynch laryngoscope
  Kleinsasser anterior commissure
    laryngoscope
  KLI rigid borescope
  laparoscope
  laser laparoscope
  Linvatec 7570R 0° 10 mm rigid
    laparoscope
  Linvatec rigid laparoscope
  Lloyd Davies sigmoidoscope
  MacIntosh laryngoscope
  Marlow rigid laparoscope
  Marlow videolaparoscope
  Medi-Vu
  Miller laryngoscope
  MIS Source sigmoidoscope
  monoscopic endoscope
  "mother-baby" dual endoscope
  Mueller 0° 5 mm rigid laparoscope
  nasolaryngopharyngoscope
  Naunton Morgan proctoscope
  Navigator flexible endoscope
  new variable stiffness (VS) colono-
    scope
  Olympus A5214 0° 10 mm
    rigid laparoscope

endoscope *(cont.)*
  Olympus A5215 rigid laparoscopic
    system
  Olympus A5254 0° 10mm rigid
    laparoscope
  Olympus A5255 30° 10 mm rigid
    laparoscope
  Olympus A5257 0° 10 mm rigid
    laparoscope
  Olympus A5258 rigid 0° 10 mm
    rigid laparoscope
  Olympus CF-1T10L flexible
    gastroscope
  Olympus CF-1T20L flexible
    gastroscope
  Olympus CF-P20L flexible gastro-
    scope
  Olympus CF-10L flexible sigmoido-
    scope
  Olympus CF-20L flexible gastro-
    scope
  Olympus CF-100S flexible
    sigmoidoscope
  Olympus CF-140I videocolono-
    scope
  Olympus CF-140L videocolono-
    scope
  Olympus CF-140S videocolono-
    scope
  Olympus CF-1TS2 flexible
    sigmoidoscope
  Olympus CF-1T100L forward-
    viewing videocolonoscope
  Olympus CF-1T10L flexible
    gastroscope
  Olympus CF-1T10L flexible
    therapeutic colonoscope
  Olympus CF-1T20L flexible
    gastroscope
  Olympus CF-1T20L flexible
    therapeutic colonoscope
  Olympus CF-1TS2 flexible
    sigmoidoscope
  Olympus CF-200Z colonoscope

endoscope *(cont.)*
Olympus CF-20L flexible
colonoscope
Olympus CF-20L flexible
gastroscope
Olympus CF-30L flexible
colonoscope
Olympus CF-P10S flexible
sigmoidoscope
Olympus CF-P20L flexible
gastroscope
Olympus CF-Q160AL/I innoflex
videocolonoscope
Olympus CF-Q160L/I/S video
sigmoidoscope
Olympus CF-V10S sigmoidoscope
Olympus CF-Q140I
Olympus CF-Q160L/I/S video-
colonoscope
Olympus CF-Q160L/I/S video-
sigmoidoscope
Olympus CHF-B20 transduodenal
choledochofiberscope
Olympus CHF-BP30 transduodenal
choledochofiberscope
Olympus CHF-CB30 choledocho-
scope
Olympus CHF-P20 choledocho-
scope
Olympus CHF-P20Q choledocho-
scope
Olympus CPF-P10-S sigmoidoscope
Olympus CV-1 endoscopic system
Olympus CV-100 endoscopic system
Olympus CYF-3 OES cystofiber-
scope
Olympus cystoscope
Olympus Evis Exera 160 endoscope
Olympus Evis 140 endoscope
reprocessing system
Olympus Evis Q-200V video
Olympus fiberoptic sigmoidoscope
Olympus flexible sigmoidoscope
Olympus GF-UM130 ultrasound
gastroscope

endoscope *(cont.)*
Olympus GF-UM3 and CF-UM20
ultrasonic
Olympus GIF-EUM2 echoendo-
scope
Olympus GIF-HM gastroscope
Olympus GIF-K gastroscope
Olympus GIF-N30 gastrofibero-
scope
Olympus GIF-100 videogastroscope
Olympus GIF-140
Olympus GIF-160
Olympus GIF-1T10 flexible thera-
peutic gastroscope
Olympus GIF-1T10 and GIF20
echoendoscope
Olympus GIF-1T10 flexible thera-
peutic gastroscope
Olympus GIF-1T140 videogastro-
scope
Olympus GIF-1TV10 flexible
gastroscope
Olympus GIF-2T10 flexible gastro-
scope
Olympus GIF-2T20 flexible thera-
peutic gastroscope
Olympus GIF-N30 gastrofibero-
scope
Olympus GIF-P140 videogastro-
scope
Olympus GIF-PQ20 flexible gastro-
scope
Olympus GIF-PV10 pediatric video-
gastroscope
Olympus GIF-Q140 videogastro-
scope
Olympus GIF-Q160 gastrointestinal
videoscope
Olympus GIF-XP20 flexible gastro-
scope
Olympus GIF-XQ140 videogastro-
scope
Olympus GIF-XQ20 flexible multi-
purpose gastroscope

endoscope *(cont.)*
    Olympus GIF-XQ30 flexible multi-purpose gastroscope
    Olympus GIF-XT30 gastrofibero-scope
    Olympus GIF-XP160 SlimSIGHT gastrointestinal videoscope
    Olympus GIF-XP20 flexible gastro-scope
    Olympus GIF-XQ140 videogastro-scope
    Olympus GIF-XQ20 flexible multi-purpose gastroscope
    Olympus GIF-XQ30 flexible multi-purpose gastroscope
    Olympus GIF-XT30 gastrofibero-scope
    Olympus GIF-XV10 videogastro-scope
    Olympus HYF-XP flexible hystero-scope
    Olympus hysteroscope
    Olympus JF-1T20 flexible thera-peutic duodenoscope
    Olympus JF-1T30 flexible thera-peutic duodenoscope
    Olympus JF-UM20 echoendoscope
    Olympus JF1T10 fiberoptic duodenoscope
    Olympus OSF flexible sigmoido-scope
    Olympus OSF-2 flexible sigmoido-scope
    Olympus OSF-235 flexible sigmoido-scope
    Olympus PCF-10 flexible pediatric colonoscope
    Olympus PCF-140I pediatric video colonoscope
    Olympus PCF-140L pediatric video colonoscope
    Olympus PCF-160AL/I video colonoscope
    Olympus PJF-7.5 pediatric duodenofiberscope

endoscope *(cont.)*
    Olympus SIF-100 video push entero-scope
    Olympus SIF-M magnifying entero-scope
    Olympus SIF10 enteroscope
    Olympus SlimSIGHT gastro-intestinal videoscope
    Olympus TGF-2D flexible gastro-scope
    Olympus TJF-100
    Olympus TJF-160F videoduodeno-scope
    Olympus TJF-M20
    Olympus URF-P2 translaparoscopic choledochofiberscope
    Olympus VU-M2 and XIF-UM3 echoendoscope
    Olympus XQ230 gastroscope
    Optik laparoscope
    Optik rigid laparoscope
    ORI electronic endoscopy system
    otoscope
    panendoscope
    Pentax EC-3430F videocolono-scope
    Pentax EC-3430L videocolon-scope
    Pentax EC-3440F videocolono-scope
    Pentax EC-3440L videocolono-scope
    Pentax EC-3830 videocolonoscope
    Pentax EC-3830L videocolono-scope
    Pentax EC-3830TL videocolono-scope
    Pentax EC-3840L videocolono-scope
    Pentax EC-3840T videocolono-scope
    Pentax ECN-1530 videochole-dochonephroscope
    Pentax ED-3430T videoduodeno-scope

endoscope *(cont.)*
    Pentax ED-3440T videoduodeno-
        scope
    Pentax EG-1840 videogastroscope
    Pentax EG-2530 gastroscope
    Pentax EG-2540 videogastroscope
    Pentax EG-2731 gastroscope
    Pentax EG-2901 flexible gastroscope
    Pentax EG-2930 gastroscope
    Pentax EG-2940 videogastroscope
    Pentax EG-3430 videogastroscope
    Pentax EG-3440 videogastroscope
    Pentax EG-3830T videogastroscope
    Pentax EG-3840T videogastroscope
    Pentax ES-3830 videosigmoido-
        scope
    Pentax ES-3840 videosigmoido-
        scope
    Pentax FC-38LX flexible gastro-
        scope
    Pentax FG-24V fiberoptic gastro-
        scope
    Pentax FG-29H flexible gastroscope
    Pentax FG-29V fiberoptic gastro-
        scope
    Pentax FG-29X flexible gastroscope
    Pentax EG-1840 videogastroscope
    Pentax EG-2530 videogastroscope
    Pentax EG-2540 videogastroscope
    Pentax EG-2731 videogastroscope
    Pentax EG-2901 flexible gastroscope
    Pentax EG-2930 videogastroscope
    Pentax EG-2940 videogastroscope
    Pentax EG-3430 videogastroscope
    Pentax EG-3440 videogastroscope
    Pentax EG-3830T videogastro-
        scope
    Pentax EG-3840T videogastro-
        scope
    Pentax ES-3830 videosigmoido-
        scope
    Pentax ES-3840 videoendoscope
    Pentax EUP-EC124 ultrasound
        gastroscope

endoscope *(cont.)*
    Pentax FCN-15H flexible chole-
        dochoscope
    Pentax FC-38LV fiberoptic colono-
        scope
    Pentax FC-38LX flexible gastro-
        scope
    Pentax FC-38MV fiberoptic colono-
        scope
    Pentax FD-34V fiberoptic
        endoscope
    Pentax fiberoptic sigmoidoscope
    Pentax flexible sigmoidoscope
    Pentax FG-24V fiberoptic gastro-
        scope
    Pentax FG-29H flexible gastroscope
    Pentax FG-29V fiberoptic gastro-
        scope
    Pentax FG-29X flexible gastroscope
    Pentax FG-36UX echoendoscope
    Pentax FS flexible sigmoidoscope
    Pentax FS-34A flexible sigmoido-
        scope
    Pentax FS-34V fiberoptic sigmoido-
        scope
    Pentax FS-38H flexible sigmoido-
        scope
    Pentax-Hitachi FG32UA endosono-
        graphic system
    Pentax SIG-E2 fiberoptic sigmoido-
        scope
    Pentax W fiberoptic endoscope
    PercScope percutaneous diskectomy
    pharyngoscope
    Pilling rigid laparoscope
    push enteroscope
    rectoscope (proctoscope)
    Reichert fiberoptic sigmoidoscope
    Reichert flexible sigmoidoscope
    Reichert MH-1 flexible sigmoido-
        scope
    Reichert SC-48 flexible sigmoido-
        scope
    REI rigid laparoscope

endoscope *(cont.)*
    resectoscope
    Rhinoline endoscopic system
    Riester economy otoscope
    rigid endoscope
    rigid-lens endoscope
    rigid sigmoidoscope
    semirigid sigmoidoscope
    Schindler semiflexible gastroscope
    self-retaining laryngoscope
    Semm rigid laparoscope
    Semm/Wisap laparoscope
    side-viewing
    SIF10 Olympus enteroscope
    sigmoidoscope
    SITEtrac
    Solos cystoscope
    Solos rigid laparoscope
    Sonde enteroscope
    SP-501 Sonoprobe endoscopy
    specialized tissue aspirating resecto-
       scope (STAR)
    Spiess
    SpineScope percutaneous
    STAR (specialized tissue-aspirating
       resectoscope)
    StereoEndoscope
    stereotaxic
    St. Mark's sigmoidoscope
    Storz bronchoscope
    Storz cystoscope
    Storz esophagoscope
    Storz hysteroscope
    Storz resectoscope
    Storz rigid laparoscope
    Storz 26003 AP 0° 10 mm rigid
       laparoscope
    Storz 26033 AP 0° 10 mm rigid
       laparoscope
    Storz 26033 BP 0° 10 mm rigid
       laparoscope
    Stryker 380-10 0° 10 mm rigid
       laparoscope

endoscope *(cont.)*
    Stryker 380-11 0° 10 mm rigid
       laparoscope
    Stryker 380-12 30° 10 mm rigid
       laparoscope
    Surgenomic
    SurgiScope
    Syringe Avitene delivery system
    3-Dscope laparoscope
    Toshiba video
    transparent cap-fitted
    Tuttle proctoscope
    two-channel
    URF-P2 choledochoscope
    variable stiffness
    VideoHydro laparoscope
    videoscope
    videoresectoscope
    videothoracoscope
    Visicath
    V. Mueller rigid laparoscope
    Weck-Baggish rigid laparoscope
    Weck 110405 0° 5 mm rigid
       laparoscope
    Weck 110800 rigid laparoscope
    Weck operating laparoscope
    Weck 0° 10 mm rigid laparoscope
    Welch Allyn flexible sigmoidoscope
    Welch Allyn videosigmoidoscope
    Wolf 8937.31 0° 10 mm rigid
       laser laparoscope
    Wolf Lumina rigid laparoscope
    Wolf 170° 12 mm rigid laparoscope
    Wolf 7732 rigid laparoscope
    Wolf 8934.40 rigid laparoscope
    Wolf rigid laparoscope
    Wolf 10/5 (L-angle) operative
       laparoscope
    Wolf videoresectoscope
    WuScope system
    Xillix LIFE-GI fluorescence
       endoscopy System
    XQ230 Olympus gastroscope

endoscope *(cont.)*
  Zeiss Endolive endoscope
  Zimmer rigid
endoscope-assisted microneurosurgery
endoscope-controlled microneuro-
  surgery
endoscopic ablation
endoscopic antireflux procedure
endoscopic argon beam plasma coagu-
  lation
endoscopic articulating (EAS) stapler
endoscopic-assisted transumbilical
  augmentation mammoplasty
endoscopic balloon sphincteroplasty
  (EBS)
endoscopic band ligation (EBL)
endoscopic BiCAP probe
endoscopic bile duct procedure
endoscopic biliary decompression
endoscopic biliary drainage
endoscopic biliary endoprosthesis
endoscopic biliary stent
endoscopic biopsy
endoscopic biopsy forceps
endoscopic biopsy surveillance
endoscopic bougienage
endoscopic catheterization
endoscopic confocal microscopy
endoscopic cryoablation
endoscopic cryotherapy
endoscopic cystogastrostomy
endoscopic decompression
endoscopic dilation
endoscopic Doppler ultrasound
endoscopic drainage
endoscopic dual tip Kittner
endoscopic forceps
endoscopic gastroplasty
endoscopic grasping forceps
endoscopic heat probe
endoscopic injection
endoscopic injection sclerosis
endoscopic injection therapy (EIT)
endoscopic intraperitoneal perforation

endoscopic laser cautery
endoscopic laser cholecystectomy
endoscopic ligation
endoscopic light source
  halogen
  strobe flash
  xenon flash
endoscopic mucosal ablation
endoscopic mucosal resection (EMR)
endoscopic mucosectomy
endoscopic multifeed (EMS) TA-90
  stapler
endoscopic optical coherence tomog-
  raphy (EOCT)
endoscopic papillectomy (EP)
endoscopic papillotomy
endoscopic polypectomy
endoscopic prosthesis
endoscopic resection
endoscopic retrograde balloon dilation
endoscopic retrograde biliary drainage
  (ERBD)
endoscopic retrograde cholangiography
  (ERC)
endoscopic retrograde cholangio-
  pancreatography (ERCP)
endoscopic retrograde cholangio-
  pancreatography/endoscopic
  sphincterotomy (ERCP/ES)
endoscopic retrograde parenchy-
  mography (ERP)
endoscopic reversal technique
endoscopic sclerotherapy
endoscopic sewing machine technique
endoscopic small bowel biopsy
endoscopic snare
endoscopic sonography
endoscopic sphincterotomy (ES)
endoscopic stent placement
endoscopic suction-cap technique
endoscopic suction cup
endoscopic surveillance
endoscopic suture-cutting forceps
endoscopic suturing

endoscopic tissue sampling
endoscopic transaxillary augmentation
   mammoplasty
endoscopic transpapillary catheteriza-
   tion of the gallbladder (ETCG)
endoscopic ultrasonography (EUS)
endoscopic ultrasound (EUS)
endoscopic ultrasound-assisted band
   ligation
endoscopic ultrasound-guided fine-
   needle aspiration (EUS-FNA)
endoscopic variceal ligation (EVL)
endoscopic washing pipe
endoscopic Water Pik
endoscopic Zenker diverticulectomy
   with cricopharyngeal myotomy
endoscopically
endoscopist, gastrointestinal
endoscopy
   biliary
   gastrointestinal
   pancreatic
   small intestinal
   surveillance
   therapeutic
   transoral
   upper gastrointestinal
endoscopy-negative reflux disease
   (ENRD)
endoscopy with tumor ablation
Endo Mini Shears
Endo Shears cutter
endosonography
Endosound endoscopic ultrasound
   catheter
endostaple
Endostatin protein
Endo Stitch knot-tying device
Endo Stitch suture device
Endo Suture introducer
Endotak C lead catheter
endothelial cells
endothelial lining
endothelium

endotherapy, pancreatic
endotoxemia, portal and systemic
endotoxin-binding protein
endotoxin concentration
endotoxin level
Endotrac cannula
Endotrac elevator
endotracheal anesthesia
endotracheal intubation
endotracheal tube
endotracheal tube intubation
Endotrac probe
Endotrac rasp
Endotrac retractor
Endotrol tracheal tube
Endotube Rae-Flex oral
Endo Universal device
endovascular coagulation of blood
   vessel
endovascular glue
endovascular stent graft
Endoview endoscopy camera
end plate
end-sigmoid colostomy
end-stage cirrhosis
end-stage diverticula
end-stage liver disease (ESLD)
end-stage renal disease (ESRD)
end-to-back bowel anastomosis
end-to-end anastomosis (EEA) stapler
end-to-end invaginating anastomosis
end-to-end jejunoileal bypass
end-to-end suture
end-to-side anastomosis
end-to-side choledochojejunostomy
end-to-side jejunoileal bypass
end-to-side portocaval shunt
end-to-side splenorenal shunt
end-to-side suture
Enecat (barium sulfate)
enema (see also *bowel prep*)
   air-contrast barium
   analeptic enema
   barium (BE)

enema *(cont.)*
   blind
   Colomed
   contrast
   Cortenema retention
   double-contrast air barium
   5-ASA (5-aminosalicylic acid)
   flatus
   Fleet
   Fleet Bisacodyl
   Fleet Mineral Oil
   full-column barium
   gastrografin
   hydrocortisone
   hydrogen peroxide
   Kayexalate
   lactulose
   mesalamine
   methylene blue
   nuclear
   oil retention
   phosphosoda
   prednisolone
   prosphate
   retention
   Rowasa
   saline cleansing
   single-contrast barium
   small bowel
   soapsuds (SSE)
   steroid foam
   sulfasalazine
   tap water
   theophylline olamine
   "3H"
   water soluble contrast
enema contrast study
enemas until clear
energy-producing respiratory processes
energy, radiofrequency
en face ("ahn fahs")
enflurane
Enforcer SDS coronary stent
Engel-May nail

Engel plaster saw
Engerix-B (hepatitis B virus vaccine,
   recombinant)
engorgement of esophageal venous
   plexus (pl. plexi)
Enhancer (barium sulfate)
enhancer, video signal
Enker brain retractor
enlarged lymph node
enlarged spleen
enlarged thymus
enlarged uterus
enlargement
   gland
   lymph node
   nodular thyroid
   pituitary
   splenic
enlarging cystic lesion
en masse ("removed en masse")
Enproct disposable anoscope
enprostil
ENRD (endoscopy-negative reflux
   disease)
ENSI syringe
ensiform appendix
EnSite cardiac catheter
ensure hemostasis
Ensure nutritional therapy
ENT (ear, nose, and throat) scissors
entamebic abscess
Entamoeba histolytica
ENTaxis nasal packing dressing
enteral administration route
enteral alimentation
enteral diarrhea
enteral feeding
enteral nutrition (EN) therapy
   Attain
   Citrotein
   Compleat Modified Formula
   Comply
   Ensure
   Entrition

enteral *(cont.)*
   Epulor
   Fiberlan
   Forta Shake
   Glucerna
   Immun-Aid
   Impact
   Introlan Half-Strength
   Introlite
   Isocal
   Isocal HCN
   Isocal HN
   Isosource HN
   Isotein HN
   Jevity
   Kindercal
   Lipisorb
   Lonalac
   Magnacal
   Meritene
   MET-Rx
   Neocate One +
   Nitrolan
   Nutraloric
   Nutren
   Nutrilan
   Osmolite
   Osmolite HN
   Peptamen
   Pre-Attain
   Precision High Nitrogen
   Precision LR
   Profiber
   Propimex-2
   Reabilan
   Reabilan HN
   Replete
   Resource
   Resource Plus
   Stresstein
   Sustacal
   Sustagen
   Tolerex
   TraumaCal

enteral *(cont.)*
   Travasorb HN
   Travasorb MCT
   Travasorb SID
   TwoCal HN
   Tyrex-2
   Ultracal
   Vital High Nitrogen
enterically transmitted non-A, non-B
   (ENANB) hepatitis (former name)
enteric bacillus
enteric-coated aspirin
enteric-coated capsule
enteric colibacillosis
enteric contents
enteric cyst
enteric drainage
enteric fever
enteric fistula
enteric orphan virus
enterinsular axis
enteritis (see also *gastroenteritis*)
   Campylobacter
   chronic ischemic
   Clostridium difficile
   Crohn regional
   graft
   granulomatous
   infectious
   ischemic
   nonspecific
   radiation
   regional
   segmental
   ulcerative
   viral
enteroadherent *E. coli* (EAEC)
Enterobacter agglomerans
Enterobacter cloacae
Enterobacter freundii
Enterobacter gergoviae
Enterobacter hafnia
Enterobacter liquefaciens
Enterobacter sakazakii

enterobacterial common antigen (ECA)
enterobiasis
enterobiliary
Enterobius vermicularis (pinworm)
enterocele sac
enterocele, vaginal
enterochromaffin cell
enterocleisis, omental
enteroclysis
enterococcus (pl. enterococci)
Enterococcus avium
Enterococcus faecalis
Enterococcus faecium
enterocolic fistula
enterocolitis (see also *colitis*)
   antibiotic-induced
   bacterial
   chronic ischemic
   fulminant
   granulomatous
   hemorrhagic
   Hirschsprung-associated (HAEC)
   ischemic
   necrotizing (NEC)
   pseudomembranous
   regional
   ulcerative
enterocutaneous fistula
enterocystoplasty
enterocyte
enterocytopathogenic human orphan
   (ECHO) virus
Enterodophilus
enteroenteral fistula
enteroenteric fistula
enteroenterostomy
enterogastritis
enterogenous cyst
enterohemorrhagic *E. coli* (EHEC)
enterohepatic circulation
enteroinsular axis
enteroinvasive *E. coli* (EIEC)
enterokinase
enterolith

enterolithotomy
enterolysis
enteropathic organism
enteropathogenic *E. coli* (EPEC)
enteropathy
   bile salt-losing
   diabetic
   exudative
   gluten
   hypercatabolic protein-losing
   lymphangiectatic protein-losing
   protein-losing
   terminal hemorrhagic
enteroperitoneal abscess
enteroptosis
enterorrhaphy
enteroscope (see *endoscope*)
   magnifying
   Olympus SIF10
   push
   SIF10 Olympus
   Sonde
   temporary
   tube
   video push
enteroscopy
enterospasm
enterostenosis
enterostomal therapist
enterostomy, cutaneous
EnteroTest
EnteroTest Pediatric
enterotomy scissors
enterotoxigenic *E. coli* (ETEC)
enterotoxin diarrhea
enterourethral fistula
enterovaginal fistula
enterovesical fistula
Enterovirus
Entero Vu (barium sulfate for
   suspension)
Enterra gastric stimulation device
Enterra gastrointestinal "pacemaker"
Enteryx biopolymer material

entire bowel wall
Entocort CR (budesonide)
Entolase (lipase; protease)
Entozyme (lipase; protease)
entrapment
   bowel
   catheter
   nerve
Entree Plus
Entree II laparoscopic trocar and
   cannula systems
Entree thoracoscopy trocar and cannula
EntriStar PEG (percutaneous endo-
   scopic gastrostomy) tube
Entrition nutritional therapy
Entrobar (barium sulfate [methyl-
   cellulose diluent])
enucleation of thrombosed hemorrhoid
enucleation of tumor
enucleation scissors
enucleator, gland
envelope, axillary
enveloping scar tissue
Enview camera
EnVision autoclavable 3CCD (three
   chip) camera head
enzyme
   brancher
   cyclophilin
   debrancher
   digestive
   DME (drug-metabolizing)
   fumarylacetoacetase parahydroxy-
      phenylpyruvic acid (p-HPPA)
      oxidase
   lactase
   lipase
   lipolytic
   liver
   liver phosphorylase
   medium chain acyl-CoA
      dehydrogenase
   pancreatic
   protease digestive

enzyme *(cont.)*
   proteinase
   proteolytic
   serum liver
enzyme-linked immunoassay (EIA-2)
enzyme linked immunosorbent assay
   (ELISA)
enzyme panel
enzyme replacement therapy
EOCT (endoscopic optical coherence
   tomography)
EORTC (European Organization for
   Research and Treatment of Cancer)
eosinophil (also eosinophile)
eosinophilic esophagitis
eosinophilic gastritis
eosinophilic gastroenteritis
eosinophilic gastroenteritis syndrome
eosinophilic granuloma
eosinophilic material
eosinophil smear
eosphagogastric orifice
EOTC (endoscopic optical coherence
   tomography)
EP (endoscopic papillectomy)
EPC pain control
EPEC (enteropathogenic *E. coli*)
"epi" (epinephrine)
Epi-C (barium sulfate)
Epic ophthalmic 3-in-1 laser
epicritic pain
epidemic gastroenteritis
epidemic gastroenteritis virus
epidemic keratoconjunctivitis virus
epidemic nonbacterial gastroenteritis
epidemic vomiting
epidermal carcinoma
epidermal growth factor (EGF)
epidermal inclusion cyst
epidermoid carcinoma
epidermoid cyst
epidermoid skin cysts and benign
   craniofacial and long bone tumors
   (Gardner syndrome)

epidermolysis bullosa dystrophica
epidural abscess
epidural anesthesia
epidural blood patch graft
epidural catheter
epidural hematoma
epidural hemorrhage
Epigard composite wound dressing
epigastralgia
epigastric angle
epigastric discomfort
epigastric distress
epigastric fold
epigastric hernia
epigastric incision
epigastric mass
epigastric pain
epigastric reflex
epigastric region
epigastric spot
epigastric tenderness
epigastric vessel
epigastrium
epiglottis
EpiLaser laser
Epi-Lock wound dressing
epinephrine ("epi")
epinephrine and cisplatin injectable gel
epinephrine level
epinephrine/norepinephrine level
epiphrenic diverticulum
epiphyseal bar, excision of
epiphyseal cartilage plate
epiphyseal ischemic necrosis
epiphyseal knife
epiphyseal staple
epiplocele
epiploectomy
epiploic appendage
epiploic appendix
epiploon abscess
epirubicin HCl
episiotomy scissors
episodic colic

episodic vomiting
epistaxis dressing
epitendineum
epithelial cell lining
epithelial cell thymoma
epithelial component
epithelial edema
epithelial hyperplasia
epithelialization
epithelioid hemangioendothelioma
epithelium
    Barrett
    bile duct
    columnar
    crypt
    glandular
    junctional
    pseudostratified
    pyramidal
    salmon-pink
    squamous
    stratified
    surface
    transitional
    villous
epithelium crypt
epitheloid leiomyoma
epitope, alpha-Gal
EpiTouch laser
Epivir-HBV (lamivudine)
Epley maneuver
EPO (epoetin alfa)
epoetin alfa
Eppendorf biopsy forceps
Eppendorf-Tischler biopsy forceps
Epstein-Barr virus (EBV) infection
Epstein bone rasp
Epstein neurological hammer
EPT (endoscopic papillotomy)
EPTFE (expanded polytetrafluoro-
    ethylene) vascular suture
Epulor nutritional therapy
Equalactin (calcium polycarbophil)
Equilet (calcium carbonate)

equivocal pancreatic cytology
equivocal primary peristalsis
ER+ (estrogen-receptor positive)
ER– (estrogen-receptor negative)
ERA (endometrial resection and
    ablation) resectoscope sheath
ERBD (endoscopic retrograde biliary
    drainage)
ERBE Endocut electrocautery generator
erbium:YAG (Er:YAG) laser
Erbotom F2 electrocoagulation unit
ERC (endoscopic retrograde cholangi-
    ography)
ERCP (endoscopic retrograde
    cholangiopancreatography)
ERCP brush sample
ERCP cannula
ERCP catheter
ERCP/ES (endoscopic retrograde
    cholangiopancreatography/
    endoscopic sphincterotomy)
ERCP-guided biopsy
ERCP-induced rupture
ERCP insertion of tube or stent
ERCP manometry
ErCr:YAG laser
Erdheim cystic medial necrosis
erect view
Ergamisol (levamisole HCl)
Ergoset (bromocriptine mesylate)
ergotamine tartrate
ER-ICA (estrogen receptor immuno-
    chemical assay)
Eriksson muscle biopsy cannula
Erlangen magnetic colostomy device
Erlangen-type papillotome
erosion
    duodenal
    gallstone
    gastric
    gastric antral
    salt and pepper duodenal
    linear
erosion into biliary tree

erosion into pericardial sac
erosion into pleural cavity
erosion or ulceration of surface
erosive duodenitis
erosive esophagitis
erosive gastritis
erosive gastroesophageal reflux disease
    (GERD)
erotic vomiting
ERP (endoscopic retrograde
    parenchymography)
eructation
erythema multiforme
erythema nodosum
erythema of abdominal wall
erythema, palmar
erythematous lesion
erythematous streak
erythrocyte sedimentation rate (ESR)
Erythroflex catheter
erythroid agenesis
erythromycin
erythromyin-induced cholecystitis
ES (endoscopic sphincterotomy)
Esberitox
Escherichia coli (E. coli)
Escherichia coli granuloma
Escherichia coli melanosis
Escherichia coli pneumatosis
Escherichia coli polyposis
Escherichia coli taeniae
Escherichia coli O157:H7 assay
E.S.I. Bite Block
ESI instrument adapter to AMCD cord
ESLD (end-stage liver disease)
Esmarch bandage
Esmarch dressing
Esmarch plaster knife
Esmarch plaster scissors
Esmarch plaster shears
esomeprazole magnesium
EsophaCoil self-expanding esophageal
    stent
esophageal A ring

esophageal achalasia
esophageal acid infusion test
esophageal adenocarcinoma
esophageal angina
esophageal aperistalsis
esophageal artery of aorta
esophageal artery of inferior thyroid
esophageal atresia
esophageal balloon
esophageal balloon technique
esophageal body
esophageal body motor function
esophageal bougie
esophageal bougienage
esophageal B ring
esophageal brushing
esophageal cancer
esophageal candidiasis
esophageal clearing
esophageal colic
esophageal contractile ring
esophageal contraction
esophageal cytomegalovirus
esophageal degeneration
esophageal dilatation
esophageal dilation
esophageal diverticulum
esophageal/duodenal decompression
   device
esophageal dyskinesia
esophageal dysmotility
esophageal dysphagia
esophageal electrocardiogram
esophageal foreign body
esophageal function test
esophageal gastric tube airways (EGTA)
esophageal gland
esophageal groove of liver
esophageal hernia
esophageal hiatal hernia
esophageal hiatus
esophageal impression
esophageal inlet
esophageal intubation

esophageal-jejunal anastomosis
esophageal lead
esophageal leiomyoma
esophageal lengthening
esophageal leukoplakia
esophageal lumen
esophageal manometry
esophageal motility disorder
esophageal motility study
esophageal mucosa
esophageal mucosal ring
esophageal muscular ring
esophageal myotomy
esophageal myotomy via thoracoscopy
esophageal obstruction
esophageal obturator airway
esophageal opening
esophageal pain
esophageal peristaltic pressure
esophageal pH
esophageal pH analysis
esophageal pH monitoring
esophageal pH test
esophageal plexus
esophageal plexus of nerves
esophageal pouch
esophageal pressure recording
esophageal reflux
esophageal reflux disease
esophageal resection
esophageal ring, distal
esophageal rupture
esophageal shunt
esophageal sling procedure
esophageal sound
esophageal spasm, diffuse
esophageal spasm mimicking angina
esophageal spasm mimicking
   myocardial infarction
esophageal sphincter
   hypertensive
   inferior
esophageal stenosis
esophageal stent

esophageal stricture
esophageal tear
esophageal temperature
esophageal temperature probe
esophageal transection with para-
    esophagogastric devascularization
esophageal transit time
esophageal tube
esophageal tumor
esophageal ulceration
esophageal variceal bleeding
esophageal variceal sclerosis
esophageal variceal sclerotherapy
esophageal varices, direct ligation of
esophageal varicosities
esophageal varix (pl. varices)
esophageal vein
esophageal venous plexus (pl. plexi)
esophageal web
esophageal window
esophageal Z-Stent with Dua antireflux
    valve
esophagectomy
    Ivor Lewis
    Ivor Lewis two-stage subtotal
    minimally invasive
    near-total
    open
    thoracoabdominal
    total
    total thoracic
    transhiatal
    transhiatal blunt
esophagitis
    acid-pepsin reflux
    alkaline
    bacterial
    Barrett
    Candida
    Candida albicans esophagitis
    candidal
    chemical
    chronic peptic
    CMV (cytomegalovirus)

esophagitis *(cont.)*
    corrosive
    eosinophilic
    erosive
    fungal
    herpetic
    infectious
    nonreflux
    peptic
    pill
    polycystic chronic
    postoperative
    radiation
    reflux (RE)
    regurgitant
    retention
    stasis
    ulcerative
esophagocele, acquired
esophagocolic anastomosis
esophagodiverticulostomy
esophagoduodenostomy
esophagoenterostomy
esophagogastrectomy
esophagogastric (EG) junction
esophagogastric anastomosis
esophagogastric complex
esophagogastric fat pad
esophagogastric fundoplasty with
    fundic patch (Thal-Nissen
    procedure)
esophagogastric intubation
esophagogastric junction
esophagogastric orifice
esophagogastric sphincter
esophagogastric tamponade
esophagogastric varices
esophagogastric vestibule
esophagogastroduodenoscopy (EGD),
    small-caliber
esophagogastroplasty
esophagogastroscopy
    Abbott
    Clagett Barrett

esophagogastroscopy *(cont.)*
    intrathoracic
    Johnson
    Thal
    Woodward
esophagogastrostomy
    cervical
    intrathoracic
esophagoglottal closure reflex
esophagogram (see *esophagram*)
esophagojejunostomy
    end-to-end
    end-to-side
    loop
    mechanical
    mediastinal
    Roux-en-Y
    Roux-Y
    stapled
    transhiatal
esophagomyotomy
    circumferential
    Heller
    laparoscopic
    modified Heller
    open
    thoracic short
    thoracoscopic
esophagoplasty
    balloon
    behind-sternum colon
    cervical
    colic patch
    colonic
    gastric patch
    gastric tube
    gastric tubular
    Grondahl-Finney
    intrathoracic
    laparoscopic
    large intestine
    one-stage posterior mediastinal
    patch
    pectoralis myocutaneous

esophagoplasty *(cont.)*
    pediatric
    peptic
    reverse gastric tube
    single-step
    subtotal
    transmediastinal posterior
esophagosalivary reflex
esophagoscope (see also *endoscope*)
    cine-esophagoscope
    double-channel
    Eder-Hufford rigid
    Holinger
    Jackson
    Jesberg
    Kelling
    Kendall esophageal sonascope
    large-bore rigid
    Negus rigid
    Olympus EF
    Schindler
    Storz
esophagospasm
esophagostenosis
esophagostomy
esophagotomy
    cervical approach
    distal
    feeding
    subtotal
    thoracic approach
    vertical
esophagotracheal (ET) junction
esophagram, barium
esophagus
    achalasia of
    aperistaltic
    Barrett
    B ring of
    columnar-lined
    corkscrew
    curling
    distal
    dyssynergic

esophagus *(cont.)*
  nutcracker
  scleroderma-like
  short-segment Barrett
  spastic
  tortuous
  tubular
esophageal dilator
Espocan needle
ESR (erythrocyte sedimentation rate)
ESRD (end-stage renal disease)
essential fatty acid (EFA)
essential mixed cryoglobulinemia
essential fatty acid deficiency
Esser skin graft
esterase stain
esterified estrogen
estimated blood loss (EBL)
Estinyl (ethinyl estradiol)
Estrace (estradiol)
estradiol
Estratab (esterified estrogen)
Estridge biopsy needle
estrogen and progesterone receptors
estrogen-induced liver disease
estrogen metabolism
estrogen receptor
estrogen-receptor-negative (ER–) tumor
estrogen-receptor-positive (ER+)
  tumor
estrogen receptor status
estrone
Estrone Aqueous (estrone)
ESWL (extracorporeal shock-wave
  lithotripsy)
ESWT (extracorporeal shock-wave
  therapy)
ET (enterostomal therapy) nurse
ETCG (endoscopic transpapillary
  catheterization of the gallbladder)
ETEC (enterotoxigenic *Escherichia
  coli*)
Ethamolin (ethanolamine oleate)
ethanolamine oleate sclerosant

ethanol consumption
ethanolism
Ethibond Excel polyester suture
Ethibond needle
Ethibond suture
Ethicon Endo-Surgery trocar
Ethicon Excel suture
Ethicon suture
Ethicon Teflon paste
Ethiflex suture
Ethiguard blunt point
Ethilon monofilament nylon suture
ethinyl estradiol
ethmoid forceps
ethmoidolacrimal suture
ethmoidomaxillary suture
ethmovomerine plate
Ethox Corporation
Ethrane (enflurane)
ethylene oxide gas
Ethyol (amifostine)
etidocaine; epinephrine
etiology, infectious
etiology undetermined
etiology unknown
etoformin HCl
EtOH, ETOH (ethanol; ethyl alcohol)
ETOH intoxication
etomoxir
etoposide injection
e-TRAIN 110 AngioJet catheter
ET tube
Eubacterium lentum
Eubacterium limosum
Eucestoda (cestoda) tapeworm
Euglucon (glyburide)
euglycemia
EU-M30S endoscopic ultrasonography
  receiver
eunuchoidism
Euro bag
Euro-Collins (EC) multiorgan perfusion
  kit
European Association for the Study
  of the Liver (EASL)

European Organization for Research
  and Treatment of Cancer (EORTC)
EUS (endoluminal ultrasound)
EUS (endoscopic ultrasonography)
EUS (endoscopic ultrasound)
EUS-FNA (endoscopic ultrasound-
  guided fine-needle aspiration)
EUS-guided cytology
EUS-guided fine-needle aspiration
  biopsy
euthymic
euthyroid goiter
euthyroid sick syndrome (ESS)
euthyroid state
Evac-Q-Kwik (bisacodyl)
Evac-Q-Mag
Evac-Q-Sert
Evac-Q-Tabs
evacuant (see *bowel prep*; *enema*)
evacuating clot
evacuation, digital rectal
evacuation disorder
evacuation proctography
Evac-U-Gen
Evac-U-Lac
Evalose (lactulose)
evanescent
Evans blue dye
Evans tissue forceps
Eve tonsil snare
evening primrose oil (EPO)
eventration of diaphragm
Everest medical bipolar instrument
everolimus
Evershears and Evershears II bipolar
  scissors
eversion, rectal
evert
Evert-O-Cath catheter
everting mattress suture
EVII endoscopic video system
evisceration
EVL (endoscopic variceal ligation)
Ewald breakfast

Ewald evacuator tube
Ewald gastric lavage tube
Ewald test meal
Ewald tube
Ewing sarcoma
Ewing tumor
Ewingella americana
ex vivo liver-directed gene therapy
Ex-Lax
Ex-Lax Extra Gentle
Ex-Lax Gentle Nature
Ex-Lax Maxium Relief
Ex-Lax Stool Softener
exacerbation of pain
ExacTech blood glucose monitor
examination
    darkfield microscopic
    digital rectal
    gross
    microscopic
    physical
eXamine cholangiography catheter
exanthematous necrosis
Excalibur Plus PC electrosurgical
  generator
excavated gastric carcinoma
excavator
    curved
    House
Excelart short-bore MRI
Excel GE electrochemical glucose
  monitoring strip
Excel irrigation system
excellent visualization
Excel polyester suture
excess fluid loss in stool
excess fluid volume
excessive bleeding
excessive cortisol production
excessive mechanical ventilation
excessive PEEP
excessive postprandial antral distension
excessive splenic sequestration of red
  cells

excess TSH stimulation
exchange
 blood
 fluid
 gas
 impaired gas
Excilon sponge dressing
excimer laser
excised scar
excision
 laser hemorrhoid
 wide
excisional biopsy
excision of branchial cleft vestige
excision of primary tumor
exclusion, wide
exclusion bypass
exclusion clamp
exclusion diet
excoriation
excreta
exemestane
exenteration
exfoliation
exfoliative gastritis
Exidine-4 chlorhexidine
exisulind
exit site of catheter
exit wound
exocrine drainage from pancreatic
 allograft
exocrine function
exocrine gland
exocrine pancreas
exocrine pancreas disorder
exocrine pancreatic cancer
exocrine pancreatic insufficiency
exocrine secretion
exogenous bicarbonate
exogenous calcium
exogenous infection
exogenously administered
exogenous obesity
exogenous thyroid hormone

exomphalos-macroglossia-gigantism
 syndrome
exophthalmic goiter
exophthalmos
exophytic adenocarcinoma
exophytic carcinoma
exophytic mass
Expand-A-Band breast binder
expandable esophageal stent (EES)
expandable metal stent
expandable olive
expanded polytetrafluoroethylene
expander, tissue
expanding reamer
expansile abdominal mass
expectoration
explantation of breast implant
exploration
 abdominal
 common bile duct (CBDE)
 surgical
exploratory celiotomy
exploratory incision
exploratory laparotomy
exploratory surgery
exploring cannula
explosive diarrhea
eXpose retractor
exposure to chemicals
Express PTCA catheter
ExpressView blood glucose monitor
exquisitely tender abdomen
exquisite pain
exquisite tenderness
exsanguinated
exsanguinating hemorrhage
exsanguination
Exserohilum rostratum
extended-field radiotherapy (EFRT)
extended right hepatectomy
extended right hepatic lobectomy
extended-survival graft
extension nail
extensive DCIS (ductal carcinoma
 in situ)

extensive florid transmural ganglio-
neuromatosis
extensive intraductal carcinoma (EIC)
extensive lymph node dissection
extensive pancreatic necrosis
extensive transmural ganglioneuroma-
tosis
exteriorization colostomy
exteriorize the colon
external anal sphincter
external beam radiotherapy and 5-FU
chemoradiotherapy
external biliary fistula
external bleeding
external clot
external fistulization of intestine
external hemorrhoid
external inguinal ring
external ligament
external oblique aponeurosis
external oblique fascia
external oblique muscle
external pancreatic fistula
external rectal sphincter
external ring
external skin tag
external spermatic fascia
external urethral orifice
external ventricular (EVD) drain
extirpation of tissue
extirpative surgery
extra-abdominal injury
extra-adrenal pheochromocytoma
extra-articular graft
extracellular concentration
extracellular fluid
extracellular material (ECM)
extracellular matrix
extracellular space
extracorporeal
extracorporeal anastomosis
extracorporeal knot
extracorporeal shock-wave lithotripsy
(ESWL)

extracorporeal shock-wave therapy
(ESWT)
eXtract specimen bag
extracting forceps
extraction balloon technique
extraction, stone
extractor
    Austin Moore
    bone
    bone plug
    break screw
    Cherry
    cloverleaf pin
    corkscrew femoral head
    endoscopic magnetic
    femoral head
    FIN
    Fox
    Glassman stone
    Jewett
    Kalish Duredge wire
    Küntscher (Kuentscher)
    Massie
    metatarsal head
    Moore prosthesis
    Murless fetal head
    Nicoll
    Rousek
    Schneider
    staple
    Sven-Johansson
Extractor three-lumen retrieval balloon
extractor-driver, Schneider
extractor-impactor, Fox
extradural abscess
extradural anesthesia
extradural hemorrhage
extrahepatic abdominal carcinoma
extrahepatic bile
extrahepatic bile duct
extrahepatic bile duct carcinoma
extrahepatic biliary atresia
extrahepatic biliary cystic dilation
extrahepatic biliary duct

extrahepatic biliary system
extrahepatic cholangiolitis
extrahepatic cholestasis
extrahepatic cirrhosis
extrahepatic duct involvement
extrahepatic malignancy
extrahepatic obstruction
extrahepatic portal venous hypertension
extrahepatic spread
extraintestinal
extraluminal retrorectal tumor
extramucosal myotomy
extramucosal stitch
extranodal extension of lymph node
    metastasis
extranodal growth
extranodal T cell lymphoma
extraparathyroidal tumor
extraperitoneal abscess
extraperitoneal approach
extraperitoneal fascia
extraperitoneal fat
extraperitoneal lymphocele
extraperitoneal organ
extraperitoneal space
extraperitoneal tissue
extrapyramidal movement disorder
extrasphincteric anal fistula
Extra Sport coronary guidewire
extrathyroidal invasion
extravasate
extravasated blood
extravasated contrast media
extravasation of contrast
extravasation of dye

extravasation of erythrocytes
extravascular fluid
Extra View balloon
ExtreSafe catheter
ExtreSafe needle
extrinsic lesion
extrinsic obstruction
extrinsic sphincter
extrude
extruding
extubate
extubation
exudate
exudation, peritoneal
exudative ascites
exudative colitis
exudative enteropathy
exudative peritonitis
ExuDerm hydrocolloid dressing
    material
Exu-Dry absorptive dressing
exulceratio simplex
eyelid edema
eye magnet
eye needle
eyepiece
eye spear sponge
eye wick sponge
EZ Detect colorectal screening test kit
E-Z Flap cranial bone plate
EZ45 thoracic linear cutter/stapler
Ez-HBT test
E-Z Tac soft tissue reattachment system
eZY WRAP abdominal binder

F, f

Fabco gauze bandage dressing
FABRase (alpha-galactosidase)
Fabrazyme (agalsidase beta)
Fabry disease
FAC (ferric ammonium citrate)
face-lift scissors
face, moon
faceplate (of ostomy appliance)
    Marlen Neoprene All-Flexible
    Torbot
    United Surgical Hypalon
faceted gallstone
facial cannula brush
facial muscle weakness
facies (surface)
    cushingoid
    moon
facies abdominalis
facies anterior corporis pancreatis
facies anterior glandulae suprarenalis
facies anterior prostatae
facies anterior renis
facies anteroinferior corporis pancreatis
facies anterosuperior corporis pancreatis
facies articularis capitis costae
facies articularis ossium
facies articularis tuberculi costae
facies colica lienis

facies colica splenis
facies costalis pulmonis
facies diaphragmatica cordis
facies diaphragmatica hepatis
facies diaphragmatica lienis
facies diaphragmatica pulmonis
facies diaphragmatica splenis
facies gastrica lienis
facies gastrica splenis
facies hepatica
facies hippocratica
facies inferior hepatis
facies inferior linguae
facies inferior pancreatis
facies inferolateralis prostatae
facies interlobaris pulmonis
facies intestinalis uteri
facies lateralis ovarii
facies lateralis testis
facies medialis ovarii
facies medialis pulmonis
facies medialis testis
facies mediastinalis pulmonis
facies posterior corporis pancreatica
facies posterior glandular suprarenalis
facies posterior hepatis
facies posterior prostatae
facies posterior renis

facies pulmonalis cordis
facies pulmonalis dextra cordis
facies pulmonalis sinistra cordis
facies renalis glandulare suprarenalis
facies renalis lienis
facies renalis splenis
facies sternocostalis cordis
facies superior hepatis
facies urethralis penis
facies vesicalis uteri
facies visceralis hepatis
facies visceralis lienis
facies visceralis splenis
FACT (Focal Angioplasty Catheter
   Technology)
FACT (focused appendix computed
   tomography)
factitial proctitis
factitious thyrotoxicosis
factor
   clotting
   coagulating
   coagulation
   growth
   intrinsic
   precipitating
   predisposing
   tissue growth (TGF)
   tumor necrosis (TNF)
factor V Leiden as a cause of
   Budd-Chiari syndrome
factor V Leiden heterozygote
factor VIII R:WF (von Willebrand
   factor)
factor VIII SQ, recombinant (ReFacto)
Factor One Medical
Fahey-Compere pin
Fahey retractor
failed nipple valve
failed shunt surgery
failing bone marrow
failure
   fulminant hepatic
   fulminant hepatocellular

failure *(cont.)*
   left-sided congestive heart
   organ
   right-sided congestive heart
failure of child to mature
failure of pancreatic ducts to fuse
failure to thrive
fair skin
falciform ligament
falciform retinal fold
falciparum malaria
Falcon coronary catheter
falling hematocrit
fallopian hiatus
false colonic obstruction
false diverticula
false-positive result
familial adenomatous polyposis (FAP)
familial adenomatous polyposis coli
familial amyloid polyneuropathy
familial chloride diarrhea
familial cholemia
familial cholestasis
familial chronic idiopathic jaundice
familial colorectal polyposis
familial dysproteinemia
familial gastrointestinal polyposis
familial hepatitis
familial hypercalcemia with nephro-
   calcinosis and indicanuria (blue-
   diaper syndrome)
familial hyperparathyroidism
familial hypocalciuric hypercalcemia
familial hypoproteinemia with lymph-
   angiectatic enteropathy
familial intestinal polyposis
familial intestinal pseudo-obstruction
familial intrahepatic cholestasis
familial Mediterranean fever
familial nonhemolytic jaundice
familial pancreatic cancer
familial pancreatitis
familial patent ductus venosus
familial polyposis coli (FPC)

familial polyposis syndrome
familial ulcerative colitis
familial visceral neuropathy
family history of breast cancer
family history, positive
FAMMM (familial atypical multiple
    mole melanoma) syndrome
famotidine
fan retractor
Fanelli guide
Fansler-Ives anoscope
Fansler proctoscope
Fansler speculum
FAP (familial adenomatous polyposis)
Farabeau-Lambotte rasp
Farabeuf bone rasp
Farabeuf bone-holding forceps
Farabeuf-Collin rasp
Farabeuf-Lambotte bone-holding
    forceps
Farabeuf periosteal elevator
Farabeuf rasp
Farabeuf raspatory
Farabeuf retractor
far-away metastasis
Fareston (toremifene citrate)
farmer's lung
Farrell cotton applicator
Farrior-Dworacek canal chisel
Farrior wire-crimping forceps
Farr spring-wire retractor
Farr wire retractor
fascia
    anterior rectus
    autologous rectus abdominis
    clavipectoral
    cribiform
    dartos
    deep
    deltopectoral
    Denonvillier
    endoabdominal
    external oblique
    external spermatic

fascia *(cont.)*
    Gerota
    internal oblique
    lateral oblique
    pectineus
    pectoral
    pectoralis
    posterior rectus
    preperitoneal
    rectus
    Scarpa
    spigelian
    transversalis
    Waldeyer
fascia anchor
fascial absorbable suture
fascia lata graft
fascia layer
fascial band
fascial bridge
fascial closure
fascial closure of trocar site
fascial defect
fascial graft
fascial layer
fascial plane
fascial-splitting incision
fascial stranding
fascia of abdomen
fascia/peritoneum funnel
fascia reapproximated
fascicular sarcoma
fasciitis, necrotizing
Fasciola gigantica
Fasciola hepatica
fasciolopsiasis
Fasciolopsis buski
Faslodex
fast-absorbing surgical gut (plain)
Fast-Cath introducer catheter
fast Fourier transform (FFT) technique
    for EGG analysis
fasting
fast smear

FASTak suture anchor
fastener
    ROC suture
    ROC XS suture
    Suture Clinch
Fastin anchor
fasting
fasting blood glucose
fasting chemistry panel
fasting diet
fasting gastric bile acid test
fasting gastrin level
fasting hyperinsulinemia
fasting hypoglycemia
fasting insulin and glucose levels
fasting serum gastrin
F.A.S.T. 1 (First Access for Shock and
    Trauma) System
FastPack test
Fastrac gastrostomy access port
FasTrac guidewire
FasTracker catheter
FastTake blood glucose monitoring
    system
fat
    abdominal
    blurred pericecal (on CT scan)
    dietary
    interposed omental
    intramuscular
    mesenteric
    omental
    paucity of
    perinephric
    perirenal
    preperitoneal
    protruding
    subcutaneous
fatal anaphylaxis
fatal hereditary tyrosinemia
fat cell
fat creeping
fat emulsion, intravenous
fatigability

fat metabolism
fat necrosis
fat necrosis of breast
fat pad, abdominal
fat pad retractor
fat plane
fat saponification
fat-soluble bilirubin
fat-soluble vitamin
fat storage disorder
fat-storing liver cell
fat towel
fatty acid bile acid conjugate
    (FABAC)
fatty acid metabolism
fatty acid
fatty ascites
fatty cirrhosis
fatty food intolerance
fatty foods
fatty infiltration of liver
fatty kidney
fatty liver
fatty liver disease
fatty liver hepatitis
fatty liver of pregnancy (obstetric
    yellow atrophy)
fatty liver relation to HAART
fatty meal
fatty meal sonogram (FMS)
fatty micromedionodular cirrhosis
fatty necrosis
fatty stools
fatty tissue
faucial thermal-tactile stimulation
Faure forceps
Favaloro-Morse rib spreader
Favaloro sternal retractor
favorable prognosis
Fazier modified suction tube
FBA (fecal bile acid)
FCIS (Flint Colon Injury Scale)
FCPA2 ultrafast laser
FCS-ML II colonoscope

FCS-ML II endoscope
FCS-ML II gastroscope
FCS (full cervical spine) view
FDA (Food and Drug Administration)
FD-43 microdissector
FDL (fluorescein dilaurate) test
FeatherTouch CO_2 laser
feathery degeneration
feathery pattern of barium in small
    bowel
febrile agglutinin panel
febrile illness
fecal alpha$_1$-antitrypsin test
fecal analysis
fecal bile acid (FBA)
fecal contamination of food or water
fecal continence
fecal fat analysis
fecal fat excretion, 24-hour
fecal fat study
fecal fistula
fecal flora
fecal impaction
fecal incontinence
fecal incontinence score
fecalith, appendiceal
fecal mass
fecal material
fecal obstruction
fecal occult blood
fecal occult blood test (FEOT)
fecal-oral route of virus transmission
fecal-oral transmission
fecal osmolarity
fecal peritonitis
fecal reservoir
fecal residue
fecal stasis
fecal stream
fecal stream diversion
fecal transmission
fecaluria
fecal urobilinogen
fecal vomitus

Fecatest
feces (see *stool*)
    impacted
    inspissated
feces smear
feculence
feculent
feculent drainage
feculent vomitus
Federici sign
fedotozine
feedback mechanism
feeding (see also *formula*)
    Amin-Aid powdered
    bolus
    Build Up enteral
    Citrotein liquid
    Clinifeed Iso enteral
    Compleat-B liquid
    continuous drip
    Criticare HN elemental liquid
    Enrich
    Ensure Plus liquid
    enteral
    Entrition Entri-Pak
    Finkelstein
    Flexical enteral
    forced
    Fortison enteral
    gastrostomy
    gavage
    half-strength
    Hepatic-Aid powdered
    HN (high nitrogen)
    hyperosmotic
    intermittent drip
    intravenous (I.V., IV)
    Isocal HCN (high calorie and
        nitrogen) liquid
    Isotein HN
    isotonic
    Jevity isotonic liquid nutrition
    lactose-free
    Lonalac

feeding *(cont.)*
  low-residue
  Magnacal
  Meritene liquid
  NJ (nasojejunal)
  Osmolite HN liquid
  parenteral
  Portagen
  Precision Isotein HN powdered
  Precision Isotonic powdered
  Precision LR powdered
  Renu
  Resource
  Stresstein
  Sustacal HC (high calorie) liquid
  Sustacal HN liquid
  TraumaCal enteral liquid
  Traum-Aid HBC
  Travasorb HN powdered
  Travasorb MCT liquid
  Travasorb STD
  tube
  Vital
  Vitaneed
  Vivonex HN powdered
  Vivonex T.E.N.
feeding gastrostomy tube
feeding jejunostomy
feeding tube
Feen-A-Mint
Fehland colon resection clamp
Fehland intestinal clamp
Feilchenfeld splinter forceps
Feild (*not* Field) blade
Feild-Lee brain biopsy needle
Felig insulin pump
FELL suction tube
Fellonet ointment gauze dressing
felt dressing
Felty syndrome
female catheter
female reamer
feminizing tumor
femoral artery

femoral canal
femoral condyle drill
femoral-cutaneous nerve
femoral guide pin
femoral head extractor
femoral head necrosis
femoral hernia repair
femoral intermedullary guide
femoral ligament
femoral lymphadenopathy
femoral neck nail
femoral plate
femoral pulse
femoral shaft reamer
femoral sheath
femoral vein
femorocrural graft
femorocutaneous nerve
femorodistal PTFE graft
FemRx Soprano cryotherapy system
Femtosecond laser keratome
FEN (fluids, electrolytes, nutrition)
FENa (fractional excretion of sodium)
fenestrated bowel grasper
fenestrated cup biopsy forceps
fenestrated drape
fenestrated grasper
fenestrated reamer
fenestrated tube
fenestration saw
fenfluramine
Fenger gallbladder probe
fenoctimine; fenoctimine sulfate
fentanyl citrate
Fentanyl Oralet (fentanyl)
Fenwick disease
FEOT (fecal occult blood test)
FEP polymer
Ferguson bone-holding forceps
Ferguson brain suction tube
Ferguson forceps
Ferguson-Frazier suction tube
Ferguson gallstone scoop
Ferguson hemorrhoidectomy

Ferguson-Moon rectal speculum
Ferguson view
Fergusson dressing scissors
Fergusson forceps
Fergusson gallstone scoops
Fergusson hemorrhoidal clamp
Fergusson speculum
Fergusson suction tube
Feridex (ferumoxides)
Feridex I.V. (ferumoxides injectable
    solution)
feritin concentration
ferric ammonium citrate (FAC)
Ferris biliary duct dilator
FerriSeltz (ferric ammonium citrate
    [FAC])
Ferris Smith intervertebral disk rongeur
Ferris Smith-Kerrison forceps
Ferris Smith-Kerrison laminectomy
    rongeur
Ferris Smith laminectomy rongeur
Ferris Smith pituitary jaw rongeur
Ferris Smith rongeur forceps
Ferris Smith-Spurling disk rongeur
Ferris Smith tissue forceps
ferrite filter
ferritin, serum
ferromagnetic tamponade
Festalan
Festal II
fetal cortical tissue graft
fetal (early, intermediate, late) death
fetal diagnosis
fetal goiter
fetal substantia nigra graft
Feth-R-Kath epidural catheter
fetor hepaticus
fever
    acute rheumatic
    aseptic
    bullous
    cat-bite
    cat-scratch
    Colorado tick

fever *(cont.)*
    dehydration
    dengue
    drug
    enteric
    familial Mediterranean
    hepatic
    herpetic
    high-grade
    intermittent
    low-grade
    Mediterranean
    parenteric
    puerperal
    rat-bite
    relapsing
    rheumatic
    San Joaquin Valley
    scarlet
    Sennetsu
    septic
    steroid
    syphilitic
    yellow
    valley
fever of unknown or undetermined
    origin (FUO)
fever spike
Festal II
FFP (fresh frozen plasma)
FFT line
FGS and FCS endoscope
FGS-ML II endoscope
FGS-ML II gastroscope
FHF (fulminant hepatic failure)
FHIT (fragile histidine triad)
FHP (familial hypofibrinogenemia)
Fiberall (calcium polycarbophil)
FiberCon (calcium polycarbophil)
fiber, dietary
Fiberlan (lactose-free formula)
Fiberlase laser
Fiber-Lax (calcium polycarbophil)
Fiber-Norm (calcium polycarbophil)

Fiber One bran cereal
fiberoptic choledochoscope
fiberoptic endoscope
fiberoptic gastroscope
fiberoptic injection sclerotherapy (FIS)
fiberoptic light cable
fiberoptic panendoscopy
fibers, circular muscle
fiberscope (see *endoscope*)
fiber-splitting incision
Fibracol collagen-alginate dressing
Fibracol Plus collagen wound dressing
Fibrijet adhesive
fibrillary bacteria
Fibrillex (NC-503)
fibrin glue
fibrin glue adhesive
fibrinogen
fibrinoid lung
fibrinoid necrosis
fibrinolysin and desoxyribonuclease
fibrinolysis
fibrinous adhesions
fibrinous polyp
fibrin sealant
fibrin sponge
fibroadenoma of breast
fibroadipose tissue
fibroblastic ingrowth
fibroblastic tissue response
fibrocartilaginous pad
fibrocartilaginous plate
fibrocongestive splenomegaly
fibrocystic breast
fibrocystic breast syndrome
fibrocystic disease of breast
fibrocystic disorder of breast
fibroepithelial papilloma
fibroepithelial polyp
fibrofatty infiltration of pancreas
fibrofatty tissue
fibrogenesis
fibroglandular tissue

fibroid degeneration
fibrolamellar carcinoma
fibrolamellar hepatocarcinoma
fibrolamellar hepatocellular carcinoma
    (HCC)
fibrolamellar hepatoma
fibroma
fibromyoma
fibromyxoma
fibronectin-repeat domains
fibroplasia
fibrosarcoma
fibrosing piecemeal necrosis
fibrosis
    alcoholic
    arachnoid
    bridging
    chronic sclerosing hyaline
    congenital hepatic (CHF)
    cystic
    diffuse lobular
    inflammatory
    lung
    noncirrhotic portal (NCPF)
    pancreatic
    periductal
    periportal
    perisinusoidal
    perivenular
    portal
    portal-to-portal
    progressive perivenular alcoholic
        (PPAF)
    retroperitoneal
    secondary biliary
    sinusoidal
    transmural
fibrosis of liver
fibrosis of lung
fibrosis of thyroid
fibrotic liver
fibrotic pattern
fibrous adhesion
fibrous capsule of kidney

fibrous change
fibrous fullness
fibrous goiter
fibrous obliterative cholangitis
fibrous septum
fibrous sheath
fibrous stroma
fibrous stromal tissue
fibrous thyroiditis
fibrous tissue
fibrous tuberosity
fibrous tumor (desmoid)
fibrovascular polyp
fiducial plate
Fiedler disease
field
  bloodless
  operative
  surgical
field block anesthesia
fifth vital sign (pain)
figure-of-8 (or figure-8) dressing
figure-of-8 interscapular bandage
figure-of-4 (or figure-4) position
filament-forming bacillus
filariasis
file, Bayonet bone
filiform bougie
filiform guide for Lefort sound
filiform papilla
filiform polyposis
filiforms and followers
filler tube
fillet local flap graft
filleted the tract open
filling defect, radiolucent
filling of gallbladder with fluid
film (see also *position, projection, view)*
  absorbable gelatin
  Accu-Flo dura
  AP (anteroposterior)
  chiropractic
  comparison

film *(cont.)*
  cross-table lateral
  decubitus
  digital subtraction
  DuPont Cronex x-ray
  Knuttsen bending
  lateral decubitus
  low-contrast
  NUVO barrier
  oblique
  overhead
  PA (posteroanterior)
  plain
  portable
  postevacuation
  preliminary
  prone
  Repel abdominal
  Repel-CV abdominal
  scout
  skull
  spot
  stress
  suboptimal
  subtraction
  supine
  upright
film-based viewing
filmless imaging
filmy adhesion
Filshie clip applier
Filshie female sterilization clip
filter
  CO_2 gas
  OmniFilter
  PFR95
Filtzer interbody rasp
fimbriated fold
final diagnosis
Fine cross-action retractor
FIN extractor
Fine-Kerrison cervical rongeurs
finely fatty foamy liver
fine needle

fine-needle aspirate
fine-needle aspiration (FNA)
fine-needle aspiration biopsy
fine-needle aspiration cytology
fine-needle biopsy
fine-needle percutaneous cholangio-
    gram
fine-needle transhepatic cholangiogram
fine-tip forceps
fine tissue forceps
fine-toothed forceps
fine-tooth fenestrated grasper
fingerbreadth
finger dissection
finger fracture dissection
finger fracture of liver
finger fracture technique
fingernail drill
finger retractor
finger ring cutter
fingerstick (see *lancet*)
fingertip dissection
fingertip lesion
Finney pyloroplasty
Finochietto forceps
Finochietto laminectomy retractor
Finochietto-Metzenbaum scissors
Finochietto needle
Finochietto retractor
Finochietto rib spreader
Finochietto thoracic scissors
FIN pin guide
FiO$_2$
Firlit drip stent
firm and rubbery gland
firm mass
firm neoplasm
First Access for Shock and Trauma
    (F.A.S.T.) system
First Aid Bandage Company
First Aid triple-antibiotic bandage
first branch of the external carotid
    artery
First Choice reagent strips

first-degree hemorrhoid
first-degree history
first-degree relative
first duodenal sphincter
first-pass effect
first rib rongeur
first rib shears
First Warning breast cancer screening
    device
FIS (fiberoptic injection sclerotherapy)
Fisch bone rongeur
Fisch dural hook
Fischer cone biopsy excisor
Fischer transfixing pin
Fischer ventricular cannula
Fisch micro hook
Fisch rectal probe
Fisch retractor
FISH (fluorescence in situ hybridiza-
    tion)
Fisher and Paykel humidifier
Fisher exact test
Fisher guide
Fisher half pin
fisherman's knot
Fisher rasp
fishhook hook
fish insulin
Fishman-Doubilet test
fishmouth incision
fishmouth suture
fish-odor syndrome (trimethylaminuria)
fish-scale gallbladder
Fiskars Softouch scissors
fissure
    anal
    azygos
    chronic fissure refractory to
        conservative treatment
    portal
    rectal
    umbilical
fissurectomy
fissure in ano

fissure *of lung*
fistula (pl. fistulae, fistulas)
   abdominal
   abdominal wall
   anal
   anoperineal
   anorectal
   anovestibular
   aortoduodenal
   aortoenteric
   aortoesophageal
   aortosigmoid
   appendiceal
   arteriovenous (AV)
   biliary
   biliary-cutaneous
   biliary-duodenal
   biliary-enteric (bilioenteric)
   bladder
   Blom-Singer tracheoesophageal
   brachioaxillary bridge graft (BAGF)
   brachiosubclavian bridge graft
     (BSGF)
   branchial
   Brescia-Cimino AV
   bronchobiliary
   bronchocavitary
   bronchoesophageal
   bronchopleural
   cholecystenteric
   cholecystocholedochal
   cholecystocolonic
   cholecystoduodenal
   cholecystoduodenocolic
   cholecystoenteric
   choledochocolonic
   choledochoduodenal
   colocutaneous
   coloenteric
   colonic
   colovaginal
   colovesical
   complex anorectal
   congenital pulmonary arteriovenous

fistula *(cont.)*
   cystic
   duodenal
   duodenocolic
   Eck
   enteric
   enterocolic
   enterocutaneous
   enteroenteral; enteroenteric
   enterourethral
   enterovaginal
   enterovesical
   external biliary
   external pancreatic
   extrasphincteric anal
   fecal
   gallbladder
   gastric
   gastrocolic
   gastrocutaneous
   gastroduodenal
   gastrointestinal
   gastrojejunal-colic
   gastrojejunocolic
   genitourinary
   graft-enteric
   hepatic
   hepatopleural
   high-output
   horseshoe
   H-type
   ileorectal
   ileosigmoid
   intersphincteric anal
   intrahepatic AV
   ischiorectal
   jejunocolic
   lactiferous duct
   Mann-Bollman
   mesenteric
   mucous
   nasolabial
   orofacial
   pancreatic cutaneous

fistula *(cont.)*
    pancreatic enteric
    pancreaticocutaneous
    pancreaticopleural
    parietal
    perineovaginal
    pilonidal
    rectal
    rectourethral
    rectovaginal
    rectovesical
    refractory pancreatic
    respiratory-esophageal
    retroperitoneal
    sigmoidovesical
    small bowel
    splanchnic AV
    splenic AV
    suprasphincteric
    thyroglossal
    tracheoesophageal (TE, TEF)
    transsphincteric anal
    urethrovaginal
    vesical
    vesicoenteric
    vesicouterine
    vesicovaginal
    vitelline
fistula formation
fistula hook
fistula in ano
fistula needle
fistula probe
fistula scissors
fistulation, spreading
fistulectomy
fistulization, cholecystobiliary
fistulization of esophagus
fistulization of sublingual salivary cyst
fistulizing Crohn disease
fistulogram
fistulography
fistulotomy, Parks staged
fistulous tract

Fitbox
Fitz-Hugh–Curtis syndrome
Fitzgerald aortic aneurysm forceps
five-hole (5-hole) plate
Fixateur Interne rod
fixation of breast mass to chest wall
fixation of breast mass to overlying skin
fixation pin
fixator-augmented nail
fixed-angle blade plate
fixed axillary lymph node
fixed segment of bowel
flabby abdomen
flagellate diarrhea
Flagyl (metronidazole)
flail chest
flail segment
Flanagan-Burem apposing hemicylin-
    dric graft
Flanagan spinal fusion gouge
flank
flank bruit
flank incision
flank pain
flank scar
flap
    abdominal
    advancement
    advancement of rectal
    anconeus muscle
    artery island
    Atasoy-Kleinert
    Atasoy palmar
    Atasoy triangular advancement
    axial flag
    axial pattern
    Bakamjian
    bilobed
    bipedicle
    bone
    bursal
    butterfly
    Chinese
    cross-finger

flap *(cont.)*

cross-leg
cross-lip
cross-lip pedicle
Dandy myocutaneous scalp
deep circumflex iliac artery-iliac
crest
deltopectoral
digital
dorsal rotation
dorsal transposition
dorsalis pedis fasciocutaneous
dorsalis pedis myofascial
double pedicle
double pedicle TRAM
DRAM (de-epithelialized rectus
abdominis) muscle
entry
extended
extensor carpi radialis longus
fascial
fasciocutaneous island
finger-fillet
free
free fasciocutaneous
free fibular harvest
free latissimus dorsi
free temporal
galeal
gastrocnemius sliding
gracilis muscle
groin
hemipulp
horseshoe-shaped
iliac osteocutaneous free
iliofemoral pedicle
interdigitating skin
island
island pedicle
Karydakis
Kutler digital
lateral transverse thigh
latissimus dorsi
latissimus dorsi island

flap *(cont.)*

latissimus dorsi musculocutaneous
free
latissimus dorsi myocutaneous
liver
lumbrical muscle
maple leaf
Martius flap and fascial sling
Martius labial fat pad
McCraw gracilis myocutaneous
microsurgical free
Moberg
modified dorsalis pedis myofascial
muscle
musculocutaneous free
musculotendinous
myocutaneous
myofascial
necrotic
neurocutaneous island
neurovascular island pedicle
nutrient
omental
Oriental V-Y
osteocutaneous free
osteoplastic
palmar advancement
parascapular
pectoralis major
pedicle
pedicled muscle-tendon
pericranial
peritoneal
peroneal island
pulp
radial-based
radial forearm
rectus abdominis
rectus abdominis musculocutaneous
free
rectus muscle
remote pedicle
rotational
rotator

flap *(cont.)*
  Rubens
  scalp
  scapular
  segmented
  single pedicle
  single pedicle TRAM
  skin
  subscapularis muscle
  Tait
  tensor fasciae latae
  thenar
  three-square
  TRAM (transverse rectus abdominis
    myocutaneous)
  transposition
  transverse rectus abdominis
    myocutaneous (TRAM)
  triangular
  triceps
  tumbler
  tummy tuck
  turned-down tendon
  vascularized
  V-Y advancement
  wraparound
flap graft, Kutler V-Y
flap knife
flapping tremor sign
flap tear
flap-valve mechanism
flap viability
flareup
flashlamp-pulsed dye laser
flashlamp-pulsed Nd:YAG laser
flashlamp-pumped pulsed dye laser
flask-shaped ulcer
flat condyloma
flat drill
flatfooted
flat grasping forceps, fenestrated,
  double-action
flat lesion
flat narrow elevator

flat-nose pliers
flat plate
flat plate of abdomen
flat Silastic suction drain
flat stick sponge
flat suture
Flatt driver
flattened duodenal fold
flattened T wave
flattened stool
flattening of ileal epithelium
flatulence
flatulent
flatulent colic
flatulent dyspepsia
Flatulex (simethicone)
flatus
flatus enema
flavin-containing mono-oxygenase
  (FMO) 2
flea-bitten kidney
fleecy mass
Fleet Babylax (glycerin)
Fleet bowel prep
Fleet Bisacodyl enema
Fleet enema
Fleet Laxative (bisacodyl)
Fleet Mineral Oil enema
Fleet Phospho-Soda (monobasic sodium
  phosphate; dibasic sodium
  phosphate)
"flesh-eating" bacteria
Fletcher's Castoria (senna concentrate)
Fletcher polypectomy forceps
fleur de lis breast reconstruction pattern
Flex Advantage kit
Flexbar Machine Corp video camera
  system
flex drill
Flex-EZ balloon dilator
Flex-Foam bandage
Flexguard Tip catheter
Flexiblade laryngoscope
flexible arm (Leyla) retractors

flexible dental suction
flexible endoscope
flexible endoscopic surgery
flexible esophagoscopy
flexible gastrointestinal cryotherapy
flexible medullary reamer
flexible operating instruments
flexible optical biopsy forceps
flexible retractor
flexible sigmoidoscope
flexible, steerable nasolaryngo-
  pharyngoscope
flexible stent
flexible ureteroscope
Flexiflo Lap G laparoscopic gastros-
  tomy kit
Flexiflo Lap J laparoscopic jejunostomy
  kit
Flexiflo Stomate low-profile gastros-
  tomy tube
Flexilite conforming elastic bandage
Flexima biliary stent system
Flexinet dressing
flexion view
Flexlase 600 laser
Flex-Master bandage
Flexon steel suture
flexor palmar plate
flexor tendon graft
FlexPack HP test
FlexPosure endoscopic retractor
Flex-T cannister
FlexTip intervertebral rongeur
FlexTube bandage
flexure
  duodenojejunal
  hepatic
  left colonic
  right colonic
  sigmoid
  splenic
Flexxicon Blue dialysis catheter
Flexzan foam wound dressing
F. L. Fischer microsurgical neurectomy
  bayonet scissors

FL-HCC (fibrolamellar hepatocellular
  carcinoma)
FLIC (Functional Living Index-Cancer)
Flint Colon Injury Scale (FCIS)
floating gallbladder
floating gallstone
floating kidney
floating liver
floating spleen
floating stool
flocculation on barium enema
Flo-Coat (barium sulfate)
FloCoil shunt
Flocor (poloxamer 188)`
Flood syndrome
floor of canal
floor of foregut
floor of inguinal region
floor, pelvic
floorstand reflector
floppy guidewire
floppy Nissen fundoplication
floppy-type Nissen fundoplication
flora
  colonic
  fecal
  intestinal
  normal
florid cirrhosis
florid duct lesion
Florinef Acetate (fludrocortisone
  acetate)
FloSeal Matrix hemostatic sealant
flow-compromising lesion
flower-shaped polypropylene mesh plug
  with multiple petal
FlowGun suction/irrigation
flow-limiting lesion
flow/pressure/resistance formula
Floxin (ofloxacin)
floxuridine (FUDR; FUdR)
flu-like syndrome
fluctuance, rectal submuscular
fluctuant abscess

fluctuant mass
fludrocortisone acetate
fluence (measurement)
fluffs dressing
Fluhrer rectal probe
fluid
   amniotic
   articular
   ascitic
   bile-stained
   bile-tinged
   bloody
   bloody peritoneal
   body
   Bouin
   cavitary
   cerebrospinal
   chylous
   clear
   cloudy
   crystalloid
   cystic
   Delafield
   dentinal
   Dialyflex dialysis
   digestive
   edema
   embalming
   extracellular
   extravascular
   free
   frothy
   gelatinous
   intercellular
   interstitial
   intracellular
   intravascular
   intravenous
   joint
   LDH level of ascitic
   loculated
   low-viscosity
   lymphatic
   meconium-stained amniotic

fluid *(cont.)*
   milky
   motor oil peritoneal
   natural body
   periappendiceal
   pericardial
   pericardial effusion
   pericholecystic
   peritoneal
   peritoneal effusion
   pleural
   pleural effusion
   prostatic
   protein-rich
   prune juice peritoneal
   sanguineous
   seminal
   serosanguineous
   serous
   spinal
   straw-colored
   subhepatic space
   synovial
   testing
   thoracentesis
   transcellular
   turbid
   turbid peritoneal
   viscous
   Zenker
fluid accumulation (from aneurysm or
   perforation)
fluid and electrolyte absorption
Fluid Alarm System (FAS) glove
   integrity system
fluid collection in pericholecystic area
fluid collection pouch
fluid-filled cleft
fluid-filled cyst
fluid-filled mass
fluid-filled papule
fluid-filled sac
fluid-filled vacuole within lens
fluid loss, gastrointestinal

fluid material
fluid overload
fluid protein
fluid resuscitation
fluid sequestration
fluid specimen, filtration of
fluid volume deficit
fluid volume excess
fluid warmer
fluid wave
fluke (trematode)
fluke, liver
flu-like syndrome
flumecino
FluMist vaccine
FLU OIA assay
fluorescein
fluorescence in situ hybridization
   (FISH)
fluorescence spectroscopy
FluoroNav virtual fluoroscopy system
Fluoropassiv thin-wall carotid patch
fluoropyrimidine
fluoroscopic control
fluoroscopic resolution
fluoroscopic stress x-ray view
fluoroscopy
fluorouracil (5-FU)
fluorouracil and leucovorin
Fluothane (halothane)
fluoxymesterone
flush port cap
flush-with-skin stoma
flushing
fluted J-Vac drain
fluted medullary rod
fluted titanium nail
FMO (flavin-containing mono-
   oxygenase) 2
FMS (fatty meal sonogram)
FNAC (fine-needle aspiration cytology)
FNH (focal nodular hyperplasia)
foam cell
foam dressing

foam gauze dressing
Foamicon (aluminum hydroxide;
   magnesium trisilicate)
foam roll bandage
foam sheet bandage
foam wound dressing
foamy esophagus
foamy liver
foamy material
foamy stool
Fobi pouch
focal biliary cirrhosis
focal calcification
focal colitis
focal colonic mucosal ulcer
focal dilation of the splenic vein
focal edema
focal goiter
focal hemorrhage
focal hepatocellular necrosis with
   hemorrhagic cyst
focal infection
focal lesion
focal necrosis
focal neurologic deficit
focal nodular hyperplasia (FNH)
focal pancreatitis
FocalSeal sealant
FocalSeal-L sealant
FocalSeal-S surgical sealant
focal small bowel obstruction
focal tenderness
focal tumor
focal ulceration and hemorrhage
foci (plural of focus)
   hypotensive
   hepatocyte dysplasia
   metastasis
   tumor
focused appendix computed
   tomography (FACT)
Foerster abdominal ring retractor
Foerster capsulotomy knife
Foerster sponge-holding forceps

Fogarty adherent clot catheter
Fogarty balloon
Fogarty balloon biliary catheter
Fogarty biliary probe
Fogarty-Chin clamp
Fogarty clamp
Fogarty embolectomy catheter
Fogarty forceps
Fogarty graft thrombectomy catheter
Fogarty Hydrogrip clamp
Fogarty irrigation catheter
Fogarty-type jaw
fogging of laparoscope
fog reduction elimination device
　(FRED)
fold
　adipose
　alar
　amniotic
　aryepiglottic
　axillary
　caval
　cecal
　cholecystoduodenocolic
　ciliary
　circular
　circulator
　costocolic
　Douglas
　duodenojejunal
　duodenomesocolic
　epigastric
　falciform retinal
　fimbriated
　flattened duodenal
　gastric
　gastropancreatic
　genital
　glossopalatine
　gluteal
　Guérin
　haustral
　hepatopancreatic
　ileocecal

fold *(cont.)*
　ileocolic
　inferior duodenal
　inferior transverse rectal
　inguinal
　interureteric
　Kerckring
　labioscrotal
　lateral umbilical
　medial umbilical
　mucosal
　Nélaton
　palatopharyngeal
　paraduodenal
　peritoneal
　rectal
　rectouterine
　sacrogenital
　semilunar
　sentinel
　sigmoid
　spiral
　superior duodenal
　superior transverse rectal
　vestigial
folded fundus gallbladder
folded gallbladder
fold pattern
Folergot-DF (belladonna alkaloids;
　phenobarbital; ergotamine tartrate)
Foley catheter
Foley catheter bladder decompression
Foley catheter gastrostomy tube
foliate papilla
F/O light carrier
F of follicular cancer (far-away
　metastasis, female, FNA-not,
　favorable prognosis)
folinic acid
follicle associated epithelium
follicular carcinoma
follicular cells of the thyroid
follicular cholecystitis
follicular gastritis

follicular goiter
follicular mucinosis
follow-up examination
Foloxatine (oxaliplatin)
Foltz catheter
Fomon chisel
Fomon periosteal elevator
Fomon rasp
Fonar Stand-Up MRI
Fonar-360 MRI Scanner
food
　bland
　blenderized
　cholecystokinetic
　fatty
　fried
　gas-producing
　greasy
　liquid
　spicy
Food and Drug Administration (FDA)
food bolus obstruction
food-borne gastroenteritis
food pipe
food poisoning, staphylococcal
food supplement
foot drape
foot plate
forage core biopsy
foramen cecum at the base
　of the tongue
foramen of Bochdalek
foramen of Winslow
Forane (isoflurane)
Forbes-Albright syndrome
Forbes disease
Force balloon dilatation catheter
forced alimentation
forced feeding
forceful retching
forceps (see also *hemostat*)
　Acland clamp-applying
　ACMI Martin endoscopy
　Acufex curved basket

forceps *(cont.)*
　Acufex rotary biting basket
　Adair-Allis
　Adson
　Adson bayonet dressing
　Adson bipolar
　Adson-Brown tissue
　Adson clip-introducing
　Adson dressing
　Adson dura protecting
　Adson hemostatic
　Adson hypophyseal
　Adson lightweight plain
　Adson lightweight toothed
　Adson microforceps
　Adson micro tissue
　Adson-Mixter neurosurgical
　Adson rongeur
　Adson tissue
　adventitial
　Aesculap bipolar cautery
　Alderkreutz
　Alexander biopsy
　Allen intestinal
　alligator
　alligator grasping
　alligator jaws
　alligator-type grasping
　Allis
　Allis atraumatic tissue
　Allis-TC tissue
　Allis-Willauer
　Anderson
　Angell James hypophysectomy
　Angell James reverse-action
　　hypophysectomy
　angled-down
　angled-up
　anterior
　AO reduction
　approximating
　Arruga-Nicetic
　artery
　arthroscopy basket

forceps *(cont.)*
   arthroscopy grasping
   Asch
   AtrauGrip
   atraumatic
   Babcock
   Babcock atraumatic tissue
   Babcock grasping, double-action
   Babcock intestinal
   Babcock-TC
   baby Allis
   baby Babcock tissue
   baby Doyen intestinal
   baby Tischler biopsy
   Backhaus
   Backhaus towel
   Bacher flexible biopsy
   Bacon rongeur
   Baer bone cutting
   Baggish
   Bailey aortic valve cutting
   Bainbridge
   Baird
   ball-and-socket towel
   Ballantine
   Ballenger
   Ballenger sponge-holding
   Bane rongeur
   Bangerter muscle
   Bardeleben bone-holding
   Barnes-Neville
   Barraquer cilia
   Barraquer Colibri
   Barraquer suture-removing
   Barrett intestinal
   Barrett placenta
   Barrett tenaculum
   Barton obstetrical
   basket
   basket-type crushing
   Bauer
   bayonet
   bayonet bipolar
   bayonet-shaped

forceps *(cont.)*
   bayonet-type
   Beasley-Babcock
   Beer cilia
   Behrend cystic duct
   Bellucci alligator
   Bengolea artery
   Berens muscle
   Berry-TC wire-twisting
   Best gallstone
   Bevan gallbladder
   Beyer rongeur
   biarticular bone-cutting
   BiCOAG bipolar
   Billingham hemorrhoidal grasping
   Billroth
   Billroth tumor
   biopsy
   biopsy cup
   bipolar
   bipolar cautery
   Bircher-Ganske cartilage
   Bishop-Harmon
   BiSure laparoscopic
   Blake gallstone
   Blakesley suction flow
   Bloodwell
   blunt
   blunt grasping, double-action
   Boettcher artery
   Boies
   bone-biting
   bone-breaking
   bone-cutting
   bone-grasping
   bone-holding
   bone punch
   bone-splitting
   Bonney
   bottle and specimen
   bottle nose
   Bozeman sponge-holding
   brain
   brain clip

forceps *(cont.)*
    brain spatula
    brain tumor
    Brand tendon-holding
    Brand tendon-passing
    Brand tendon-tunneling
    Braun tenaculum
    Bridge
    Brigham brain tumor
    bronchoesophageal
    bronchus
    Brown-Adson
    Brown-Adson tissue
    Brown-Cushing
    Brown tissue
    Brunner intestinal
    Brunschwig artery
    Buie pile
    bulldog
    bulldog clamp-applying
    bullet-nose, tissue-well, double-action
    Burke biopsy
    Butler bayonet
    Cairns
    Cairns hemostatic
    Caparosa wire-crimping
    capsular release
    Carmalt
    Carmalt artery
    Carroll bone-holding
    Carroll dressing
    Carroll tendon-pulling
    Carroll tissue
    cartilage
    Caspar alligator
    Castroviejo-Colibri
    catheter-introducing
    cervical punch
    Chandler spinal perforating
    Charnley
    Charnley suture
    Charnley wire-holding
    Cheatle sterilizing
    Cheron polypus and dressing

forceps *(cont.)*
    Cherry-Kerrison laminectomy
    Childe approximating
    Children's Hospital intestinal
    Childs intestinal
    cholecystectomy
    Citelli punch
    clamp-applying
    claw
    claw-grasping, 2 x 3 teeth, double-
        action
    Cleveland bone-cutting
    clip-applying
    clip-bending
    clip-cutting
    clip-inserting
    clip-introducing
    clip-removing
    Cloward punch
    Cloward rongeur
    coagulating
    coaptation bipolar
    cobra-grasping, double-action
    Cobra rat-tooth grasping
    Colibri
    Collin-Duval lung grasping
    Collin tissue-grasping
    Collingwood Stewart hernia ring
    Collins intestinal
    Collison
    Colver tonsil-seizing
    cone-nose
    cone skull punch
    cone wire-twisting
    Cooley-Baumgarten aortic
    Cooley vascular
    Crafoord
    cranial rongeur
    Crile artery
    Crile curved
    Crile gall duct
    Crile hemostatic
    Crile-Rankin
    cup

forceps *(cont.)*
> cupped-jaw
> curved
> curved Crile
> curved Kelly
> curved mosquito
> Cushing bayonet
> Cushing bipolar
> Cushing-Brown
> Cushing delicate
> Cushing dressing
> Cushing monopolar
> Cushing rongeur
> Cushing tissue
> cutting
> CV
> cystic duct
> Dale
> Dandy scalp hemostatic
> Davis
> Davis coagulating
> Davis monopolar
> Dawson-Yuhl-Kerrison rongeur
> Dawson-Yuhl-Leksell rongeur
> DeBakey-Adson tissue
> DeBakey arterial
> DeBakey AtrauGrip
> DeBakey-Bainbridge atraumatic
>> intestinal
> DeBakey-Bainbridge intestinal
> DeBakey-Cooley dissecting
> DeBakey-Diethrich atraumatic tissue
> DeBakey-Diethrich vascular
> DeBakey dissecting
> DeBakey double-action grasping
> DeBakey-Mixter artery
> DeBakey-Semb
> DeBakey tissue
> DeBakey vascular
> Decker alligator
> Decker microsurgical
> Deddish-Potts intestinal
> DeLee
> DeMartel appendix

forceps *(cont.)*
> DeMartel scalp flap
> Demel wire-tightening
> Demel wire-twisting
> Denis Browne intestinal holding
> depilatory
> D'Errico bayonet pituitary
> D'Errico hypophyseal
> D'Errico pituitary
> D'Errico tissue
> Desjardins gall duct
> Desjardins gallstone
> DeTakats-McKenzie brain clip
> DeVilbiss rongeur
> Dewey obstetrical
> diathermy
> dilating
> Dingman bone-holding
> DirectBite coated disposable biopsy
> disk
> dissecting
> dissecting and grasping
> dolphin nose-grasping
> double-spoon
> Doughty
> Doyen intestinal
> dressing
> dual-cup grasping
> duckbill
> Dumont dissecting
> Dumont micro-dissecting
> Dunhill artery
> dura protecting
> Durmont-style dissecting
> Duval-Crile lung
> Duval-Scheie hemorrhoidal
> Duval tissue-grasping
> eagle's beak bone-cutting
> ear
> Echlin rongeur
> Edna towel
> Effler-Groves
> electrocoagulating biopsy
> Elliot

forceps *(cont.)*
    Elliott gallbladder
    Emmett cotton swab
    end-biting
    Endo Dissect
    endoscopic
    endoscopic biopsy
    endoscopic grasping
    endoscopic suture-cutting
    Eppendorf biopsy
    Eppendorf-Tischler biopsy
    ethmoid
    Evans tissue
    extracting
    Farabeuf bone-holding
    Farabeuf-Lambotte bone-holding
    Farrior wire-crimping
    Faure
    Feilchenfeld splinter
    fenestrated cup biopsy
    Ferguson bone-holding
    Fergusson
    Ferris-Smith rongeur
    Ferris-Smith tissue
    fine-tip
    fine tissue
    fine-toothed
    Finochietto
    Fitzgerald aortic aneurysm
    flat grasping, fenestrated
    Fletcher polypectomy
    flexible optical biopsy
    Foerster sponge-holding
    Fogarty
    foreign body
    Foss
    Fox bipolar
    Fraser artery
    Friedman rongeur
    Fujinon biopsy
    gall duct
    gallstone
    Gardner bone
    Gavin-Miller intestinal

forceps *(cont.)*
    Gemini Finochietto artery
    Gemini gall duct
    Gemini thoracic
    George
    Gerald bipolar
    Gerald-Brown tissue
    Gerald dissecting
    Gerald dressing
    Gerald tissue
    Gerbode
    Gilbert cystic duct
    Gildenberg biopsy
    Gillies diathermy
    Gillies lightweight
    Gillies tissue
    gland
    Glassman-Allis intestinal
    Glenn diverticulum
    glenoid-reaming
    Gomel micro tying
    Graefe dissecting
    grasping
    Gray cystic duct
    Green-Armytage hemostasis
    Greene
    Greenwood bayonet
    Greenwood bipolar and suction
    Greven
    Gruenwald ear
    Gruppe wire-crimping
    Gunderson bone
    Gunderson muscle
    Gunnar-Hey roller
    Haberer intestinal
    Hajek-Koffler bone punch
    Halsted artery
    Halsted hemostatic mosquito
        (straight/curved)
    Halsted mosquito
    Hardy bipolar
    Hardy dressing
    Hardy microbipolar
    Hardy sella punch

forceps *(cont.)*
    Harrington-Mixter thoracic
    Harrington thoracic
    Harrison bone-holding
    Harrison Cripp
    Harrison sterilizing
    Hartmann hemostatic mosquito
    Hartmann nasal dressing
    Haugh
    Hayes Martin
    Hayton Williams wire-twisting
    Healy intestinal
    Heaney
    Heath-Richter clip-removing
    Heermann alligator
    Heiss artery
    Heiss Finochietto
    hemoclip-applying
    hemostatic
    Henahan extracting
    Hendrin
    Herget rectal biopsy
    hernia ring
    Herrmann alligator
    Heywood-Smith hemorrhoidal
    Hibbs bone-cutting
    Hildebrandt uterine hemostatic
    Hinderer cartilage
    Hirsch hypophysis punch
    Hoen angular
    Hoen scalp hemostatic
    Hopkins aortic
    Horsley bone-cutting
    Horsley-Stille bone-cutting
    Hosemann
    hot biopsy
    hot flexible
    Hot Sampler disposable hot
    House cup
    Housepan clip-applying
    Howard Kelly
    Howmedica Microfixation System
    Hudson
    Hulka tenaculum

forceps *(cont.)*
    Hunt tumor
    Hunt-Yasargil pituitary
    Hunter
    Hunter splinter
    Hurd bone-cutting
    hypophyseal
    hypophysectomy
    hypophysis punch
    Ingraham skull punch
    intervertebral disk
    intestinal-grasping
    Iowa
    Iowa membrane
    Iselin
    Jackson grasping polyp
    Jackson tendon-seizing
    Jacobson-Adson artery
    Jacobson dressing
    Jacobson hemostatic
    Jacobson micro mosquito
    Jacobson mosquito
    Jaffee capsulorrhexis
    Jannetta alligator
    Jannetta bayonet
    Jansen-Middleton septal
    Jansen monopolar
    jar
    Jarell
    Jarit brain
    Jarit tendon-pulling
    Jarvis hemorrhoid
    Jawz biopsy
    Jawz endomyocardial biopsy
    jeweler's bipolar
    Johns Hopkins
    Johns Hopkins gallbladder
    Johnson brain tumor
    Johnson thoracic
    Johnson tumor
    Jones IMA
    Judd-Allis intestinal
    Judd-DeMartel gallbladder
    Juers-Lempert rongeur

forceps *(cont.)*
    Julian splenorenal
    Julian thoracic
    jumbo biopsy
    Kalman-Mixter
    Kantrowitz
    Karp aortic punch
    Kelly hemostatic
    Kelly placenta
    Kelly artery
    Kern bone-holding
    Kern-Lane bone
    Kevorkian-Tischler biopsy
    Kevorkian-Younge biopsy
    kidney stone
    Kielland
    Kleinert-Kutz bone-cutting
    Kleinert-Kutz rongeur
    Kleinert-Kutz tendon
    Knight bone-cutting
    Knight septum-cutting
    knotting
    Kocher
    Kocher artery
    Kocher intestinal
    Koeberlé
    Koehne cover glass
    Koerte gallstone
    Kraff-Utrata tear capsulotomy
    Kuehne cover glass
    Lahey dissecting
    Lahey Finochietto dissecting
    Lahey gall duct
    Lahey thyroid traction
    Lalonde delicate hook
    Lambotte bone-holding
    laminectomy punch
    lancet-shaped biopsy
    Landolt spreading
    Lane bone-holding
    Lane intestinal
    Lane screw-holding
    Lane self-retaining bone-holding
    Lane tissue

forceps *(cont.)*
    Lange approximation
    Langenbeck bone-holding
    Larsen tendon-holding
    laser tenaculum
    laser vulsellum
    Laufe
    Laurer
    Lees artery
    Leibinger Micro System
        plate-holding
    Lejeune thoracic
    Leksell rongeur
    Lempert rongeur
    LeRoy scalp clip-applying
    Lester muscle
    Lewin bone-holding
    Lewin spinal-perforating
    ligamentum flavum
    ligature-holding
    Lillehei valve
    Lillie intestinal
    lion
    lion-jaw
    Lister sinus
    Liston
    Liston bone-cutting
    Liston-Key bone-cutting
    Liston-Littauer bone-cutting
    Liston-Stille bone-cutting
    Littauer-Liston bone-cutting
    Littlewood tissue
    Livernois lens-holding
    Livernois-McDonald
    Llorente dissecting
    Lloyd Davies rectal biopsy
    Lloyd Davies rectal occlusion
    Lockwood-Allis intestinal
    Lockwood tissue
    London College
    long grasping
    Long
    loop
    loop-type snare

forceps *(cont.)*
    loop-type stone-crushing
    Lore suction tube and tip-holding
    Lorna towel
    Love-Gruenwald alligator
    Love-Gruenwald intervertebral disk
    Love-Gruenwald pituitary
    Love-Kerrison rongeur
    Lovelace lung grasping
    Lovelace thyroid traction
    Lowman bone-holding
    Lucae dressing
    Lucae ear
    Luer hemorrhoid
    Luer rongeur
    Luer-Whiting rongeur
    Luhr Microfixation System
        plate-holding
    Magill catheter introducing
    Malis angled-up bipolar
    Malis bipolar cautery
    Malis bipolar coagulation
    Malis irrigation
    Malis-Jensen microbipolar
    Malis jeweler bipolar
    Markwalder rib
    Martin
    Martin cartilage
    Martin tissue
    Maryland dissecting
    Mathieu
    Max Fine tying
    Mayfield
    Mayo-Blake gallstone
    Mayo-Péan
    Mayo-Robson intestinal
    Mayo-Russian tissue
    Mayo towel
    Mazzariello-Caprini
    McCain TMJ
    McClintock
    McGee
    McGee-Priest wire
    McGee wire-crimping

forceps *(cont.)*
    McGill
    McGivney
    McGivney hemorrhoidal-seizing
    McIndoe diathermy
    McIndoe dressing
    McIndoe rongeur
    McKenzie brain clip
    McKenzie clip-applying
    McKenzie clip-bending
    McKenzie clip-introducing
    McKernan-Adson
    McKernan-Potts
    McLean-Tucker obstetrical
    McNealey-Glassman-Mixter
    McPherson
    Medco
    Medco Adson tissue
    Medco Allis tissue
    Medco Babcock
    Medco Bozeman uterine
    Medco Brown Adson
    Medco Carmalt splinter
    Medco Crile
    Medco eye dressing
    Medco Foerster sponge
    Medco Halsted mosquito
    Medco Schroder tenaculum
    Medco splinter
    Medco thumb dressing
    Medco tissue thumb
    Medicon-Jackson rectal
    Meeker
    membrane-puncturing
    meniscus
    Meriam dissecting
    Michel applying and removing
    Michel clip-applying and
        clip-removing
    micro
    microartery
    microbipolar
    Micro dissecting
    micro Halsted mosquito

forceps *(cont.)*
    Micro Jaw rotatable Kelly
    Micro-One dissecting
    Micro-optical
    microsurgery
    Micro-Two
    microvascular
    MIC Thermal Option disposable
      biopsy
    Mikulicz peritoneal
    Miller rectal
    Millin ligature-holding
    Miltex tendon-pulling
    Mixter artery
    Mixter dissecting
    Mixter gallstone
    Mixter-O'Shaughnessy artery
    Mixter thoracic
    modified Allis grasping
    MOLLY bipolar
    monopolar grasping
    Moolgaoker
    Moorfield stitch
    Morrison tissue
    Moynihan artery
    Moynihan gall duct
    Muir hemorrhoid
    Multibite biopsy
    Mya hook
    Nadler coaptation bipolar
    nail-pulling
    needle-nose dissecting
    needle-pulling
    Nelson tissue
    Neville-Barnes
    Nicola
    NIH mitral valve
    Niro bone-cutting
    Niro wire-twisting
    Nissen gall duct
    Noyes alligator
    Nussbaum intestinal
    Ochsner
    Oehler tissue and needle-pulling

forceps *(cont.)*
    Officer sigmoidoscope biopsy
    Officer tissue
    Ogura tissue and cartilage
    Oldberg pituitary
    Olivecrona clip-applying and
      removing
    Olivecrona-Toennis clip-applying
    Olympus alligator-jaw endoscopic
    Olympus basket-type endoscopic
    Olympus FBK-13 endoscopic biopsy
    Olympus hot biopsy
    Olympus magnetic extractor
    Olympus mini-snare
    Olympus pelican-type endoscopic
    Olympus rat-tooth endoscopic
    Olympus reusable biopsy
    Olympus reusable hot biopsy
    Olympus rubber-tip endoscopic
    Olympus shark-tooth endoscopic
    Olympus tripod-type endoscopic
    Olympus W-shape endoscopic
    Ombredanne
    optical
    optical biopsy
    Orr gall duct
    Oschner artery
    Overholt artery
    Overholt clip-applying
    Overholt thoracic
    O'Shaughnessy artery
    paddle
    Paterson biopsy
    Payr pylorus
    Péan
    peapod intervertebral disk
    Peers towel
    Peet
    Peet splinter
    Pennington grasping
    Pennington tissue
    Percy intestinal
    perforating
    Perman cartilage

forceps *(cont.)*

    Phaneuf artery
    pickup
    Pierce
    Pierse micro dissecting
    Pierse tip
    Pilling Weck Y-stent
    pinch
    pinch-band
    Piper OB
    pituitary
    plain splinter
    plain tissue
    plate-holding
    polyp-grasping
    Poppen
    Porter duodenal
    Potts bronchus
    Potts bulldog
    Potts-Smith
    Potts-Smith dressing
    Potts-Smith tissue
    Potts thumb
    Potts vascular
    Pratt rectal
    Pratt tumor
    Preston ligamentum flavum
    Price-Thomas bronchial
    Providence Hospital artery
    pulpiform nucleus
    punch
    Quadripolar cutting
    Radial Jaw single-use biopsy
    Radolf
    Raimondi hemostatic
    Raimondi scalp
    Rampley sponge-holding
    Ramsay tissue
    Randall stone
    Raney clip-applying
    Raney coagulating
    Raney rongeur
    Raney scalp clip-applying
    ratchet-on-demand grasping

forceps *(cont.)*

    rat-tooth or rat-toothed
    Ratliff-Blake gallstone
    Ratliff-Mayo
    Re-New
    rectal biopsy
    Reddick Olsen
    Rees-Martel flap
    Reich-Nechtow
    Remington Hobbs diathermy
    retrograde grasping, double-action
    Rhoton bipolar
    Rhoton cup
    Rhoton-Cushing
    Rhoton dissecting
    Rhoton-Tew bipolar
    rib
    Riches artery
    Riches diathermy artery
    Richter-Heath clip-removing
    Richter laminectomy punch
    ring
    Ritebite biopsy
    Robbers
    Roberts artery
    Robson intestinal
    Rochester-Carmalt artery
    Rochester gallstone
    Rochester-Mixter artery
    Rochester-Ochsner
    Rochester-Péan artery
    Rochester-Péan hemostatic
    roller
    rongeur
    rotary
    round cup
    Rowe disimpaction
    Rowe glenoid-reaming
    Rowe-Harrison bone-holding
    Rowe modified-Harrison
    Rudd Clinic hemorrhoidal
    Ruel
    Rumel artery
    Rumel thoracic

forceps *(cont.)*
    Ruskin bone-cutting
    Ruskin bone-splitting
    Ruskin-Liston bone-cutting
    Ruskin rongeur
    Ruskin-Rowland bone-cutting
    Russian tissue
    Rutherford-Morrison tissue
    Samuels
    Sarot artery
    Sauerbruch rib
    Sawtell artery
    Sawtell tonsil hemostatic
    scalp clip
    scalp flap
    Scharff microbipolar and suction
    Scheicker laminectomy punch
    Schindler peritoneal
    Schlesinger cervical punch
    Schlesinger rongeur
    Schnidt artery
    Schnidt gall duct
    Schnidt thoracic
    Schoenberg intestinal
    Schroeder tenaculum
    Schubert biopsy
    Schumacher biopsy
    Schwartz clip-applying
    Schwartz temporary clamp-applying
    Scoville brain clip-applying
    Scoville brain spatula
    screw-holding
    Scudder intestinal
    Seitzinger tripolar cutting
    seizing
    self-centering bone-holding
    sella punch
    Selman vessel
    Selverstone rongeur
    Semb bone
    Semb rib
    Semken (also Semkin)
    Semken bipolar
    Semken delicate

forceps *(cont.)*
    Semken tissue
    septal
    sequestrum
    serrated
    Sewall brain clip
    Sewall clip-applying
    Shea alligator
    Shutt Mantis retrograde
    Simpson A6635
    Simpson-Luikart
    Singley intestinal
    Singley-Tuttle tissue
    Skene tenaculum
    skull punch
    Smithwick clip-applying
    smooth-tipped jeweler's
    smooth tissue
    Snowden-Pencer
    Somer
    spatula
    SpectraScience reusable biopsy
    Spence rongeur
    Spencer Wells artery
    spinal perforating
    spiral basket
    splinter
    sponge
    sponge-holding
    spoon
    spoon-grasping
    spreading
    Spurling-Kerrison rongeur
    standard Allis grasping
    standard endoscopic
    Steinmann intestinal
    Steinmann tendon
    sterilizing
    Stevenson alligator
    Stevenson grasping
    St. George hemorrhoid-seizing
    Stieglitz splinter
    Stiles seizing
    Stille-Barraya intestinal

forceps *(cont.)*
   Ward approximating
   Waugh diathermy
   Waugh dissecting
   Weller cartilage
   Westphal
   Westphal gall duct
   Wiet cup
   Wikstroem artery
   Wilde dressing
   Wilde ethmoid
   Wilde rongeur
   Wilfred Adams diathermy artery
   Williams intestinal
   Wilson-Cook
   wire
   wire-crimping
   wire-cutting
   wire-extracting
   wire-holding
   wire-pulling
   wire-tightening
   wire-twisting
   Wittner biopsy
   Wrigley
   W-shaped
   Yankauer
   Yasargil artery
   Yasargil bayonet
   Yasargil clip-applying
   Yasargil hypophyseal
   Yasargil knotting
   Yasargil micro
   Yasargil tumor
   Yeoman biopsy
   Yeoman rectal biopsy
   Yeoman-Turrell rectal biopsy
   Yeoman-Wittner rectal
   Young
   Young intestinal
   Z-Clamp
   Zenker artery
forceps speculum
forceps with needle bayonet/stylet

Ford-Dixon hemorrhoid ligator
Ford Hospital ventricular cannula
foregut
foreign body forceps
foreign body infiltrate
foreign body sensation
foreign body trauma
foreign material
forensic pathology
foreshortening of mesentery
forestomach
fork
   carotid
   double-prong
   Gardiner-Brown tuning
   Hardy three-prong
   implant application
   Jannetta
   Rhoton
   three-prong
   tuning
Formad kidney
formal laparotomy
Forman nasal elevator
Forman nasal rasp
Forman rhinoplasty scissors
formation
   bezoar
   gallstone
   gas
   gastric pouch
   Gothic arch
   hernia
   intestinal pouch
   pouch
   stone
formed stool
formula (see also *feeding*)
   Advance
   Deliver 2.0
   Enfamil with iron
   Ensure Plus
   flow/pressure/resistance
   Harris-Benedict mathematical

formula *(cont.)*
    I-Soyalac
    Impact enteral
    infant
    Isomil SF (sucrose-free)
    Lofenalac
    Lonalac
    Nursoy
    Nutramigen
    Peptamen liquid diet
    Perative
    Portagen
    PreCare Conceive nutritional
        supplement
    predigested protein
    Pregestimil
    Prosobee
    RCF (Ross carbohydrate-free)
    Similac PM 60/40 low iron
    Similac with iron
    SMA
    soy-based
    Soyalac
    Travasorb MCT (medium chain
        triglyceride) food supplement.
Foroblique lens (in cystoscope)
Forrest classification of gastroduodenal
    ulcer
Forta Shake nutritional therapy
Forte distal radius plate
fortification
fortisan fabric (cellulose) graft
Fortison enteral feeding
Forvade (cidofovir) gel dressing
forward-cutting knife
forwarding probe
forward oblique telescope
forward-viewing endoscope
Foscan (temoporfin, mTHPC) mediated
    photodynamic therapy
fossa (pl. fossae)
    adipose (of breast)
    axillary
    Broesike

fossa *(cont.)*
    duodenal
    epigastric
    gallbladder
    Gruber-Landzert
    hypogastric
    ileocecal
    infraduodenal
    inguinal
    Jobert
    Jonnesco
    Landzert
    mesentericoparietal
    mesogastric
    paraduodenal
    parajejunal (Broesike)
    retroduodenal
    Scarpa
    sigmoid
    subsigmoid
    Treitz
    umbilical
    Waldeyer
Foss bifid gallbladder retractor
Foss biliary duct retractor
Foss forceps
Foss intestinal clamp
Foster needle holder
Foster-TC needle holder
fotemustine
Fouchet test
foul-smelling stools
four-channel water-perfused system
four Fs (female, fat, forty, fertile)
four-flanged nail
four-gland hyperplasia
four-hole (4-hole) plate
four-hour glucose tolerance test
four-lumen tube
Fourneau 309 (suramin sodium)
Fournier gangrene after hemor-
    rhoidectomy
Fournier One-Piece cannula
Fournier Toomey syringe cannula

four-quadrant hemorrhoidectomy
four-strand Savage suture
four-strand suture
fourth bronchial pouch
fourth intercostal space
fourth pharyngeal pouch
four-wire basket
foveal gastric mucosa
foveolar gastric mucosa
foveolar hyperplasia
foveolosulciolar gastric mucosa
Fowler position
Fox bipolar forceps
Fox curette
Fox sign
Foxy Pouch Cover
FPC (familial polyposis coli)
fractional epidural anesthesia
fractional spinal anesthesia
fractionated diet
fractionation of bilirubin
fraction, plasma protein
Fractura Flex bandage
fracture, basilar skull
fracture-reducing elevator
fragile histidine triad (FHIT)
fragmented tissue
fragment of tissue
Fragmin (dalteparin sodium injection)
fraise, DFDR diamond
Framer tendon-passing needle
Francis test
Francisella tularensis (formerly
    Pasteurella tularensis)
frank blood
frank blood in stool
frank cirrhosis
Frankenfeldt cotton applicator
Frankfeldt rectal diathermy snare
Frankfeldt rectal swab holder
frank gangrene of bowel
frank hemorrhage
Franklin-Silverman biopsy cannula
Franklin-Silverman biopsy needle

frank necrosis
frank perforation
frank pulmonary edema
frank pus
frank rigors
Frank-Starling curve
Frank-Starling mechanism
frank ulceration
Franseen needle
Franz abdominal retractor
Fraser artery forceps
Frater suture guide
Frazier Baron-style
Frazier brain-exploring cannula
Frazier Britetrac suction tube
Frazier cordotomy knife
Frazier dural elevator
Frazier dural hook
Frazier dural scissors
Frazier dural separator
Frazier hook
Frazier laminectomy retractor
Frazier lighted brain retractor
Frazier nerve hook
Frazier-Paparella suction tube
Frazier pituitary knife
Frazier scissors
Frazier suction tip
Frazier suction tube
Frazier suction tube obturator
Frazier ventricular cannula
Frazier ventricular needle
FreAmine amino acid solution
FreAmine HBC 6.9%
FreAmine III 3% (8.5%) with
    Electrolytes
freckle-like lesion
Fredet-Ramstedt pyloromyotomy
FRED (fog reduction/elimination
    device)
FRED Lite alcohol-free solution
free air
free air in abdomen
free air in colon

free air in GI tract
free band of colon
Freedom knife
free fat graft
free flap
free flap breast reconstruction
    (gluteus maximus to internal
    mammary vessels)
free flap transfer
free-floating testis
free fluid
freeform prosthetic mesh
free graft
freehand CT-guided biopsy
free hepatic venous pressure
free hormone
freeing up of adhesion
free intestinal graft
free intraperitoneal air
free jejunal graft
free jejunum transfer
free jejunum transfer with
    microvascular anastomosis
freely movable nodule
Freeman cookie cutter areola marker
free muscle graft
free nipple graft
free nipple transposition technique
    reduction mammoplasty
free perforation
free radical
Freer chisel
Freer dissector
free reflux
Freer periosteal elevator
Freer septal elevator
Freer septum elevator
Freer skin hook
Freer-Swanson ganglion knife
free skin graft
FreeStyle glucose monitoring device
free thyroxine (T_4)
free thyroxine index (FT_4I or FTI)
free tie (individual ligature)

free/total PSA (prostate-specific
    antigen) index
free transplanted graft
free water
free water infusion
freeze-dried bone graft
Freezor cryocatheter catheter
Freiberg biopsy set
Freiberg cartilage knife
Freiberg meniscectomy knife
French bougie
French dilator
French eye needle
French mushroom-tip catheter
French stent
French T-tube
frenectomy
frenoplasty
frenulectomy
frenum, lingual
frequency of stools
fresh blood clot
fresh frozen graft
fresh frozen plasma (FFP)
fresh frozen section
Fresh Start breast support
fresh whole blood
friability
friable bowel
friable clot
friable lesion
friable mass
friable mucosa
friable papilloma
friable tissue
friction knot
friction rub
fried food
Friedland scissors
Friedländer bacillus
Friedman bone rongeur
Friedman perineal retractor
Friedman rongeur forceps
Friedman rongeur

FRIEND (foreign body, radiation, infection, epithelialization, neoplasm, distal obstruction)
Frigitronics probe
Fritsch abdominal retractor
frog-leg (adj.)
frog-leg lateral view
frog-leg position
Fröhlich (Froehlich) syndrome
frondlike filling defect
frondlike pattern
frontal abscess abscess
frontal plate
frontal region
frontal suture
frontal view
front and side wire cutter
front lifting hood rectoscope tube
frontoethmoidal suture
frontolacrimal suture
frontomaxillary suture
frontonasal suture
frontoparietal suture
frontosphenoid suture
frontozygomatic suture
frosted liver
Frost stitch
frothy fluid
frown incision
frozen section
frozen section diagnosis
Frykholm bone rongeur
FTI (free thyroxine index)
FTSG (full-thickness skin graft)
fucosylated alpha-fetoprotein (AFP)
fucosylation index of alpha-fetoprotein (AFP)
FUDR; FUdR (5-fluorouracil deoxyribonucleoside) (floxuridine)
Fujinon biopsy forceps
Fujinon colonoscope
Fujinon duodenoscope
Fujinon endoscope
Fujinon EVC-M videocolonoscope

Fujinon EVD-XL videoduodenoscope
Fujinon EVE videoendoscope
Fujinon EVG-F upper GI video-endoscope
Fujinon EVS-E flexible sigmoidoscope
Fujinon FG-100FP flexible gastroscope
Fujinon FG-100PE flexible gastroscope
Fujinon flexible sigmoidoscope
Fujinon PRO-PC flexible sigmoido-scope
Fujinon SIG-E2 flexible sigmoidoscope
Fujinon SIG-EK flexible sigmoidoscope
Fujinon SIG-ET flexible sigmoidoscope
Fujinon SIG-PC flexible sigmoidoscope
Fujinon sigmoidoscope
Fujinon UGI-FP endoscope
Fujinon UGI-PE flexible gastroscope
Fujita snake retractor
Fujita suction retractor
Fukushima C-clamp
Fukushima-Giannotta curette
Fukushima-Giannotta dissector
Fukushima-Giannotta needle holder
Fukushima-Giannotta scissors
Fukushima retractor
Fukushima teardrop suction
fulgurate
fulguration, electrosurgical
fulguration of tumor
fulguration of ulcerative lesion
full activity
full backboard
full-blown bacterial peritonitis
full-blown syndrome
full-column barium enema
full-curve blade
Fuller rectal shield
Fuller shield
Fuller shield dressing
full lateral position
full length view
full-liquid diet
full Magill curve
fullness, abdominal

full-radius resector knife
full-thickness involvement
full-thickness reconstruction
full-thickness rectal biopsy
full-thickness skin graft (FTSG)
fulminant bacteremia
fulminant colitis
fulminant enterocolitis
fulminant hepatic failure (FHF)
fulminant hepatitis
fulminant liver failure or end-stage
   chronic liver disease
fulminant viral hepatitis (FVH)
fulminant Wilson disease
fulminating appendicitis
fulminating pancreatitis
fulminating ulcerative colitis
Fulton laminectomy rongeur
fumarylacetoacetase parahydroxy-
   phenylpyruvic acid (p-HPPA)
   oxidase
FUMIR (5-fluorouracil, Mitomycin C,
   radiation)
functional anatomical mapping
functional bowel disease
   irritable bowel disease (IBD)
   irritable colon
functional bowel obstruction
functional bowel syndrome
functional colitis
functional constipation
functional cystic duct obstruction
functional death
functional diarrhea
functional disorder
functional dyspepsia
functional gastrointestinal disorder
   (FGID)
functional hyperinsulinism
functional hypoglycemia
functional intestinal obstruction
Functional Living Index–Cancer
   (FLIC)
functional material

functional pain
functional shrunken colon
functional spleen
functioning adrenocortical tumor
functioning allograft
functioning neoplasm
functioning thyroid tissue
fundal plication
fundal varices
fundic-antral junction
fundic gland gastritis
fundic mobilization in Nissen fundo-
   plication
fundic mucosa
fundic patch
fundoplasty (see also *operation*)
   anterior
   Belsey IV
   Dor
   esophagogastric
   Gomez
   Hill
   laparoscopic esophagogastric
   Nissen
   posterior
   Thal-Nissen
   Toupet
fundoplasty with fundic patch
fundoplication (see also *operation*)
   Belsey Mark IV
   Belsey partial
   Belsey two-thirds wrap
   Collis-Nissen
   endoscopic
   floppy-type of Nissen
   herniated
   high-resistance
   Hill gastropexy
   intrathoracic Nissen
   laparoscopic
   laparoscopic anterior partial
   laparoscopic Nissen and Toupet
   ligamentum teres cardiopexy
   low-resistance

fundoplication *(cont.)*
   Nissen
   Nissen 360° wrap
   re-do
   Rossetti modification of Nissen
   slipped Nissen
   Toupet hemifundoplication
   transthoracic Nissen
   twisted
   videoscopic
fundus
   bald gastric
   gallbladder
   gastric
   stomach
   uterine
fungal abscess
fungal esophagitis
fungal infection
fungal smear
fungating mass
fungiform papilla
fungus

fungus-like bacteria
funicular inguinal hernia
funicular suture
funisitis
funnel, fascia/peritoneum
FUO (fever of unknown or
   undetermined origin)
Furacin gauze dressing
Furamide (diloxanide furoate)
furazolidone
Furniss anastomosis clamp
Furniss-Clute clamp
furodazole
furosemide
furrier suture
fused kidney
fusiform bacillus
fusiform widening of duct
fusion graft
fusion plate
fusion protein
FVH (fulminant viral hepatitis)
FyBron alginate wound dressing

G, g

Gabriel hemorrhoidal needle
Gabriel proctoscope
Gabriel rectal speculum
GAD (glutamic acid decarboxylase)
gadodiamide
Gadolite oral suspension
gadopentetate dimeglumine
Gaenslen split-heel incision
gag (see *mouth gag*)
gagging without emesis
gag reflex
gag response
Gail breast cancer model
gait plate
galactocele
galactogram
galactorrhea
galactose-1-phosphate uridyltransferase
galactosemia
Galeati gland
Galencia disposable anoscope
Gallagher rasp
Gallannaugh bone plate
gallbladder
   bilobed
   body of
   calcified
   chronically inflamed
   Courvoisier

gallbladder *(cont.)*
   dilated
   distended
   double
   edematous
   fish-scale
   floating
   folded fundus
   fundus of
   hourglass
   inflamed
   mobile
   multiseptate
   neck of
   painful palpable
   partially intrahepatic
   perforated
   porcelain
   robin's egg–blue
   sandpaper
   stasis
   strawberry
   thick-walled
   thin-walled
   totally intrahepatic
   wandering
gallbladder adenoma
gallbladder bag positioner
gallbladder bed

gallbladder bile
gallbladder calculus (pl. calculi)
gallbladder carcinoma
gallbladder colic
gallbladder contractility, impaired
gallbladder contraction
gallbladder-cystic duct junction
gallbladder disuse
gallbladder emptying
gallbladder empyema
gallbladder fistula
gallbladder fossa
gallbladder fundus
gallbladder hydrops
gallbladder ileus
gallbladder inflammation
gallbladder infundibulum
gallbladder lift
gallbladder mucosa
gallbladder polyp
gallbladder scan
gallbladder scoop
gallbladder sludge
gallbladder stasis
gallbladder stone
gallbladder trocar
gallbladder villi
gallbladder wall abscess
gallbladder wall thickening
gall duct
gall duct forceps
gall duct spoon
Gallego method
Gallie needle
gallium-arsenide (GaA) laser
gallium 67 (^{67}Ga)
gallium scan
gallows-type retractor
gallstone (see also *stone*)
  asymptomatic
  bilirubin pigment
  black pigment
  brown pigment
  cholesterol

gallstone *(cont.)*
  common bile duct
  dissolution of
  faceted
  floating
  impacted
  innocent
  large
  mixed-cholesterol
  mulberry
  opacifying
  pigmented
  radiolucent
  radiopaque
  retained
  silent
  spilled
  symptomatic
gallstone erosion
gallstone forceps
gallstone formation
gallstone ileus
gallstone ileus syndrome
gallstone in common bile duct
gallstone migration
gallstone obstruction of main pancreatic
  duct
gallstone pancreatitis
gallstone probe
GALT (gut-associated lymphoid tissue)
Galt cranial trephine
galvanic probe
Galzin (zinc acetate)
Gambee suture
gamma alcoholism
gamma brachytherapy
gamma globulin
gamma-glutamyl transferase (GGT)
gamma-glutamyl transpeptidase
  (GGTP)
gamma locking nail
Gamma radiosurgical knife
gamma transverse colon loop
Gamna disease

Gandhi knife
ganglion hook
ganglion knife
ganglionated plexus
ganglioneuroma
ganglioneuromatosis
    diffuse transmural
    diffuse transmural intestinal
    extensive florid transmural
    extensive transmural
gangrene
    appendiceal
    arteriosclerotic
    cold
    cutaneous
    decubital
    diabetic
    dry
    embolic
    emphysematous
    Fournier
    gas
    hemorrhagic
    hospital
    hot
    Meleney
    moist
    nosocomial
    Pott
    pressure
    primary
    progressive bacterial synergistic
    secondary
    static
    thrombotic
    traumatic
    venous
    wet
    white
gangrenous appendicitis
gangrenous appendix
gangrenous bowel
gangrenous cholangiolitis
gangrenous cholecystitis

gangrenous colitis
gangrenous hernia
gangrenous necrosis
gangrenous pulp necrosis
Ganser diverticulum
Gant clamp
Gantrisin
gaping wound
Garcia aorta clamp
Gardiner-Brown tuning fork
Gardner forceps
Gardner elevator
Gardner neurosurgical skull clamp
Gardner skull clamp pin
Gardner syndrome
Gardner-Wells tongs
Gardnerella vaginitis (formerly
    Haemophilus vaginalis or
    Corynebacterium vaginale)
garment hook
Garren-Edwards balloon
Garren-Edwards gastric (GEG) bubble
Garren gastric bubble
Garrett dilator
Garrett retractor
gas
    colonic
    compressed carbon dioxide
    free subphrenic
    paucity of colon
    periappendiceal
    subcutaneous
Gas-Ban (calcium carbonate;
    simethicone)
gas bloating
gas-bloat syndrome
gas cupula
gas density line (on x-ray)
gas embolism
gaseous cholecystitis
gaseous distention
gas exchange
gas formation
gas-forming bacteria

gas-forming liver abscess
gas-forming organism in bowel wall
GasFree Omni-Lift retractor
gas insufflation
gasless laparoscopic-assisted colostomy
gasless laparoscopy
gas pattern
gas-producing food
Gas Relief (simethicone)
gassiness
gassy
gastrectomized patient
gastrectomy
    Billroth I
    Billroth II
    distal
    distal with excision of ulcer
    hand-assisted laparoscopic
    high subtotal
    Horsley
    limited
    Maki pylorus-preserving
    near-total
    palliative
    pancreatic-preserving total
    partial
    partial, distal
    Polya
    proximal
    segmental
    subtotal
    total
    video-assisted total
gastric achlorhydria
gastric acid
gastric acid hypersecretion
gastric acid production
gastric acid secretion, decreased
gastric acid test
gastric adenocarcinoma
gastric air bubble (on x-ray)
gastric algid malaria
gastric analysis
gastric antral erosion

gastric antral mucosa
gastric antral vascular ectasia (GAVE)
gastric antrum
gastric antrum G cell
gastric artery
gastric aspirate
gastric aspiration tube
gastric atony
gastric atrophy
gastric balloon (see *balloon*)
gastric band
gastric banding, laparoscopic
gastric baseline
gastric B cell lymphoma
gastric bile acid test
gastric bubble
gastric bypass
gastric calculus
gastric calibration tube
gastric canal
gastric capacity
gastric carcinoma (linitis plastica)
gastric cardia
gastric channel
gastric colic
gastric content test
gastric contents
gastric cuff
gastric cytology
gastric decompression
gastric diet
gastric dilatation
gastric dilatation/volvulus (GDV)
gastric distention
gastric-duodenal coordination
gastric duplication cyst
gastric dyspepsia
gastric dysrrhythmia
gastric emptying
    decreased
    delayed
gastric emptying scan
gastric emptying test
gastric erosion

gastric fistula
gastric fold
gastric follicle
gastric function test
gastric fundus
gastric fundus wrap
gastric gland
gastric groove
gastric hemorrhage
gastric hypersecretion
gastric hypersecretion of hydrochloric
   acid
gastric hypersensitivity
gastric hypoacidity
gastric impression on liver
gastric inhibitory polypeptide (GIP)
gastric integrity
gastric juice
gastric Kaposi sarcoma
gastric lavage
gastric lavage tube
gastric leiomyoma
gastric leiomyosarcoma
gastric loop-type bypass
gastric lymph node
gastric lymphatic follicle
gastric membrane vesicle
gastric motility disorder
gastric motility study
gastric motor disorder
gastric mucin
gastric mucosa
gastric mucosa atrophy
gastric mucosa ischemia
gastric mucosal barrier
gastric mucosal fold
gastric mucosal hypertrophy
gastric mucosal pattern classification:
   A, AB, B, BC, C, etc.
gastric myoelectrical activity
gastric neobladder procedure
gastric NK-like T cell lympho-
   proliferative disorder
gastric obstruction

gastric omentum
gastric outflow obstruction
gastric outlet, dilation of
gastric outlet obstruction (GOO)
gastric outlet stricture
gastric outline (on x-ray)
gastric pacemaker
gastric pacemaker cell
gastric pacemaker region
gastric parietal cell
gastric partition
gastric partitioning
gastric perforation
gastric phase of acid secretion
gastric pit
gastric plexus
gastric polyp
gastric polyposis
gastric pool
gastric pouch
gastric protection
gastric reconstruction
   Longmire-Gutgemann
   Roux
   Turbinger
gastric remnant
gastric resection
gastric reservoir
gastric restrictive procedure
gastric retention (GR)
gastric rupture
gastric sclerosis
gastric secretion
gastric secretion rate
gastric secretory test
gastric stapling
gastric stasis and postprandial fullness
gastric stump
gastric stump cancer
gastric surface
gastric T-cell lymphoma
gastric tear
gastric tissue patch, vascularized
gastric transit time

gastric ulcer
gastric ulceration
gastric variceal bleeding
gastric varices
gastric vein
gastric venacaval shunt
gastric volvulus
gastric washing
gastric window
Gastrimmune (gemcitabine) vaccine
gastrin cell hyperfunction
gastrin, fasting serum
gastrin hormone
gastrin-induced excessive gastric acid
   production
gastrin inhibition
gastrinoma
   duodenal
   metastatic
   pancreatic
   primary
   recurrent
gastrinoma triangle
gastrin-producing tumor
gastrin-secretin stimulation
gastrin-secretin stimulation test
gastrin-secreting cell
gastrin-secreting non-beta islet cell
   tumor
gastrin-secreting tumor (gastrinoma)
gastrin-stimulated intestinal motility
gastrin stimulation test
gastrin test
gastritis
   acute
   acute erosive (AEG)
   acute hemorrhagic
   alcoholic
   alkaline reflux
   allergic
   antral
   aspirin-induced
   atrophic
   autoimmune chronic

gastritis *(cont.)*
   bile-induced
   bile reflux
   catarrhal
   chemical
   chronic
   chronic atrophic
   chronic cystic
   chronic erosive
   chronic follicular
   chronic (type B)
   cirrhotic
   corrosive
   cystica polyposa
   diffuse varioliform
   drug-induced
   emphysematous
   eosinophilic
   erosive
   exfoliative
   follicular
   fundic gland
   giant hypertrophic
   granulomatous
   Helicobacter pylori-associated
      (HPAG)
   hemorrhagic
   hypersecretory chronic
   hypertrophic
   idiopathic chronic erosive
   interstitial
   irritant
   necrotizing
   nonerosive nonspecific
   phlegmonous
   polypous
   proliferative hypertrophic
   pseudomembranous radiation
   radiation
   reflux bile
   stress
   stress-induced
   superficial
   toxic

gastritis *(cont.)*
    type A (autoimmune chronic)
    type B (hypersecretory chronic)
    type AB (idiopathic chronic
      [environmental])
    ulcerative
    varioliform
    viral
    zonal
gastritis varioliformis
gastroadenitis
gastroalbumorrhea
gastroanastomosis
gastroatonia
gastroblennorrhea
gastrocamera, Olympus GTF-A
gastrocardiac syndrome
Gastroccult test
gastrocele
gastrochronorrhea
gastrocolic fistula
gastrocolic ligament
gastrocolic omentum
gastrocolic reflex
gastrocolic ulcer
gastrocolitis
gastrocolonic response
gastrocoloptosis
gastrocolostomy
gastrocutaneous fistula
gastrodialysis
gastrodiaphragmatic ligament
Gastrodiscoides hominis
Gastrodiscus hominis
gastroduodenal anastomosis
gastroduodenal artery
gastroduodenal artery complex
gastroduodenal fistula
gastroduodenal lumen
gastroduodenal lymph node
gastroduodenal orifice
gastroduodenal ulcer
gastroduodenitis
gastroduodenopancreatectomy

gastroduodenoscopy
gastroduodenostomy
    Billroth I
    Jaboulay
    laparoscopic
    tube
gastrodynia
gastroenteric
gastroenteritis (see also *enteritis*)
    acute (AGE)
    acute infectious
    astrovirus
    bacterial
    calicivirus
    Campylobacter
    coronavirus
    endemic nonbacterial
    eosinophilic
    epidemic
    epidemic nonbacterial
    food-borne
    infantile
    infectious
    nonbacterial
    Norwalk
    porcine transmissible
    rotavirus
    toxic
    viral
    water-borne
    winter
gastroenteritis virus type A
gastroenteritis virus type B
gastroenteroanastomosis
gastroenterocolitis
gastroenterocolostomy
gastroenterologist
gastroenterology
gastroenteropathy
gastroenteroplasty
gastroenteroptosis
gastroenterostomy
    anterior gastric
    Balfour

gastroenterostomy *(cont.)*
  Billroth I
  Billroth II
  Braun-Jaboulay
  Courvoisier
  Finney
  Heineke-Mikulicz
  Hofmeister
  laparoscopic
  Polya
  prophylactic
  Roux
  Roux-en-Y
  Schoemaker
  short-limb Roux-en-Y
  side-to-side
  transomental posterior
  Von Haberer
  Wolfler
gastroepiploic arcade
gastroepiploic artery
gastroepiploic gland
gastroepiploic vein
gastroepiploic vessel
gastroesophageal (GE)
gastroesophageal hernia
gastroesophageal incompetence
gastroesophageal junction
gastroesophageal laceration
gastroesophageal laceration-hemorrhage
  syndrome
gastroesophageal reflux (GER)
gastroesophageal reflux disease
  (GERD)
gastroesophageal scintiscan
gastroesophageal sphincter
gastroesophageal variceal bleed
gastroesophageal variceal plexus
gastroesophageal vestibule
gastroesophageal window
gastroesophagitis
gastroesophagostomy
gastrogastrostomy
gastrogavage

gastrogenic
gastrogenous diarrhea
Gastrografin contrast medium
Gastrografin enema
Gastrografin swallow
gastrograph
gastrohepatic bare area
gastrohepatic ligament
gastrohepatic omentum
gastrohydrorrhea
gastroileac reflex
gastroileal reflex
gastroileitis
gastroileostomy
gastroinoma triangle
gastrointestinal (GI)
gastrointestinal bleeding
gastrointestinal cross
gastrointestinal cross artifact
gastrointestinal decompression
gastrointestinal dysmotility syndrome
gastrointestinal electrolytes
gastrointestinal endoscopist
gastrointestinal fistula
gastrointestinal fluid loss
gastrointestinal hemorrhage
gastrointestinal hormone
gastrointestinal hyperacidity
gastrointestinal inhibitory hormone
gastrointestinal losses
gastrointestinal manifestations
  of Zollinger-Ellison syndrome
gastrointestinal motility
gastrointestinal mucosa
gastrointestinal mucosal hemorrhage
gastrointestinal needle
gastrointestinal peptide
gastrointestinal perforation
gastrointestinal peristalsis
gastrointestinal plaque
gastrointestinal polyposis
gastrointestinal polyp
gastrointestinal quality of life index
  (GIQLI)

gastrointestinal regularity peptide
gastrointestinal series
gastrointestinal stasis
gastrointestinal stoma
gastrointestinal telangiectasia
gastrointestinal therapeutic system
   (GITS)
gastrointestinal toxicity
gastrointestinal tract
gastrointestinal tract bleeding
gastrointestinal tract perforation
gastrointestinal tumor
gastrointestinal ulcer
gastrointestinal ulceration
gastrojejunal anastomosis
gastrojejunal constipation
gastrojejunal loop obstruction syndrome
gastrojejunal ulcer
gastrojejunocolic fistula
gastrojejunostomy
   antecolic long-loop isoperistaltic
   Billroth II
   loop
   percutaneous endoscopic
   prophylactic
   Roux-en-Y
   Roux-Y
   stapled
gastrokinesograph
gastrolavage
gastrolienal ligament
gastrolith
gastrolithiasis
gastrologist
gastrology
gastrolysis
Gastrolyte oral solution
gastromalacia
GastroMARK (ferumoxsil) imaging
   agent
gastromegaly
gastromyxorrhea
gastronesteostomy
gastro-omental artery

gastropancreatic fold
gastropancreatic ligament
gastropancreatic reflex
gastroparalysis
gastroparesis
   diabetic
   idiopathic
   nondiabetic
   postvagotomy
   transient
gastroparesis diabeticorum
gastropathic
gastropathy
   benign hyperplastic
   chemical
   diabetic
   drug-induced
   hemorrhagic erosive
   hyperplastic
   hypersecretory
   hypertrophic
   idiopathic hypertrophic
   NSAID-induced
   portal hypertensive
   prolapse
   protein-losing
gastropexy
   anterior
   Belsey-Mark IV
   belt loop
   Boerema anterior
   circumcostal
   Hill posterior
   incisional
   laparoscopic-assisted
   laparoscopic-assisted percutaneous
     anterior
   percutaneous anterior
   posterior
   posterior diaphragmatic
   prophylactic
   T-fastener
   T-tack
gastropexy to diaphragm

gastrophrenic ligament
gastroplasty (GP)
   adjustable ring
   Albert-Lembert
   Collis
   Collis-Nissen
   Eckhout vertical
   endoscopic
   fundoplication
   fundus rotation
   Gomez horizontal
   greater curvature banded
   horizontal
   Kuzmak gastric banding
   laparoscopic
   laparoscopic horizontal
   Laws
   layer-to-layer
   Mason vertical banded
   mini
   O'Leary lesser curvature
   silicone elastomer ring vertical
     (SRVG)
   Stamm
   tubular vertical
   unbanded
   V-banded
   vertical banded (VBG)
   vertical ring (VRG)
   vertical Silastic ring
gastroplication
gastropneumonic
Gastroport
gastroptosis
gastroptyxis
gastropulmonary
gastropylorectomy
gastropyloric
gastrorrhagia
gastrorrhaphy
gastrorrhea
gastrorrhexis
gastroschisis, Silastic silo reduction

gastroscope (see also *endoscope*)
   FCS-ML
   Fujinon FG-100FP flexible
   Fujinon FG-100PE flexible
   Fujinon UGI-PE flexible
   MIS Source
   Olympus CF-1T10L flexible
   Olympus CF-1T20L flexible
   Olympus CF-20L flexible
   Olympus CF-P20L flexible
   Olympus GF-UM130 ultrasound
   Olympus GIF-100 video
   Olympus GIF-1T10 flexible
   Olympus GIF-1T10 flexible
     therapeutic
   Olympus GIF-1T140 video
   Olympus GIF-1TV10 flexible
   Olympus GIF-2T10 flexible
   Olympus GIF-2T20 flexible
     therapeutic
   Olympus GIF-HM
   Olympus GIF-K
   Olympus GIF-N30 gastrofibroscope
   Olympus GIF-P140 video
   Olympus GIF-PQ20 flexible
   Olympus GIF-PV10 pediatric video
   Olympus GIF-Q140 video
   Olympus GIF-XP20 flexible
   Olympus GIF-XQ140 video
   Olympus GIF-XQ20 flexible
     multipurpose
   Olympus GIF-XQ30 flexible
     multipurpose
   Olympus GIF-XT30 gastrofibro-
     scope
   Olympus TGF-2D flexible
   Pentax EG-1840 video
   Pentax EG-2530
   Pentax EG-2540 video
   Pentax EG-2731
   Pentax EG-2901 flexible
   Pentax EG-2930
   Pentax EG-2940 video
   Pentax EG-3430 video

Gaviscon (aluminum hydroxide;
　magnesium carbonate)
Gaviscon-2
gay bowel syndrome
Gay gland
Gaymar blanket
Gaymar Industries
Gaynor-Hart position
Gazayerli endoscopic retractor
Gazayerli knot tier
GBP (gastric bypass procedure)
GBS (group B streptococcus)
G cell
GCS (Glasgow Coma Scale)
GCT (giant cell transformation)
GD DTPA compound for MRI scan
GDM (gestational diabetes mellitus)
GDV (gastric dilatation volvulus)
GEA (gastroepiploic artery) graft
GE (gastroesophageal)
Gee-Herter disease
Gee-Herter-Heubner disease
Gee-Herter-Heubner syndrome
Geenan Endotorque guidewire
Gee-Thaysen disease
GEG (Garren-Edwards gastric) bubble
Geiger rongeur
GE junction
gel (see *dressing*; *medication*)
gelatin-resorcin-formalin glue
gelatin sponge
gelatinous carcinoma
gelatinous fluid
gelatinous material
gelatinous polyp
gelbe cell
gel-filled breast implant
Gelfilm (absorbable gelatin film)
Gelfoam (absorbable gelatin sponge)
Gelfoam cookie (pad)
Gelfoam soaked in sodium tetradecyl
　sulfate
gel-like material
Gelpi pediatric retractor

Gelpi perineal retractor
Gelpi self-retaining retractor
Gelusil (aluminum hydroxide; magne-
　sium hydroxide; simethicone)
Gelusil-M
Gelusil-II
Gely suture
gemcitabine HCl
Gemella morbillorum
Gemini artery forceps
Gemini Finochietto artery forceps
Gemini gall duct forceps
Gemini thoracic forceps
Gemzar (gemcitabine HCl)
Genasense
Genasoft Plus (casanthranol; docusate
　sodium)
Genaton; Genaton Extra Strength
　(aluminum hydroxide; magnesium
　carbonate)
gene
　adenomatous polyposis coli (APC)
　adenoviral p53
　APC (adenomatous polyposis coli)
　beta
　beta-globin
　BRCA1
　BRCA2
　DNA repair
　HER-2/neu
　IFN-alpha 2
　MCC (mutated in colon cancer)
　MDR3
　multidrug resistance (MDR) 3
　mutant
　p53 adenoviral
　RhoC
　RhoC CTPase
　tumor suppressor
gene amplification
gene mutation
gene promoter methylation
general endotracheal anesthesia
general mask

general pathology
generalized edema (anasarca)
generalized glycogenosis
generalized gut dysmotility
generalized inflammatory state
generalized peritonitis
General Surgical Innovations (GSI)
generation, islet cell
generator
Genesis container
Genesis 2000 laser
Genestone 190 lithotriptor
gene therapy program
genetic counseling
genetic death
genetic diagnosis
genetic disorders, major causes of
  complex
  cytogenic
  environmental
  polygenic/multifactorial
  single gene (mendelian)
genetic engineering
genetic evaluation
genetic hemochromatosis
genetic heterogenicity
genetic marker
genetic material
genetic screening
genetic trait
  autosomal dominant
  autosomal recessive
Gengraf (cyclosporine)
geniculum
genital branch of genitofemoral nerve
genital carcinoma
genital fold
genital infection
genital nerve
genital ridge
genital ulcer
genitofemoral cutaneous nerve
genitofemoral nerve
genitourinary fistula

Genotropin (somatropin lyophilized
  powder)
Genotropin MiniQuick
Genotropin Pen 12
genotype, HCV (1-6)
Gentell wound dressing
Gentlax (senna concentrate)
GentleLASE Plus laser
gentle sump action
Gentle Touch postoperative colostomy
  appliance
genu of pancreatic duct
Genz-Arm pneumatic retractor
Genzyme Surgical Products
George artery forceps
Georgia (GA) law (glucose, age, LDH,
  AST, WBC)
Gerald bipolar forceps
Gerald-Brown tissue forceps
Gerald dissecting forceps
Gerald dressing forceps
Gerald tissue forceps
Gerbode forceps
Gerbode patent ductus clamp
GERD (gastroesophageal reflux
  disease)
Geref (sermorelin acetate)
GE (gastroesophageal) reflux
GE RT 3200 ADV II ultrasound system
GE Senographe 20001 digital
  mammography system
geriatric constipation
GeriMend dressing
Geriplex-FS
Germanin (suramin sodium)
germinal infection
germinating basal cell layer
germline RET proto-oncogene point
  mutations
Gerota fascia
Gerson therapy protocol
Gerzog bone mallet
gestational diabetes
gestational edema

gestational sac
GFX 2 coronary stent
GGT (gamma-glutamyl transferase)
GGTP (gamma-glutamyl transpepti-
    dase)
Ghajar guide
Gherini-Kauffman endo-otoprobe laser
Ghon primary lesion
GI (see *gastrointestinal*)
GIA (gastrointestinal anastomosis)
GIA Auto Suture apparatus
Giampapa suturing technique
Gianotti-Crosti syndrome
giant anorectal condyloma acuminatum
giant cell
giant cell adenocarcinoma
giant cell carcinoma
giant cell hepatitis
giant cell monstrocellular sarcoma
giant cell sarcoma
giant cell thyroiditis
giant cell tumor
giant colon
giant congenital nevus (pl. nevi)
giant hypertrophic gastritis
giant peptic ulcer
Gianturco expandable (self-expanding)
    metallic biliary stent
Gianturco prosthesis
Gianturco-Rösch Z-stent
Gianturco-Roubin flexible coil stent
Gianturco wool-tufted wire coil
Giardia intestinalis
Giardia lamblia
giardial colitis
giardiasis
GIA stapler
Gibberella fujikuroi
gibbous deformity
Gibney bandage
Gibson-Balfour abdominal retractor
Gibson bandage
Giebel blade plate
Gierke disease

Giertz rongeur
Giertz-Shoemaker rib shears
Giertz-Stille scissors
Gifford mastoid retractor
gift-wrap suture technique
gigantism
Gigli saw
Gigli saw blade
Gigli saw guide
Gigli wire saw
Gilbert cholemia
Gilbert classification of groin hernias
    (types 1–5)
Gilbert cystic duct forceps
Gilbert disease
Gilbert free-formed umbrella-shaped
    plug
Gilbert-Rutkow-Robbins classification
    of groin hernias (types 1–7)
Gilbert sign
Gilbert syndrome
Gilchrist ileocecal bladder
Gildenberg biopsy forceps
Gillette joint
Gillies bone graft
Gillies bone hook
Gillies diathermy forceps
Gillies-Dingman hook
Gillies-Finochietto needle holder
Gillies hook
Gillies horizontal dermal suture
Gillies lightweight forceps
Gillies needle
Gillies needle holder
Gillies skin hook
Gillies suture
Gillies-TC needle holder
Gillies tissue forceps
Gilliland etching cannula
Gilvernet retractor
gingival gland
gingival mucosa
gingivectomy
Gingrass and Messer pin

Giordano sphincter
GIP (gastric inhibitory polypeptide)
GIP (glucose-dependent insulinotropic
    polypeptide)
girdle anesthesia
girth, increased abdominal
GITS (gastrointestinal therapeutic
    system)
Given Diagnostic Imaging System
glabellar rasp
glabrous cirrhosis
glancing wound
gland
    absorbent (lymph)
    accessory thyroid
    accessory parotid
    accessory suprarenal
    acid
    adrenal
    anal
    apocrine
    areolar
    arytenoid
    Aselli
    Bartholin
    Bauhin
    bile duct
    biliary
    Blandin
    Brunner
    buccal
    bulbocavernous
    bulbourethral
    cardiac (stomach)
    celiac
    cervical
    Ciaccio
    circumanal
    Cloquet
    Clobelli
    coil
    compound
    Cowper
    ductless

gland *(cont.)*
    duodenal
    Duverney
    Ebner
    endocrine
    esophageal
    exocrine
    fundic
    Galeati
    gastric
    Gay
    gingival
    Gley
    gustatory
    hepatic
    hyperplastic
    hypothalamus
    intermediate
    interstitial
    intestinal
    lacrimal
    lactiferous
    lenticular
    Lieberkühn (Lieberkuehn)
    lymph
    mandibular
    mesenteric
    mesocolic
    Montgomery
    Morgagni
    mucus-secreting
    multinodular
    nabothian
    oxyntic
    parathyroid
    paraurethral
    parotid
    peptic
    Peyer
    pharyngeal
    pineal
    pituitary
    Poirier
    pregnancy

gland *(cont.)*
    prehyoid
    prostate
    pyloric
    salivary
    Sand
    Sandström
    sentinel
    solitary (of large intestine)
    splenoid
    substernal thyroid
    suprarenal
    Suzanne
    sweat
    Theile
    thymus
    thyroid
    urethral
    Virchow
    Weber
    Wölfler (Woelfler)
gland atrophy
gland enlargement
gland enucleator
gland forceps
gland scissors
glandular carcinoma
glandular organ
glandular swelling
glans intraepidermal
Glaser automatic laminectomy retractor
Glasgow classification of choledocho-
    lithiasis
glass pH electrode
Glasscock ear dressing
Glasser gastrostomy tube
Glasser gastrotomy
Glassman-Allis intestinal forceps
Glassman atraumatic bowel clamp
Glassman clamp
Glassman dissecting scissors
Glassman gastrostomy
Glassman grasper
Glassman stone extractor

Gleason score
Glenn diverticulum forceps
glenoid-reaming forceps
Gley gland
gliadin, wheat
GliaSite implantable radiation therapy
    system
Glidewire
glimepiride tablets
glioblastoma multiforme
glipizide
Glisson capsule
Glisson cirrhosis
glistening mass
glitazone classification of diabetes drugs
global inhibition of GI function
globoid material
globular tumor
globulin
    alpha$_1$-antitrypsin
    cortisol-binding globulin
    hepatitis B hyperimmune
    thyroid-binding
globus hystericus
globus sensation
glomerular filtration rate (GFR)
glomerulopathy associated with infec-
    tious hepatitis (HB$_S$Ag-positive)
glomerulopathy associated with visceral
    abscess
glomerulus (pl. glomeruli)
glossectomy
glossitis
glossopalatine fold
glossopharyngeal afferent
glottic adduction
glottic closure during deglutition
glottic thyroid
glove
    antivibratory
    Bio-Form
    Biobrane
    carpal tunnel
    Handeze fingerless

glove *(cont.)*
  Isotoner
  Jobst
  SoftFlex computer
  Tubigrip
  Valeo lifting
glove-and-stocking anesthesia
  distribution
glove anesthesia
glovelike distribution
Glover bulldog clamp
Glover coarctation clamp
Glover patent ductus clamp
Glover vascular clamp
GLS suture anchor
GlucaGen (glucagon)
glucagon-secreting tumor
  (glucagonoma)
glucagonoma syndrome
Glucerna
Gluck rib shears
Gluco-Pro nutritional supplement
Gluco-Protein OTC self-test
Glucochek Pocketlab II blood glucose
  system
glucocorticoid production
glucocorticosteroid-induced side effects
Glucofilm reagent strips
Glucometer DEX blood glucose
  monitor
Glucometer Elite R blood glucose
  monitor
Glucometer Encore reagent strips
Glucometer II blood glucose monitor
Gluconate skin prep tray
gluconeogenesis
Glucophage (metformin HCl)
Glucophage XR (metformin HCl
  extended-release)
glucose
  blood
  intravenous (I.V., IV)
  liquid
  plasma

glucose *(cont.)*
  serum
  urine
glucose administration, I.V., IV
  (intravenous)
glucose-dependent insulinotropic
  polypeptide (GIP)
glucose-galactose malabsorption
glucose intolerance
glucose metabolism
glucose meter
glucose monitor (see *blood glucose
  monitor*)
glucose-6-phosphatase deficiency
glucose-6-phosphate dehydrogenase
  (G6PD) deficiency
glucose tolerance, impaired
glucose tolerance test (GTT)
Glucostix reagent strips
glucosuria
glucosylceramide lipids
Glucotrol XL (glipizide)
Glucovance (glyburide; metformin
  HCl)
GlucoWatch blood glucose monitor
glucuronide
glucuronosyltransferase (liver enzyme)
glue (see also *adhesive*)
  biomedical
  cyanoacrylate
  endovascular
  fibrin
  HemaMyst aerosol adhesive
  Hemaseel APR fibrin adhesive
  Hemaseel HMN biological tissue
    glue
  HemaSyst sealant
  Krazy Glue
  LiquiBand topical wound closure
  percutaneous fibrin
  skin
  Superglue
  Tissucol fibrin
glutamic acid

glutamic acid decarboxylase (GAD)
    antibody
glutamine and somatropin
glutamine test
glutaraldehyde-tanned bovine collagen
    tubes
glutaraldehyde-tanned porcine heart
    valve
Glutasorb diet
gluteal fold
gluteal region
gluten, dietary
gluten enteropathy
gluten-free diet
gluten intolerance
Glutose
Gluzinski test
glyburide
glyburide/metformin hydrochloride
Glycacor assay
glycemic control
glycemic index
glycerin (Fleet Babylax)
glycerol
glycerol monoctanoate (GMOC)
    solution
glycine extended gastrin
glycocalix
glycogen infiltration of liver
glycogen storage disease
glycogen store
glycogenic acanthosis
glycogenolysis
glycogenosis
    brancher deficiency
    generalized
    hepatophosphorylase deficiency
    hepatorenal
glycopyrrolate
glycopyrronium bromide
Glycosal diabetes monitoring device
glycosuria
glycosylated hemoglobin
glycyltryptophan test

Glynase Pres Tab (glyburide)
Glypressin (terlipressin)
Glyset (miglitol)
Gmelin test
GMOC (glycerol monoctanoate)
    solution
gnawing pain
Go-Evac (polyethylene glycol-
    electrolyte solution electrolytes)
goblet cell
goblet cell hyperplasia
Godina double hook
Goelet retractor
goiter
    aberrant
    adenomatous
    Basedow
    colloid
    congenital
    cystic
    diffuse
    diffuse colloid
    diffuse multinodular
    diffuse toxic non-nodular
    diving
    dyshormonogenic
    endemic (colloid)
    euthyroid
    exophthalmic
    fetal
    fibrous
    focal
    follicular
    hyperplastic
    intrathoracic
    iodide
    iodine deficiency
    lingual
    lithiumogenic
    lymphadenoid
    multinodular
    multiple colloid adenomatous
    nodular
    nontoxic

goiter *(cont.)*
  nontoxic diffuse
  nontoxic nodular
  parenchymatous
  perivascular
  plunging
  retrovascular
  simple
  smooth
  soft
  sporadic
  substernal
  suffocative
  thyroid
  toxic
  toxic diffuse
  toxic multinodular
  toxic nodular
  toxic uninodular
  uninodular
  vascular
  wandering
goitrogen
goitrous cretinism
Golaski graft
gold (Au); gold-198 (^{198}Au)
Goldberg Anorectic Attitude Scale
Goldberg-Maxwell syndrome
Goldblatt clamp
Goldblatt kidney
Goldman-Fox dissecting scissors
Gold Probe bipolar hemostasis catheter
Gold Series
Goldstein Microspike approximator clamp
Goldstein Microspike clamp
golf-hole ureteral orifice
Goligher abdominal scissors
Goligher extraperitoneal ileostomy
Goligher retractor
GoLYTELY (polyethylene glycol-electrolyte solution) bowel prep
Gomco suction
Gomco suction tube

Gomel blade
Gomel micro tying forceps
gomer (acronym for pejorative, "get out of my emergency room")
Gomez fundoplasty
Gomez gastroplasty
Gomez horizontal gastroplasty with reinforced stoma
gonadal neoplasm
Gonadimmune
gonococcal perihepatis pelvic inflammatory disease
gonococcal perihepatitis
gonococcal peritonitis
gonorrheal proctitis
Gonzalez, meandering artery of
GOO (gastric outlet obstruction)
good prognosis
good renal function
Good rasp
Goodsall rule
Good Sam adult breathing circuit
gooseneck gouge
gooseneck rongeur
Gopalan syndrome
GORD (British/European spelling of GERD)
Gordon disease
Gore cast liner
Gore 1.5-T Torso Array
Gore-Tex banding of sigmoid colon to abdominal wall
Gore-Tex DualMesh Plus
Gore-Tex FEP-Ringed vascular graft
Gore-Tex graft
Gore-Tex MycroMesh Plus
Gore-Tex nonabsorbable surgical suture
Gore-Tex SAM (subcutaneous augmentation material) facial implant
Gore-Tex shunt
Gore-Tex soft tissue patch
Gore-Tex stretch vascular graft
Gore-Tex strips
Gore-Tex surgical membrane

Gore-Tex surgical mesh
Gore-Tex tapered vascular graft
Gore-Tex vascular graft
gorge
gorging
Gorney scissors
goserelin acetate
Gosset appendectomy retractor
Gosset retractor
gossypiboma (cotton)
Gothic arch formation
Gottron papule
Gott shunt
Gott tube
Gottschalk Nasostat
Gouffon hip pin
gouge (see also *chisel*)
   Abbott
   Acufex
   Alexander
   Andrews
   Army bone
   arthroplasty
   Aufranc
   Bishop
   bone
   Buck-Gramcko
   Campbell
   Capner
   Cobb spinal
   curved
   Dawson-Yuhl
   Duray-Read
   Flanagan spinal fusion
   gooseneck
   Guy
   Hibbs spinal fusion
   Hoen
   Hoen lamina
   Jewett
   Killian
   Lexer
   Lucas
   Metzenbaum

gouge *(cont.)*
   Meyerding curved
   mini-Lexer
   Moe
   motorized
   Murphy
   oscillating
   Partsch
   Read
   Ruben
   Sheehan
   Smith-Petersen curved
   Smith-Petersen straight
   Smith-Peterson gooseneck
   spinal fusion
   Stille bone
   straight
   swan-neck
   tendon
   USA pattern
   U.S. Army
   Watson-Jones bone
   West
   West bone
   Zielke
   Zimmer
Gould polygraph
Goulet retractor
Goulian mammoplasty
gourmand syndrome
GP (gastroplasty)
GR (gastric retention)
GR II coronary stent
gracilis muscle graft
gracilis muscle transposition
graciloplasty
grade, grading (see *classification*)
graded compression ultrasonography
graded esophageal balloon distention
   test
gradient
   biliary-duodenal pressure
   duodenobiliary pressure
   gastrosphincteric pressure
   hepatic venous pressure

grading neoplasm
grading of malignancy
grading tumor
Gradle scissors
gradual volume loss
graduated metal cup
Graefe dissecting forceps
Graefe dissecting hook
Graefe skin hook
Grafco all-nylon Y connector
graft
    ACL
    adipose
    adrenal medulla
    advancement flap
    Albee bone
    AlloDerm processed tissue
    allogenic (allogencic) bone
    allogenous bone
    allograft
    AlloMatrix injectable putty bone
      graft substitute
    AneuRx stent
    anterior iliac crest
    anterior sliding tibial
    aortofemoral bypass (AFBG)
    aortohepatic arterial
    Apligraf (graftskin)
    Aria coronary artery bypass
    articular cartilage autograft
    autochthonous
    autogenous bone
    autogenous dermal
    autogenous fascial heterograft
    autogenous inlay
    autogenous soft tissue graft
    autologous crest bone
    autologous fat
    autologous reverse
    BAGF (brachioaxillary bridge graft
      fistula)
    Banks bone
    Bard Composix mesh
    Bard Sperma-Tex preshaped mesh

graft *(cont.)*
    Bard Visilex mesh
    batten
    bicortical iliac bone
    bicortical ilial strip
    bifurcated vascular graft
    Biobrane/HF skin substitute
    Biograft bovine heterograft
    BioPolyMeric
    bone chip
    bone graft substitute
    bone peg
    BonePlast
    bone-retinaculum-bone autograft
    bone-tendon-bone
    Bonfiglio bone
    bovine heterograft
    bovine pericardium
    Boyd dual-onlay bone
    BPB (bone-patellar ligament-bone)
      autologous
    BPB (bone-patellar tendon-bone)
      autologous
    brachiosubclavian bridge
    Braun skin
    Brennen biosynthetic surgical mesh
    bridge
    BSGF (brachiosubclavian bridge
      graft fistula)
    C
    CABG (coronary artery bypass)
    cable
    Calcitite
    calvarial free bone
    Campbell onlay
    cancellous and cortical bone
    cancellous chip bone
    Capset (calcium sulfate) bone graft
      barrier
    Carbo-Seal
    carbon fiber
    carbon fiber synthetic ligament
    cardiovascular patch
    cartilage

graft *(cont.)*
    cavum conchal cartilage
    CHAG (coralline hydroxyapatite
       Goniopora)
    chip
    Chuinard autogenous bone
    clothespin spinal fusion
    Codivilla bone
    Collagraft bone graft matrix
    composite
    Composite Cultured Skin (CCS)
    Composix mesh
    consolidated
    cortical strut
    corticocancellous bone
    corticocancellous chip
    Cotton cartilage
    Cragg endoluminal
    cranial bone
    cultured epithelial autograft
    cutaneous
    cymba conchal cartilage
    Cymetra tissue replacement material
    Dacron
    Dacron synthetic ligament material
    Daniel iliac bone
    Dardik Biograft
    Davis muscle-pedicle
    delayed xenograft rejection (DXR)
    demineralized bone
    denatured homograft
    Dermagraft human-based dermal
       replacement
    Dermagraft-TC (transitional
       covering)
    dermal collagen
    devitalized bone
    diamond inlay
    Diastat vascular access
    discordant cellular xenograft
    discordant organ xenograft
    Distaflo bypass
    double mesh
    doubled semitendinosus and gracilis
       autograft (DST&G)

graft *(cont.)*
    Douglas skin
    dowel
    Dragstedt skin
    DST&G (doubled semitendinosus
       and gracilis) autograft
    DTAFA (descending thoracic aorta-
       to-femoral artery) bypass
    dual onlay bone
    DualMesh biomaterial
    DuraGen
    dural
    Durapatite
    E-CABG (endoscopic coronary
       artery bypass graft)
    Edwards woven Teflon aortic
       bifurcation
    endovascular stent
    epidural blood patch
    Esser skin
    extended survival
    extra-articular
    fascia lata
    fascial
    femorocrural
    femorodistal PTFE
    fetal cortical tissue
    fetal substantia nigra
    fillet local flap
    Flanagan-Burem apposing
       hemicylindric
    flap
    flexor tendon
    Fluoropassiv thin-wall carotid patch
    fortisan fabric (cellulose)
    free
    free fat
    free intestinal
    free jejunal
    free muscle
    free nipple
    free skin
    free transplanted
    freeze-dried

graft *(cont.)*

    freeze-dried bone
    fresh frozen
    full-thickness skin
    fusion
    GEA (gastroepiploic artery)
    Gillies bone
    glutaraldehyde-tanned bovine collagen tubes
    glutaraldehyde-tanned porcine heart valve
    Golaski
    Gore-Tex
    Gore-Tex DualMesh Plus
    Gore-Tex FEP-Ringed vascular
    Gore-Tex MycroMesh Plus
    Gore-Tex stretch vascular
    Gore-Tex tapered vascular
    Gore-Tex vascular
    gracilis muscle
    Grafton DBM (demineralized bone matrix) bone
    Graftpatch
    Haldeman bone
    Hapset bone graft plaster
    Harris superior acetabular
    harvesting of
    Healos synthetic bone-grafting material
    Hedrocel bone substitute material
    Hemashield
    Hemashield enhanced
    hemicylindrical bone
    Henderson onlay bone
    Henry bone
    Herniamesh surgical mesh
    heterogeneous (heterogenous)
    heterograft
    Hey-Groves-Kirk bone
    Hoaglund bone
    homogeneous (homogenous)
    homologous
    H-shaped
    human meniscal allograft

graft *(cont.)*

    Huntington bone
    hydroxyapatitite
    IEA (inferior epigastric artery)
    iliac crest bone
    iliotibial band
    IMA (inferior mammary artery)
    impaction
    in situ vein
    Inclan bone
    infrarenal aortobifemoral bypass
    inlay
    inlay bone
    intercalary
    interfascicular nerve
    InterGard Knitted collagen coated
    Interpore
    interposition bone
    interposition Dacron
    interposition saphenous vein
    intramedullary
    Ionescu-Shiley pericardial xenograft
    irradiated
    Isotec patellar tendon
    ITA (internal thoracic artery)
    Judet
    jump
    keystone
    Kimura cartilage
    Krause-Wolfe skin
    Kutler V-Y flap
    Langenskiöld bone
    Lee bone
    Leibinger Micro Dynamic mesh
    LIMA (left internal mammary artery)
    lyophilized bone
    Marlex
    Marlex mesh
    Marlex PerFix plug
    Marlex synthetic
    Martius
    Massie sliding
    matchstick

graft *(cont.)*
  McFarland bone
  McMaster bone
  MD-111 bone allograft
  Meadox Microvel arterial
  medullary bone
  Microknit vascular
  mitral valve homograft
  morselized (morcellized) bone
  MycroMesh biomaterial
  myocutaneous
  Ne-Osteo bone morphogenic protein
     (BMP)
  nerve
  neuroplasty fat
  neurovascular island
  Nicoll
  Nicoll cancellous bone
  nontubed closed distant flap
  nontubed open distant flap
  nylon mesh
  Ollier thick split free
  Ollier-Thiersch skin
  onlay
  onlay cancellous iliac
  onlay mesh
  OP-1 implant
  open weave mesh
  Opteform 100HT bone
  osteoarticular
  osteocartilaginous
  osteochondral
  osteoperiosteal
  Osteoset bone graft substitute
  Overton dowel
  pancreatic allograft
  Papineau
  Parietex composite mesh
  Paritene mesh
  particulate
  patellar tendon
  pedicle
  pedicle bone
  peg

graft *(cont.)*
  PepGen P-15 (peptide-enhanced)
  percutaneous autogenous dowel bone
  PerioGlas bone graft material
  Perma-Flow coronary bypass
  PermaMesh
  Perma-Seal dialysis access
  peroneus brevis
  PFTE (polyfluorotetraethylene)
  Phemister onlay bone
  pigskin
  polyester tripled hamstring
  polyfluorotetraethylene (PTFE)
  polyglactin mesh dural
  polytetrafluoroethylene mesh
  polyvinyl sponge
  porcine dermal collagen
  porcine xenograft
  porous polyethylene
  portacaval H
  portocaval synthetic H-graft
  postage stamp
  postage-stamp type skin
  powdered bone
  PowerLink endoluminal
  ProOsteon 500 bone implant
  Proplast
  prosthetic femorodistal
  proud
  PTFE (polytetrafluoroethylene)
  pulmonary autograft (PA)
  Pyrost
  Rapidgraft arterial vessel substitute
  Repliform
  Reverdin epidermal free
  Russe bone
  Ryerson bone
  sandwiched iliac bone
  saphenous vein extracranial-
     intracranial bypass
  Sauvage
  segmental
  semitendinosus
  sentinel skin paddle

graft *(cont.)*
    Sepramesh biosurgical composite
      mesh
    seromuscular intestinal patch
    short vessel
    silicon-velvet composite
    single onlay cortical bone
    skin
    skull bone
    sliding inlay
    slit-cut mesh
    Solvang
    Soto-Hall bone
    Sperma-Tex preshaped mesh
    split calvarial bone
    split-thickness skin
    spreader
    stem cell autograft
    strut bone
    subclavian-external carotid artery
    Sure-Closure skin-stretching system
    Surgipro Prolene mesh
    SurgiSis sling/mesh
    Synergraft
    Tait
    temporal fascia
    Thiersch
    Thiersch medium split free
    Thiersch thin split free
    Thomas extrapolated bar
    Thoralon biomaterial
    three-strand semintendinosus tendon
    TransCyte skin substitute
    transplanted stamp
    Trelex mesh
    tricortical bone
    tricortical ilial strip
    tube flap
    tumbler
    Unigraft bone
    Unilab Surgibone
    Vascu-Guard bovine pericardial
      surgical patch
    vascularized fibula

graft *(cont.)*
    Vascutek
    Vectra vascular access (VAG)
    vein
    Venaflow vascular
    Visilex mesh
    Weaveknit vascular
    Wesolowski vascular
    Wilson bone
    Wolfe
    Wolfe full-thickness free
    Wolfe hand surgery
    Wolfe-Kawamoto bone
    wraparound flap bone
    XenoDerm
    xenograft
    Y-shaped graft
    Zenith AAA (abdominal aortic
      aneurysm) endovascular
    Zenotech
    Z-plasty local flap
GraftAssist vein and graft holder
graft copolymer
GraftCyte gauze wound dressing
graft delamination
graft elongation
graft enhanced with collagen
graft-enteric fistula
graft enteritis
graft fracture
grafting
grafting suction tube
graft irradiation
graft loading pattern
graft loosening
graft morselizer
graft necrosis
Graftpatch
graft rejection
graft survival
Grafton DBM (demineralized bone
    matrix) bone graft
Graftskin human skin product
graft-versus-host disease (GVHD)

graft-versus-host reaction
graft-versus-tumor activity
Graham closure with omental pouch
Graham-Cole cholecystography
Graham dural hook
Graham muscle hook
Graham nerve hook
Graham omental pouch
Graham patch
Graham plication
Graham scale for drug-induced gastric
  damage
Graham test
Graham-Field Inc.
grain handler's lung
gram-negative bacillus
gram-negative bacteria
gram-negative diplococci
gram-negative organism
gram-negative rod
gram-negative sepsis
gram positive
gram-positive bacillus
gram-positive bacteria
gram-positive organism
Gram stain
Gram stain and culture
Gram stain of stool
granddaughter cyst
GraNee grasper needle
granisetron HCl
granny knot
Granocyte (lenograstim)
Grant aneurysm clamp
Grant gallbladder retractor
granular appearance
granular-cell tumor
granular kidney
granularity
granulation tissue
Granulderm (trypsin; Peruvian balsam)
granule
  DiPAS-positive
  hemosiderin
  Weibel-Palade

Granulex (trypsin; Peruvian balsam)
granulocyte colony stimulating factor
  (G-CSF)
granulocyte-macrophage colony
  stimulating factor
granulocytic sarcoma
granulocytopenia
granuloma (pl. granulomas,
    granulomata)
  amebic
  calcified
  ceroid-like histiocytic granuloma
  eosinophilic
  hepatic
  inflammatory
  noncaseating tubercle-like
  portal zone
  rectal
granuloma inguinale
granulomatosis, intestinal lipophagic
granulomatous cholangitis
granulomatous colitis
granulomatous disease
granulomatous enteritis
granulomatous enterocolitis
granulomatous gastritis
granulomatous hepatitis
granulomatous ileitis
granulomatous infection
granulomatous mastitis
granulomatous thyroiditis
granulomatous transmural colitis
granulomatous ulcer
granulosa cell carcinoma
granulosa cell tumor
GranuMed (trypsin; Peruvian balsam)
grapefruit diet
Graser diverticulum
grasper
  alligator grasper/forceps
  atraumatic
  blunt-nose
  bottle-nose
  bowel
  bullet-nose

grasper *(cont.)*
  dolphin-nose
  duck-nose micrograsper
  Endo Babcock
  Endo Cinch
  Endo Grasp
  fenestrated
  fenestrated bowel
  fine-tooth fenestrated
  four-pronged polyp
  Glassman
  Hasson
  Hunter style double-action bowel
  laparoscopic
  long dolphin nose
  MetraGrasp
  Pivotal
  pointed-nose
  Pollock
  Questus Leading Edge
  Reddick
  Reddick-Saye suture
  reusable
  Riza-Ribe
  round-nose
  stationary
  Storz dolphin-nose
grasper needle
grasping forceps (see *forceps*)
grasping loop
Grassi test
grater reamer
Graves disease
Graves speculum
gravity drainage
gravity, specific
gray tumor
Gray bone drill
Gray cystic duct forceps
gray foam bandage
Gray reamer
gray-scale ultrasonography
gray-scale ultrasound
Grayson ligament in hand

greasy food
great imitator
Great Smokies intestinal permeability
  test kit
greater curvature banded gastroplasty
greater curvature of stomach
greater curvature ulcer
greater omentum (omentum majus)
greater peritoneal sac
greater trochanter
great vessel injury
Green-Armytage hemostasis forceps
Greenberg clamp
Greenberg Universal retractor
green-brown drainage
Greene biopsy needle
Greene forceps
Greene retractor
green liver
Green muscle hook
green stools
Green thyroid retractor
Greenville gastric bypass
Greenwald cutting loop
Greenwald flexible endoscopic
  electrode
Greenwich catheter
Greenwood bayonet forceps
Greenwood bipolar and suction forceps
Greer EZ Access drainage pouch
Greer's goo dressing (hydrocortisone,
  nystatin, zinc oxide)
Gregory baby profunda clamp
Gregory carotid bulldog clamp
Gregory DeBakey bulldog clamp
Gregory external clamp
Gregory stay suture
Grenoble-Paris-Rennes (GPR) robot
  microscope
Greven forceps
Grey Turner sign of retroperitoneal
  hemorrhage
GRFoma pancreatic endocrine tumor
gridiron incision

Griffen Roux-en-Y bypass
Grinfeld cannula
Gripper needle
gritty material
gritty tumor
Grocco sign
groin dissection
groin flap
groin hernia
groin incision
groin mass
Grollman catheter
Grondahl-Finney esophagogastroplasty
groove
    esophageal (on liver)
    gastric
    Liebermeister
    oval-form colonic
    radial
    spindle colonic
grooved dissector
grooved titanium rod
groove pancreatitis
grooving reamer
Groshong PICC catheter
gross blood
gross blood in stool
gross blood with small clots
Gross coarctation occlusion clamp
Gross disease
gross diagnosis
Grosse and Kempf locking nail system
Grosse-Kempf interlocking medullary
    nail
gross lesion
Gross operation
Gross test
gross tumor
gross tumor involvement
grounded patient
ground-glass appearance (on x-ray)
ground-glass body of Hadziyannis
ground-glass cell
ground-glass pattern

group B streptococcus (GBS)
Grover clamp
Grover meniscus knife
growth, extranodal
growth plate
growth plate abscess
growth retardation
Gruber-Landzert fossa
Gruber suture
Gruentzig balloon catheter
Gruenwald ear forceps
Gruenwald neurosurgical rongeur
grumous material
Grüntzig (Gruentzig)
Grüntzig balloon
Grüntzig balloon catheter
Gruppe wire-crimping forceps
Grynfeltt hernia
Grynfeltt triangle
GS (Gardner syndrome)
GSI (General Surgical Innovations)
GSI balloon dissector
GSI Spacemaker II
GSRS (gastrointestinal symptom rating
    scale)
GSW (gunshot wound)
G6PD deficiency
G-suit external counterpressure device
G-34 ("big gastrin")
GII EasyAnchor
GII Snap-Pak anchor
G tube
guaiac-negative stool
guaiac-positive nipple discharge
guaiac-positive stool
guaiac test of occult blood in stool
Guardian ring bracket
Guardian suction cannister
guarding
    involuntary
    muscle
    voluntary
guarding of abdomen
guarding sign

Guardsman femoral screw
gubernaculum
Gudebrod, Inc., instruments
Guedel disposable airway
Guedel plastic airway
Guedel rubber airway
Guenzberg test
Guérin fold
Guibor Silastic tube
guidance
   sonographic
   ultrasound
Guidant Origin system
guide
   Accu-Line
   acetabular
   ACL drill
   Acufex tibial
   adjustable angle
   Adson drill
   Adson dural protector
   Adson saw
   alignment
   Arthrex femoral
   Arthrex tibial
   Bailey-Gigli saw
   ball-tipped Küntscher (Kuentscher)
   barrel
   Blair saw
   bone wire
   Bullseye
   calibrated pin
   Cloward drill
   Cushing-Gigli saw
   Cushing saw
   Davis saw
   DePuy femoral acetabular overlay
   drill
   Duopress
   eccentric drill
   Fanelli
   femoral intramedullary
   FIN pin
   Fisher

guide *(cont.)*
   Ghajar
   Gigli saw
   Guyon catheter
   Hall-Dundar drill
   Hewson cruciate
   Hewson drill
   Hoffmann pin
   Howell tibial
   intercondylar drill
   intramedullary
   Iowa trumpet needle
   Lebsche saw
   ligature
   long axial alignment
   Lunderquist-Ring torque
   nail rotational
   needle
   neutral and load drill
   neutral drill
   patellar drill
   PCA cutting
   PCA medullary
   picket fence
   Pilot suture
   Pinn.ACL
   Poppen Gigli saw
   Raney saw
   Reese osteotomy
   Richards angle
   saw
   stationary angle
   Synthes wire
   T-bar
   telescopic wire
   tibial cutter
   tibial cutting
   tibial drill
   Todd-Wells
   trocar
   Trumpet needle
   tube
   tunnel drill
   wire

guide *(cont.)*
   XMB tibial reaming
   Yasargil ligature
guide bushing
guide catheter
guided imagery
guided microsurgery
guided-needle aspiration cytology
guided-needle biopsy
guided transcutaneous biopsy
guideline
   Böhler (Boehler)
   Hartel
   Letournel
guide pin
   ball-point
   ball-tip
   calibrated
guide sleeve
guide tube
guidewire
   ACS (Advanced Catheter Systems)
   ACS Hi-Torque Balance
     Middleweight
   Amplatz Super Stiff
   angiographic
   atherolytic
   atherolytic reperfusion
   Athlete coronary
   Bentson floppy-tip
   Critikon
   Director biliary
   Extra Sport coronary
   FasTrac
   Flex
   flexible
   flexible J
   floppy
   floppy-tipped
   Geenan Endotorque
   Glidewire
   high-torque floppy
   Hi-Per Flex
   Hi-Torque Flex-T

guidewire *(cont.)*
   Hi-Torque Floppy (HTF)
   Hi-Torque Intermediate
   Hi-Torque Standard
   HPC
   hydrophilic
   Hyperflex
   Iguana
   J
   J-tip
   J-tipped exchange
   J-tipped hydrophilic
   J-tipped spring
   Linx exchange
   long taper/stiff shaft Glidewire
   Lumina
   Lunderquist
   Magnum
   Medrad
   Microvasive Glidewire
   Microvasive stiff piano wire
   Mustang steerable
   PDT
   preformed
   QuickSilver hydrophilic-coated
   Radiofocus Glidewire
   Redifocus
   Rosen
   ROTACS
   Schwarten LP
   shapeable
   Silk
   Sof-T
   soft-tipped
   Sones
   SOS
   steerable
   straight
   TAD
   Teflon-coated
   Terumo
   TherOx 0.014 infusion
   Tracer hybrid
   transluminal angioplasty

guidewire *(cont.)*
USCI
VeriFlex
WaveWire
Wholey Hi-Torque Floppy
Wholey Hi-Torque Modified J
Wholey Hi-Torque Standard
Zebra exchange
guidewire exchanged
guidewire exchange technique
guidewire for needle localization
guidewire introducer
guiding catheter
Guidor barrier
Guidor surgical mesh
Guilford-Wiet foot plate pick
Guilford-Wright double-edged sickle
knife
Guilford-Wright duckbill elevator
Guilford-Wright flap knife
Guilford-Wright micro bone curette
Guilford-Wright stapes pick
Guilford-Wright suction tube
Guillain-Barré syndrome
guillotine blade
Guleke bone rongeur
gullet
gull-wing incision
gum, karaya
gum rubber Martin bandage
gun (see *stapler*)
Gunderson bone forceps
Gunderson muscle forceps
Gunnar-Hey roller forceps
gunshot wound (GSW)
GunSlinger shoulder orthosis
gurgle (bowel sound)
gurgling bowel sounds
Gusberg hysterectomy clamp

Gussenbauer suture
gusseted arm board
gustatory anesthesia
gustatory gland
gut
artificial
caffeine
catgut
nervous
plain
Gutaform
gut-associated lymphoid tissue (GALT)
gut dysmotility
Gutgemann clamp
Gutgemann-Longmire gastric recon-
struction
gut-hormone profile
Guthrie fixation hook
gut suture
gutter
lateral
left
paracolic
right
gutter wound
Guy gouge
Guyon catheter guide
Guyon catheter introducer
Guyon-Péan kidney clamp
guy suture
GVAX pancreatic vaccine
GVHD (graft-versus-host disease)
Gwilliam clamp
gynecologic pain
gynecologic tumor
gynecomastia
Gynex angle hook
Gynex Emmett tenaculum
Gynex extended-reach needle

H, h

H$_2$ (histamine 2)
HAART (highly active antiretroviral
  therapy)
Haberer abdominal spatula
Haberer forceps
Haberer intestinal clamp
habit (pl. habits)
  bowel
  change in bowel
  dietary
  drinking
  drug
  eating
  smoking
habitus
  asthenic
  body
  gracile
  large
HACA (human antichimeric antibody)
Hadefield-Clarke syndrome
Hadziyannis, ground-glass body of
HAEC (Hirschsprung-associated
  enterocolitis)
Haemonetics Cell Saver 5
Haemonetics red blood cell collection
  protocol
Haemophilus ducreyi

Haemophilus haemolyticus
Haemophilus influenzae
Haemophilus influenzae type B
Haemophilus parahaemolyticus
Haemophilus parainfluenzae
Haemophilus vaginalis
Hafnia alvei (formerly *Enterobacter
  hafniae*)
Hafter diet trick
Hagedorn needle
Hagie hip pin
Hagie pin nail
Hagie sliding nail plate
Hahn bone nail
HAI (histologic activity index)
Haid cervical plate
Haight-Finochietto rib retractor
Haimovici arteriotomy scissors
hairy cell leukemia
Hajek antrum rongeur
Hajek-Ballenger septal elevator
Hajek chisel
Hajek-Koffler bone punch forceps
Hajek-Koffler laminectomy rongeur
Hajek-Koffler punch
Hajek laminectomy punch
Hajek mallet
Hakansson bone rongeur

Hakim-Cortis ventriculoperitoneal
shunt
HAL (hemorrhoid arterial ligation)
Haldane-Priestley tube
Haldeman bone graft
Haley's M-O (magnesium hydroxide;
mineral oil) (now Phillips' M-O)
half-and-half nail
half-circle microplate
half-circle plate
half-hitch knot
halflife of circulating thyroid hormone
half pin
half-strength feeding
Halifax clamp
Halifax interlaminar clamp
Hall air drill
Hall air-driven oscillating saw
Hallberg biliointestinal bypass
Hall driver
Hall-Dundar drill guide
Halle dura knife
Halle infant speculum
Hall large bore drill
Hall Micro E drill
Hall Micro E oscillating saw
Hall Micro E reciprocating saw
Hall Micro E sagittal saw
Hall rod
Hall sternal saw
Hall Surgairtome drill
Hall Versipower drill
Hall Versipower oscillating saw
Hall Versipower reamer
Hall Versipower reciprocating saw
hallux nail
halo effect (on x-ray)
halofuginone
halogen endoscopic light source
halogen exam lamp
halo melanoma
halo pin
Halotestin (fluoxymesterone)
halothane

halothane-induced hepatitis
halothane poisoning
HALS (hand-assisted laparoscopic
surgery)
Halsey nail scissors
Halsey needle holder with tungsten
carbide inlay
Halsey-TC needle holder
Halsted artery forceps
Halsted-Bassini herniorrhaphy
Halsted hemostat
Halsted mosquito forceps
Halsted hemostatic mosquito forceps
(straight/curved)
Halsted inguinal herniorrhaphy
Halsted mosquito forceps
Halsted operation
Halsted radical mastectomy
Halsted suture
HALT-C (hepatitis C antiviral long-
term treatment to prevent cirrhosis)
study
Halverson classification of groin hernias
(types 1–4)
Halverson-McVay classification of groin
hernias (class 1–4)
hamartoma
benign
bile duct
duodenal wall
pancreatic
hamartomas throughout the GI tract
hamartomatous gastric polyp
hamartomatous intestinal polyposis
hamartomatous lesion
hamartomatous polyp
hamartomatous polyposis
hamburger sign
Hamel test
Hamilton bandage
Hamman sign
hammer
Berliner percussion
Buck neurological

hammer *(cont.)*
    Buck percussion
    Cloward
    Davis percussion
    Dejerine-Davis percussion
    Dejerine percussion
    Epstein neurological
    Küntscher (Kuentscher)
    neurological
    percussion
    Rabiner neurological
    slotted
    Taylor percussion
    Traube neurological percussion
    Trömner (Troemner) percussion
Hampton air
Hampton line (on x-ray)
Hancke/Vilmann biopsy handle
    instrument
Handages dressing
hand-assisted laparoscopic colectomy
hand-assisted laparoscopic gastrectomy
hand-assisted laparoscopic hemicolec-
    tomy
hand-assisted laparoscopic surgery
    (HALS)
hand-assisted laparoscopy
hand-assisted sigmoidectomy
hand drill
hand elevator
H&H (hemoglobin and hematocrit)
handheld retractor
handheld ultrasonic nebulizer
handheld UV light
hand instrument
handle
    Bill axis traction
    Bill traction
    blade
    DeBakey ring
    elevator, T
    E-Z off reusable plastic knife
    Gigli saw
    Gigli-Strully saw

handle *(cont.)*
    Hancke-Vilmann biopsy
    Hunstad infiltration
    knife
    Kollman dilator
    laryngeal mirror
    Lysonics
    Medi-Vac Flexi-Clear suction
    Medi-Vac Yankauer suction
    octagon-threaded
    pistol-grip spring
    reinsulate "U" style
    ring
    scalpel
    Siegel knife
    standard laparoscopic
    Strully Gigli saw
    Take-Apart
    T, elevator
    thumb
    Tip-Trol
    Townsend
    Turner
    Turner Warwick diathermy scalpel
    type reamer
    U
    universal
    universal chuck
handle-type reamer
hand-operated drill
hand piece bandage
HandPort hand-assist device
hand retractor
hand roller
hand-sewn anastomosis
Hands Free knee retractor
Hanger test
hanging panniculus (also see *apron*)
Hanks Balanced Salt Solution (HBSS)
Hanot-Chauffard syndrome
Hanot cirrhosis
Hansen-Street nail
Hansen-Street pin
Hansen-Street plate

H_2 antagonist
Ha1A human monoclonal antibody
Hapset bone graft plaster
haptoglobin, serum
HAR (hyperacute rejection)
Hara classification of gallbladder
    inflammation
hard adhesion
hard fixed mass
hard stool passage
hard stools
Hardy bipolar forceps
Hardy dressing forceps
Hardy microbipolar forceps
Hardy sella punch
Hardy sella punch forceps
Hardy spinal retractor
Hardy suction tube
Hardy three-prong fork
Hare pin
Hariri-Heifetz needle
Harken auricle clamp
Harlow plate
Harm posterior cervical plate
Harmonic hemorrhoidectomy
Harmonic Scalpel Ultracision
Harpenden caliper
Harpoon suture anchor
Harrell Y stent (airway)
Harrington compression rod
Harrington distraction rod
Harrington esophageal diverticulectomy
Harrington hook
Harrington hook clamp
Harrington hook driver
Harrington-Mayo thoracic scissors
Harrington-Mixter thoracic forceps
Harrington retractor
Harrington rod
Harrington rod clamp
Harrington scissors
Harrington spinal elevator
Harrington splanchnic retractor
Harrington thoracic forceps

Harris band
Harris-Beath axial hindfoot view
Harris-Benedict energy requirement
    equation
Harris center-cutting acetabular reamer
Harris condylocephalic nail
Harris condylocephalic rod
Harris hip nail
Harris medullary nail
Harrison bone-holding forceps
Harrison Cripp artery forceps
Harrison knife
Harrison-Nicolle polypropylene peg
Harrison spot test
Harrison sterilizing forceps
Harris plate
Harris superior acetabular graft
Harris tube
Harris view
Hartley breast prosthesis
Hartmann bone rongeur
Hartmann closure of rectum
Hartmann hemostatic mosquito forceps
Hartmann mosquito forceps
Hartmann nasal dressing forceps
Hartmann nasal speculum
Hartmann point
Hartmann pouch
Hartmann procedure
Hartmann resection of bowel
Hartmann tonsil punch
Hartnup disease
Hartshill rectangle rod
Hartzler ACX-II or RX-014 balloon
    catheter
Hartzler angioplasty balloon
Hartzler Micro II balloon
Hartzler rib retractor
Harvard infusion pump
Harvard 2 dual syringe pump
harvesting of graft
harvesting of organ
Harvey hospital prognostic nutritional
    index

Harvey Stone clamp
Harvey suture scissors
Harvey wire-cutting scissors
Hashimoto struma
Hashimoto thyroiditis
Hassall corpuscles
Hasson blunt-end cannula
Hasson grasper
Hasson laparoscopy cannula
Hasson open laparoscopy cannula
Hasson SAC (stable access cannula)
Hasson technique
Hasson trocar
Hastings frame
HAT (hepatic artery thrombosis)
Hatcher pin
hatching test
Haugh forceps
haustra (pl. of haustrum)
haustral blunting
haustral fold
haustral indentation
haustral markings
haustral pattern
haustral pouch
haustrum (pl. haustra)
HAV (hepatitis A virus)
Haverfield-Scoville hemilaminectomy
  retractor
Havrix (hepatitis A vaccine, inactivated)
Hawkeye suture
Hawkeye suture needle
Hawkins breast localization needle
Hayes anterior resection clamp
Hayes Martin forceps
Haynes brain cannula
Haynes pin
Haynes retractor
Haynes scissors
Hays hand retractor
Hay test
Hayton Williams wire-twisting forceps
Hb (hemoglobin)

HB (hepatitis B)
HbAg, HBAg ("H-bag") (hepatitis B
  antigen)
HB$_c$Ab (hepatitis B core antibody)
HB$_c$Ag (hepatitis B core antigen)
HB$_e$Ab (hepatitis B "e" antibody)
HB$_e$Ag (soluble "e" antigen in hepatitis
  B)
HB$_e$Ag-negative wild-type precore
  HBV
HBIG (hepatitis B immune globulin)
HB$_s$Ab (hepatitis B surface antibody)
HB$_s$Ag (hepatitis B surface antigen)
HB$_s$Ag carrier
H$_2$ blocker
H$_2$ breath test
HBSS (Hanks Balanced Salt Solution)
HBV (hepatitis B virus)
HCA (hepatocellular adenoma)
HCC (hepatocellular carcinoma) nodule
HCl (hydrochloride)
HCO$_3^-$ (bicarbonate)
hCS (human chorionic somato-
  mammotrophin)
HCS (hematocystic spot)
Hct (hematocrit)
HCV (hepatitis C virus)
HCV co-infection
HCV RNA
HDAg (delta antigen)
HD5 (human defensin 5)
HD5 immunoreactivity
HD 85 (barium sulfate)
HDI 3000 ultrasound system
HDL (high-density lipoprotein)
HDL cholesterol
HD 200 Plus (barium sulfate)
HD II (or 2) total hip prosthesis
HDV (hepatitis D virus)
HE (hepatic encephalopathy)
headache
head CT
head drape

headlight
  Burton
  Clar 55
head of pancreas
headrest, Malcolm-Rand radiolucent
head trauma
healed erosive GERD (gastroesophageal
  reflux disease)
healed per primam
healed yellow atrophy
Healey revision acetabular component
healing (or healed) by primary intention
healing (or healed) by secondary
  intention
healing ulcer
Healos synthetic bone-grafting material
Health Buddy monitoring device
HealthCheck monitor
health-related quality of life (HRQOL)
HealthShield antimicrobial mediastinal
  wound drainage catheter
Healy intestinal forceps
Heaney biopsy curette
Heaney clamp
Heaney forceps
Heaney hysterectomy retractor
Heaney needle
Heaney needle holder
Heaney needle holder with tungsten
  carbide inlays
Heaney retractor
Heaney-TC needle holder
heart block
heartburn (pyrosis)
Heart Laser (for transmyocardial revas-
  cularization)
heat edema
heater probe
heater probe ablation
heater probe coagulation
Heath-Richter clip-removing forceps
Heath ligature scissors
Heath mallet
Heath suture scissors

heaves, dry
heavy alcohol use
heavy-duty femur plate
heavy-duty two-tooth retractor
heavy side plate
heavy silk suture
heavy wire suture
Hebra blade
Hectorol (doxercalciferol)
Hedblom rib retractor
Hedrocel bone substitute material
heel ulcer
Heerferdt-Waldenstrom syndrome
Heermann alligator forceps
Heffington lumbar seat
Hegar-Baumgartner needle
Hegar bougie
Hegar rectal dilator
Hegemann-Diethrich vascular scissors
Hegenbarth clip forceps
Heidenhain cell
Heidenhain pouch
Heifitz clamp
Heimlich maneuver for choking
Heine G series loupe
Heineke-Mikulicz gastroenterostomy
Heineke-Mikulicz pyloroplasty
Heine K series loupe
Heine sigmoidoscope
Hein rongeur
Heinz bodies
Heiss artery forceps
Heiss Finochietto artery forceps
Heiss soft tissue retractor
Heister valve
helical bacteria
helical computed tomography (CT)
helical suture
Helicide (bismuth subnitrate;
  metronidazole; tetracycline)
Helicobacter hepaticus
Helicobacter pylori-associated gastritis
  (HPAG)
Helicobacter pylori bacteria in vitro

Helicobacter pylori breath test
Helicobacter pylori gastritis
Helicosol (synthetic ^{13}C-urea)
 lyophilized powder
Helidac (bismuth subsalicylate,
 metronidazole, and tetracycline)
Heliodorus bandage
Helisal rapid blood test
Helistat absorbable collagen hemostatic
 sponge
Helitene absorbable hemostatic agent
Helivax vaccine
HeliX knot pusher
helle cell
Heller-Belsey operation for achalasia of
 esophagus
Heller cardiomyotomy
Heller-Dor operation for achalasia of
 esophagus
Heller esophagomyotomy
Heller myotomy
HELLP (hemolysis, elevated liver
 enzymes, and low platelets)
 syndrome
HELLP (hemolysis with a microangio-
 pathic blood smear, elevated liver
 enzymes, and low platelet count)
 syndrome
helminth
helminthic appendicitis
helminthic disorder
helper T cell
Hema-Check test
hemagglutination inhibition/inhibiting
 (HI)
hemagglutination titer for MSA
HemaMyst aerosol adhesive
hemangioendothelial sarcoma
hemangioendothelioma, epithelioid
hemangioma
 capillary
 cavernous
 congenital
 hepatic

hemangioma *(cont.)*
 sclerosing
 strawberry
 vascular
 venous
hemangioma angioma
hemangioma of liver
hemangiomatosis, splenic capillary
hemangiopericytoma
Hemaquet catheter introducer
Hemaquet sheath introducer
Hemarrest patch
Hemaseel APR fibrin adhesive
Hemaseel HMN biological tissue glue
Hemashield enhanced graft
HemAssist blood substitute
Hemasure r/LS red blood cell filtration
 system
HemaSyst sealant
hematemesis, post-retching
Hematest
hematocellular jaundice
hematochezia
hematochezia PR (per rectum)
hematocrit (Hct)
hematocystic spot (HCS)
hematogenous dissemination of tumor
hematogenous dissemination of virus
hematogenous dissemination to distant
 organs
hematogenous route
hematogenous seeding
hematogenous spread of micro-
 organisms
hematologic dyscrasia
hematologic malignancy
hematoma
 bowel-wall
 intramural
 nasal septal
 pelvic
 perianal
 postoperative
 rectus sheath

hematoma *(cont.)*
  subcapsular
  subdural
  subfascial
  submucosal
  vestibule of mouth
hematoma aspiration
hematoma evacuation
hematopoiesis
hematopoietic disorder
hematopoietic malignancy
hematoxylin and eosin (H&E) stain
HemDetect three-field occult blood test
heme-negative stool
hemeostatic balance
heme-positive NG aspirate
heme-positive stool
HemeSelect reagent and collection kit
hemiaxial view
hemicolectomy (also see *operation*)
  Duecollement
  extended right
  hand-assisted laparoscopic
  laparoscopic
  laparoscopic left
  left
  standard right
hemicolon
hemicylindrical bone graft
hemidiaphragm
hemigastrectomy
hemiglossectomy
hemilaminectomy knife
hemilaminectomy retractor
Hemi Sling
hemispherical contact probe
hemispherical reamer
Hemobahn endovascular stent/graft
hemobilia
Hemoccult SENSA test
Hemoccult II test
hemochromatosis, precirrhotic
hemochromatotic cirrhosis
Hemochron high-dose thrombin time
  (HiTT)

Hemoclip-applying forceps
Hemoclip ligating clip
hemoconcentration
Hemocor HPH
HemoCue photometer
hemodialyzer
Hemo-Drain needle
Hemo-Drain wound tube
hemodynamically significant lesion
hemodynamically stable
hemodynamically unstable
hemodynamic monitoring
hemodynamic status
hemofiltration, continuous arterio-
  venous (CAVH)
hemoglobin (Hb, Hgb)
hemoglobin concentration
hemoglobin crosfumaril blood substi-
  tute
hemoglobin electrophoresis
hemoglobin, glycosylated
hemoglobinopathy
Hemolink blood substitute
Hem-o-lok clamp
Hem-o-lok ligating clip
hemolysis
  chronic
  intravascular
hemolytic jaundice
hemolytic malaria
hemolytic splenomegaly
hemolytic strep (streptococcus)
hemolytic uremic syndrome (HUS)
hemolyzed blood
HemoMatic monitor
Hemopad absorbable collagen hemostat
Hemopad microfibrillar collagen
  hemostat
hemoperitoneal
hemoperitoneum
hemoporphyrin derivative, photo-
  sensitizing
hemoptysis
Hemopump
Hemopure blood substitute

Hemopure (hemoglobin glutamer-250
[bovine]) oxygen therapy system
HemoQuant fecal occult blood test
Hemorid for Women (pramoxine HCl;
phenylephrine HCl)
hemorrhage
bilateral adrenal
concealed
epidural
exsanguinating
external
extradural
focal
frank
gastric
gastrointestinal (GI)
internal
interstitial
intestinal
intra-abdominal
intra-alveolar
intracranial
intratumoral
massive
nasopharyngeal
oropharyngeal
postoperative
punctate
retroperitoneal
salmon-patch
severe
stromal
subarachnoid
subdural
submucosal
subserosal
hemorrhagic ascites
hemorrhagic colitis
hemorrhagic consolidation of lung
hemorrhagic cyst
hemorrhagic cystitis
hemorrhagic dengue
hemorrhagic diarrhea
hemorrhagic effusion

hemorrhagic encephalitis
hemorrhagic enterocolitis
hemorrhagic fever
hemorrhagic gastritis
hemorrhagic infarct
hemorrhagic intestinal infarction
hemorrhagic malaria
hemorrhagic material
hemorrhagic mucosa
hemorrhagic myelitis
hemorrhagic necrosis of alveolar septum)
hemorrhagic necrosis of intestine
hemorrhagic necrotizing pancreatitis
hemorrhagic nephritis
hemorrhagic pancreatitis
hemorrhagic pericarditis
hemorrhagic plague
hemorrhagic pleurisy
hemorrhagic salpingitis
hemorrhagic shock
hemorrhagic speck
hemorrhagic telangiectasia
hemorrhagic tendency
hemorrhoid (pl. hemorrhoids)
arterial ligation (HAL)
combined
external
first-degree
fourth-degree
internal
large refractory
mixed
mucocutaneous
necrotic
prolapsed
prolapsing internal
second-degree
strangulated
third-degree
thrombosed
thrombosed external
hemorrhoid arterial ligation (HAL),
Doppler-guided
hemorrhoid artery

hemostatic agent
  acetylhydrolase
  Amicar
  Aquamephyton
  argatroban
  Avitene
  calcium alginate
  cellulose, oxidized
  collagen sponge, absorbable
  Collastat
  CoStasis
  DynaStat
  EndoAvitene
  Ethamolin
  ethanolamine oleate
  gelatin film
  gelatin powder
  gelatin sponge
  Gelfilm
  Gelfoam
  Helistat sponge
  Helitene absorbable
  Hemaseel HMN
  Hemopad
  Hemotene
  InStat
  InStat MCH
  MCH (microfibrillar collagen hemostat)
  Myphyton
  Novastan
  Oxycel
  phytonadione (vitamin K_1)
  Sorbsan
  Surgicel
  Surgicel Nu-Knit
  Surgifoam
  thrombin
  Thrombin-JMI
  Thrombogen topical thrombin
  Thrombostat
  Tissucol
  Trasylol
hemostatic clamp

hemostatic forceps
hemostatic sponge (see *hemostatic agent*)
hemostatic suture
Hemotene absorbable collagen hemostat
Hemotherapies Liver Dialysis Unit
hemothorax, massive
hemotympanum
Hemovac drain
Hemovac Hydrocoat drain
Hemovac suction tube
Hem-Prep (phenylephrine HCl; zinc oxide)
Hemril Uniserts (bismuth subgallate; bismuth resorcin compound; benzyl benzoate; peruvian balsam; zinc oxide)
Henahan elevator
Henahan extracting forceps
Henderson onlay bone graft
Henderson skin incision
Hendrin ductus clamp
Hendrin ductus forceps
Hendrin forceps
Henke-Sass rigid laparoscope
Henke-Sass Wolf laparoscope
Henke triangle
Henle, jejunal interposition of
Henle loop
Henley carotid retractor
Henley vascular clamp
Henner T-model endaural retractor
Hennig plaster cast spreader
Henning mallet
Henning meniscal retractor
Henning sign
Henoch-Schönlein (Schoenlein) purpura
Henry bone graft
Henry incision
hepadna virus (hepatitis B-like DNA)
Hepafix low-allergy adhesive tape dressing
Hepagene (hepatitis B vaccine)

Hepamed-coated Wiktor stent
heparin
  beef lung
  pyrogen-free
heparin anticoagulant
heparin calcium
heparin-induced thrombocytopenia
  (HIT)
heparin infusion prior to stentint (HIPS)
heparinize
heparinized solution
heparin lock (hep lock)
Heparin Lock Flush solution (heparin
  sodium)
heparin lock introducer
heparin/protamine infusion
heparin sodium & sodium chloride
heparin sulfate
heparin therapy, monitoring of
heparin whole blood
HepatAmine nutrient solution
HepatAssist bioartificial liver
hepatectomy
  cadaveric donor
  donor
  extended right
  hemi-
  laparoscopic
  left
  limited
  local
  partial
  recipient
  regional
  right
  right lobe
  segmental
  simultaneous segmental
  subsegmental
  total left
  wedge
hepatic abscess
hepatic adenoma
Hepatic-Aid powdered feeding

Hepatic-Aid II Instant Drink (multiple
  branched-chain amino acids)
hepatic amyloid
hepatic architecture
hepatic arterial infusion (HAI)
hepatic arterial infusion chemotherapy
hepatic arterial supply
hepatic arteriogram
hepatic artery ligation
hepatic artery portal vein fistula
hepatic artery system
hepatic artery thrombosis (HAT)
hepatic atrophy
hepatic bed
hepatic bifurcation
hepatic calculus
hepatic capsular vasculitis
hepatic capsule
hepatic carcinoma
hepatic cell carcinoma
hepatic cirrhosis
hepatic colic
hepatic coma
hepatic cord
hepatic degeneration
hepatic duct
hepatic duct calculus
hepatic dullness
hepatic encephalopathy (HE)
hepatic failure
hepatic fever
hepatic fibrosis
hepatic fistula
hepatic flexure of colon
hepatic function test
hepatic gland
hepatic glycogen
hepatic glycogen storage
hepatic glycogen stores
hepatic granuloma
hepatic hemangioma
hepatic hilum
hepatic Hodgkin disease

hepatic hydrothorax
hepatic infarction
hepatic insufficiency
hepatic iron stores
hepatic ligament
hepatic lithiasis
hepatic lobectomy
hepatic lobular parenchyma
hepatic lobule
hepatic lymph node
hepatic necrosis
hepatic nerve plexus
hepatico- (see *hepato-* entries)
hepaticoenterostomy (also hepato-
     enterostomy)
hepaticojejunostomy (see *hepato-
     jejunostomy*)
hepatic obstruction
hepaticoportoenterostomy
hepatic osteomalacia
hepaticostomy
hepaticotomy
hepatic outflow tract
hepatic parasitic cyst
hepatic parenchyma
hepatic parenchymal cell
hepatic perfusion index (HPI)
hepatic phosphorylase deficiency
hepatic plexus
hepatic porphyria
hepatic-renal angle
hepatic resection
hepatic reserve
hepatic rupture
hepatic sclerosis
hepatic segmentectomy
hepatic segment of liver
hepatic sinusoid
hepatic stem cell
hepatic tenderness
hepatic transaminase
hepatic triad
hepatic vein
hepatic vein occlusion

hepatic vein thrombosis
hepatic vein outflow
hepatic vein stent
hepatic vein thrombosis
hepatic vein vena cava thrombosis
hepatic veno-occlusive disease
hepatic venous drainage
hepatic venous isolation by direct hemo-
     perfusion (HVI-DHP)
hepatic venous outflow
hepatic venous outflow block
hepatic venous outflow obstruction
     (HVOO)
hepatic venous pressure gradient
hepatic venous web disease
hepatic web
hepatic web dilation
hepatic wedge pressure
hepatitis (pl. hepatitides)
     acute mononucleosis-like
     acute parenchymatous
     acute viral (AVH)
     alcoholic
     amebic
     anesthetic
     anicteric
     anti-HBe-positive
     autoimmune
     cholestatic viral
     chronic
     chronic active (CAH)
     chronic active viral (CAVH)
     chronic active viral, non-A,
          non-B (CAVH-NAB)
     chronic active viral, type B
          (CAVH-B)
     chronic aggressive
     chronic fibrosing
     chronic interstitial
     chronic lobular (CLH)
     chronic persistent (CPH)
     chronic persisting
     chronic progressive
     coinfection with

hepatitis G virus (HGV)
hepatitis serologic marker
hepatization
hepatobiliary disease
hepatobiliary hepatitis
hepatobiliary scan
hepatobiliary scintigraphy
hepatobiliary tree
hepatoblastoma
hepato- (also *hepatico-*)
hepatocarcinogenic pesticide
hepatocarcinoma, fibrolamellar
hepatocellular adenoma (HCA)
hepatocellular ballooning
hepatocellular carcinoma (HCC)
hepatocellular cholestasis
hepatocellular disease
hepatocellular iron storage
hepatocellular jaundice
hepatocellular necrosis
hepatocerebral intoxication
hepatocholangiolitic carcinoma
hepatoclavicular view
hepatocolic ligament
hepatocystic
hepatocystocolic ligament
hepatocyte
    ballooning degeneration of
    cobblestone pattern of
    lipid-laden
    periportal
hepatocyte dysfunction
hepatocyte nuclear factor-1 alpha
    (HNF-1 alpha)
hepatodiaphragmatic interposition
    of colon (Chilaiditi syndrome)
hepatoduodenal ligament compression
hepatoduodenal-peritoneal reflection
hepatoduodenal reflection
hepatoduodenoperitoneal reflection
hepatoenteric anastomosis
hepatoerythropoietic porphyria (HEP)
hepatoesophageal ligament
hepatofugal flow

hepatogastric duodenal ligament
hepatogastric ligament
hepatogenous jaundice
hepatogenous pigment
hepatoiminodiacetic acid (HIDA)
hepatojejunostomy (also hepatico-
    jejunostomy)
    complex
    high
    hilar
    intracystic
    laparoscopic
    left
    palliative
    pediatric
    peripheral
    right
    right and left
    Roux-en-Y
    side-to-side
    simple
hepatojejunostomy with cutaneous
    stoma
hepatojugular reflux (HJR)
hepatolenticular degeneration
hepatolenticular disease
hepatolienal cirrhosis
hepatolithiasis with biliary stricture,
    complicated residual
hepatologist
hepatology
hepatoma, fibrolamellar
hepatomegaly
    congestive
    painful
hepatopancreatic ampulla sphincter
hepatopancreatic fold
hepatopancreatoduodenectomy
hepatopathy, radiation
hepatopetal flow
hepatophosphorylase deficiency
    glycogenosis
hepatophrenic ligament
hepatopleural fistula
hepatoportal sclerosis

hepatoportoenterostomy, Kasai-type
hepatoptosis
hepatopulmonary syndrome
hepatorenal angle
hepatorenal ligament
hepatorenal pouch
hepatorenal recess
hepatorenal syndrome (HRS)
hepatorrhaphy
hepatosplenic infestation
hepatosplenomegaly
hepatotomy
hepatotoxic effect
hepatotoxicity
hepatotoxic range
hepatoumbilical ligament
Hep-B-Gammagee
hep lock catheter
Hep-Lock (heparin sodium) flush
Hep-Lock U/P (heparin sodium) flush
Heprofile ELISA (enzyme-linked
    immunosorbent assay)
heptadecapeptide
Heptalac lactulose solution
Heptavax-B vaccine
Heptazyme
Heptodin (lamivudine)
Heptovir (lamivudine)
herald bleed
herbal therapy
Herbert bone screw
Herbert saw
Herbert-Whipple bone screw
HercepTest
Herceptin (trastuzumab) monoclonal
    antibody
Hercules Nd:YAG laser system
Hercules plaster and bandage scissors
Hercules plaster shears
Hercules 7000 mobile x-ray unit
Herculink biliary stent
Herculink 14 biliary stent system
Herculon suture

Herczel rasp
Herczel rib elevator
hereditary angioedema
hereditary angioneurotic edema
hereditary cancer
hereditary carcinoma
hereditary elliptocytosis
hereditary hemorrhagic telangiectasia
    (HHT)
hereditary MEA (multiple endocrine
    adenomatosis) syndrome
hereditary MTC (MEN 2A and MEN
    2B, and familial non-MEN MTC)
hereditary nonpolyposis colorectal
    cancer (HNPCC)
hereditary pancreatitis
hereditary tyrosinemia
heredofamilial disease
Herget rectal biopsy forceps
Hering canal
Hering duct
Hermansky-Pudlak syndrome
HERMES surgery monitoring unit
Hermesh-3 polypropylene mesh
hermetic external shunt
Hermitage Hospital Products
Hernandez-Ros bone staple
hernia (pl. hernias, herniae)
    abdominal wall
    acquired
    axial hiatal
    Barth
    Béclard
    bilateral
    bilateral incarcerated scrotal
    bilateral inguinal
    bilocular femoral
    Bochdalek
    cecal
    Cheatle-Henry
    Cloquet
    combined hernia
    complete
    concealed

hernia *(cont.)*
    concentric hiatal
    congenital
    contralateral
    Cooper
    crural
    diaphragmatic
    direct inguinal
    double
    double-loop
    dry
    duodenal jejunal
    easily reducible
    epigastric
    esophageal
    extrasaccular
    fascial
    fat
    fatty
    femoral
    funicular inguinal
    gangrenous
    gastroesophageal
    gluteal
    groin
    Grynfeltt
    Hesselbach
    Hey
    hiatal
    Holthouse
    iliacosubfascial
    incarcerated
    incisional
    incomplete
    indirect inguinal
    infantile
    inguinal
    inguinal with scrotal extension
    inguinocrural
    inguinofemoral
    inguinolabial
    inguinoscrotal
    inguinosuperficial
    internal

hernia *(cont.)*
    intersigmoid
    interstitial
    intestinal
    intra-abdominal
    intraepiploic
    intrailiac
    intraparietal
    intrapelvic
    irreducible
    ischiatic
    ischiorectal
    Krönlein (Kroenlein)
    Larrey
    Laugier
    Lesgaft
    levator
    Littré
    lumbar
    Malgaigne
    Maydl
    mesenteric
    mixed hiatal
    Morgagni
    nontraumatic
    oblique
    obturator
    obturator hernia
    pannicular
    pantaloon
    paracolostomy
    paraesophageal
    paraesophageal hiatal
    paraesophageal hiatus
    parahiatal
    paraileostomal
    paraperitoneal
    parasaccular
    parasternal
    parastomal
    paraumbilical
    parietal
    pediatric
    perineal

hernia *(cont.)*
   peritoneal
   Petit
   postoperative
   postoperative paraesophageal hiatus
   properitoneal inguinal
   pudendal
   recurrent
   recurring
   reducible
   retrograde
   retroperitoneal
   retropubic
   retrosternal
   Richter
   Rieux
   Rokitansky
   rolling hiatal
   sciatic
   scrotal
   sliding esophageal
   sliding hiatal
   slipped
   spigelian
   spontaneous lateral ventral
   spontaneous ventrolateral
   stoma
   strangulated
   strangulated paraesophageal
   strangulation
   transthoracic diaphragmatic
   traumatic
   Treitz
   trocar
   type I hiatal
   type II hiatal
   umbilical
   unilateral
   uterine broad ligament
   Velpeau
   ventral
   ventrolateral
   vesical
   "W"

hernia defect
hernia dissector
hernia en bissac
hernia knife
hernial lipoma
hernial orifice
hernial sac
Herniamesh surgical mesh graft
hernia pouch
hernia repair
hernia ring forceps
hernia rupture
hernia sac does not traverse the internal
   ring
hernia spoon
herniated preperitoneal fat
herniation of bowel
herniation, physiological gut-loop
hernioplasty (also see *herniorrhaphy;*
   operation)
   double-buttress laparoscopic
   LAP-TAPP (laparoscopic trans-
     abdominal preperitoneal)
   laparoscopic
   mesh plug
   modified Shouldice
   modified TAPP
   open mesh-plug
   preperitoneal
   TAPP (transabdominal preperito-
     neal) laparoscopic
   tension-free
   TEP (totally extraperitoneal) laparo-
     scopic
   totally (or total) extraperitoneal
     laparoscopic
   transabdominal preperitoneal
     laparoscopic
herniorrhaphy (see also *hernioplasty;*
   operation)
   Bassini inguinal
   elective
   emergent
   Halsted-Bassini

herniorrhaphy *(cont.)*
   Halsted inguinal
   Hill-type hiatus
   Lichtenstein
   Macewen
   Madden incisional
   McVay
   open
   pants-over-vest
   Ponka
   Shouldice inguinal
   umbilical
   ventral
   vest-over-pants
Herp-Check
herpes mucositis
herpes simplex virus (HSV)
herpes type 5 virus (cytomegalovirus)
herpes ulcer
herpesvirus
herpes whitlow infection
herpes zoster virus (HZV)
herpetic esophagitis
herpetic hepatitis
herpetic vesicle
Herplex Liquifilm (idoxuridine)
Herrick kidney pedicle clamp
Hers disease
Herter-Gee disease
Herter-Heubner disease
Hertra-2 polypropylene mesh
HER-2/neu gene
Hertzler rib retractor
Herzberg test
Herzyme
Hespan (hetastarch) plasma volume
   expander
Hesselbach hernia
Hesselbach ligament
Hesselbach triangle
Hessel-Nystrom pin
Hessert triangle
hetastarch plasma volume expander
heterogeneous (heterogenous) graft

heterogeneous parenchyma
heterograft
   arterial
   bone
   bovine
   porcine
   stentless
heteroplasmy
heterotopia, gastric
heterotopic pancreas
heterotopic pancreatic tissue
heterotopic tissue
heterotopic transplantation
Hetrazan (diethylcarbamazine citrate)
HEV (hepatitis E virus)
Hewlett-Packard ultrasound system
Hewson cruciate guide
Hewson drill guide
Hexabrix (ioxaglate meglumine;
   ioxaglate sodium)
hexafluoropropylene-VDF suture
hexocyclium
Hextend blood substitute
Hextend plasma volume expander
Heyer-Schulte neurosurgical shunt
Heyer-Schulte Pour-Safe bag
Heyer-Schulte tissue expander
Heyer-Schulte wound drain
Hey hernia
Hey-Groves-Kirk bone graft
Heywood-Smith hemorrhoidal forceps
HF infrared laser
"H. flu" (slang for *Haemophilus
   influenzae*)
Hgb (hemoglobin)
HGD (high-grade dysplasia)
HGH (human growth hormone)
HGV (hepatitis G virus)
HHT (hereditary hemorrhagic
   telangiectasia)
HHV-8 (human herpesvirus-8)
hiatal hernia
hiatal stenosis
hiatus
   aortic

hiatus *(cont.)*
  diaphragmatic
  esophageal
  fallopian
  semilunar
  sternocostal
hiatus hernia
Hibbs blade
Hibbs bone-cutting forceps
Hibbs chisel
Hibbs chisel elevator
Hibbs mallet
Hibbs retractor
Hibbs spinal fusion gouge
Hibbs-Spratt curette
Hibiclens (chlorhexidine gluconate;
  alcohol)
HIB polysaccharide vaccine
Hib (*Haemophilus influenzae* type b)
  vaccine
hiccup (pl. hiccups)
hiccuping
Hickman catheter
Hicks lugged plate
HIC wire guide
HIDA (hepato-iminodiacetic acid)
HIDA Kinevac
HIDA/PRIDA scan
HIDA scan
HIDA sincalide
hidradenitis suppurativa
Hieshima coaxial catheter
HIFU (high-intensity focused
  ultrasound)
Higgins technique for ureterointestinal
  anastomosis
high-bulk, low-fat diet
high-calcium bath dialysis
high-carbohydrate diet
High Definition Imaging (HDI) 3000
  ultrasound system
high-density lipoprotein (HDL)
high-dose dexamethasone suppression
  test

high-energy gunshot wound
high-energy laser
high failure rate
high fever, shock, and death
high-fiber diet
high-flow cannula
high-flow electronic insufflator
high-frequency cutting loop
high-frequency miniprobe
high-frequency probe
high-grade angioinvasive follicular
  carcinoma
high-grade dysplasia (HGD)
high-grade fever
high-grade lesion
high-grade malignancy
high-grade obstruction
high-grade obstructive lesion
high imperforate anus
high index of suspicion
high-intensity focused ultrasound
  (HIFU)
high intracellular concentration
high ligation
high ligation of hernia sac
high lipase
highly active antiretroviral therapy
  (HAART)
highly selective vagotomy
highly vascular tumor
Highmore abscess
high-output fistula
high-pitched bowel sounds
high-protein diet
high-pressure catheter
high-pressure shunt
high-pressure zone
high recurrence rate
high-residue diet
high-resistance fundoplication
high-resolution computed tomography
high-resolution ultrasound
high-resolution video monitor
high-riding ballotable prostate

high-riding prostate
high-risk population
high-roughage diet
high small bowel obstruction
high-speed twist drill
high spinal anesthesia
high sphincter pressure
high subtotal gastrectomy
high torque dermabrader
high-velocity gunshot wound
high-volume/low-pressure cuff
high volume reflux
hilar involvement
hilar lesion
hilar obstruction
hilar plate
hilar stricture
hila of kidney
Hildebrandt uterine hemostatic forceps
Hill antireflux operation
Hill cluster harvest technique
Hill-Ferguson rectal retractor
Hill fundoplasty
Hill gastropexy
Hill gastropexy fundoplication
Hill hiatus hernia repair
Hill median arcuate repair
Hill operation
Hill posterior gastropexy
Hill procedure
Hill rectal retractor
Hill repair for esophageal reflux
Hill-Sachs lesion
Hi-Lo Evac endotracheal tube
Hi-Lo Jet tracheal tube
Hi-Lo tracheal tube
hilum (pl. hila)
   hepatic
   kidney
   lung
   pulmonary
   renal
   splenic
hilus, kidney

Himmelstein sternal retractor
Hinchey diverticulitis grading system
Hinderer cartilage forceps
hindgut (distal colon and rectum)
hindgut dysfunction
hinge rod
Hinkle-James rectal speculum
hip fracture compaction drill
hip pin
Hippocrates bandage
Hippuran
HIPS (heparin infusion prior to
   stenting)
hip spica cast
hip-to-ankle view
Hirsch hypophyseal punch
Hirsch hypophysis punch forceps
Hirschman anoscope
Hirschman pile clamp
Hirschman proctoscope
Hirschman rectal speculum
Hirschsprung-associated enterocolitis
   (HAEC)
Hirschsprung disease
Hirschsprung enterocolitis
hirsutism
Hirulog (bivalirudin)
His, angle of
Histalog stimulation test
histamine blocker
histamine-resistant achlorhydria
histamine test
histamine-2 (H_2) receptor agonist
histamine-2 (H_2) receptor antagonist
Histerone 100 (testosterone)
Histoacryl Blue (HAB) tissue adhesive
Histoacryl glue (cyanoacrylate) tissue
   adhesive
Histoacryl glue adhesive
histologic activity index (HAI)
histologic diagnosis
histologic grading
histologic involvement of axillary
   lymph node

histologic lesion
histologic type
histology
histopathological diagnosis
histopathologic examination
histopathologic preparation
histopathology
Histoplasma capsulatum polysaccharide
  antigen (HPA)
history of radiation therapy to the neck
HIT (heparin-induced thrombo-
  cytopenia
Hitachi Model 737 multichannel
  analyzer
Hitachi 2.0 diagnostic ultrasound
  system
HI VAC tubing
Hi-Vegi-Lip (pancreatase; lipase;
  protease; amylase)
HLA (human lymphocyte antigen)
HLA crossmatch
HLA haplotype
HME Intertech
HM4 lithotriptor
HMTV (human mammary tumor virus)
HNB angiographic catheter
HNF-1 alpha (hepatocyte nuclear
  factor-1 alpha)
HNKC (hyperosmolar nonketotic coma)
HNPCC (hereditary nonpolyposis
  colorectal carcinoma)
H_2O absorption
Hoaglund bone graft
hoarseness
hoarse voice
Hobbs balloon dilator
Hobb view
hobnail cirrhosis
hobnailed appearance of liver surface
hobnail liver
hockey-stick appearance of catheter tip
hockey-stick incision
Hodge intestinal decompression tube
Hodgkin disease

Hodgkin lymphoma
hoe, Joe (retractor)
Hoen angular forceps
Hoen clamp
Hoen gouge
Hoen hemilaminectomy retractor
Hoen intervertebral disk rongeur
Hoen lamina gouge
Hoen laminectomy rongeur
Hoen nerve hook
Hoen periosteal elevator
Hoen scalp hemostatic forceps
Hoen scalp retractor
Hoen skull plate
Hoen ventricular needle
Hoffmann pin guide
Hofmeister anastomosis
Hofmeister gastroenterostomy
Hofmeister technique
Hohmann bone retractor
Hohn central venous catheter
Hoke osteotome
Holihesive Skin Barrier (for ostomy
  skin)
Holinger esophagoscope
Holinger open-end aspirating tube
Hollander test
Hollister Convex Insert
Hollister First Choice pouch
Hollister gastrostomy tube
Hollister Guardian F Skin Barrier
Hollister Holligard pouch
Hollister Karaya 5 ostomy pouch
Hollister Karaya Seal pouch
Hollister Premium paste
Hollister Premium pouch
hollow chisel
hollow mill reamer
hollow needle
hollow viscus
holmium (Ho) laser
holmium laser resection of the prostate
  (HoLRP)
holmium:YAG (yttrium-argon-garnet)
  laser

HoLRP (holmium laser resection of the
   prostate)
Holscher knee retractor
Holscher nerve root retractor
Holt nail
Holt nail plate
Holter tube
Holter valve
Holthouse hernia
Holzheimer retractor
Homans sign
home parenteral nutrition (HPN)
Home Access Hepatitis C Check kit
homeostasis, glucose
HomMed Sentry/Observer monitor
homogeneous graft
homogeneous material
homologous graft
homosexual rectal trauma
homovanillic acid (HVA)
homozygotes
honeycombed appearance
honeycomb lung
honeycomb mucosa
honeycomb pattern
hood forceps
Hood stoma stent
hook
   Acufex nerve
   Adson
   Adson dissecting
   Adson dural
   Adson nerve
   André
   APRL (Army Prosthetics Research
      Laboratory)
   Austin Moore
   Barr
   Barr crypt
   Barr fistula
   Barsky skin
   bayonet-shaped
   bifid
   Blair palate

hook *(cont.)*
   blunt
   blunt nerve
   Bobechko
   bone
   Boyes-Goodfellow
   Braun
   button
   buttressed
   Cairns-Oliver
   Carroll skin
   caudal
   cautery
   C-D (Cotrel-Dubousset)
   clawed pedicle
   Cloward cautery
   Cloward dural
   compression
   cordotomy
   corkscrew dural
   Cotrel-Dubousset (C-D)
   Crile
   Crile nerve
   crypt
   Culler
   Cushing angular
   Cushing dural
   Cushing gasserian ganglion
   Cushing nerve
   Dandy nerve
   DePuy nerve
   dissecting
   distraction
   double
   Drummond
   DTT (dynamic transverse traction)
   dura
   dural
   Edwards
   Edwards-Levine
   Effler-Groves
   Emmett fistula
   Emmett tenaculum
   Fisch dural

hook *(cont.)*
- Fisch dural
- Fisch micro
- fishhook
- fistula
- Frazier dural
- Frazier nerve
- Freer skin
- ganglion
- garment
- Gillies bone
- Gillies-Dingman
- Gillies skin
- Godina double
- Graefe dissecting
- Graefe skin
- Graham muscle
- Graham nerve
- Green muscle
- Guthrie fixation
- Gynex angle
- Harrington
- Hoen nerve
- House crura
- House foot plate
- House oval window
- House strut
- Isola
- Iterson trachea
- Jackson trachea
- Jameson muscle
- Jannetta
- jig
- Jordan
- Joseph skin
- Keene compression
- Kennerdell-Maroon
- Kilner skin
- Kirby muscle
- Kleinert-Kutz skin
- Knodt
- Kocher
- Krayenbuehl (Krayenbühl) vessel
- Küntscher nail extracting

hook *(cont.)*
- Lahey Clinic dural
- Lahey Clinic nerve
- Lambotte bone
- laminar
- laser
- Leatherman
- Love nerve root
- Lucae nerve
- Malis nerve
- malleable
- Marino transsphenoidal
- Martin rectal
- meniscus
- micro
- micro dural
- micro nerve
- Micro-One
- Miltex tissue twist
- Moe spinal
- Moe square-ended
- Moss
- muscle
- Mya
- nail-extracting
- Neivert polyp
- nerve
- O'Brien rib
- pedicle
- Pratt
- Pratt crypt
- Pratt rectal
- prosthetic
- Rhoton
- rib
- right-angle
- Rogozinski
- Rosser crypt
- Sachs dural
- Saunders-Paparella stapes
- Scoville nerve
- Selby II
- Selverstone cordotomy
- Shambaugh fistula

hook *(cont.)*
   Shambaugh microscopic
   sharp
   shoe of the
   side-opening
   skin
   sliding barrel
   Smillie
   Smithwick button
   Smithwick nerve
   Smithwick sympathectomy
   Speare dural
   spring
   Starion thermal cautery
   Stewart crypt
   straight dural
   Strully dural
   suture
   sympathectomy
   Take-Apart nerve
   tendon
   T-handled
   Toennis dural
   tracheal
   traction
   transsphenoidal
   transverse
   transverse process
   Trautman Locktite prosthetic
   TSRH (Texas Scottish Rite Hospital)
   twist
   Tyrell
   Valleylab electrocautery inter-
      changeable
   valve
   vessel
   Volkmann bone
   Weary nerve
   Yankauer
   Yasargil spring
   Zielke
   Zimmer caudal
   Zuelzer
hook clamp

hooked intramedullary nail
hooked medullary nail
hook electrocautery
hook-end intramedullary pin
hook knife
hook-lying position
hook pin
hook scissors, single-action
hook wire localization, CT-directed
hookworm
Hopkins aortic forceps
Hopkins clamp
Hopkins lens system
Hopkins plaster knife
Hopkins rigid glass lens endoscope
Hopkins rod-lens system for rigid
   choledochoscope
Hopkins II forward oblique telescope
Hopkins II telescope
Hopmann papilloma
Hopmann polyp
Horizon stent (temporary/urinary)
Horizons C-13 urea breath test for
   H. pylori
horizontal gastroplasty
horizontal incision
horizontal mattress suture
horizontal position
horizontal retractor
horizontal suture
horizontal transmission
hormonally active
hormonal therapy
hormone
   counter-regulatory
   endocrine pancreas
   endogenous parathyroid
   exogenous thyroid
   free
   gastrointestinal
   GI inhibitory
   HGH (human growth)
   human growth (HGH)
   inhibiting
   long-acting thyroid-stimulating
      (LATS)

hormone *(cont.)*
   parathyroid (parathormone)
   recombinant human thyroid-
     stimulating
   thyroglobulin thyroid
   thyroid (TH)
   thyrotrophic
   thyrotropin-releasing (TRH)
   TSH (thyroid-stimulating)
hormone-dependent
hormone-induced hypopituitarism
hormone-induced pancreatitis
hormone receptor site
hormone-refractory disease
hormone-sensitive breast cancer
Horn endo-otoprobe laser
Horn sign
horseshoe abscess
horseshoe fistula
horseshoe kidney
horseshoe-shaped incision
Horsley anastomosis
Horsley bone-cutting forceps
Horsley bone rongeur
Horsley gastrectomy
Horsley-Stille bone-cutting forceps
Horsley-Stille rib shears
Horsley suture
hose-pipe appearance of terminal ileum
Hosemann forceps
host cell membrane
host constituent
host defense mechanism
host immune mechanism
host immune responsiveness
hot appendix
hot biopsy
hot biopsy forceps
hot defect
hot flexible forceps
hot knife
hot laser
hot nodule
Hot Sampler disposable hot biopsy
   forceps

hot-shot PCR (polymerase chain
   reaction) test
hot spot
Hotsy Cautery
Houget maneuver
Hough ("huff") hoe
Hounsfield unit
hourglass constriction of gallbladder
hourglass contraction of the stomach
hourglass deformity
hourglass gallbladder
hourglass pattern
hourglass-shaped lesion
hourglass stomach
House-Barbara shattering needle
House crura hook
House cup forceps
House endaural elevator
House excavator
House-Fisch dural retractor
House foot plate hook
House knife
House needle
House oval window hook
Housepan clip-applying forceps
House-Paparella stapes curette
House-Radpour suction-irrigator
House-Rosen needle
House separator
House stapes curette
House stapes elevator
House stapes speculum
House strut hook
House suction-irrigation tube
Houston, valve of
Howard Kelly artery forceps
Howarth dissector
Howel-Evans syndrome
Howell coronary scissors
Howell-Jolly body
Howell tibial guide
Howmedica Microfixation cranial plate
Howmedica Microfixation System
   forceps

Howmedica Microfixation System pliers
Howmedica Universal compression
   screw
Howmedica Vitallium staple
Howship-Romberg sign
Ho:YAG (holmium:yttrium-argon-
   garnet) laser
Ho:YAG LTK (holmium: YAG laser
   thermal keratoplasty), noncontact
HPAG (*Helicobacter pylori*-associated
   gastritis)
HPC guidewire
hpf (high-power field)
HPI (hepatic perfusion index)
HPN (home parenteral nutrition)
HR (heart rate)
H$_2$ receptor agonist
H$_2$ receptor antagonist
H$_2$ receptor-blocker
H$_2$ receptor-blocking drug
HRN (Hepatitis Resource Network)
HRQOL (health-related qualify of life)
HRS (hepatorenal syndrome)
HRT (hormone replacement therapy)
   patch
H-shaped capsular incision
H-shaped configuration
H-shaped graft
H-shaped ileal pouch
H-shaped microplate
H-shaped plate
HSP (heat shock protein) antigen
H-TRON plus V100/V40 insulin
   infusion pump
H-type fistula
Hubbard plate
hubbed needle
Huber needle
Huckstep nail
Hudson brace drill
Hudson cranial drill
Hudson cranial rongeur
Hudson forceps
Huebner-Herter disease

Hueter bandage
Hufnagel clamp
huge stools
Hughston view
huHMFG1
Huibregtse-Katon papillotome
Hulka clip applicator
Hulka tenaculum forceps
Humalog insulin
Humalog Mix 75/25
Humalog Pen (insulin delivery device)
human antichimeric antibody (HACA)
human cell transplantation
human chorionic gonadotropin
human defensin 5 (HD-5)
human growth hormone (HGH)
human hemoglobin cross-linked with
   glutaral
human herpesvirus 1 (HHV-1)
human herpesvirus 2 (HHV-2)
human herpesvirus 3 (HHV-3)
human herpesvirus 4 (HHV-4)
human herpesvirus 5 (HHV-5)
human herpesvirus 6 (HHV-6)
human herpesvirus 7 (HHV-7)
human immunodeficiency virus (HIV)
human insulin
human islet allograft
human islets
human lymphocyte antigen (HLA)
human mammary tumor virus (HMTV)
human meniscal allograft
human papillomavirus (HPV) infection
human T-cell leukemia virus
human T-cell lymphoma virus (HTLV I
   and II)
human T-cell lymphotropic virus type I
   (HTLV-I)
Humatrix Microclysmic gel
Humatrope (somatropin)
Humatro-Pen (growth hormone delivery
   device)
humeral head retractor
humeral mechanism

humeral rod
Humicade
humidifier lung
Hummingbird wand
humoral host defense mechanism
humpback Weitlaner retractor
hump, buffalo
Humphries clamp
Humulin L (human insulin zinc
 [rDNA])
Humulin R (human insulin [recombi-
 nant])
Humulin R pen (insulin delivery device)
Humulin 30/70 (insulin; isophane
 insulin)
Humulin 50/50 (isophane human
 insulin [rDNA]; human insulin
 [rDNA])
Humulin 70/30 (isophane human
 insulin [rDNA]; human insulin
 [rDNA])
Humulin-U (extended insulin zinc)
Humulin U Ultralente (extended insulin
 human zinc [rDNA])
hum, venous
hunger pain
Hunner ulcer
Hunstad infiltration handle
Hunstad punch
Hunter forceps
Hunter-Sessions balloon
Hunter Silastic rod
Hunter splinter forceps
Hunter-style double-action bowel
 grasper
Hunter tendon rod
Huntington bone graft
Huntington disease
Hunt-Lawrence pouch
Hunt-Reich trocar
Hunt tumor forceps
Hunt-Yasargil pituitary forceps
Huppert test
Hupp trachea retractor

Hurd bone-cutting forceps
Hurd tonsil dissector and pillar retractor
Hurst bullet-tip dilator
Hurst mercury bougie
Hurst-Tucker pneumatic dilator
Hürthle (Huerthle)
Hürthle cell carcinoma
Hürthle cell neoplasm
Hürthle cell tumor
Hurwitz dialysis catheter
Hurwitz esophageal clamp
Hurwitz thoracic trocar
HUS (hemolytic uremic syndrome)
Huschke ligament
Husk bone rongeur
Hutchinson freckle
Hutchinson-Weber-Peutz syndrome
Hutinel disease
HVA (homovanillic acid)
HVI-DHP (hepatic venous isolation by
 direct hemoperfusion)
HVOO (hepatic venous outflow
 obstruction)
HVS (herpesvirus simplex)
hyalin
 alcoholic
 Mallory
hyaline necrosis
hyaluronidase
Hybrid Capture CMV DNA test
Hybrid Capture cytomegalovirus DNA
 test
Hybrid Capture HPV DNA test
hybrid sphincterotome
Hybritech Tandem PSA ratio (free PSA/
 total PSA) (PSA, prostate-specific
 antigen)
Hycamtin (topotecan hydrochloride)
hyCURE collagen hemostatic wound
 dressing
hyCURE G hydrogel dressing
hyCURE protein powder wound-filler
 dressing
hydatid cyst

hydatid cyst disease
hydatidiform mole (molar pregnancy)
hydatid liver cyst
hydatid, Morgagni
hydatid polyp
hydatid sand
Hyde shunt
hydragogue
HydraGran absorbent dressing
hydralazine
Hydrapak
Hydrasorb foam wound dressing
Hydrate (dimenhydrinate)
hydrated
hydration
hydration status
hydrazine sulfate
hydremic ascites
Hydrocel bone substitute
hydrocelectomy
hydrocele of the cord
hydrocele, postoperative
hydrocele trocar
hydrochloretic drug
hydrochloric acid test
hydrochloride (HCl)
hydrocholeretic
Hydrocil Instant (psyllium hydrophilic
    mucilloid)
Hydrocol (hydrocolloid dressing)
Hydrocollator heating unit
hydrocolloid dressing
hydrocortisone
hydrocortisone acetate
hydrocortisone enema
hydrocortisone foam
Hydrofiber dressing
hydrogel dressing
hydrogel sheet
hydrogen breath test
hydrogen ion
hydrogen peroxide enema
Hydrolyser microcatheter
Hydromer Aquatrix II

Hydromer coated bipolar coagulation
    probe
Hydron burn bandage
hydrophilic guidewire
    J-tipped
    straight
hydrophilic powder dressing
hydrophilic semipermeable absorbent
    polyurethane foam dressing
hydrops of gallbladder
hydrostatic balloon
hydrostatic balloon catheter
hydrostatic decompression
HydroSurg laparoscopic irrigator
Hydro-Temp probe
hydrothorax
    chylous
    hepatic
hydroxyapatite adhesive
hydroxyapatite-coated pin
hydroxyapatitite graft
hydroxylation
hydroxymethylacyfulvene (HMAF)
hydroxyurea tablet
HyFil hydrogel dressing
Hyfrecator 2000
Hyfrecator pencil sheath
Hyfre-Fav
hygroscopic condensor
Hylaform (hylan polymer) viscoelastic
    gel
Hylagel-Nuro viscoelastic gel
Hylasine viscoelastic gel
Hylin rasp
hyoid bone
hyoscyamine sulfate
Hyosophen (atropine sulfate; scopol-
    amine hydrobromide; hyoscyamine
    hydrobromide; phenobarbital)
Hypafix dressing
Hypafix nonwoven tape
Hypaque contrast medium
Hypaque-Cysto contrast medium
Hypaque Meglumine (diatrozoate
    meglumine iodine)

Hypaque Sodium (diatrozate
sodium iodine)
Hypaque-76 (diatrozate meglumine;
diatrozate sodium)
Hypaque swallow
hyperacidity
gastric
gastrointestinal
hyperactive bone marrow
hyperactive bowel sounds
hyperactive sphincter
hyperacute rejection (HAR)
hyperacute rejection of porcine
xenograft
hyperadrenocorticalism
hyperal (hyperalimentation)
hyperaldosteronism
hyperalimentation
central
intravenous (I.V., IV)
parenteral
peripheral
hyperamylasemia
hyperbaric anesthesia
hyperbaric spinal anesthesia
hyperbilirubinemia
conjugated
idiopathic unconjugated
neonatal
unconjugated (UCB)
hypercalcemia, familial hypocalciuric
hypercalcemia with nephrocalcinosis
and indicanuria
hypercalcitoninemia
hypercalciuric
hypercaloric diet
hypercapnia
hypercatabolic protein-losing
enteropathy
hypercellular gland
hypercellularity
hyperchloremia
hyperchloremic acidosis
hyperchlorhydria

hypercholesterolemia
hypercortisolism
hyperdistention of abdomen
hyperemesis gravidarum
hyperemia
hyperemic mucosa
hyperestrogenism
hyperfunction
adrenal cortex
medulloadrenal
pituitary
thyroid
hyperfunction of adrenal medulla
hyperfunctioning adenoma
hyperfunctioning spleen
hypergastrinemia with acid
hypersecretion
Hypergel hydrogel dressing
hyperglobulinemic hepatitis
hyperglobulinemic purpura
hyperglycemia
diabetic
postpancreatectomy
symptomatic
Hyper-Had camera
HyperHep (hepatitis B immune
globulin)
hyperinsulinar obesity
hyperinsulinemia
hyperinsulinemic-euglycemic glucose
clamp
hyperinsulinism
ectopic
functional
iatrogenic
hyperinterrenal obesity
Hyperion LTK laser
hyperkalemia
hyperkeratosis, esophageal
hyperkinetic circulatory state
hyperlipidemia
hyperlipoproteinemia
hyperlucent lung
hypermagnesemia

hypermetabolic state
hypermetabolism
hypermobile kidney
hypermotility of bowel
hypernatremia
hypernephroid carcinoma
hyperosmolar coma
hyperosmolarity
hyperosmolar nonketotic coma (HNKC)
hyperosmotic feeding
hyperoxaluria, enteric
hyperparathyroidism
  ectopic
  familial
  primary
  secondary
  tertiary
hyperparathyroid state
hyperpepsinogenemia
hyperperistalsis
hyperphosphatemia
hyperpigmentation of the skin
hyperplasia
  adrenal
  antral G cell
  appendiceal
  basal cell
  benign
  benign prostatic
  Brunner gland
  chief cell
  congenital adrenal
  congenital virilizing adrenal
  crypt
  cystic breast
  ductal
  epithelial
  focal epithelial
  focal nodular (FNH)
  four-gland
  foveolar
  gastric mucosal
  giant lymph node
  giant of gastric mucosa

hyperplasia *(cont.)*
  goblet cell
  islet cell
  lipomatous
  long-standing adenomatous
  lymphoid
  lymphonodular
  nodular lymphoid (NLH)
  nodular regenerative (NRH)
  physiologic
  primary thyroid
  refractory
  squamous
  thyroid
  transmissible murine colonic
  unilateral
  verrucous
hyperplasmic obesity
hyperplastic adenomatous polyp
hyperplastic alveolar mucosa
hyperplastic gastric polyp
hyperplastic gland
hyperplastic goiter
hyperplastic-hypertrophic obesity
hyperplastic lesion
hyperplastic mucinous cystadenoma
hyperplastic mucosal diverticula
    in gallbladder
hyperplastic obesity
hyperplastic polyp
hyperplastic polyposis of the colon
hyperprotidic diet
hyperpyrexia
hyperresonance
hyperresonant abdomen
hyperrugosity
hypersecretion
  acid
  aldosterone
  colonic
  gastric acid
  glucagon
  pituitary
  vasoactive intestinal peptide

hypersecretory gastropathy
hypersensitivity, gastric
hypersplenism
hyper-TBG-nemia (thyroid-binding
    globulin)
hypertension
    adrenal
    benign
    borderline
    essential
    extrahepatic portal venous
    idiopathic portal (IPH)
    labile
    malignant
    noncirrhotic portal
    portal
    presinusoidal intrahepatic portal
    primary
    renal
    renovascular
    splenoportal
    surgically correctable
    systemic venous
hypertensive crisis
hypertensive ischemic ulcer
hypertensive LES (lower esophageal
    sphincter)
hyperthermia catheter
hyperthyroidism
    apathetic
    classic
    Graves disease
    iodine-induced
    masked
    primary
    secondary
    silent thyroiditis
    subacute thyroiditis
    thyrotoxicosis factitia
    toxic adenoma
    toxic diffuse
    toxic multinodular goiter
    transient (Jod-Basedow phenomenon)

hypertonic plasma
hypertonic saline
hypertonic state
hypertrophic cirrhosis
hypertrophic gastritis
hypertrophic gastropathy
hypertrophic obesity
hypertrophic papilla
hypertrophic pyloric stenosis
hypertrophied mucosa
hypertrophied muscular layer
hypertrophy (see *hyperplasia*)
hyperuricemia
hyperventilation
hypervitaminosis
hypnosis anesthesia
hypoacidity, gastric
hypoactive bowel sounds
hypoalbuminemia
hypobaric anesthesia
hypobetalipoproteinemia
hypocalcemia, postoperative
hypocalcemic tetany
hypocalciuria
hypochloremia
hypochloremic metabolic acidosis
hypochlorhydria
hypochondriac fossa
hypochondriac region
hypochondriasis
hypochondrium (pl. hypochondria)
hypodermic needle
hypoechoic area (on ultrasound)
hypofibrinogenemia, familial (FHP)
hypofunction, adrenal cortex
hypofunctioning
hypogammaglobulinemia
hypoganglionosis of colon
hypogastric artery ligation
hypogastric fossa
hypogastric region
hypogastric vessel
hypogastrium

hypothyroid obesity
hypotonic duodenography
hypotonic fluid
hypovolemia secondary to acute hemor-
rhage
hypovolemia-induced metabolic acidosis
hypovolemic shock
hypoxemia

hypoxia
Hyrtl sphincter
hysterical anesthesia
hysterical colic
hysterical vomiting
hysteroscope
Hy-Tape latex-free surgical tape

I, i

Iamin (prezatide copper acetate)
Iamin gel wound dressing
Iamin hydrating gel (Blue Goo)
Iamin-IB solution (prezatide copper
  acetate)
I&D (incision and drainage)
I&O, I/O (intake and output)
IAP (International Association of
  Pancreatology)
IAS (intra-abdominal sepsis)
iatrogenic cause
iatrogenic Cushing syndrome
iatrogenic hyperinsulinism
iatrogenic hypopituitarism
iatrogenic hypothyroidism
iatrogenic infection
iatrogenic malabsorption
iatrogenic pituitary disorder
iatrogenic thyroiditis
iatrogenic trauma
IBC (inflammatory breast cancer)
IBD (inflammatory bowel disease)
IBD (irritable bowel disease)
IBS (irritable bowel syndrome)
IBW (ideal body weight)
Icar (carbonyl iron)
iced lactated Ringer solution
iced saline lavage

Ice hair trimming shears
ice water swallow
ICF (intracellular fluid)
ICHOP (intractability, cancer, hemor-
  rhage, obstruction, perforation)
icing liver
icodextrin
ICP (intrahepatic cholestasis of
  pregnancy)
ICP (intracranial pressure) catheter
icteric leptospirosis
icteric phase of hepatitis
icteric sclerae
icteric skin
icterohemorrhagic leptospirosis
icterus
    conjunctival
    scleral
icterus gravidarum
icterus gravis
Idealbind bandage
IDD (intraluminal duodenal
  diverticulum)
IDDM (insulin-dependent diabetes
  mellitus)
ideal body weight (IBW)
identified, suture-ligated, clamped, and
  cut

identify the appendix
identify the inguinal anatomy
idiopathic anal fissures
idiopathic and diabetic gastroparesis
idiopathic autoimmune hemolytic
   anemia
idiopathic bile acid malabsorption
idiopathic chronic erosive gastritis
idiopathic colitis
idiopathic Cushing syndrome
idiopathic gastrointestinal bleeding
idiopathic gastroparesis
idiopathic hypertrophic gastropathy
idiopathic hypoglycemia
idiopathic hypoproteinemia
idiopathic inflammatory bowel disease
idiopathic intestinal pseudo-obstruction
idiopathic megacolon
idiopathic obstruction
idiopathic pancreatitis
idiopathic poor fixation of the right
   colon
idiopathic portal hypertension (IPH)
idiopathic proctocolitis
idiopathic steatorrhea
idiopathic thrombocytopenic purpura
   (ITP)
idiopathic unconjugated hyper-
   bilirubinemia
idoxifene
IDST (intraductal secretin test)
IEA (inferior epigastric artery) graft
IECRT (intraoperative endoscopic
   Congo red test)
I-Flow nerve block infusion kit
IFN-alpha 2 gene
IgA (immunoglobulin A)
   mesangial
   polymeric
IgA antigen complex
IgA deficiency
IgD (immunoglobulin D)
IgE (immunoglobulin E)
IgE-mediated immune reaction (type 1)

IgE-mediated injury
IgF-1 (insulin-like growth factor 1)
IgG (immunoglobulin G)
IgG-2A monoclonal antibody
Iglesias fiberoptic resectoscope
IgM anti-HAV antibody
IgM anti-HB$_c$ antibody
IgM antibody
IgM (immunoglobulin M)
Iguana guidewire
IHA (intrahepatic atresia)
IHOP (intractability, hemorrhage,
   obstruction, perforation)
ILA surgical stapler
ILC (interstitial laser coagulation)
ileal conduit
ileal crypt
ileal inflow tract
ileal J pouch
ileal lesion
ileal neobladder
ileal pouch anal anastomosis (IPAA)
   H-shaped
   J-shaped
   S-shaped
   W-shaped
ileal primary tumor
ileal pull-through procedure
ileal resection
ileal reservoir
ileal secretion
ileal S pouch
ileal stasis
ileal varices
ileal villous atrophy in the absence
   of jejunal villous atrophy
ileal W pouch
ileectomy
ileitis
   allergic
   backwash
   Crohn
   dietetic
   distal

ileitis *(cont.)*
  granulomatous
  infectious
  obstructive dysfunctional
  prestomal
  regional
  segmental
  terminal
ileoanal anastomosis
ileoanal endorectal pull-through
ileoanal pouch
ileoanal pull-through procedure
ileoanal reservoir
ileoascending colostomy
ileocecal edema
ileocecal fat pad
ileocecal fold
ileocecal fossa
ileocecal junction
ileocecal orifice
ileocecal pouch
ileocecal recess
ileocecal valve
  competent
  incompetent
ileocecitis, infectious bacterial
ileococcygeus muscle
ileocolectomy
ileocolic arcade
ileocolic artery
ileocolic cecal artery
ileocolic disease
ileocolic fold
ileocolic plexus
ileocolic resection
ileocolic vein
ileocolic vessel
ileocolitis
  Crohn
  regional
  transmural
  ulcerative
ileocolonoscopy

ileocolostomy
  end-loop
  LeDuc-Camey
ileoconduit
ileocystoplasty
  Camey
  LeDuc-Camey
ileogastric reflex
ileogastrostomy
ileogram
ileo-ileal anastomosis
ileoproctostomy
ileorectal anastomosis (IRA)
ileorectal fistula
ileorectostomy
ileoscopy, retrograde
ileoscopy through stoma
ileosigmoid colostomy
ileosigmoid fistula
ileosigmoid knot
ileosotomy closure
ileostomate
ileostomist
ileostomogram
ileostomy
  blowhole
  Brooke
  continent
  Dennis-Brooke
  diversionary
  diverting
  diverting loop
  double-barrel
  end
  end-loop
  Goligher extraperitoneal
  incontinent
  J-loop
  Kock continent
  Kock reservoir
  loop
  loop-end
  permanent loop

ileostomy *(cont.)*
  pouched
  split
  temporary loop
  terminal
ileostomy appliance
ileostomy bag
ileostomy closure
ileostomy diarrhea
ileostomy effluent
ileostomy stoma
ileotransverse colon anastomosis
ileotransverse colostomy
ILE-SORB absorbent gel
ileum
  antimesenteric border of distal
  mesentery of
  terminal
ileus
  adhesive
  adynamic
  adynamic
  decreased
  duodenal
  dynamic
  gallbladder
  gallstone
  mechanical
  meconium
  occlusive
  paralytic
  postoperative
  spastic
ileus subparta
iLEX skin protectant paste dressing
iliac colon
iliac crest biopsy
iliac crest bone aspiration
iliac crest bone graft
iliac lymph node
iliac node
iliac vein
iliac vessel
iliofemoral triangle

iliohypogastric nerve
ilioinguinal ligament
ilioinguinal nerve
ilioinguinal ring
iliopectineal arch
iliopectineal line
iliopsoas ring
iliopsoas sign
iliopsoas test
iliopubic tract
iliotibial band graft
Ilizarov telescoping rod
illicit drug
illness, febrile
Illumen-8 guiding catheter
Illumina PROSeries laparoscopy system
Ilopan-Choline (dexpanthenol; choline
  bitartrate)
Ilozyme
ILS (intraluminal stapler)
ILUS (intraluminal ultrasound) catheter
IM (intramedullary) rod
IMA (inferior mammary artery) graft
IMA (inferior mesenteric artery)
  retractor
IMA (internal mammary artery)
ImageChecker M1000
image-guided pancreatic core biopsy
image-guided surgery
Imagent GI (perflubron)
Imager ac rectal suspension (barium
  sulfate)
imagery, guided
IMAGE TEC video camera system
image, video
imaging (also *image; scan; scanner;*
  ultrasound)
  ACAT (automated computerized
    axial tomography)
  acoustical shadowing
  Acuson Aspen ultrasound system
  AddOn-Bucky
  Airis II open MRI system
  Aloka 650 ultrasound system

imaging *(cont.)*
    Aspen ultrasound system
    Atlas 2.0 diagnostic ultrasound
        system
    ATL UM 9 HDI Colorflow
        ultrasound system
    AU5 Harmonic ultrasound system
    Aurora MR breast imaging system
    AutoSonix system
    B-mode acquisition and targeting
        (BAT)
    barium enema
    barium swallow
    BAT (B-mode acquisition and
        targeting) system
    BI-RADS (Breast Imaging Reporting
        and Data System)
    Bisound AP 3000 Colorflow
        ultrasound system
    breast
    Bruel & Kjaer 3535 ultrasound
        system
    Bucky
    computed tomography laser
        mammography (CTLM)
    Computerized Thermal Imaging
        system
    cross-sectional
    CTLM (computed tomography laser
        mammography)
    diffraction-enhanced
    digital x-ray detector
    Digitizer Director
    DirectRay device
    dual-phase spiral CT scan
    Dynamic PACSPlus
        system
    E.CAM+ coincidence-imaging
    E.CAM dual-head emission imaging
    EBCT (electron-beam computed
        tomography)
    electron-beam computed
        tomography (EBCT)
    endoanal ultrasound

imaging *(cont.)*
    endoscopic optical coherence
        tomography (EOCT)
    endoscopic ultrasonography
    endosonography
    EOCT (endoscopic optical
        coherence tomography)
    EU-M30S endoscopic ultra-
        sonography receiver
    evacuation proctography
    FACT (focused appendix computed
        tomography)
    fluorescence spectroscopy
    FluoroNav virtual fluoroscopy
        system
    focused appendix computed
        tomography (FACT)
    FONAR-360 MRI scanner
    galactogram
    GE RT 3200 ADV II ultrasound
        system
    Given Diagnostic Imaging System
    Gore 1.5-T Torso Array
    graded compression ultrasonography
    helical computed tomography
    Hercules 7000 mobile x-ray unit
    Hewlett-Packard ultrasound system
    High Definition Imaging (HDI)
        3000 ultrasound system
    Hitachi 2.0 diagnostic ultrasound
        system
    iiRAD DR1000C
    ImageChecker M1000
    IMiG-MRI
    intraoperative laparoscopic
        cholangiography
    IsoStent radioisotope stent
    LAST (large-area sensing
        technology) imager
    Longport Digital Scanner (LDS)
    magnetic resonance cholangio-
        pancreatography (MRCP)
    magnetic resonance neurography
        (MRN)

imaging *(cont.)*
  Enhancer (barium sulfate)
  Entrobar (barium sulfate [methyl-
    cellulose diluent])
  Epi-C (barium sulfate)
  FAC (ferric ammonium citrate)
  Feridex (ferumoxides)
  ferric ammonium citrate (FAC)
  FerriSeltz (ferric ammonium citrate
    [FAC])
  ferumoxsil
  Flo-Coat (barium sulfate)
  gadodiamide
  Gadolite oral suspension
  Gastrografin (diatrizoate
    meglumine; diatrizoate sodium)
  GastroMARK (ferumoxsil)
  glucagon
  gold Au-198 (^{198}Au)
  HD 85 (barium sulfate)
  HD 200 Plus (barium sulfate)
  Hexabrix (ioxaglate meglumine;
    ioxaglate sodium)
  Hypaque-Cysto contrast medium
  Hypaque Meglumine 30%; 60%
    (diatrozoate meglumine iodine)
  Hypaque Sodium 25%; 50%
    (diatrozate sodium)
  Hypaque Sodium; Hypaque Sodium
    20% (diatrozate sodium [59.87%
    iodine])
  Hypaque-76 (diatrozate meglumine;
    diatrozate sodium)
  Imagent GI (perflubron)
  Imager ac (barium sulfate)
  ImmuRAID-AFP
  ^{123}I murine MAb to alpha-
    fetoprotein (AFP)
  ^{131}I murine MAb to alpha-
    fetoprotein (AFP)
  ^{131}I 6B-iodomethyl-19-
    norcholesterol
  ^{111}In altumomab pentetate
    (monoclonal antibody)

imaging *(cont.)*
  indocyanine green
  ^{111}In satumomab pendetide
    (monoclonal antibody)
  insulin ^{125}I
  insulin ^{131}I
  Intropaste (barium sulfate)
  iobenzamic acid
  iocetamic acid
  iodipamide meglumine
  iodixanol
  Iodotope (sodium iodide ^{131}I)
  ioglycamic acid
  iohexol
  iopanoic acid
  iothalamate meglumine
  iothalamate sodium
  Iotrex
  ioversal
  ipodate calcium
  ipodate sodium
  Isovue-370 (iopamidol)
  Kinevac (sincalide)
  LeuTech
  Liqui-Coat HD (barium sulfate)
  LumenHance (manganese chloride
    tetrahydrate)
  Magnevist (gadopentetate
    dimeglumine)
  manganese chloride tetrahydrate
  mangofodipir trisodium
  MD-Gastroview (diatrozoate meglu-
    mine; diatrozoate sodium)
  Medebar Plus (barium sulfate)
  Medescan (barium sulfate)
  meglumine diatrizoate
  meglumine iocarmate
  meglumine iothalamate
  meglumine ioxaglate
  methylene blue
  Miraluma (technetium ^{99m}Tc
    sestamibi kit)
  MS-325
  NeoTect disease-specific

imaging *(cont.)*
  nofetumobab
  nonionic contrast media
  Novopaque (barium sulfate)
  OctreoScan 111 (^{111}In pentetreotide)
  Omnipaque (iohexol)
  Omniscan (gadodiamide)
  OncoScint CR/OV ([111]In
    satumomab pendetide)
  OptiMARK (gadoversetamide
    injection)
  Optiray 350 (ioversal)
  Optison
  Oragrafin sodium (ipodate sodium)
  pentagastrin
  Peptavlon (pentagastrin)
  perflenapent
  perflisopent
  perflutren
  Prepcat (barium sulfate)
  Quantison
  ReVele
  sincalide
  Sitzmarks (polyvinyl chloride)
  sodium amidotrizoate
  sodium iothalamate
  sodium ioxaglate
  sodium ipodate
  sodium mitrizoate
  sodium tyropanoate
  Sonazoid ultrasound
  SonoRx (simethicone-coated
    cellulose suspension)
  stannous sulfur colloid
  technetium ^{99m}Tc ethylene dicysteine
    (EC)
  technetium ^{99m}Tc sestamibi
  Telepaque (topanoic acid)
  Teslascan (mangafodipir trisodium)
  Tomocat (barium sulfate)
  Tonopaque (barium sulfate)
  tyropanoate sodium
  Vascoray (iothalamate meglumine;
    iothalamate sodium)

imaging *(cont.)*
  Verluma (nofetumobab)
  Visipaque (iodixanol)
imaging workup
IMAGN 2000 cellular analysis test
Imagyn clip applier
imbibe
imbricated posterior wall closure
imbricating suture
imbrication of diaphragm
IMED infusion device
imidoacetic acid radioactive agent
imiglucerase
immature neutrophils (bands)
immediate decompression
Immergut suction coagulation tube
imminent cardiac collapse
Immix bioabsorbable implant
IMMIX CB implant
immobilize, immobilization
immobilizing bandage
ImmTher (disaccharide tripeptide
    glycerol tripalmitoyl)
ImmTher (disaccharide tripeptide)
Immun-Aid
immune complex
immune deficiency
immune electron microscopy
immune mechanism
immune response
immunity, cell-mediated
immunizing agent
immunoassay, PP-CAP IgA enzyme
immunoblastic lymphoma large cell
immunoblastic sarcoma
immunoblot analysis
ImmunoCard STAT! Rotavirus test
immunocompetency
immunocompromised patient
immunodeficiency, severe combined
    (SCID)
immunoelectrophoresis
immunogenicity
immunoglobulin A (IgA)

immunoglobulin D (IgD)
immunoglobulin E (IgE)
immunoglobulin G (IgG)
immunoglobulin I (IgI)
immunoglobulin M (IgM)
immunohistochemical detection
immunohistochemical staining
immunohistochemistry
immunoinflammatory sequelae
immunologic deficiency disorder
immunologic insulin resistance
immunologically mediated disease
immunomodulation
immunomodulator
immunomodulatory protocol
immunoproliferative small intestinal
    disease (IPSID)
immunoreactive parathyroid hormone
    (iPTH)
immunosuppressant cocktail
immunosuppression, corticosteroid-
    based
immunosuppressive agent
immunosuppressive drug
immunosuppressive protocol
immunosuppressive steroid weaning
ImmuRAID-AFP (technetium ^{99m}Tc
    murine MAb to human alpha-
    fetoprotein)
Immurait (IgG-2A monoclonal
    antibody)
Immodium, Imodium A-D (loperamide)
Impact enteral formula
impacted calculus
impacted feces
impacted gallstone
impacted stool
impaction
    basket
    fecal
    intestinal
    stone
impaction graft
impaction lesion

impactor, Browne pneumatic
impactor rod
impaired cellular defense mechanism
impaired esophageal peristalsis
impaired excretion of conjugated
    bilirubin
impaired fat metabolism
impaired gallbladder contractility
impaired gas exchange
impaired glucose tolerance
impaired nutritional state
impaired regeneration syndrome (IRS)
impaired skin integrity
impaired thymic development
impaired wound healing
impalement injury
    abdominal
    anorectal
    transcorpus
IMP-Capello arm support
impedance, bioelectrical
imperforate anus
impervious drape
implant (also see *breast implant*;
        prosthesis)
    carcinomatous
    Duros drug delivery
    Gore-Tex SAM (subcutaneous
        augmentation material) facial
        implant
    Gore-Tex strips
    Immix bioabsorbable
    IMMIX CB
    iridium-192 wire
    islet cell
    lumbar anterior-root stimulator
        (LARSI)
    Macroplastique bladder
    peritoneal
    Restore orthobiologic soft tissue
    saline
    silicone gel
implant application fork
Implast bone cement adhesive

Import vascular-access port with
  BioGlide
impregnated sponge
Impress instrument tracking
impression
  cardiac, on the liver
  colic
  digastric
  duodenal
  esophageal
  gastric
  liver
  renal
  suprarenal
impromidine
impromidine HCl
improved gas exchange
ImuLyme vaccine
Imuran (azathioprine)
IMV (inferior mesenteric vein)
IMV (intermittent mandatory
  ventilation)
Inactivin
inadequate bowel prep
inadequate cardiac output
inadequate circulating blood volume
inadequate hemostasis of the splenic
  pedicle
inadequate perfusion of organ
Inamed technique
inanition
Inapsine (droperidol)
inborn error in liver bilirubin uptake
  and glucuronyl transferase
inborn error of metabolism
incarcerated hernia
incarcerated omentum
incarcerated sepsis
incarceration of hernia
incarceration of inguinal hernia
incarceration of loop of intestine
Incel (biricodar dicitrate)
incentive spirometry, postoperative
Incert bioabsorbable implantable
  sponge

In Charge diabetes control system
incidence
incidental abdominal radiograph
incidental appendectomy
incised in the direction of its fibers
Incise drape
incised ulcer
incised wound
incision
  abdominal
  Amussat
  anterolateral thoracotomy
  anteromedial
  Battle
  Battle-Jalaguiere-Kammerer
  battledore (racquet-shaped)
  bayonet-type
  Bevan abdominal
  bifrontal
  bikini skin
  bilateral subcostal
  Brunner modified
  Brunner palmar
  Bruser skin (knee)
  capsular
  celiotomy
  cervical
  Charnley
  Cherney
  Chernez
  chevron
  choledochotomy
  Cincinnati
  circumareolar
  circumferential
  circumlinear
  circumscribing
  circumumbilical
  clamshell
  coronal
  cross-tunneling
  cruciate
  C-shaped
  Cubbins

incision *(cont.)*
- Curtin
- curved
- curvilinear
- Deaver
- deltoid-splitting
- diamond-shaped
- dorsal linear
- dorsomedial
- double
- DuVries
- elliptical
- epigastric
- exploratory
- fascial-splitting
- fiber-splitting
- fishmouth
- flank
- frown
- Gaenslen split heel
- gridiron
- groin
- gull-wing
- Heineke-Mikulicz
- Henderson skin
- Henry
- hernia
- hockey-stick
- horizontal
- horseshoe-shaped
- H-shaped capsular
- infraclavicular
- inframammary
- infraumbilical
- inguinal
- intercartilaginous
- intraperitoneal
- inverted-U abdominal
- J-shaped skin
- Kammerer-Battle
- Kehr
- keyhole
- Kocher
- Kocher collar (thyroidectomy)

incision *(cont.)*
- LaRoque herniorrhaphy
- lateral
- lateral utility
- lazy H
- lazy S
- lazy Z
- L-curved
- longitudinal
- low transverse
- L-shaped
- Ludloff
- Mayfield
- Maylard
- McBurney
- medial
- medial parapatellar
- median
- median parapatellar
- midabdominal transverse
- midaxillary line
- midline
- midline abdominal
- minilaparotomy
- muscle-splitting
- Nagamatsu
- oblique
- Ollier
- omega-shaped
- palmar
- paramedial
- paramedian
- parapatellar
- pararectus
- paraumbilical
- Penduloff
- periareolar
- Pfannenstiel
- posterior
- puncture
- racquet-shaped
- recently healed surgical
- rectus sheath
- relaxing

incision *(cont.)*
  relief
  relieving
  Rethi
  right subcostal
  Rockey-Davis
  S
  saber-cut
  scoring
  semilunar
  serpentine
  S-flap
  skin
  skin crease
  smile (or smiling)
  smiling
  spindle-shaped
  split
  S-shaped
  stab
  stab wound
  standard
  standard Kocher
  steri-stripped
  sternal-splitting
  sternotomy
  straight
  subcostal
  subumbilical
  tangential
  thoracoabdominal
  through-and-through
  transverse
  T-shaped
  U-shaped
  vertical
  vertical midline
  volar
  V-shaped
  Wagner skin
  Warren
  Watson-Jones
  web space
  Wilde

incision *(cont.)*
  Willy Meyer mastectomy
  xiphoid to umbilicus
  Y
  Yorke-Mason
  Y-shaped
  Z-plasty
  zigzag
  zigzag finger
incisional biopsy
incisional hernia
incisional scar
incision and drainage (I&D) of abscess
incision extended laterally
incision extended superiorly and
    inferiorly
incision into rectus sheath
incision line
incision made from xiphoid to
    umbilicus
incision of labial frenum (frenotomy)
incisive bone
incisive canal
Incisor arthroscopic blade
incisura angularis of stomach
incisura dextra of Gans
Inclan bone graft
inclusion body
incompetent ileocecal valve
incompetent sphincter
incompetent valve
incomplete colonoscopy
incomplete hernia
incomplete UES (upper esophageal
    sphincter) relaxation
incontinence
  bladder
  bowel
  exercise-induced
  fecal
  ischemic fecal
  rectal
  stool
  stress
  urge

incontinent ileostomy
incontinent of stool
increased abdominal girth
increased alveolar ventilation
increased BUN
increased catecholamines
increased collateral blood flow
increased colonic phasic contractions
increased concentration of liver
   enzymes
increased contractility
increased direct bilirubin
increased end-tide CO_2
increased estrogen
increased gastric acid and pepsin
   production
increased gastric pressure
increased granularity and friability
   of mucosa
increased heart rate
increased intra-abdominal pressure
increased intracranial pressure
increased intraluminal pressure
increased intravascular volume
increased lactic acid
increased LFTs
increased morbidity and mortality
increased PCO_2
increased PEEP
increased portal pressure
increased preload
increased pulmonary compliance
increased renin to angiotensin
increased respiratory rate
increased secretion of PTH
increased serum sodium
increased shunt fraction
increased surface lubricity
increased telomerase activity
increased thyroid hormone synthesis
increased tidal volume
increased turnover of red blood cells
increased vascularity
increased venous capacitance

increased WBCs
increase in angiotensin
increase in metabolic rate
increase in oxygen consumption
incuTemp monitoring device
independence, insulin
independent parallel circuits
Indermil topical tissue adhesive
index (pl. indexes, indices) (see also
   classification)
  biliary saturation
  body mass (BMI)
  Bouchard
  Broder
  Crohn disease activity (CDAI)
  free thyroxine
  free/total PSA (prostate-specific
    antigen) index
  Harvey hospital prognostic
    nutritional index
  hepatic perfusion (HPI)
  nutritional
  obesity
  parietal cell
  PATI (Penetrating Abdominal
    Trauma Index)
  Prognostic Nutritional (PNI)
  saturation (SI)
  spleen
in diameter
Indian childhood cirrhosis
Indiana pouch procedure
Indiana reamer
indicanuria
indices (see *index*)
Indiclor (^{111}In radioimaging agent)
indigestion
indigo carmine dye
indigo carmine stain
Indigo LaserOptic treatment system
indirect bilirubin
indirect hemagglutination antibody test
indirect hemagglutination titer
indirect hepatic vein wedge pressure

infection *(cont.)*
    airborne
    animal bite
    apical
    bacterial
    biliary tract
    Bunyavirus
    Campylobacter
    candidal
    cat-bite
    catheter tunnel
    cat-scratch
    chronic
    CMV (cytomegalovirus)
    colonization
    community-acquired
    cross
    cryptogenic
    cytomegalovirus (CMV)
    disseminated gonococcal
    dog-bite
    droplet
    dust-borne
    EBV (Epstein-Barr virus)
    ECHO (enterocytopathogenic
      human orphan) virus
    endogenous
    Epstein-Barr virus
    exogenous
    Fasciola hepatica
    focal
    fungal
    genital
    germinal
    Giardia
    gram-positive bacterial
    granulomatous
    human ehrlichial, Sennetsu-type
    human papillomavirus (HPV)
    iatrogenic
    latent
    local
    mass
    mixed

infection *(cont.)*
    nosocomial
    ocular
    opportunistic
    pelvic
    postoperative
    preexisting
    primary
    protozoal
    pulmonary
    pyogenic
    recurrent upper respiratory tract
      (RURTI)
    regional spread of
    rickettsial
    Salinem
    scalp
    secondary
    secondary bacterial
    skin
    subclinical
    suppurative
    surgical site
    systemic
    systemic fungal
    terminal
    tick-borne
    TORCH (toxoplasmosis, rubella,
      cytomegalovirus, herpes simplex)
    tunnel
    upper respiratory (URI)
    upper respiratory tract (URTI)
    urinary tract (UTI)
    vector-borne
    Vincent
    viral
    viral respiratory (VRI)
    water-borne
    wound
infection due to gram-positive bacteria
infectious arthritis
infectious avian nephrosis
infectious bacterial ileocecitis
infectious colitis

infectious disease
 communicable
 contagious
 transmissible
infectious eczematous dermatitis
infectious enteritis
infectious esophagitis
infectious etiology
infectious gastroenteritis
infectious granuloma
infectious hepatitis
infectious ileitis
infectious jaundice
infectious jejunitis
infectious mononucleosis (IM)
infectious myocarditis
infectious myositis
infectious pancreatic necrosis virus
infectious pancreatitis
infectious sigmoiditis
infectious splenomegaly
infectious stomatitis
infectious wart virus
infective colitis
infective splenomegaly
Infergen (interferon alfacon-1)
inferior border of liver
inferior central pedicle reduction
 mammoplasty
inferior constrictor muscle
inferior duodenal fold
inferior duodenal recess
inferior epigastric artery
inferior epigastric vessel
inferior esophageal sphincter
inferior hemorrhoidal artery
inferior hemorrhoidal vein
inferior laryngeal nerve
inferior lumbar triangle
inferior mesenteric artery
inferior mesenteric vein
inferior MI (myocardial infarction)
inferior myocardial infarction
inferior pancreaticoduodenal artery

inferior parathyroid gland
inferior pedicle of breast
inferior pedicle technique reduction
 mammoplasty
inferior surface of diaphragm
inferior surface of pancreas
inferior thyroid artery
inferior thyroid vein
inferior transverse rectal fold
inferior vena cava
inferior vena cava obstruction
inferior venacavography
inferolateral surface of prostate
inferomedial
infestation, parasitic
infiltrate (see *infiltration*)
infiltrate lymphoma
infiltrating adenocarcinoma
infiltrating ductal carcinoma of breast
infiltrating lesion
infiltrating lobular carcinoma
infiltration (also *infiltrate*)
 cavitary
 consolidated
 diffuse
 eosinophilic
 foreign body
 glycogen
 interstitial
 leukocytic
 lymphocytic
 mesenteric
 mononuclear
 nodular
 pulmonary
 tumor
infiltration anesthesia
infiltration of nodule
infiltrative carcinoma
infiltrative disorder
Infiniti catheter
Infinity hip system
inflamed appendicitis
inflamed appendix

inflamed gallbladder
inflamed stenosis of the sigmoid colon
inflammation
  acute
  active chronic
  adhesive
  appendiceal
  appendix
  atrophic
  caseous
  catarrhal
  cavitating
  chronic
  chronic jejunal
  circumscribed
  cirrhotic
  colonic
  confluent
  diffuse
  diffuse acute
  diffuse chronic
  erosive
  esophageal
  exudative
  fibrinous
  fibrocaseous
  fibrosing
  gallbladder
  gangrenous
  granulomatous
  hemorrhagic
  hyperplastic
  hypertrophic
  interstitial
  ischemic
  localized
  metastatic
  miliary granulomatous
  mucosal
  multifocal
  necrotic
  necrotizing granulomatous
  obliterative
  pancreatic

inflammation *(cont.)*
  pelvic
  periesophageal
  perirectal
  portal
  proliferative
  pseudomembranous
  psoas
  purulent
  recurrent
  sanguineous
  serofibrinous
  splenic
  subacute
  suppurative
  thyroidal
  transmural
  transudative
  traumatic
  ulcerative
inflammation of pouch of ileoanal
  pull-through
inflammation of thyroid
inflammation spleen
inflammatory bowel disease (IBD)
inflammatory breast cancer (IBC)
inflammatory cancer
inflammatory carcinoma of breast
inflammatory cascade (leading to sepsis
  syndrome)
inflammatory cytokine
inflammatory diarrhea
inflammatory disease of small bowel
inflammatory edema
inflammatory fibroid polyp
inflammatory fibrosis
inflammatory granuloma
inflammatory intra-abdominal process
inflammatory lesion
inflammatory mediator
inflammatory myopathy
inflammatory polyp
inflammatory process
inflammatory response

insufflate the peritoneum
insufflation
  blind needle
  gas
insufflation anesthesia
insufflation gas source
  "E" tank
  "H" tank
insufflation needle
insufflation tank room
insufflator
  carbon dioxide
  high-flow electronic
  Karl Storz N_2O Endoflator
  nitrous oxide
  Storz high-speed
Insuflon indwelling insulin delivery
  system
insular cirrhosis
insulated cautery
insulated coagulation suction
insulated coatings: nylon, Kynar, Teflon
  or ceramic
insulated Foman ball retractor
insulated instrument
insulated outer tube with Luer lock
insulation on flexible, semirigid shafts
insulation-tipped (IT) diathermic knife
insulin
  AC137 analog
  biphasic
  biphasic isophane
  dalanated
  globin zinc
  exogenous
  Humalog
  human
  isophane human
  Humulin
  Humulin L (human insulin zinc
    [rDNA])
  Humulin R (human insulin [recom-
    binant])
  Humulin 30/70

insulin (cont.)
  Humulin 50/50
  Humulin 70/30
  Humulin-U (extended insulin zinc)
  Humulin U Ultralente (extended
    insulin human zinc [rDNA])
  intermediate-acting
  isophane
  Lente Insulin
  long-acting
  neutral
  neutral protamine Hagedorn (NPH)
  Novolin 70/30 PenFill
  Novolin 70/30 Prefilled
  Novolin 85/15 PenFill
  Novolin L
  Novolin N
  Novolin N PenFill
  Novolin N Prefilled
  Novolin R
  Novolin R PenFill
  Novolin R Prefilled
  NovoRapid
  NPH (neutral protamine Hagedorn)
  NPH Iletin II
  NPH-N
  Oralgen oral aerosol
  protamine zinc (PZI)
  rapid-acting
  regular
  Regular Iletin II
  Regular Iletin II U-500
    (concentrated)
  Regular Purified Pork
  Semilente
  short-acting
  Ultralente
  Velosulin BR
  Velosulin BR human buffered
    regular
  Velosulin Human BR
insulin allergy
insulin argine
insulin aspart

intercalary graft
intercapillary glomerulosclerosis
intercartilaginous incision
Interceed surgical adhesion barrier
Interceed TC7
intercellular fluid
Intercept Platelet System
interceptive conditioning
intercondylar drill guide
intercostal anesthesia
intercostal arteries
intercostal nerve block
intercostal space
intercostal veins
intercostal vessels
intercostobrachial nerve
interfascicular nerve graft
interferometry
interferon
   lymphoblastoid
   pegylated
interferon alfacon-1
interferon alfa-n1
interferon alfa-n3
interferon alfa-2a
interferon alfa-2b
interferon alfa-2b and ribavirin
interferon alfa-2b recombinant
interferon-ribavirin therapy for
   hepatitis C
interferon beta (IFN-B)
interferon beta-1a
interferon gamma-1b
interferon monotherapy
interfoveolar ligament
interfragmentary plate
InterGard Knitted collagen-coated graft
InterGard patch
Intergel adhesion prevention solution
interjugular node
interlaminar clamp
interleukin-4 receptor (IL-4R)
interleukin 10 (IL-10)
interlobular artery of kidney

interlobular bile duct
interlocking intramedullary nail
interlocking ligature
interlocking nail
interloop abscess
intermediate gland
intermediate Hi-Lo tracheal tube
intermediate Hi-Lo with Brandt
intermesenteric abscess
intermittent diarrhea
intermittent drainage
intermittent drip feeding
intermittent dysphagia
intermittent malaria
intermittent melena
intermittent open system
intermittent pain
intermittent suture
internal abdominal ring
internal anal sphincter (IAS)
internal biliary drainage
internal clot
internal hemorrhage
internal hemorrhoid
internal hernia
internal inguinal ring
internal mammary artery (IMA)
internal mammary lymph node
internal mammary vein
internal oblique fascia
internal oblique muscle
internal procidentia
internal rectal sphincter
internal ring
internal spermatic fascia
internal sphincterotomy
internal urethral orifice
International Association of
   Pancreatology (IAP)
International Islet Transplant Registry
   (ITR)
International Pancreas Transplant
   Registry
International System of Units (SI)

International Transplant Registry
Intern Line "Boston Style"
Intern Line "Physician Style"
interosseous knife
interparietal fascia
interparietal suture
interpectoral lymph node
Interpore graft
interposed omental fat
interposition bone graft
interposition Dacron graft
interposition graft
interposition of colon between liver and
    diaphragm
interposition saphenous vein graft
interrupted near-far, far-near suture
interrupted pledgeted suture
interrupted suture
intersphincteric abscess
intersphincteric anal fistula
intersphincteric rectal dissection
interspinous line
interstitial catheter
interstitial cells of Cajal
interstitial fluid
interstitial gastritis
interstitial gland
interstitial hemorrhage
interstitial hernia
interstitial laser coagulation (ILC)
interstitial nephritis
interstitial pancreatitis
interstitial pattern
intertrochanteric plate
interureteric fold
interval resection of redundant sigmoid
intervention
    medical
    operative
    surgical
    therapeutic
intervertebral disk forceps
intervertebral disk punch
intervertebral disk rongeur

intestinal allograft
intestinal amebiasis
intestinal anastomosis
intestinal angiodysplasia
intestinal atony
intestinal atresia
intestinal bacteria
intestinal bag
intestinal bypass
intestinal calculus
intestinal candidiasis
intestinal clamp
intestinal cleansing
intestinal colic
intestinal concretion
intestinal contents
intestinal crushing clamp
intestinal decompression
intestinal diverticulum
intestinal dysmotility and stasis
intestinal failure due to short-
    bowel syndrome
intestinal flora
intestinal ganglioneuromatosis
intestinal gland
intestinal glucose transport
intestinal graft radiation
intestinal-grasping forceps
intestinal hemorrhage
intestinal hernia
intestinal impaction
intestinal intussusception
intestinal invagination
intestinal juice
intestinal lipodystrophy
intestinal lipophagic granulomatosis
intestinal loop
intestinal lumen
intestinal lymphangiectasia
intestinal lymphoma
intestinal M cells
intestinal metaplasia
intestinal motility disorder
intestinal mucosa

intestinal muscle contractions
intestinal necrosis
intestinal neuronal dysplasia (IND)
intestinal obstruction
intestinal perforation
intestinal perfusion study
intestinal permeability
intestinal phase of acid secretion
intestinal plication
intestinal polyposis
intestinal polyposis II
intestinal polyposis-cutaneous
   pigmentation syndrome
intestinal prolapse
intestinal pseudo-obstruction
intestinal secretion
intestinal sepsis
intestinal stasis
intestinal stenosis
intestinal strangulation
intestinal stricturoplasty
intestinal torsion
intestinal tract
intestinal transplant
intestinal transplantation (ITx)
intestinal trichomoniasis
intestinal ulcer
intestinal urinary conduit
intestinal villous architecture
intestinal villous atrophy
intestinal web
intestine
   blind
   empty (jejunum)
   iced
   jejunoileal
   large
   mesenteric
   segmented
   small
   straight
intestinointestinal reflex
intestinum crasum
intestinum caecum

intestinum ileum
intestinum jejunum
intestinum rectum
intestinum tenue mesenteriale
in the midaxillary line
intolerance
   gluten
   heat
   lactose
   sucrose
in toto
intoxication, hepatocerebral
intra-abdominal abscess
intra-abdominal adhesion
intra-abdominal bleeding
intra-abdominal fluid collection
intra-abdominal hemorrhage
intra-abdominal hernia
intra-abdominal ileal reservoir
intra-abdominal mass
intra-abdominal pressure
intra-abdominal sepsis (IAS)
intra-abdominal sheer stress
intra-abdominal wall
intra-abdominal wall musculature
intra-alveolar hemorrhage
intra-anal pressure
intra-anal wart
intra-aortic balloon (IAB)
intra-aortic endovascular sonography
intra-arterial bolus injection
intra-arterial chemotherapy catheter
intra-articular shaver
intracanalicular papilloma
Intracath catheter
Intracath needle
intracellular bacteria
intracellular compartment
intracellular fluid (ICF)
intracellular organism
intracellular protein
intracellular space
intracellular water
IntraCoil

intracolonic Kaposi sarcoma
Intracone intramedullary reamer
intracorporeal anastomosis
intracorporeal shock-wave lithotripsy
    (ISWL)
intracranial clamp
intracranial mass lesion
intracranial tumor
intracrural fiber
intractability, cancer, hemorrhage,
    obstruction, perforation (ICHOP)
intractable abscess
intractable diarrhea
intractable leg ulcer
intractable ulcer
intractable ulcerative colitis
intractable vomiting
intracuticular suture
intracystic papilloma
intradeglutitive phase of swallowing
intradermal suture
IntraDose (cisplatin/epinephrine) gel
intraductal carcinoma of breast
intraductal papilloma
intraductal pressure
intraductal secretin test (IDST)
intradural abscess
intraepidermal carcinoma
intraepithelial carcinoma
intraepithelial nonkeratizing carcinoma
intraesophageal acid test
intraesophageal peristaltic pressure
intraesophageal pH test
intraesophageal stent
Intraflex intramedullary pin
intragastric balloon
intragastric bubble
intragastric pH mapping
intragastric pressure
intragraft polymerase chain reaction
    (PCR) assay
intrahaustral contraction ring
intrahepatic abscess
intrahepatically

intrahepatic atresia
intrahepatic AV fistula
intrahepatic bile duct
intrahepatic biliary cystic dilation
intrahepatic biliary duct
intrahepatic cholangiocarcinoma
intrahepatic cholangioenterostomy
intrahepatic cholangiolitis
intrahepatic cholestasis of pregnancy
    (ICP)
intrahepatic cirrhosis
intrahepatic disease
intrahepatic duct
intrahepatic hepatitis of pregnancy
intrahepatic radicle
intrahepatic sclerosing cholangitis
intrahepatic stone
intrahepatic stricture
intrahepatic transjugular portosystemic
    shunt
intralesional therapy
Intralipid fat emulsion
intralobular biliary canal
intralobular fibrosis
intraluminal (ILS) stapler
intraluminal acid
intraluminal contents
intraluminal cyst
intraluminal esophageal pressure
intraluminal manometry
intraluminal occluding suture
intraluminal pH electrode test
intraluminal shelf (infolding of the
    media)
intraluminal Silastic esophageal stent
intraluminal stone
intramammary sulcus
intramedullary (IM)
intramedullary anesthesia
intramedullary graft
intramedullary guide
intramedullary nail
intramedullary pin
intramedullary rasp

intramedullary reamer
intramesenteric abscess
intramucosal development
intramural abscess
intramural bowel mass
intramural colonic air
intramural duodenal hematoma after
    blunt abdominal trauma
intramural edema
intramural esophageal rupture
intramural fistulous tract
intramural hematoma
intramuscular abscess
intranasal anesthesia
Intran disposable pressure measurement
    catheter
intraocular malignancy
intraocular melanoma
Intra–Op autotransfusion
intraoperative autologous transfusion
    (IOAT)
intraoperative bile spillage
intraoperative chemical splanchnic-
    ectomy
intraoperative cholangiogram
intraoperative cholangiography (IOC)
intraoperative endoscopic Congo red
    test (IECRT)
intraoperative laparoscopic cholangi-
    ography
intraoperative pancreatography
intraoperative trauma
intraoperative ultrasound
intraoperative view
intraoral anesthesia
intraosseous anesthesia
intraosseous abscess
intraosseous probe
intraosseous suture anchor
intrapapillary terminus
intraparenchymal liver injury
intraperitoneal abscess
intraperitoneal adhesion
intraperitoneal air

intraperitoneal blood
intraperitoneal cavity
intraperitoneal drain placement
intraperitoneal hyperthermic
    chemotherapy (IPHC)
intraperitoneal incision
intraperitoneal onlay mesh (IPOM)
    hernia repair technique
intraperitoneal viscus
intrapulmonary shunting
intrarectal ultrasound
intrarenal reflux
IntraSite (graft T starch copolymer)
IntraSite gel
IntraSite hydrogel dressing
intraspinal anesthesia
IntraStent DoubleStrut biliary
    endoprosthesis
IntraStent DoubleStrut XS stent
IntraStent LP biliary stent
intrathoracic esophagogastroscopy
intrathoracic goiter
intrathoracic injury
intrathoracic Nissen fundoplication
intratracheal anesthesia
intratumoral catheter
intravariceal sclerotherapy
intravascular compartment
intravascular fluid
intravascular stent
intravascular ultrasound (IVUS)
    catheter
intravascular volume
intravascular volume status
intravenous (I.V., IV)
intravenous alimentation
intravenous administration of fluids
intravenous administration of
    medications
intravenous amino acids
intravenous anesthesia (IVA)
intravenous calcium gluconate
intravenous cholangiogram (IVC)
intravenous extension of tumor

intravenous feeding (IVF)
intravenous fluid
intravenous fluid bolus
intravenous fluid therapy
intravenous glucose administration
intravenous hydration
intravenous hyperalimentation
intravenous Instant Timer
intravenous line sepsis
intravenous nutritional therapy (also see
    feeding formula)
    FreAmine HBC 6.9%
    FreAmine III 3% (8.5%)
        with Electrolytes
    HepatAmine (multiple branched-
        chain essential and nonessential
        amino acids; electrolytes)
    Iodo-Pak (sodium iodide)
    Iodopen (sodium iodide)
    Molypen
    MulTE-Pak-5 (multiple trace
        elements [metals])
    Neotrace-4
    PedTE-Pak-4
    Pedtrace-4 (multiple trace elements)
    Zinca-Pak
intravenous piggyback
intravenous pole
intravenous push
intravenous regional anesthesia
intravenous sedation anesthesia
intravenous sponge
intravenous tolbutamide
intravenous vasopressin
intraventricular cannula
intraventricular catheter
intrepid PTCA angioplasty catheter
intrinsic factor
intrinsic muscles of the larynx
intrinsic plus position
intrinsic stenotic lesion
introducer
    Bard Safety Excalibur catheter
    Becton-Dickinson

introducer *(cont.)*
    Check-Flo
    Ciaglia
    Cook
    Czaja-McCaffrey rigid stent
    Desilets-Hoffman catheter
    electrode
    Endosuture
    Fast-Cath
    guidewire
    Guyon catheter
    Hemaquet catheter
    Hemaquet sheath
    heparin lock
    Key-Med Nottingham
    laparoscopic
    Littleford-Spector
    LPS Peel-Away
    Micropuncture Peel-Away
    Moss G-tube PEG kit
    Mullins catheter
    Naviguide
    Nottingham
    Nottingham semirigid
    Oasis One Action stent
    Pacesetter
    peel-away
    percutaneous lead
    percutaneous tracheostomy
    permanent lead
    Dumon-Gilliard prosthesis
    Swartz SL Series Fast-Cath
    Tuohy-Borst
    Wilson-Cook prosthesis
introducer sheath
introduction of endoprosthesis by ERCP
    (endoscopic retrograde cholangio-
    pancreatography)
Introlan Half-Strength
Introlite (lactose-free formula)
Intron A (interferon alfa-2b, recombi-
    nant)
Intropaste (barium sulfate)
intubate

Ioban Vi-Drape
iobenzamic acid
IOC (intraoperative cholangiogram)
iocetamic acid contrast medium
iodide goiter
iodinated contrast agent
iodinated contrast media
iodine
    ^{123}I murine MAb to alpha-
      fetoprotein (AFP)
    ^{125}I
    ^{131}I 6B-iodomethyl-19-
      norcholesterol
iodine-deficiency goiter
iodine hypothyroidism
iodixanol
iodocholesterol scanning
Iodoflex absorptive dressing
Iodoflex solid gel pad dressing
iodoform gauze dressing
iodoform gauze pack
Iodo-Pak (sodium iodide)
Iodopen (sodium iodide)
iodophor-impregnated adhesive drape
iodophor scrub
iodoquinol
Iodosorb absorptive dressing
Iodosorb wound cleansing gel dressing
Iodotope (sodium iodide ^{131}I)
IoGen
ioglycamic acid
iohexol
Ionescu-Shiley pericardial xenograft
ion-exchange resin
ion laser
IontoDex (dexamethasone sodium
   phosphate)
iontophoresis
IOP (intraoperative pressure)
iopamidol
iopanoic acid contrast medium
IOS immunoassay system
Iotec cannula
Iotec trocar

iothalamate sodium
Iotrex radioisotope
ioversal
Iowa membrane forceps
Iowa trumpet needle guide
Iowa University periosteal elevator
IPAA (ileal pouch-anal anastomosis)
ipecac-induced cardiotoxicity
ipecac-induced myopathy
ipecac-induced vomiting
ipecac syrup
IPH (idiopathic portal hypertension)
IPHC (intraperitoneal hyperthermic
   chemotherapy)
IPHP (intraperitoneal hyperthermic
   perfusion)
ipodate (also iopodate)
ipodate calcium
ipodate contrast medium
ipodate sodium
IPOM (intraperitoneal onlay mesh)
ipoxygenase
IPPB (intermittent positive pressure
   breathing)
iprofenin
IPSID (immunoproliferative small
   intestine disease)
ipsilateral arm lymphedema
ipsilateral brain mass
ipsilateral breast
ipsilateral internal mammary lymph
   node
ipsilateral lymph node
ipsilateral pneumoscrotum
ipsilateral side
ipsilateral supraclavicular node
ipsilateral thyroid lobe
ipsilateral thyroid lobectomy
ipsilateral vocal cord paralysis
iPTH (immunoreactive parathyroid
   hormone)
IRA (ileorectal anastomosis)
Iressa
iridium-192 (^{192}Ir)

iridium-loaded stent
iridium ribbon
iridium seed
iridium wire implant
irinotecan HCl injection
IRIS coronary stent
Irish node
Iris Medical EndoProbe
iris scissors
IRMA blood analysis system
IRMA-M test
IRMA SL test
irofulven
iron-binding capacity of blood
iron-deficiency anemia
iron liver
iron-overload syndrome
iron storage disease
iron store
irradiated graft
irradiation, graft
irradiation injury
irradiation of donor organ
Irravac irrigator
irreducible hernia
irregular amputated mucosal pattern
irregular mass
irregularity
irreversible chronic graft rejection
irrigant, Renacidin
irrigate and aspirate until clear
irrigated with warm saline
irrigating solution, physiological
irrigating syringe, Toomey
irrigation, irrigator
 Asepto
 closed-system
 Coloplast
 Conseal
 copious
 Dansac
 Endo-AID suction
 End-Flo laparoscopic
 Endo-Flo

irrigation *(cont.)*
 Excel
 FlowGun
 House suction
 HydroSurge laparoscopic
 Irravac
 IrrigaTORR
 Irrijet DS
 Lap Vacu-Irrigator
 Nibbler
 Orthotec
 Pathfinder
 pressurized pulsatile
 Ringer
 Shambaugh
 Squirt wound
 StrykeFlow suction
 suction
 Surgilav
 tissue
 United Ostomy
 Vozzle Vacu-Irrigator
irrigation instrument
irrigation of colostomy
irrigation pump
irrigation tubing
irrigator (see *irrigation*)
IrrigaTORR device
Irrijet DS debridement and irrigation
 system
Irrijet DS wound irrigation system
irritability
irritable bowel disease (IBD)
irritable bowel syndrome (IBS)
 constipation-predominant
 diarrhea-predominant
irritable colon
irritable stricture
irritant gastritis
irritation, peritoneal
irritative diarrhea
irritative lesion
IRS (impaired regeneration syndrome)

isolation drape
Isolex 300i stem cell selection system
Isolyser
IsoMed implantable drug pump
Isomil DF (soy protein formula)
Isomil SF (sucrose-free) formula
isoniazid-induced hepatitis
Isopan (magaldrate)
Isopan Plus (magaldrate; simethicone)
isoperistaltic anastomosis
isoperistaltic ileal reservoir
isoprene strap
isopropyl alcohol
isoproterenol
Iso-Seal drape
isosexual virilization
isosorbide dinitrate (ID)
isosorbide mononitrate
Isosource HN
Isospora belli
Isospora hominis
Isospora natelenis
IsoStent radioisotope stent
Isotec patellar tendon graft
Isotein HN enteral feeding
isotomic fluid secretion
Isotoner glove
isotonic feeding
isotope meal
isotope tracer
isovaleric acid
isovaleric acid CoA dehydrogenase
 deficiency
isovaleric acidemia (IVA)
isovaleryl CoA carboxylase deficiency
Isovue-370 (iopamidol)
I-Soyalac formula
Israel rasp
Israel retractor
ISSE optical dissecting and suction
 cannula
isthmectomy
isthmus

isthmus of thyroid
isthmusectomy
ISWL (intracorporeal shock-wave
 lithotripsy)
ITA (internal thoracic artery) graft
ITC balloon catheter
ITC radiopaque balloon catheter
itching
Iterson trachea hook
ITI (Instrument Technology, Inc.)
 0.5 mm rigid endoscope
ITI rigid borescope
Ito cell
Ito cell sarcoma
ITR (International Islet Transplant
 Registry)
itraconazole (Sporanox)
ITx (intestinal transplantation)
I.V., IV (intravenous)
IVA (isovaleric acidemia)
IVAC Core·Check thermometer
IVAC electronic thermometer
IVAC MedSystem III multichannel
 infusion pump
IVAC SmartSite needleless system
IVAC Space·Saver volumetric pump
IVAC Vital·Check device
IVAC volumetric infusion pump
Ivalon rectopexy
Ivalon sponge
Ivalon sponge rectopexy
Ivalon sponge-wrap operation
IVC (intravenous cholangiogram)
IVC stenosis
IVC venous sampling for
 catecholamines
Ivemark syndrome
ivermectin
Ives anoscope
Ives-Fansler anoscope
IVF (intravenous feeding)
IVF (intravenous fluids)
Ivor Lewis esophagectomy

Ivor Lewis esophagogastrectomy
Ivor Lewis two-stage subtotal
esophagectomy

IVUS (intravascular ultrasound)
catheter
Ivy Biomedical Systems
Ivy bleeding time (BT)

J, j

Jaboulay gastroduodenostomy
Jaboulay pyloroplasty
jackknife position
Jackman orthogonal catheter
Jackson battery
Jackson bone extension clamp
Jackson esophageal bougie
Jackson esophagoscope
Jackson grasping polyp forceps
Jackson, inside curve
Jackson intervertebral disk rongeur
Jackson laryngeal atomizer
Jackson laryngectomy tube
Jackson Open-End aspirating tube
Jackson-Pratt (JP)
Jackson-Pratt catheter
Jackson-Pratt drain
Jackson-Pratt gold branch Hemaduct
    wound drain
Jackson retractor
Jackson scissors
Jackson tendon-seizing forceps
Jackson trachea hemostat
Jackson trachea hook
Jackson trachea tenaculum
Jackson trachea tube
Jackson tracheal bistoury
Jackson Velvet eye aspirating tube

jackstone calculus
Jacobs distraction rod
Jacobson-Adson artery forceps
Jacobson bulldog clamp
Jacobson dressing forceps
Jacobson hemostatic forceps
Jacobson micro mosquito forceps
Jacobson microneurosurgical scissors
Jacobson micro probe
Jacobson microvascular knife
Jacobson microvascular needle holder
    with tungsten carbide inlays
Jacobson mosquito forceps
Jacobson-Potts vascular clamp
Jacobson probe
Jacobson-TC needle holder
Jacobson vessel knife
Jacobs-Palmer laparoscope
Jacoby test
Jacuzzi
Jaeger lid plate
Jaffee capsulorrhexis forceps
Jahnke anastomosis clamp
Jako laryngeal suction tube
Jamaican vomiting sickness
Jameson dissecting scissors
Jameson muscle hook
Jameson scissors

Jamestown Canyon virus
Jamshidi biopsy needle
Jamshidi liver biopsy needle
J&J Medical (Johnson & Johnson)
Janeway lesion
Janeway procedure
Jannetta alligator forceps
Jannetta aneurysm neck dissector
Jannetta bayonet forceps
Jannetta dissector
Jannetta duckbill elevator
Jannetta forceps
Jannetta fork
Jannetta hook
Jannetta knife
Jannetta-Kurze dissecting scissors
Jannetta posterior fossa retractor
Jannetta probe
Jansen curette
Jansen mastoid retractor
Jansen-Middleton septal forceps
Jansen monopolar forceps
Jansen rasp
Jansen retractor
Jansen rongeur
Jansen scalp retractor
Jansen-Wagner retractor
Japanese classification of gastric
　　carcinoma
jar forceps
Jarcho self-retaining uterine cannula
Jarell forceps
Jarit brain forceps
Jarit cystoscope
Jarit-Kerrison laminectomy rongeur
Jarit laparoscope
Jarit-Liston bone rongeur
Jarit P.E.E.R. retractor
Jarit rigid laparoscope
Jarit Rotator
Jarit-Ruskin bone rongeur
Jarit tendon-pulling forceps
Jarit 0° 5 mm rigid laparoscope
Jarit 0° 10 mm rigid laparoscope

Jarvis clamp
Jarvis hemorrhoid forceps
Jasan flexible fiberoptic sigmoidoscope
Jasan JFE choledochoscope
Jasan rigid proctoscope
jaundice
　　acholuric
　　acquired hemolytic
　　anhepatic
　　benign postoperative
　　breast milk
　　Budd
　　choleric
　　cholestatic
　　chronic acholuric
　　chronic familial
　　chronic idiopathic
　　congenital familial nonhemolytic
　　congenital hemolytic
　　familial chronic idiopathic
　　familial nonhemolytic
　　hematogenous
　　hemolytic
　　hepatocellular
　　hepatogenous
　　infectious
　　leptospiral
　　malignant
　　malignant obstructive
　　mechanical
　　neonatal
　　newborn
　　nonhemolytic
　　obstructive
　　painless
　　parenchymal
　　physiologic (newborn)
　　retention
　　scleral
　　spirochetal
　　yellow
jaundiced plasma
jaundiced skin
Javid carotid artery clamp

Javid shunt
Javorski test
jaw gib
jaw thrust
Jawz biopsy forceps
Jawz endomyocardial biopsy forceps
JC DNA virus
JDM (juvenile diabetes mellitus) (now
    classified as type 1)
Jegher syndrome
jejunal angiodysplasia
jejunal aspirate
jejunal atresia
jejunal biopsy
jejunal feeding tube
jejunal limb
jejunal loop
jejunal loop interposition of Henle
jejunal pouch
jejunal rupture
jejunal syndrome
jejunal ulcer
jejunectomy
jejunitis
    allergic
    dietetic
    infectious
    nongranulomatous
jejunocolic fistula
jejunoileal bypass (JIB)
    Payne-DeWind
    Scott
jejunoileitis
jejunoileostomy, Roux-en-Y distal
jejunojejunostomy
jejunostomy
    afferent
    decompression
    endoscopic
    feeding
    laparoscopic
    loop
    needle catheter
    percutaneous endoscopic (PEJ)

jejunostomy (cont.)
    subserosal needle catheter
    Witzel
jejunostomy catheter
    Baker
    decompression
    feeding
    Flexiflo Lap J
    laparoscopic
    loop
    MIC
    needle
    Witzel
jejunostomy tube
jejunum
    arterial arcades of
    coils of
    mesentery of
    proximal
    windows of
Jelco I.V. catheter
Jelco needle
Jelco winged I.V. catheter
jelly
    Wharton
    Xylocaine
jelly-like material
Jelonet (paraffin-soaked tulle) dressing
Jenckel cholecystoduodenostomy
Jennings mouth gag
Jensen sarcoma
Jergesen I-beam plate
Jergesen tapered plate
Jergesen tube
Jesberg aspirating tube
Jesberg esophagoscope
jet lesion
jet pilot position
Jeter lag screw
Jeter position screw
Jevity isotonic liquid nutrition
jeweler's bipolar forceps
Jewett driver
Jewett extractor

Jewett gouge
Jewett nail
Jewett nail overlay plate
JFB III endoscope
J-hook cannula
J-hook electrode
J-hook ElectroProbe
JIB (jejunoileal bypass)
jig, cutting
jig hook
J ileal reservoir
Jimmy dissector
JL4 (Judkins left 4 cm curve) catheter
JL5 (Judkins left 5 cm curve) catheter
J needle
J needle technique
Jober fossa
Jobson Horne probe
Jobst glove
Jobst stockings
Jod-Basedow phenomenon (transient
    hyperthyroidism)
JODM (juvenile-onset diabetes
    mellitus) (now classified as type 1)
Joe hoe retractor
Johannesberg staple
Johannson hip nail
Johns Hopkins bulldog clamp
Johns Hopkins coarctation clamp
Johns Hopkins forceps
Johns Hopkins gallbladder forceps
Johns Hopkins gallbladder retractor
Johnson & Johnson Medical
Johnson brain tumor forceps
Johnson esophagogastrostomy
Johnson retractor
Johnson thoracic forceps
Johnson tumor forceps
joint fluid
joker (slang for instrument)
joker periosteal elevator
Joll thyroid retractor
Jolles test
Jones compression pin

Jones compression plate
Jones dressing
Jones IMA forceps
Jones position
Jones thoracic clamp
Jones towel clip
Jones view
Jonnesco fossa
Jordan-Bookwalter retractor
Jordan hook
Jordan needle
Jorgenson scissors
Joseph button-end knife
Joseph dissecting scissors
Joseph hook
Joseph nasal rasp
Joseph nasal scissors
Joseph periosteal elevator
Joseph skin hook
joule (J)
Joule-Thompson effect in endoscopic
    cryotherapy
Joystick
J periosteal elevator
J pouch, two-loop ileal
J-shaped ileal pouch
J-shaped reservoir
J-shaped skin incision
J-shaped tube
J-tipped hydrophilic guidewire
J tube
J-turn maneuver with endoscope
Judd-Allis intestinal forceps
Judd-DeMartel gallbladder forceps
Judd ventral hernia repair
Judet graft
Judet radius view
Judkins 4 diagnostic catheter
Juers-Lempert rongeur forceps
jugal suture
jugular line
jugular venous distention
jugular versus peripheral ACTH levels

juice
   acid-peptic
   appetite
   gastric
   intestinal
   pancreatic
Julian splenorenal forceps
Julian thoracic forceps
jumbo biopsy forceps
jump graft
jumper's knee position
junction
   anorectal
   cardioesophageal (CE)
   choledochopancreatic ductal
   cystic-choledochal
   cystocholedochal
   esophagogastric (EG)
   fundic-antral
   gastroesophageal (GE)
   ileocecal
   duodenojejunal
   mucocutaneous
   pancreaticobiliary ductal
   pyloroduodenal
   squamocolumnar
   tracheoesophageal (TE; TEF)
   ureteropelvic

junction of papillary and reticular
   dermis
junction of right and left hepatic
   ducts
junction of second and third portions
   of duodenum
Juven nutritional supplement
juvenile angiofibroma
juvenile cirrhosis
juvenile diabetes mellitus (JDM) (now
   classified as type 1)
juvenile embryonal carcinoma
juvenile hypothyroidism
juvenile melanoma
juvenile-onset diabetes mellitus
   (JODM) (now classified as type 1)
juvenile pattern
juvenile polyp
juvenile polyposis
juvenile polyposis coli
juxtacortical osteogenic sarcoma
juxtaglomerular cells
juxtahepatic venous injury
juxtapyloric ulcer
J-Vac closed wound drainage
J-Vac suction reservoir
J wire
J-wire guide

K, k

K (potassium)
Kader gastrostomy
Kaessmann nail
Kahn dissecting scissors
Kahn-Frazier suction tube
Kahn uterine trigger cannula
Kahre-Williger periosteal elevator
Kaletra (lopinavir/ritonavir)
Kalginate alginate wound dressing
Kalginate calcium alginate dressing
Kalish Duredge wire extractor
Kalman-Mixter forceps
Kalman needle holder with tungsten
    carbide inlay
Kalt needle
Kaltostat calcium alginate dressing
Kaltostat Fortex high-absorbent wound
    dressing
Kaltostat pad (high-absorbent) dressing
Kaltostat rope dressing
Kaltostat wound packing material
Kam Vac suction tube
Kanavel brain-exploring cannula
Kaneda plate
Kaneda rod
Kantor-Berci videolaryngoscope
Kantor sign
Kantrowitz artery forceps

Kantrowitz thoracic clamp
Kantrowitz vascular scissors
Kanulase
Kaodene Non-Narcotic (kaolin; pectin;
    bismuth subsalicylate)
Kao Lectrolyte
kaolin
Kaopectate
Kao-Spen (kaolin; pectin)
Kapectolin (kaolin; pectin)
Kaplan PenduLaser 115 surgical laser
    system
Kaposi sarcoma, intracolonic
Kapp-Beck-Thomson clamp
Kapsinow test
karaya powder
Karaya 5 paste
Karaya 5 seal
Karaya ring ileostomy appliance
Karl Storz endoscope
Karl Storz endoscopy video camera
    system
Karl Storz N$_2$O Endoflator
Karl Storz rigid laparoscope
Karl Storz Take-Apart instruments
Karmody venous scissors
Karnofsky rating scale
Karp aortic punch forceps

Kartchner carotid artery clamp
Kartush insulated retractor
Karuse nasal snare
Karydakis flap
Karydakis pilonidal cyst excision
karyotype determination
Kasai peritoneal venous shunt
Kasai portoenterostomy
Kasdan retractor
Kashiwado test
Kaslow intestinal tube
Kasof (docusate potassium)
Kasugai classification of chronic
    pancreatitis
Kato test
Kay aorta clamp
Kaycel towel
Kayer-Fleischer ring
Kaye scissors
Kaye tamponade balloon catheter
Kaye-TC scissors
Kayexalate enema
Kay-Lambert clamp
Kayser-Fleischer ring
K blade
K-C (kaolin; pectin; bismuth
    subcarbonate)
kcal (kilocalorie, calorie)
KDF-2.3 catheter
K-dissector sponge
K-Dur (potassium chloride)
Keel Cobra One-Piece cannula
Keel Cobra Toomey syringe cannula
Keene compression hook
Kefzol
Kehr incision
Kehr sign
Keith abdominal needle, straight,
    triangular point
Keith abdominal triangle
Keith needle
Kelling esophagoscope
Kelling test
Kelly abdominal retractor

Kelly anoscope
Kelly artery forceps
Kelly clamp
Kelly dissecting scissors
Kelly fistula scissors
Kelly forceps, curved
Kelly hemostat
Kelly hemostatic forceps
Kelly-Locklin scissors
Kelly-Paterson syndrome
Kelly placenta forceps
Kelly plication suture
Kelly proctoscope
Kelly rectal speculum
Kelly retractor
Kelly scissors
Kelly sphincteroscope
Kelly straight proctoscope
Kelly tapered proctoscope
keloid scar
Kelsey pile clamp
Kemerovo virus
Ken sliding nail
Kendall esophageal sonascope
Kendall Healthcare Company
Kendall sontatemp
Kennerdell-Maroon elevator
Kennerdell-Maroon hook
Kennerdell-Maroon orbital retractor
Keofeed feeding tube
ketoacidosis
keratome
keratome blade
keratosis
    actinic
    lacelike
    pharyngeal
    seborrheic
    senile
Kerckring duodenal fold
Kerlix bandage
Kerlix disposable laparotomy sponge
Kerlix dressing
Kern bone-holding clamp

Kern bone-holding forceps
Kern-Lane bone forceps
kernicterus
Kerrison down-biting rongeur
Kerrison forceps
Kerrison laminectomy rongeur
Kerrison punch
Kerrison rongeur
KESS constipation scoring system
Kessel plate
Kessler suture
Kestrone 5 (estrone)
Ketek (telithromycin)
ketoacidosis
   alcoholic
   diabetic
ketoconazole
kctone
ketonuria
ketoprofen
ketorolac tromethamine
ketosis, benign dietary
ketosis-prone diabetes mellitus
ketosis-resistant diabetes mellitus
KetoSite test for status of ketoacidosis
ketotic hypoglycemia
Kevorkian biopsy tip
Kevorkian-Tischler biopsy forceps
Kevorkian-Townsend biopsy curette
Kevorkian-Younge biopsy curette
Kevorkian-Younge biopsy forceps
Keyes cutaneous punch
Keyes dermal punch
Key hernia director
Key-Med Atkinson endoprosthesis
Key-Med Nottingham introducer
Key periosteal elevator
Key rasp
keyhole incision
keyhole surgery
keystone graft
kidney
   abdominal
   afferent vessels of

kidney *(cont.)*
   amyloid
   arcuate artery of
   Armanni-Ebstein
   arteriosclerotic
   artificial
   Ask-Upmark
   atrophic
   biopsy of
   cake
   cicatricial
   congested
   contracted
   cow
   crush
   cyanotic
   cystic
   disk
   donor
   doughnut
   dromedary
   duplex
   edematous
   fatty
   fibrous capsule of
   flea-bitten
   floating
   Formad
   fused
   Goldblatt
   granular
   hila of
   horseshoe
   hypermobile
   interlobular artery of
   ischemic
   large red
   medullary sponge
   mortar
   movable
   mural
   myelin
   myeloma
   pancake

kidney *(cont.)*
  pelvic
  polycystic
  putty
  pyelonephritic
  Rose-Bradford
  sacciform
  sclerotic
  sigmoid
  sponge
  supernumerary
  thoracic
  wandering
  waxy
kidney calculus
kidney cancer
kidney abscess
kidney colic
kidney function test
kidney laceration
kidney stone
kidney stone forceps
kidney transplant
Kidney Internal Splint/Stent (KISS)
  catheter
kidney-shaped placenta
kidney tubule
kidney tumor
Kielland forceps
Kiernan space
Kifa catheter
killer T cell
Killian antrum cannula
Killian gouge
Killian-Lynch laryngoscope
Killian rectal speculum
Killian septum speculum
Killian suction tube
Kilner catspaw retractor (cat's paw)
Kilner cheek retractor
Kilner dissecting scissors
Kilner hook
Kilner insulated retractor
Kilner skin hook

Kilner-TC needle holder
kilocalorie (kcal, calorie)
Kimberly Clark Ballard Medical
Kimmelstiel-Wilson syndrome
Kimura cartilage graft
Kinberg test
Kindercal nutritional therapy
Kindt carotid artery clamp
Kinesed
kinetic gallbladder study
Kinevac (sincalide)
King Systems
kinked intestine
kinked ureter
kink in bowel
kinking of CNS catheter
kink in intestine
kinky hair syndrome (Menkes disease)
Kinnier Wilson disease
Kinsella-Buie lung clamp
Kinsey atherectomy catheter
Kirby muscle hook
Kirchner diverticulum
Kiricuta breast reconstruction
Kirklin atrial retractor
Kirk mallet
Kirmission periosteal elevator
Kirmission periosteal rasp
Kirsch laser welding technique
Kirschner abdominal retractor
Kirschner hand drill
Kirschner wire drill
Kish urethral illuminated catheter
KISS (Kidney Internal Splint/Stent)
  catheter
kissing balloon
kissing ulcer
kit
  Adenovirus EIA test
  Alatest Latex-specific IgE allergen
  B-D Easy A1c test
  CdTOX A OIA
  Circulon System Step 2 venous ulcer
    dressing

kit *(cont.)*
   CloseSure procedure
   Daxor quantitative injection syringe
   Decon Mini-Plus
   Dulcolax Bowel Prep Kit (bisacodyl)
   Duraprep
   Euro-Collins (EC) multiorgan
     perfusion
   EZ Detect colorectal screening test
   Flex Advantage
   Flexiflo Lap G laparoscopic
     gastrostomy
   Flexiflo Lap J laparoscopic
     jejunostomy
   Great Smokies intestinal
     permeability
   hematopoietic progenitor assay
   HemeSelect reagent and collection
   I-Flow nerve block infusion
   Isletest and Isletest-ICA
   LeuTech radiolabeled antibody
   Matritech NMP22 test
   Moss G-tube PEG
   NeoTect
   Nerve Block Infusion
   NuMA
   NuMA test
   PainBuster infusion pain
     management
   PAK (percutaneous access kit)
   PathVysion HER-2 DNA probe
   Quick AC Enema
   Riba 3.0 SIA reagent kit for
     hepatitis C
   Russel gastrostomy
   standard bunny
   Surgi-Start Kit single basin set
   Three-Spring Reservoir Wound
     Suction Drainage
   Tridrate Bowel Evacuant
   Trinity adenovirus EIA test
   Virgo antimitochondrial antibody)
   V-scan test
Kitano knot

Kittner blunt dissector
Kittner clamp
Kittner dissecting scissors
Kittner retractor
Kittner sponge
Klatskin liver biopsy needle
Klatskin tumor
Klear-Temp probe
Klebanoff common duct sound
Klebanoff gallstone scoop
Klebsiella
KleenSpec dispenser
KleenSpec disposable anoscope
Kleihauer-Betke acid elution test
Kleinert-Kutz bone rongeur
Kleinert-Kutz bone-cutting forceps
Kleinert-Kutz periosteal elevator
Kleinert-Kutz rasp
Kleinert-Kutz rongeur forceps
Kleinert-Kutz skin hook
Kleinert-Kutz synovectomy rongeur
Kleinert-Kutz tendon forceps
Kleinert-Ragdell retractor
Klein pump
Kleinsasser anterior commissure
   laryngoscope
Kleinschmidt appendectomy clamp
Klemme laminectomy retractor
Klemm sign
Klemperer disease
Kleppinger bipolar forceps
KLI rigid borescope
Klima-Schleicher biopsy needle
Klinefelter syndrome
Kling adhesive dressing
Kling elastic bandage
Kling fluff roll and sponge
Klintmalm clamp
Klippel-Trenaunay syndrome
KLS Centre-Drive screw
Knapp scissors
knee-chest position
knee-elbow position
kneeling position

knee retractor
knife (see also *blade; scalpel*)
   A-K diamond
   A-OK ShortCut
   acetabular
   Adson dural
   Adson right-angle
   amputation
   angular
   arachnoid
   arthroscopic
   Ayre
   backward-cutting
   Bailey-Glover-O'Neill commis-
      surotomy
   Ballenger swivel
   banana
   Bard-Parker
   bayonet
   Beaver
   Beaver-DeBakey
   beveled
   Bircher meniscus
   bladebreaker
   Blount
   Bovie
   Braithwaite
   Brock commissurotomy
   Bucy chordotomy (or cordotomy)
   cartilage
   Catlin amputating
   cautery
   chondroplasty
   chordotomy (cordotomy)
   Cobalt Knife
   cobalt-60 gamma
   Cobbett
   Collin amputating
   commissurotomy
   cordotomy (chordotomy)
   crescent
   Crile gasserian ganglion
   Culbertson canal
   Cushing dural hook

knife *(cont.)*
   deep blade
   DeMarneffe meniscotomy
   Derlacki capsule
   Derra commissurotomy
   Desmarres paracentesis
   double-bladed
   Down epiphyseal
   Downing cartilage
   dural
   Edgeahead phaco slit
   electrocautery
   electrosurgical cutting
   epiphyseal
   Esmarch plaster
   flap
   Foerster capsulotomy
   forward-cutting
   Frazier cordotomy
   Frazier pituitary
   Freedom
   Freer-Swanson ganglion
   Freiberg cartilage
   Freiberg meniscectomy
   full-radius resector
   Gamma radiosurgical
   Gandhi
   ganglion
   Grover meniscus
   Guilford-Wright double-edged sickle
   Guilford-Wright flap
   Halle dura
   Harmonic Scalpel
   Harrison
   hemilaminectomy
   hernia
   hook
   Hopkins plaster
   hot
   House
   insulation tipped diathermic
   interosseous
   intimectomy
   Jacobson microvascular

knife *(cont.)*

    Jacobson vessel
    Jannetta
    Joseph button-end
    Knifelight surgical knife and light
    Koos microvascular
    Krull acetabular
    Langenbeck flap
    Langenbeck resection
    LaserSonics Nd:YAG LaserBlade
      scalpel
    LaserSonics SurgiBlade
    Lebsche sternal
    left-cutting
    Leksell cobalt-60 gamma
    Leksell Gamma
    Lempert paracentesis
    L hook
    Lindvall-Stille
    Liston amputating
    Liston amputation
    Liston phalangeal
    Lorenz PC/TC scissors ultra-sharp
    Lowe-Breck cartilage
    Lowe-Breck meniscectomy
    Maltz cartilage
    McCabe canal
    McHugh facial nerve
    McHugh flap
    McKeever cartilage
    meniscotomy
    meniscus
    MicroKnife XL triple-lumen
      needleknife
    microvascular
    Midas Rex
    Mori
    myelotomy
    needle
    Neff meniscus
    Neoflex bendable
    NeoKnife electrosurgical
    Olivecrona trigeminal
    Oretorp

knife *(cont.)*

    Paparella canal
    Paparella drum elevator
    Paparella incudostapedial
    Paparella sickle
    Parasmillie double-bladed
    Parker
    Paufique
    pituitary
    plaster
    Premium dissecting
    Questrus Leading Edge sheathed
    Rayport
    Reiner plaster
    resection
    retrograde
    Ridlon plaster
    right-angle
    right-cutting
    roentgen
    roentgen radiosurgical
    Rosen incision
    Salenius meniscus
    SatinCrescent
    SatinShortcut
    semilunar cartilage
    sharp
    Shaw I and Shaw II
    Sheehy round
    ShortCut
    sickle
    skin
    skin blade
    Smart Scalpel
    Smillie-Beaver
    Smillie cartilage
    Smillie meniscus
    Smith cartilage
    specimen
    standard dissecting
    Stecher arachnoid
    Stryker cartilage
    swivel
    Tabb double-ended flap

knife *(cont.)*
    Tabb myringoplasty
    Take-Apart
    tenotomy
    Tiemann Meals tenolysis
    Toennis dura
    201-source cobalt-60 gamma
    Typhoon microdebrider
    UltraCision ultrasonic
    vessel
    Virchow
    Visitec circular
    Visitec crescent
    Visitec stiletto
    Watson
    Weary cordotomy
    Weck
    Yamada myelotomy
    Yankauer
    Yasargil arachnoid
    Yasargil microvascular
knife blade
Knifelight illuminated retractor
Knifelight surgical knife and light
knifelike pain
Knight bone-cutting forceps
Knight needle
Knight septum cutting forceps
knife/sleeve device
Knighton hemilaminectomy retractor
Knighton laminectomy retractor
knitted Dacron graft
knitted double velour Dacron patch
    graft
knitted tantalum
knobby process
Knodell classification of chronic
    hepatitis C
Knodell periportal inflammation score
Knodt compression rod
Knodt hook
Knodt rod
knot
    Aberdeen
    arthroscopic

knot *(cont.)*
    convertible slip
    extracorporeal
    fisherman's
    friction knot
    half-hitch
    heliX knot pusher
    ileosigmoid knot
    Kitano
    LapTie endoscopic
    lockable arthroscopic
    Nicky
    ratchet
    Roeder loop
    sailorman's
    slip
    square
    surfer's
    surgeon's
    Tennessee slider
    Topel
knot geometry
knotless suture anchor
knotless anchor suture
knot of Henry
knot pusher
    Arrequi
    heliX
    MetraTie
knot tied with throws
knot tier and ligature carrier, Retter
knot tier, Gazayerli
knot tightener, Nordt
knotting forceps
Knowles bandage scissors
Knowles nail
Knowles pin
knuckle of bowel
knuckle of colon
knurled rod
Knuttsen bending view (x-ray)
Ko-Airan maneuver
Koala pressure catheter
Koala vascular clamp
Kobak pudendal block needle

Kocher anastomosis
Kocher artery forceps
Kocher bladder spatula
Kocher bronchocele sound
Kocher clamp
Kocher collar incision (in thyroidectomy)
Kocher dilatation ulcer
Kocher director
Kocher elevator
Kocher forceps
Kocher gallbladder retractor
Kocher hemostat
Kocher hook
Kocher incision
Kocher intestinal forceps
Kocher-Langenbeck ilioinguinal
    approach
Kocher maneuver
Kocher pylorectomy
Kocher pyloromyotomy
Kocher retractor
Kocher thyroid dissector
Koch-Mason dressing
Koch nucleus hydrolysis needle
Kock ("coke")
Kock continent ileostomy
Kock ileal reservoir
Kock ileostomy
Kock pouch modified procedure
Kock reservoir ileostomy
Kodsi scale of Candida esophagitis
Koeberlé forceps
Koenig (König)
Koenig nail-splitting scissors
Koenig rasp
Koenig small director
Koenig syndrome
Koerte gallstone forceps
Koerte rake retractor
Kogan-Burke speculum
Kogan speculum
KOH (potassium hydroxide)
KOH colpotomizer system
KOH smear

Kolantyl
Kollman urethral dilator
kombucha (yeast/bacteria/fungus
    symbiont)
Komprex bandage
Komprex-Binde bandage
König (Koenig) syndrome
Konsyl (psyllium)
Konsyl-D
Konsyl Orange (psyllium hydrophilic
    mucilloid)
Konsyl Fiber (calcium polycarbophil)
Konton catheter
Kontron intra-aortic balloon
Koos microvascular knife
Kopans breast lesion localization needle
Kostuik rod
K-Pek (attapulgite)
Krackow suture
Kraff-Utrata tear capsulotomy forceps
Krankendonk pin
K-ras gene
Kraske jackknife position in surgery
Kraske position
Kraske transsacral proctectomy
KRAS mutation (gene implicated in
    cancer)
Krause biopsy tip
Krause nasal snare
Krause suture
Krause-Wolfe skin graft
Krayenbuehl (Krayenbühl) vessel hook
Krazy Glue sclerosant
Kreuscher scissors
Krimpt sponge
Kristeller specula
Krokiewicz test
Kronecker aneurysm needle
Kron gall duct dilator
Krukenberg tumor
Krull acetabular knife
krypton (red) laser
K-Sponge
K.T. Medical

KTP (potassium titanyl phosphate) laser
KTP/532 laser
KTP/YAG surgical laser system
K-Tube
Kuehne cover glass forceps
Kugel approach
Kugel hernia patch
Kugel patch repair
Kulchitsky cell
Kulchitsky cell carcinoma
Kunkel syndrome
Küntscher (Kuentscher)
Küntscher awl
Küntscher condylocephalic rod
Küntscher drill
Küntscher extractor
Küntscher hammer
Küntscher intramedullary reamer
Küntscher medullary nail
Küntscher nail driver
Küntscher nail extracting hook
Küntscher pin
Kupffer cell
Kupffer cell recovery (in obstructive
 jaundice)

Kupffer cell sarcoma
Kurze dissecting scissors
Kussmaul sign
Kutler V-Y flap graft
Kutrase (amylase; protease; lipase;
 cellulase; hyoscyamine sulfate;
 phenyltoloxamine citrate) digestive
 enzymes
Küttner (Kuettner)
Küttner blunt dissector
Kuzmak gastric banding technique
Kuz-Medics total knee retractor
Ku-Zyme HP (amylase; protease;
 lipase; cellulase) digestive enzymes
kwashiorkor protein-energy under-
 nutrition
Kwik-Kits
K-wire driver
Kyasanur Forest hemorrhagic fever
 virus
Kynar insulated coating
Kytril (granisetron hydrochloride)

L, l

LA (left atrial)
LABA (laser-assisted balloon
    angioplasty)
Labbe triangle
Laborde trachea dilator
lacelike keratosis
lacerated wound
laceration
    gastroesophageal
    kidney
    spleen
    through-and-through
    V-shaped
    wound
La Crosse virus
Lactaid
lactase deficiency
lactase enzyme
lactate dehydrogenase (LDH)
lactated Ringer (LR) solution
lactation
lacteal vessel
lactic acid
lactic acid bacillus
lactiferous duct
lactiferous duct fistula
lactiferous gland

Lactinex
Lactobacillus acidophilus
lactoferrin
Lactomer absorbable subcuticular skin
    staple
lactose-associated diarrhea
lactose breath hydrogen test
lactose deficiency
lactose enzyme
lactose-free diet
lactose-free feeding
lactose intolerance
lactose, undigested
Lactrase
lactulose enema
lactulose-mannitol test
lactulose/rhamnose permeability
    (L/R ratio)
lactulose solution
lacunar ligament
Ladd band
Ladd correction of malrotation
    of the bowel
Ladd procedure
Ladd syndrome
Laënnec cirrhosis
Laënnec pearl

Lafora body
LAGB (Lap-Band adjustable gastric
   banding) system
lag screw
Lahey bag
Lahey clamp
Lahey Clinic dural hook
Lahey Clinic nerve hook
Lahey dissecting forceps
Lahey Finochietto dissecting forceps
Lahey gall duct forceps
Lahey gland forceps
Lahey liver transplant bag
Lahey retractor
Lahey scissors
Lahey thoracic forceps
Lahey thyroid retractor
Lahey thyroid traction forceps
Lahey tissue retractor
Laing plate
Laird-McMahon anorectoplasty
LAIS excimer laser
LAK (lymphokine activated killer) cell
lake, bile
laky blood
Lalonde delicate hook forceps
LAMA (laser-assisted microvascular
   anastomosis or laser-assisted
   microanastomosis)
Lambda Plus dye laser
Lambda Plus PDL 1 (and PDL 2) laser
lambdoid suture
lambdoidal cranial suture
Lambert aortic clamp
Lambert-Kay aorta clamp
Lambert-Kay vascular clamp
Lambert-Lowman bone clamp
Lambert-Lowman chisel
lambliasis
lambliosis
Lambotte bone-holding forceps
Lambotte bone hook
Lambotte elevator
Lambotte osteotome

Lambotte rasp
lamellated pattern
lamina elevator
lamina of the aponeurosis
lamina propria
lamina retractor
laminar hook
laminated clot
laminectomy blade
laminectomy chisel
laminectomy punch
laminectomy punch forceps
laminectomy retractor
laminectomy rongeur
Lamis adapter
Lamis patella clamp
Lamis tubing set
Lamis Y tubing
lamivudine therapy
lamp, Wood
Lancereaux-Mathieu-Weil spirochetosis
lancet
   Autoclix
   auto-Lancet
   ExacTech pen
   Laser Lancet
   Lasette
   Microlet Vaculance
   Microtainer
   Softclix
   Vaculance
lancet-shaped biopsy forceps
lancinating pain
Landau trocar
landmark
   anatomic
   anatomical
   bony
Landolt spreading forceps
Landon retractor
Landzert fossa
Lane band
Lane bone-holding clamp
Lane bone-holding forceps

Lane cleft palate, 1/2 circle, cutting
edge
Lane disease
Lane elevator
Lane intestinal clamp
Lane intestinal forceps
Lane operation
Lane periosteal elevator
Lane plate
Lane point
Lane procedure
Lane screw-holding forceps
Lane self-retaining bone-holding
forceps
Lane tissue forceps
Lane twin stomach clamps
Lang Stevenson intestinal clamp
Lange approximation forceps
Lange-Hohmann bone retractor
Langenbeck bone-holding forceps
Langenbeck elevator
Langenbeck flap knife
Langenbeck-Kocher retractor
Langenbeck metacarpal saw
Langenbeck periosteal elevator
Langenbeck rasp
Langenbeck resection knife
Langenbeck retractor
Lange skinfold calipers
Langenskiöld bone graft
Langerhans cell
Langer line
lansoprazole
Lantus (insulin glargine)
Lanza scale for drug-induced gastric
mucosal damage
Lanz low-pressure cuff endotracheal
tube
Lanz pressure-regulating valve
LAO (left anterior oblique) view
lap (brief form for laparotomy)
laparoendoscopic room
Laparofan device
LaparoLift gasless laparoscopy system

LaparoLift retractor system
LaparoSAC single-use obturator and
cannula
laparoscope (see also *endoscope*)
ACMI rigid
Adler Eagle Vision
Adler P.L.U.S.
Arthrotek rigid
Bryan rigid
Cabot rigid
Circon rigid
Comeg rigid
Concept rigid
CorTek semirigid microlaparoscope
Cuda 0° 10 mm rigid
Demir rigid
diagnostic
Dyonics 0° 10 mm rigid
Dyonics 3625
Dyonics 7208130 rigid
Dyonics 8007 rigid
Eder 180 10 mm rigid
Effner rigid
ElMed rigid
Endolap rigid
Endolase rigid
50° Foroblique optic
flexible video
Henke-Sass rigid
Henke-Sass Wolf
Inspex rigid laparoscope
InstrumentMakar
Jacobs-Palmer
Jarit 0° 5 mm rigid
Jarit 0° 10 mm rigid
Jarit rigid
Karl Storz rigid
laser
Linvatec
Linvatec 7570R 0° 10 mm rigid
Linvatec rigid
Marlow rigid
Marlow video
Medilas

laparoscope *(cont.)*
   MicroLap Gold microlaparoscope
   MiniSite
   Mueller 0° 5 mm rigid
   Olympus A5214 0° 10 mm rigid
   Olympus A5254 0° 10 mm rigid
   Olympus A5254 0° 10mm rigid
   Olympus A5255 30° 10 mm rigid
   Olympus A5257 0° 10 mm rigid
   Olympus A5258 rigid 30° 10 mm
   operating
   operative
   Optik rigid
   Pilling rigid
   REI rigid
   Schoelly
   Semm rigid
   Solos rigid
   Storz 26033 AP 0° 10 mm rigid
   Storz 26033 BP 0° 10 mm rigid
   Storz AP 26003 0° 10 mm rigid
   Storz Hopkins
   Storz rigid
   Stryker
   Stryker 380-10 0° 10 mm rigid
   Stryker 380-11 0° 10 mm rigid
   Stryker 380-12 30° 10 mm rigid
   Surgitech
   Surgiview
   10° operating
   3Dscope
   VerreScope
   VideoHydro
   V. Mueller rigid
   Weck-Baggish rigid
   Weck operating
   Weck 0° 10 mm rigid
   Weck 110405, 0° 5 mm rigid
   Weck 110800 rigid
   Wisap
   Wolf Lumina rigid
   Wolf rigid
   Wolf 10/5 (L-angle) operative
   Wolf 170 12 mm rigid

laparoscope *(cont.)*
   Wolf 7732 rigid
   Wolf 8934.40 rigid
   Wolf 8937.31 0° 10 mm rigid
   0° forward optic
   Zimmer rigid
laparoscope camera
laparoscopic adrenalectomy
laparoscopically assisted colorectal
   resection
laparoscopically assisted sigmoid
   resection
laparoscopically assisted vaginal
   hysterectomy (LAVH)
laparoscopic anterior fundoplication
laparoscopic antireflux surgery (LARS)
laparoscopic appendectomy
laparoscopic approach
laparoscopic-assisted procedure
laparoscopic-assisted vaginal hysterec-
   tomy
laparoscopic bile duct exploration
laparoscopic biopsy of liver
laparoscopic bladder neck suture
   suspension procedure
Laparoscopic Bowel Registry
laparoscopic bowel resection
laparoscopic Burch procedure
laparoscopic cardiomyotomy
laparoscopic cholecystectomy
   ("lap chole")
laparoscopic colectomy
laparoscopic colorectal cancer surgery
laparoscopic common bile duct
   exploration
laparoscopic contact ultrasonography
   (LCU)
laparoscopic cholecystectomy
laparoscopic dissection and
   manipulation
laparoscopic distal pancreatectomy
laparoscopic Doppler probe
laparoscopic duct exploration

laparoscopic esophagogastroplasty with Nissen fundoplication
laparoscopic exploration of common bile duct
laparoscopic extracorporeal knot
laparoscopic extraperitoneal sacrospinous suspension
laparoscopic fundoplication
laparoscopic gallbladder removal
laparoscopic gastric banding
laparoscopic gastrostomy
laparoscopic grasper
laparoscopic Heller myotomy
laparoscopic hernia repair
laparoscopic hernioplasty
laparoscopic herniorrhaphy
laparoscopic intracorporeal ultrasound (LICU)
laparoscopic introducer
laparoscopic irrigation pump
laparoscopic jejunostomy
laparoscopic Kittner device
laparoscopic laser-assisted autoaugmentation
laparoscopic laser cholecystectomy (LLC)
laparoscopic liver biopsy
laparoscopic lysis of adhesions
laparoscopic micro scissors
laparoscopic myotomy
laparoscopic Nissen and Toupet fundoplication
laparoscopic Nissen fundoplication with esophageal lengthening
laparoscopic paraesophageal hernia repair (LPHR)
laparoscopic pelvic lymph node dissection and extraperitoneal pelvioscopy
laparoscopic placement of peritoneal dialysis catheter
laparoscopic pneumodissection
laparoscopic posterior hemi-fundoplication
laparoscopic radical prostatectomy

laparoscopic repair of paraesophageal hernia (LRPH)
laparoscopic retractor
laparoscopic retroperitoneal lymphadenectomy
laparoscopic Roux-en-Y gastric bypass
laparoscopic sleeve
laparoscopic surgeon's thumb
laparoscopic surgery for peptic ulcer disease
laparoscopic telescope
   30° angle
   0° straight forward
   Storz
laparoscopic Toupet fundoplication
laparoscopic transcystic duct exploration
laparoscopic transcystic lithotripsy (LTCL)
laparoscopic transcystic papillotomy
laparoscopic trocar
laparoscopic trocar sleeve
laparoscopic tubal ligation
laparoscopic ultrasound (LUS)
laparoscopic urinary diversion procedure
laparoscopic uterine nerve ablation
laparoscopy
   diagnostic
   double-puncture
   hand-assisted
   laser
   needle
   single-port
   single-port, double-puncture
   single-puncture
   THL (Transvaginal Hydro Laparoscopy) system
   video
laparoscopy needle (see *needle*)
   Core
   Maciol
laparoscopy under local anesthesia (LULA)
LaparoSonic coagulating shears for autograft harvesting

laparotomy
   emergency
   exploratory
   mini-
   open
   second-look
   staging
laparotomy (lap)
laparotomy pad cover
laparotomy pad, sponge, and needle
   counts
laparotomy ring
laparotomy with splenectomy
laparotomy with splenorrhaphy
Lap-Band adjustable gastric banding
   (LAGB) system
Lap-Band closure tool
lap Nissen (laparoscopic Nissen fundo-
   plication)
lap pad
Lapra-Ty absorbable suture clip
Lapro-Clip ligating clip system
LaproFlator device, Storz
Laprotek
Lap Sac
lap sponge
lap, sponge, and needle counts
lap tape (pad or sponge)
LAP-TAPP (laparoscopic transabdomi-
   nal preperitoneal) hernioplasty
LAP (leucine aminopeptidase) test
LapTie endoscopic knot-tying
   instrument
Lap Vacu-Irrigator
Lapwall laparotomy sponge
Lapwall laparotomy sponge and wound
   protector
LAR (low anterior resection)
LAR/CAA (low anterior resection
   in combination with coloanal
   anastomosis)
LARA analyzer
lardaceous degeneration of liver
lardaceous liver

large aperture
large benign thymus gland
large bladder rupture
large-bore bile duct prosthesis
large-bore gastric feeding lavage
large-bore inflow cannula
large-bore I.V.'s (or IVs)
large-bore needle
large-bore rigid esophagoscope
large-bore silicone drains
large-bore slotted aspirating needle
large-bore Tygon tubing
large bowel
large bowel obstruction
large bowel torsion
large bowel volvulus
large-caliber tube
large cell carcinoma
large cell, immunoblastic lymphoma
large-diameter bougie
large-droplet fatty liver
large egress cannula
large gallstone
large hernia defect
large intestine
large intestine gland
large loop excision of the transformation
   zone (LLETZ)
large luminal diameter
large-needle biopsy
large-particle biopsy
large, noncompressible appendix
large pharyngeal diverticulum
large red kidney
large, refractory hemorrhoids
large sharp curet
large-volume crystalloid and blood
   resuscitation
large-volume nebulizer
large-volume paracentesis
larger-gauge polypropylene ring
largyneal polyp
LaRoque herniorrhaphy incision
Larrey hernia

Larry probe director
Larry rectal probe
LARS (laparoscopic antireflux surgery)
Larsen tendon-holding forceps
LARSI (lumbar anterior-root stimulator
  implant)
laryngeal abductor
laryngeal carcinoma
laryngeal edema
laryngeal mirror
laryngeal mirror with handle
laryngoflex laryngectomy tube
laryngopharyngectomy
laryngopharynx
laryngoscope (see *endoscope*)
laryngoscope blade
laryngoscopy, direct
larynx
Las Vegas One-Piece cannula
LAS (lymphadenopathy syndrome)
LASE (laser-assisted spinal endoscopy)
laser
  AccuLase excimer
  acupuncture
  alexandrite (solid-state)
  AlexLazr or AlexLAZR
  Apex Plus excimer
  ArF (argon fluorine) excimer
  argon
  argon/krypton
  argon laser
  ArthroProbe
  Aura desktop ENT
  Aurora diode-based dental
  Aurora diode soft tissue
  biocavity
  Candela 405 nm pulsed dye
  Candela SPTL
  carbon dioxide (CO_2)
  CB erbium/2.94
  Centauri Er:YAG
  CHRYS CO_2
  ClearView CO_2
  CO_2 (carbon dioxide)

laser *(cont.)*
  Coherent CO_2 surgical
  Coherent UltraPulse 5000C
  cold
  Cooper
  copper-vapor pulsed
  CorneaSparing LTK system
  coumarin pulsed-dye
  CrTMHo:YAG crystal
  CTE:YAG (CrTmEr:YAG)
  Derma K
  DermaLase ErCr:YSGG laser
    system
  Derma 20
  diode
  dye
  Eclipse TMR
  ELCA
  endoscopic
  Epic ophthalmic 3-in-1
  EpiLaser
  EpiTouch
  erbium:YAG (Er:YAG)
  ErCr:YAG
  excimer
  FCPA2 ultrafast
  FeatherTouch CO_2
  Femtosecond laser keratome
  Fiberlase
  flashlamp pulsed dye
  flashlamp pulsed Nd:YAG
  flashlamp-pumped pulsed dye
  Flexlase 600
  "flying spot" excimer
  gallium-arsenid (GaA)
  Genesis 2000
  GentleLASE Plus
  Gherini-Kauffman endo-otoprobe
  Heart Laser (for transmyocardial
    revascularization)
  He-Ne (helium-neon)
  Hercules Nd:YAG
  HF infrared
  high-energy

laser *(cont.)*
    Ho:YAG (holmium:yttrium-argon-
      garnet) laser
    holmium (Ho)
    holmium:YAG (yttrium-argon-
      garnet)
    Horn endo-otoprobe
    hot
    Hyperion LTK
    Indigo LaserOptic
    ion
    Kaplan PenduLaser 115 surgical
    Kirsch laser welding technique
    KPT
    krypton (red)
    KTP (potassium-titanyl-phosphate)
    KTP/532
    LAIS excimer
    Lambda Plus dye
    Lambda Plus PDL 1 (and PDL 2)
    laparoscopic
    Laser Lancet
    Lasermedic Microlight 830
    LaserPen
    LaserSonics EndoBlade
    LaserSonics Nd-YAG Laser Blade
    LaserSonics SurgiBlade
    Laserthermia
    LaserTripter MDL 3000
    Lasertrolysis
    LaserTweezers
    LightSheer (and LightSheer SC)
      diode
    Lightstic 180 and Lightstic 360
    low-energy (LEL)
    low intensity laser therapy (LILT)
    low-power
    LPI (Laser Photonics, Inc.)
    LTK (laser thermal keratoplasty)
    LX 20
    Lyra
    Mainster retina
    Maloney endo-otoprobe
    Max FiberScan
    Microlase transpupillary diode

laser *(cont.)*
    Microlight 830
    Microprobe
    midinfrared
    Multi-Operatory Dentalaser (MOD)
    Nd:YAG (neodymium: yttrium-
      aluminum-garnet)
    neodymium:YAG (Nd:YAG)
    neodymium:yttrium-aluminum-
      garnet (Nd:YAG)
    Nidek EC-5000 excimer
    NovaLine Litho-S DUV excimer
    NovaPulse CO_2
    Nuvolase 660
    OcuLight
    OcuLight SL diode
    OLM (ophthalmic laser micro-
      endoscope)
    OmniPulse holmium pulsed
    OmniPulse-MAX holmium
    Opmilas 144 Plus
    Opmilas 144 Plus Nd:YAG
    Opmilas CO_2 multipurpose
    OtoLam
    Palomar E2000 ruby
    Paragon CO_2
    PDT
    Pegasus Nd:YAG surgical
    PenduLaser 115 surgical
    PerioLase
    PhotoPoint
    Polaris 1.32 Nd:YAG
    Prima
    Prostalase
    Pulsar CO_2
    PulseMaster
    PulseMaster Nd:YAG
    Pulsolith (coumarin pulsed-dye)
    Q-switched neodymium:YAG
    Q-switched ruby
    red light neon
    RevitaLase erbium cosmetic
    ScleroLaser
    ScleroPlus

laser *(cont.)*
    ScleroPLUS HP
    Selecta 7000
    Sharplan SilkTouch flashscan
      surgical
    Silhouette
    Silk Laser aesthetic carbon dioxide
    Silk Touch laser skin resurfacing
    Skinlight erbium YAG
    Skinscan
    SLP1000 (super long-pulse) diode
    SLS (Spectranetics laser sheath)
    SLS Chromos 694 long pulse ruby
    soft
    SoftLight
    Softscan
    Spectranetics laser sheath (SLS)
    STATLase-SDL diode endoscopic
    SPTL-1b vascular lesion
    STAR excimer
    stereotaxically guided interstitial
    Surgilase 150
    Surgilase CO_2
    Surgilase Nd:YAG
    THC (thulium, holmium,
      chromium):YAG
    Topaz CO_2
    Topaz 30 CO_2
    TruPulse CO_2
    2040 erbium SilkLaser
    UltraFine erbium
    UltraPulse CO_2
    Unica CO_2
    Urolase fiber
    Vbeam
    VersaLight
    VersaPulse
    VersaPulse holmium
    VersaPulse Select holmium
    Versatome
    Visulas Nd:YAG
    VISX excimer laser
    VISX Star S2 excimer
    Vitesse Cos

laser *(cont.)*
    Xanar 20 Ambulase CO_2
    XeCl (xenon-chloride)
    YAG (yttrium-aluminum-garnet)
    YagLAZR or YagLazr
    yttrium-aluminum-garnet (YAG)
    Zeiss Visulas 690s
    Zyoptix
laser ablation
laser-assisted balloon angioplasty
    (LABA)
laser-assisted laparoscopic chole-
    cystectomy
laser-assisted microanastomosis
    (LAMA)
laser-assisted microvascular anasto-
    mosis (LAMA)
laser-assisted spinal endoscopy (LASE)
laser-assisted tissue-welding technique
laser-assisted uvulopalatoplasty (LAUP)
laser ball retractor
laser biomicroscopy
"Laser Bra" procedure (see *L.I.F.T.*)
laser coagulation instrument
laser correlational spectroscopy (LCS)
laser Doppler flowmetry (LDF)
laser Doppler probe
Laser-Flex tracheal tube
Laserflo blood perfusion monitor
    (BPM)
Laserflo Doppler probe
laser guard shield
laser hemorrhoidectomy
laser hook
laser image custom arthroplasty (LICA)
laser-induced thermotherapy (LITT)
laser laparoscope
laser laparoscopy
laser laryngeal suction tube
Laser Lancet
laser lithotripsy
laser mammography system
Lasermedic Microlight 830 laser
laser myringotomy

laser nucleotomy
laser photoablation
laser photocoagulation
laser plume
Laser plume filter
laser probe
LaserPen laser
laser reduction mammoplasty
laser scalpel and quartz rod
LaserScissors
laser sclerosis
Laserscope device
LaserSonics EndoBlade laser
LaserSonics Nd:YAG LaserBlade
   scalpel
LaserSonics Surgiblade
laser stylus profilometer
laser tenaculum
laser tenaculum forceps
laser therapy, OtoLam
laser thermal keratoplasty (LTK)
laser trabeculodissection (LTD)
laser tube
Laserthermia
LaserTripter MDL 3000
Lasertrolysis
LaserTweezers
LaserTweezers 100 (LT100)
laser uterosacral nerve ablation
   (LUNA)
laser vaporization
laser vulsellum forceps
laser welding
Lasette lancet
Lasette laser finger perforator
Lash hysterectomy technique
lashing suture
Lasix (furosemide)
LAST (large-area sensing technology)
   imager
Latarjet, nerve of
late hypercapnia
late menopause
latent cancer

latent infection
lateral anterior drawer stress view
lateral bending view
lateral border of rectus sheath
lateral cervical lymphadenectomy
lateral cervical node dissection
lateral cervical spine film
lateral collateral ligament retractor
lateral compression of the iliac crest
lateral crural steal (LCS)
lateral decubitus film
lateral decubitus position
lateral decubitus view
lateral extension of laceration
lateral film
lateral fixation of arytenoid cartilage
lateral flexion and extension C-spine
   film
lateral gutter
lateral hypopharyngeal pouch (LHP)
lateral incision
lateral internal pelvic reservoir
lateral internal sphincterotomy
lateralizing extremity movement
lateralizing sensory deficit
lateral-lateral pouch
lateral lobe of prostate
lateral oblique fascia
lateral oblique view
lateral park bench position
lateral pectoral nerve
lateral peritoneal reflection
lateral pharyngeal diverticula
lateral reflection of colon
lateral thoracic artery
lateral tilt stress ankle view
lateral to pectoral minor muscle
lateral transverse thigh flap
lateral umbilical fold
lateral utility incision
lateral view
late stoma closure
latex allergy
latex fixation test

LCU (laparoscopic contact ultrasonog-
  raphy)
L-curved incision
LDF (laser-Doppler flowmetry) probe
LDH (lactate dehydrogenase)
LDH (serum lactate dehydrogenase)
LDH-isoenzyme 5
L-diamond electrode
LDL (low-density lipoprotein)
LDL cholesterol
LDL/HDL ratio
LDS digital scanner
LDS stapler
LDS surgical stapler
Le Dentu suture
LE arterial insufficiency ulcer
lead colic
lead-filled mallet
lead pipe appearance
lead pipe colon
lead poisoning
Lead hand
Leadbetter-Politano ureterovesicoplasty
leading bar
leading cord method of colono-
  fiberoscopy
Leading Lady breast prosthesis
leaflet retractor
leak, leakage
  anastomotic
  bile
  pancreatic
  stomal
leakage of cyst
leakage of tracer
leaky gut syndrome
lean body mass
leapfrog position
leather bottle stomach
Leatherman hook
leaves of diaphragm
leaves of mesentery
LeBag ileocolic urinary reservoir
Lebsche knife

Lebsche rongeur
Lebsche saw guide
Lebsche sternum knife
Lebsche wire saw
lecithin
lecithin synthesis, impaired
Lecythophora hoffmannii
Lecythophora mutabilis
LeDuc anastomosis
LeDuc-Camey ileocolostomy
LeDuc-Camey ileocystoplasty
Lee bone graft
leeches (*Hirudo medicinalis*)
Leech Wilkinson cannula
Lee cutting biopsy needle
Lee microvascular clamp
LEEP (loop electrosurgical excision
  procedure)
Lees artery forceps
Lee-White clotting time
Lee-White coagulation time
Lefferts rib shears
LeFort urethral sound
LeFort uterine prolapse repair
left adrenal vein
left arm weakness
left colic artery
left colon
left colonic flexure
left-cutting knife
left decubitus position
left gastric artery
left gastroepiploic artery
left gastroepiploic vein
left gutter
left hepatic artery
left hepatic duct
left hepatic lobectomy
left hepatic vein (LHV)
left internal mammary artery (LIMA)
left lateral decubitus abdominal film
left lateral decubitus position
left lobe
left lobe of liver

left lobe of thyroid
left lower quadrant (LLQ)
left pleural effusion
left pneumothorax
left renal vein
left shift
left-sided colitis
left-sided congestive heart failure
left-sided lesion
left-sided nail
left-sided segmental portal stenosis
left-sided ulcerative colitis
left subdiaphragmatic space
left supraclavicular fossa
left-to-right subtotal pancreatectomy
left upper outer quadrant
left upper quadrant (LUQ)
leg of suture
Leibinger 3-D plate
Leibinger Micro Dynamic mesh graft
Leibinger Micro Plus plate
Leibinger Micro System cranial fixation
   plate
Leibinger Micro System plate-holding
   forceps
Leibinger Micro System pliers
Leica Aristoplan laser-scanning micro-
   scope
Leigh disease
Leiner disease
leiomyoma (pl. leiomyomata)
   epithelioid
   esophageal
   gastric
   uterine
leiomyosarcoma
   gastric
   renal
   small intestine
Leishmania brasiliensis
Leishmania donovani
Leishmania tropica
leishmaniasis
Lejeune thoracic forceps

LeJour technique of reduction mammo-
   plasty
LeJour-type breast reduction, modified
Leksell cobalt-60 gamma knife
Leksell Gamma knife
Leksell laminectomy rongeur
Leksell rongeur
Leksell rongeur forceps
Leksell-Stille thoracic rongeur
Leland-Jones vascular clamp
LEL (low-energy laser)
LeMaitre biliary catheter
Lembert suture
Lemmon rib contractor
Lempert bone rongeur
Lempert fine curette
Lempert malleus cutter
Lempert narrow elevator
Lempert paracentesis knife
Lempert periosteal elevator
Lempert rongeur
Lempert rongeur forceps
lenercept tumor necrosis factor (TNF)
lengthening, esophageal
Lennhoff sign
Lente Iletin II (insulin zinc [pork])
Lente Insulin
Lente L (insulin zinc [pork])
lenticular carcinoma
lentigo maligna melanoma
lentigo-polypose-digestive syndrome
Leonard Arm pneumatic action support
   device
Leonard catheter
Leo test
LE (lupus erythematosus) panniculitis
Lepley-Ernst tube
leptomeningeal carcinoma
leptospiral jaundice
leptospirosis
   icteric
   icterohemorrhagic
LeRoy clip-applying forceps
LES (lower esophageal sphincter)
   pressure

LES incompetence
LESA (lower esophageal sphincter
   augmentation)
Leser-Trelat sign
Lesgaft hernia
Lesgaft space
Lesgaft triangle
lesion
   acanthotic
   accessible
   acquired
   aneurysmal
   angiocentric immunoproliferative
   angulated
   aortic arch
   aphthous-type
   apple-core
   areolar
   Armanni-Ebstein
   atherosclerotic
   Baehr-Lohlein
   Bankart
   benign lymphoepithelial
   benign pigmented
   bifurcation
   bird's nest
   blastic
   bleeding
   Blumenthal
   Bracht-Wachter
   bull's-eye
   calcified
   cardiac valvular
   caviar
   central
   cherry-red endobronchial lesion
      of Kaposi sarcoma
   choristoma
   circular cherry-red
   coin
   complex
   concentric
   congenital
   constrictive

lesion *(cont.)*
   coronary artery
   Councilman
   critical
   cryosurgical
   culprit
   cystic
   de novo
   depigmented
   Dieulafoy
   diffuse
   discrete
   duct
   Duret
   Ebstein
   eccentric
   eccentric restenosis
   endobronchial
   enlarging cystic
   erythematous
   extrinsic
   fingertip
   flat
   florid duct
   flow-compromising
   flow-limiting
   fluctuant
   focal
   Forrest gastroduodenal
   freckle-like
   friable
   Ghon primary
   gross
   hamartomatous
   hemodynamically significant
   high-grade
   high-grade obstructive
   hilar
   Hill-Sachs
   histologic
   hourglass-shaped
   hyperplastic
   ileal
   impaction

lesion *(cont.)*
    indiscriminate
    infiltrating
    inflammatory
    intracranial mass
    intrinsic stenotic
    invasive
    irritative
    Janeway
    jet
    left-sided
    lichenoid
    linear cutaneous
    local
    Löhlein-Baehr
    lower motor neuron
    lymphoepithelial
    lytic
    macroscopic multicentric
    malignant
    Mallory-Weiss
    mesenteric vascular
    microscopic multicentric
    mixed
    molecular
    mongolian spotlike
    multifocal
    multiverrucous friable
    napkin-ring
    napkin-ring annular
    necrotic
    nodular
    noninfective endocardial
    occlusive
    occult
    onion scale
    onionskin
    organic
    ostial
    oval cherry-red raised
    papillary
    papular
    papulonecrotic
    partial

lesion *(cont.)*
    peripheral
    photon-deficient
    pigmented (melanotic)
    pigmented satellite
    polypoid
    precancerous
    precursor
    premalignant
    preneoplastic intraductal
    primary
    punctate keratotic
    purpuric
    purulent
    radial sclerosing
    raised, slightly pigmented
    regurgitant
    rheumatic
    right-sided
    ring-wall
    satellite
    scirrhous
    secondary
    segmental
    serial
    sessile
    skin
    skip
    solitary
    space-occupying
    spherical
    squamous anal intraepithelial
    squamous intraepithelial
    stenotic
    structural
    subtotal
    supranuclear
    suspicious
    systemic
    tandem
    target
    telangiectatic
    tight
    tortuous

lesion *(cont.)*
   total
   traumatic
   trophic
   tuberculoid
   tubular
   type A, B, or C
   ulcerated
   ulcerative
   unstable
   upper motor neuron
   valvular regurgitant
   vascular
   vasculitic
   vegetative
   vulvar
   wire-loop
LESP (lower esophageal sphincter pressure)
lesser curvature of stomach
lesser curvature ulcer
lesser esophageal sphincter (LES)
lesser multangular bone
lesser omentum
lesser palatine artery
lesser palatine foramina
lesser palatine nerve
lesser pancreas
lesser peritoneal sac
lesser sac of peritoneal cavity
Lester Martin modification of Duhamel operation
Lester muscle forceps
lethal neoplasm
lethargy
Letournel plate
letrazuril
letrozole
leucine aminopeptidase (LAP) test
leucine-induced hypoglycemia
leucovorin and fluorouracil
leukapheresis, ALPS (autologous l., processing, and storage)
leukemia

Leukine (sargramostim)
leukocyte, fecal
leukocytic infiltrate
leukocytosis
leukopenia
leukoplakia
   esophageal
   hairy
   oral
leukotrienes
LeuTech infection imaging agent
LeuTech radiolabeled antibody kit
LeuTech radiolabeled imaging agent
leuvectin
levamisole HCl
Levaquin (levofloxacin)
levator ani muscle
levator ani syndrome
levator muscle imbrication
levator span
Levbid (hyoscyamine sulfate)
LeVeen catheter
LeVeen inflator
LeVeen peritoneal shunt
LeVeen valve
level
   air-fluid
   Albarran deflecting
   blood glucose
   CA 19-9
   metabolite
   plasma glucose
   serum complement
   serum transaminase
   suppressed thyrotropin
level I axillary lymph node (low; lateral to pectoral minor)
level II axillary lymph node (middle; deep to pectoral minor)
level III axillary lymph node (high; medial to pectoral minor)
level of cricoid cartilage
level of fluid
level of nipple

Levin tube
levobupivacaine
levofloxacin
Levo-T (levothyroxine sodium)
Levothroid (levothyroxine sodium)
levothyroxine sodium (T$_4$)
Levovist ultrasound contrast agent
Levoxyl (levothyroxine sodium)
Levsin PB drops (hyoscyamine sulfate; phenobarbital; alcohol)
Levsin/SL (hyoscyamine sulfate)
Levsin with Phenobarbital (hyoscyamine sulfate; phenobarbital)
Levsinex (hyoscyamine sulfate)
Levsinex Timecaps
Levulan photodynamic therapy (PDT)
levulose test
Lewin bonc-holding clamp
Lewin bone-holding forceps
Lewin spinal-perforating forceps
Lewis laryngeal tube
Lewis laryngectomy tube
Lewis nail
Lewis periosteal elevator
Lewis periosteal rasp
Lewis rasp
Lewis-Tanner subtotal esophagectomy and reconstruction
Lewy-Holinger Teflon injection needle
Lewy-Rubin Teflon glycerine mixture injection needle
Lewy Teflon glycerine mixture syringe
Lexan quick connect
Lexer chisel
Lexer gouge
lexipafant
Lexirin
Leyden disease
Leyla brain retractor
LFT (liver function test)
LGT laryngectomy tube
LGV (lymphogranuloma venereum)
LHMT (low-range heparin management test)

L hook knife
LHP (lateral hypopharyngeal pouch)
LHV (left hepatic vein)
Li, Lm, Ls location of esophageal varices
liarozole fumarate
Liazal (liarozole fumarate)
liberator elevator
libido, decreased
Librax
LICA (laser image custom arthroplasty)
Lich-Gregoire kidney transplant surgery
Lich ureteral implantation in transplantation surgery
lichenoid lesion
lichenoid papule
lichen planus
Lichtenberg needle
Lichtenstein hernia repair
Lichtenstein Hernia Institute
Lichtenstein herniorrhaphy
Lichtenstein onlay patch repair
Licox monitoring device
LICU (laparoscopic intracorporeal ultrasound)
Liddle aorta clamp
lidocaine topical anesthetic
Lidoject-2 (lidocaine HCl)
LIE (latissimus dorsi, iliac crest, external oblique)
Lieberkühn (Lieberkuehn)
Lieberkühn crypt
Lieberkühn gland
lienogastric ligament
lienorenal ligament
lienteric diarrhea
lienteric stool
life expectancy, limited
lifelong constipation
lifelong obesity
lifelong suppressive therapy
LIFE OxygenPac
LifeShirt monitoring system
Lifestream coronary dilatation catheter

linitis plastica
Linnartz intestinal clamp
lint-free drape
Linton-Nachlas tube
Linton shunt
Linvatec autoclavable camera
Linvatec driver
Linvatec laparoscope
Linvatec microdebrider
Linvatec rigid laparoscope
Linvatec 7570R 0° 10 mm rigid
    laparoscope
lion forceps
lion-jaw forceps
liothyronine sodium
liotrix
lip lift
lip shave
lipancreatin
lipase (also see *enzyme*)
    pancreatic
    serum
lipase enzyme
lipase test for liver function
lipemia, alimentary
lipid emulsion
lipid infusion
lipid island
lipid-laden hepatocytes
lipid panel
lipid profile
lipidosis, cerebroside
lipids, serum
lipiodol CT
Lipisorb nutritional therapy
Lipitor (atorvastatin calcium)
lipoatrophic diabetes
lipoblastic sarcoma
lipodystrophy, intestinal
lipofuscin
lipolytic enzyme
lipoma
    cord
    hernial
    pancreatic

lipoma of spermatic cord
lipomatosis of pancreas, congenital
lipomatous ileocecal valve
lipomatous-like tissue
lipomatous polyp
lipopolysaccharide binding protein
    (LBP)
lipopolysaccharide (LPS) receptor
lipoprotein
    high-density (HDL)
    low-density (LDL)
    very low-density (VLDL)
lipoprotein X level
liposarcoma
liposhaver
liposome encapsulated doxorubicin
    citrate complex
Lipostructure technique
Liposyn II fat emulsion solution
liquefaction necrosis
liquefied argon gas
LiquiBand topical wound-closure glue
Liqui-Char (activated charcoal)
Liqui-Coat HD (barium sulfate)
liquid antacid
Liquiderm liquid adhesive bandage
liquid diarrhea
liquid diet
liquid food dysphagia
liquid material
Liqui-Doss (mineral oil)
liquid stools
Lister bandage scissors
Lister bougie
Lister scissors
Lister sinus forceps
Liston amputation knife
Liston bone cutter
Liston bone-cutting forceps
Liston bone rongeur
Liston forceps
Liston-Key bone-cutting forceps
Liston-Key-Horsley rib shears
Liston-Littauer bone rongeur

liver *(cont.)*
 alcoholic fatty
 ballotable
 bare area of
 biliary cirrhotic
 black
 blue
 brimstone
 bronze
 cadaveric
 capsule of
 cardiac impression on
 caudate lobe of
 centrilobular region of
 cholestatic
 cirrhosis of
 cirrhotic
 degenerative
 degraded
 diaphragmatic surface of
 dome of
 duodenal impression on
 echogenic
 end-stage
 esophageal groove of
 fatty
 fatty infiltration of
 fibrotic
 finely fatty foamy
 finger fracture of
 floating
 foamy
 frosted
 gastric impression on
 "golfball"
 green
 HepatAssist bioartificial
 hobnail
 icing
 infantile
 iron
 lardaceous
 large-droplet fatty
 left lobe of

liver *(cont.)*
 lobectomy of
 metastasis to
 nodular
 noncirrhotic
 nutmeg
 pigmented
 polycystic
 polylobar
 potato
 pyogenic
 quadrate lobe of
 renal impression on
 right lobe of
 sago
 shock
 shrunken
 small-droplet fatty
 stasis
 sugar-icing
 SYBIOL (synthetic bio-liver)
 tender
 trisegmentectomy of
 undersurface of
 visceral surface of
 wandering
 waxy
 wedge biopsy of
liver abscess
liver adenocarcinoma
liver allotransplantation
liver and peritoneum biopsy needle
liver and spleen were congested
liver bed, surface of
liver bile
liver biopsy
liver biopsy needle (see also *needle*)
 Colapinto transjugular
 Franklin-Silverman
 Jamshidi
 Klatskin
 Menghini
 Tru-Cut
 Tru-Cut/Vim Silverman

lobe *(cont.)*
  lateral
  left
  lower
  median
  pyramidal
  quadrate
  Riedel
  right
  upper
lobectomy
  contralateral subtotal thyroid
  hepatic
  ipsilateral thyroid
  left liver
  partial liver
  right liver
  thyroid
lobucavir
lobular architecture of liver
lobular carcinoma
lobular carcinoma in situ (LCIS)
lobular carcinoma of breast
lobular hepatitis
lobular panniculitis
lobular pattern
lobulated mass
lobulated tumor
lobulation
lobule
local and systemic capillary leak
local anesthesia (see *anesthesia*)
local control
local death
local edema
local epinephrine injection
local infection
local infiltration technique
local invasion by primary lesion
localization-compression grid plate
localization of infection
localization, preoperative
localized abscess
localized bleeding

localized irritation
localized necrosis
localized pain
localized resection
localizing tenderness
localizing test
local lesion
locally invasive tumor
local node
local peritoneal irritation
locating pin
LoCholest Light (cholestyramine resin)
Locilex (pexiganan acetate)
Locke clamp
Locke elevator
locked intramedullary nail
locked suture
locker room syndrome
Lockhart Mummary fistula director
locking loop suture
locking nail
locking pliers
locking suture
lock-stitch suture
Lockwood-Allis intestinal forceps
Lockwood tissue forceps
Lockwood underminer
locomotor
Lo-Contour tube with Murphy tip
locoregional cancer recurrence
locoregional residual disease
loculated fluid
locus of infection
Lofgren syndrome
logroll the patient
Löhlein-Baehr lesion
loin pain hematuria syndrome (LPHS)
lollipop-tree sign (on x-ray)
Lomanate (diphenoxylate HCl; atropine
  sulfate)
Lonalac feeding
Lonalac powder
London College forceps
Lone Star retractor

long-acting thyroid stimulator (LATS)
long-acting thyroid-stimulating
    hormone (LATS) test
long axial alignment guide
long axial oblique view
long axis of spleen
long-axis parasternal view
long axis view
long chain acyl-CoA dehydrogenase
    deficiency (LCAD)
long chain 3-hydroxyacyl-coenzyme A
    dehydrogenase deficiency (LCHAD)
long chain triglycerides (LCT)
long dolphin-nose grasper
longer-acting anesthetic
longer halflife
Long forceps
long grasping forceps, aggressive teeth,
    single-action
long grasping forceps, wavy teeth,
    tissue well, single-action
long intestinal tube
longitudinal esophageal stricture
longitudinal filleting of the pancreas
longitudinal incision
longitudinal muscle contraction
longitudinal myotomy
longitudinal orientation
longitudinal suture
long-limb gastric bypass
Longmire-Gutgemann gastric
    reconstruction
long-nose retriever snare
Longo hemorrhoidectomy
Lonox (diphenoxylate HCl; atropine
    sulfate)
long Péan clamp
Longport Digital Scanner (LDS)
long-segment intrahepatic biliary
    stricture
long segment region
long-standing adenomatous hyperplasia
long-standing stimulation of the thyroid
long splenic pedicle

long taper/stiff shaft Glidewire
long-term duodenobiliary reflux
long-term side effects of chemotherapy
long-term thyroxine therapy
long-term treatment
long thermistor
long thoracic nerve
loop
    afferent
    air-filled
    alpha sigmoid
    bowel
    colonic
    contiguous
    Cutting LOOP
    diathermic
    double reverse alpha sigmoid
    duodenal
    efferent
    gamma transverse colon
    intestinal
    ischemic bowel
    jejunal
    N-shaped sigmoid
    puborectalis
    sentinel
    sigmoid
    smart
    Surg-I-Loop
    vessel
    V+Loop
loop choledochojejunostomy
loop colostomy
loop diuretic
looped cautery
loop electrosurgical excision procedure
    (LEEP)
loop-end ileostomy
loop esophagojejunostomy
loop forceps
loop gastrojejunostomy
loop ileostomy
loop jejunostomy
loop mattress suture

loop of jejunum, efferent
loop of redundant colon
loopogram
loop ostomy bridge
loop suture
loop-type snare forceps
loop-type stone-crushing forceps
loose stools
loperamide
lopinavir/ritonavir
Lo-Pro tracheal tube
Lo-Pro tube with Murphy tip
LORAD StereoGuide stereotactic
　　breast biopsy system
Lorain-Levi dwarfism
Lord dilatation of hemorrhoids
Lord hemorrhoidectomy
lordotic view
Lore suction tube and tip-holding
　　forceps
Lorenz cranial plate
Lorenz PC/TC scissors ultra-sharp
　　knife
Lorenz shears
Lorna towel forceps
Lortat-Jacob hepatic resection
Losec (omeprazole)
loss of acidic environment
loss of aortic contour
loss of appetite
loss of energy
loss of heterozygosity (LOH)
loss of pulmonary vascular
　　autoregulation
loss of sigmoid curve
loss of splenic function
loss of urethral tethering
Lotronex (alosetron HCl)
Lottes pin
Lottes triflanged medullary nail
lotus position
Louis mastopexy
Louis plate
Loumanen airway (or Luomanen)

loupe (also see *microscope*)
　　Berger magnifying
　　binocular
　　binocular magnifying
　　fiberoptic (also fibreoptic)
　　Heine G series
　　Heine K series
　　low-power
　　Miltex
　　optical
　　Scanlan
　　SheerVision
　　surgical
loupe magnification
Love-Adson periosteal elevator
Love-Gruenwald alligator forceps
Love-Gruenwald intervertebral disk
　　forceps
Love-Gruenwald intervertebral disk
　　rongeur
Love-Gruenwald pituitary forceps
Love-Gruenwald pituitary rongeur
Love-Kerrison cervical rongeur
Love-Kerrison laminectomy rongeur
Love-Kerrison rongeur forceps
Lovelace lung grasping forceps
Lovelace thyroid traction forceps
Love nerve root hook
Love nerve root retractor
Lovenox (enoxaparin)
Love uvula retractor
low amino acid level
low anterior resection (LAR)
low anterior resection in combination
　　with coloanal anastomosis
　　(LAR/CAA)
low-calorie diet
low cardiac output
low-compliance hydrostatic balloon
low-contact dynamic compression
　　(LC-DCP) plate
low-contrast film
low-current electrocautery
low-density lipoprotein (LDL)

low-density beta lipoprotein deficiency
low-dose dexamethasone suppression
   test
Lowe-Breck cartilage knife
Lowe-Breck meniscectomy knife
low-energy laser (LEL)
lower airway sounds
lower border of the pancreas
lower esophageal sphincter (LES)
lower esophageal sphincter augmenta-
   tion (LESA)
lower esophageal sphincter pressure
   (LESP)
lower esophageal sphincter resting
   pressure
lower gall duct forceps
lower gastrointestinal tract
lower hand retractor
lower leg saphenous vein
lower motor neuron lesion
lower panendoscopy
lower pole of the thyroid
lower respiratory tract smear
lower soft tissue attenuation of the
   accordion sign
lower tract obstruction
low-fat diet
low-fiber diet
low-grade encapsulated follicular
   carcinoma
low-grade fever
low-grade malignancy
low intensity pulsed ultrasound
low imperforate anus
low intensity laser therapy (LILT) laser
low intermittent suction
low-level endotoxemia
low lung compliance
Lowman bone-holding clamp
Lowman bone-holding forceps
Lowman-Gerster bone clamp
Lowman hand retractor
Lowman-Hoglund bone-holding clamp
Lowman-Hoglund chisel

low pelvic anastomosis
low pH
low phosphorus
low-pitched bowel sounds
low-power diet
low-power laser
low-power loupe
low-pressure catheter
low-pressure shunt
Low Profile PMV 2001 Purple
   tracheostomy
low-protein diet
low-range heparin management test
   (LHMT)
low-residue diet
low-residue feeding
low-resistance fundoplication
low-roughage diet
Lowsium Plus (magaldrate; simethi-
   cone)
Lowsley prostatic tractor
low-sodium diet
low-stage disease
low transverse incision
low urethral pressure (LUP)
low urine calcium
low-viscosity fluid
low-voltage harness
LPHS (loin pain hematuria syndrome)
LPI (Laser Photonics, Inc.) laser
LPPS hydroxyapatite adhesive
LPS (lipopolysaccharide)
LPS balloon
LPS Peel-Away introducer
LR (lactated Ringer) solution
LRT (living related transplant)
LRYGBP (laparoscopic Roux-en-Y
   gastric bypass procedure)
L-shaped incision
L-shaped microplate
L-shaped plate
LSTAT (life support trauma and
   transport) system
LTD (laser trabeculodissection)

L-thyroxine
LTK (laser thermal keratoplasty)
LT.01 lithotriptor
LT.02 piezoelectric lithotriptor
LTS (Liquid Treatment System)
Lubri-Flex stent
Lucae bone mallet
Lucae dressing forceps
Lucae mallet
Lucae nerve hook
Lucas chisel
Lucas gouge
Lucey-Driscoll syndrome
Luck-Bishop bone saw
Lucké carcinoma
Ludloff incision
Luekosilk bandage
Luer bone rongeur
Luer-Friedman bone rongeur
Luer-Hartmann rongeur
Luer hemorrhoid forceps
Luer-Koerte gallstone scoop
Luer lock
Luer-Lok syringe
Luer retractor
Luer rongeur forceps
Luer trachea retractor
Luer-Whiting rongeur forceps
Lugol solution
Lugol stain
Luhr Microfixation cranial plate
Luhr Microfixation System plate-
   holding forceps
Luhr Microfixation System pliers
Luhr microplate
Luhr miniplate
Luhr pan plate
Lukens PGA synthetic absorbable
   suture
Lukens trachea retractor
Lukes-Collins classification of
   lymphoma
LULA (laparoscopy under local
   anesthesia)

lumbar anterior-root stimulator implant
   (LARSI)
lumbar appendicitis
lumbar arachnoid peritoneal shunt
lumbar drain
lumbar epidural abscess
lumbar epidural anesthesia
lumbar hernia
lumbar lamina retractor
lumbar puncture needle
lumbar region
lumbar thecoperitoneal shunt
lumbar vein
lumbocostoabdominal triangle
lumboperitoneal (LP) shunt
lumbosacral fusion elevator
lumen (pl. lumina)
   appendiceal
   bile duct
   bowel
   cystic duct
   duct
   duodenal
   esophageal
   gastroduodenal
   intestinal
   monitoring
   scalloped bowel
lumenal antigen
LumenHance (manganese chloride
   tetrahydrate) imaging agent
Lumina guidewire
luminal bacteria
luminal colonic pH
luminal diameter
luminal microorganisms
luminal narrowing
lumpectomy and radiation
lumpectomy of breast
lumpiness in breast
lumpy material
LUNA (laparoscopic uterine nerve
   ablation)

LUNA (laser uterosacral nerve
  ablation)
Lund Browder burn diagram, modified
Lunderquist guidewire
Lunderquist-Ring torque guide
Lundh meal
Lundholm plate
Lundh test
lung
  airless
  atelectatic
  bird-breeder's
  black
  cardiac
  cheese handler's
  coal-miner's
  drowned
  dull purple
  emphysematous
  farmer's
  fibrinoid
  fissures of
  grain handler's
  hemorrhagic consolidation of
  hilum of
  honeycomb
  humidifier
  hyperlucent
  hypoplastic
  liverlike
  malt worker's
  mason's
  meat wrapper's
  miner's
  normal gas exchange in
  pigeon-breeder's
  rudimentary
  shock
  shrunken
  silo-filler's
  silver finisher's
  smoker's
  thresher's
  vanishing

lung *(cont.)*
  welder's
  wet
  white
lung abscess
lung adenocarcinoma
lung apex
lung base
lung cancer
lung capacity
lung flukes
lung-grasping forceps (see *forceps*)
lung mass
lung metastasis
lung parenchyma
lung plague
lung retractor
lung root
lung stone
lung tumor
lung tumor resection
lung volume reduction surgery (LVRS)
Luongo hand retractor
LUP (low urethral pressure)
lupoid hepatitis
LUQ (left upper quadrant)
Luque II plate
Luque rod
Luque rod scissors
Luque-Galveston plate
Lurz hemorrhoidal suction ligator
LUS (laparoscopic ultrasound)
Lusk instruments for pediatric
  endoscopic sinus surgery
luteinizing hormone
Lu-Tex
Lutkens sphincter
Lutrin photosensitizer
Luttke test
Luxtec fiberoptic system
LVEDP (left ventricular end diastolic
  pressure)
LVRS (lung volume reduction surgery)
L-wedge electrode

lymphadenopathy syndrome (LAS)
lymphangiectasia
  intestinal
  primary intestinal
  intestinal
lymphangiectatic protein-losing
  enteropathy
lymphangioma
lymphangioma of mesentery
lymphangioma of small bowel
lymphangiomatous cyst
lymphangiosarcoma
lymphangitis
lymphapheresis
lymphatic and hematogenous distant
  metastasis
lymphatic channel
lymphatic compression
lymphatic drainage
lymphatic edema
lymphatic flow
lymphatic fluid
lymphatic invasion
lymphatic medulla
lymphatic obstruction
lymphatic sarcoma
lymphatic spread
lymphatics
  abdominal
  inguinal
  mediastinal
  perirectal
Lymphazurin (isosulfan blue) dye
Lymphedema Alert Bracelet
lymphedema edema
lymphedema, neonatal
lymphoblastoid interferon, human
  (L-IFN)
lymphocele, extraperitoneal
lymphocyte-depleted Hodgkin disease
lymphocyte immune globulin
lymphocyte invasion
lymphocyte, sinusoidal
lymphocytic choriomeningitis virus
  (LCMV)

lymphocytic colitis
lymphocytotoxic antibody
lymphoepithelial lesions
lymphogenous
lymphogranuloma inguinale
lymphogranuloma venereum (LGV)
lymphoid cell thymoma
lymphoid cholangitis
lymphoid hyperplasia
lymphoid polyp
lymphoid tumor
lymphoma
  African Burkitt
  Burkitt
  diffuse
  extranodal T-cell
  follicular
  follicular center cell
  gastric B-cell
  gastric T-cell
  GI tract
  histiocytic
  Hodgkin
  immunoblastic
  infiltrate
  infiltrative
  intestinal
  large cell
  large cleaved cell
  large noncleaved cell
  Lennert
  lymphoblastic
  lymphocytic
  malignant
  mantle cell
  Mediterranean
  mixed lymphocytic-histiocytic
  mixed small and large cell
  nodular
  non-African Burkitt
  non-Hodgkin
  plasmacytoid
  polypoid
  primary GI tract

lymphoma *(cont.)*
   Rappaport classification of gastric
   small cell
   small cleaved cell
   small intestinal malignant
   small lymphocytic
   small noncleaved cell
   stomach
   U-cell
   ulcerative
lymphomatosis, struma
lymphonodular hyperplasia
lymphoproliferative disorder
lymphoproliferative syndrome
lymphosarcoma
lymphoscintigraphy
Lynch syndrome I
Lynch syndrome II

LYOfoam A dressing
LYOfoam C dressing
LYOfoam T dressing
LYOfoam tracheostomy dressing
lyophilized aortic homograft
lyophilized bone graft
lyophilized liposomal delivery system
lypressin
Lyra laser system
Lyrelle patch
lyse, lysed ("adhesions were lysed")
lysis of adhesions
Lysonics handle tubing
Lysonix 2000 soft tissue aspirator
"lytes" (electrolytes)
lytic lesion
lytic virus
Lytren electrolyte solution

M, m

Maalox (aluminum hydroxide;
    magnesium hydroxide)
Maalox Plus
Maalox TC
Maalox Whip
MAAP scan
MAA shunt fraction
MAb monoclonal antibody
MAb-170 monoclonal antibody
MAC (monitored anesthesia care)
Macewen hernia operation
Macewen herniorrhaphy
Machado-Guerreiro test
Machida choledochoscope
MacIntosh laryngoscope
Maciol laparoscopic suture needle set
Mackenrodt, ligament of
MacKenty periosteal elevator
Mackenzie point
MacLean test
macroaggregated albumin (MAA) lung
    perfusion scan
macroamylasemia
macrogenitosomia praecox
macroglobulinemia, Waldenstrom
Macrokine (WF10)
macrolobular cirrhosis
macronodular cirrhosis

macrophage function
macrophages, ceroid-laden
Macroplastique implant
macroscopic appearance
macroscopic damage
macroscopic island
macroscopic multicentric lesions
Madayag biopsy needle
Maddacrawler
Madden herniorrhaphy
Madden repair of incisional hernia
Madigan prostatectomy
Madurella mycetomatis
mafenide acetate
magakaryocytosis
magaldrate
Magaldrate Plus (magaldrate;
    simethicone)
Magalox Plus (aluminum hydroxide;
    magnesium hydroxide; simethicone)
Magerl screw placement in lower
    cervical spine
maggots (*Lucilia caesar; Phaenicia
    sericata; Pharmia regina*)
Magill catheter-introducing forceps
Magill curve
Magill forceps
Magill insulated suction tube

Magill suction tube
Magnacal liquid feeding
Magnalox (aluminum hydroxide;
    magnesium hydroxide)
Magnatril
MAGneedle controller
magnesia, milk of
magnesium (Mg)
magnesium citrate
magnesium, serum
magnesium sulfate
magnesium trisilicate
magnet, eye
magnetic-controlled suturing (MCS)
magnetic endoscope imaging (MEI)
magnetic positional imaging (MPI)
magnetic resonance cholangiography
    (MRC)
magnetic resonance cholangiography
    with HASTE
magnetic resonance cholangio-
    pancreatography (MRCP)
magnetic resonance imaging (MRI)
magnetic resonance mammography
    (MRM)
magnetic resonance neurography
    (MRN)
magnetic resonance pancreatography
    (MRP)
magnetic resonance splenoportography
magnetic susceptibility test
Magnevist (gadopentetate dimeglumine)
magnification, power
magnifying loupe
Magnox (aluminum hydroxide;
    magnesium hydroxide)
Magnum guidewire
MAGPI (meatal advancement, glanulo-
    plasty, penoscrotal junction
    meatotomy) operation
Magrina-Bookwalter vaginal retractor
mahogany-colored stools
MAI (*Mycobacterium avium-intracellu-
    lare*)

Maingot clamp
main pancreatic duct (MPD)
main route of drainage
Mainstay urologic soft tissue anchor
Mainster retina laser
maintaining equilibrium
maintenance fluids
main tumor
Mainz pouch urinary reservoir
Maison retractor
major crossmatch
major duodenal papilla
major organ injury
major water loss
Maki pylorus-preserving gastrectomy
malabsorption
    congenital lactose
    congenital sucrose-isomaltose
    glucose-galactose
    sucrose-isomaltose, congenital
    tryptophan
malabsorption and weight loss
malabsorption of fats
malabsorption of vitamin B_{12}
malabsorption state
malabsorption syndrome
malabsorptive diarrhea
malaise
malaise and fever
malaria
    acute
    algid
    autochthonous
    avian
    benign tertian
    bilious remittent
    cerebral
    congenital
    double tertian
    dysenteric algid
    falciparum
    gastric algid
    hemolytic
    hemorrhagic

malaria *(cont.)*
   induced
   intermittent
   malignant tertian
   nonan
   ovale
   pernicious
   quartan
   quotidian
   relapsing
   remittent
   tertian
   therapeutic
   transfusion
   vivax
malarial cachexia
malarial cirrhosis
malarial granuloma
malarial hepatitis
malaria-like illness
malarial knobs
malarial necrosis
malarial pigment
malarial pneumonitis
malaria smear
Malarone (atovaquone/proguanil)
Malassezia furfur
Malassezia pachydermatis
Malcolm-Lynn C-RXF cervical
   retractor frame
Malcolm-Lynn rongeur
Malcolm-Rand radiolucent headrest
Malcolm-Rand retractor
maldigestive diarrhea
male breast cancer
male gynecomastia
male Luer lock
male reamer
male Undies
Malecot catheter
Malecot drain, two-wing
Malecot drain, four-wing
Malecot gastrostomy tube

malformation
   anorectal
   arteriovenous (AVM)
   congenital cardiac
   congenital cavernous of splenic vein
   Dieulafoy vascular
malignancy
   aggressive
   borderline
   colorectal
   extrahepatic duct
   grading of
   hematologic
   hematopoietic
   high-grade
   intrahepatic duct
   intraocular
   low-grade
   metastatic
   neuroendocrine
   pancreatic
   primary
   prostatic
   staging of
   thyroid
   unresectable
malignancy of extrahepatic ducts
malignancy of intrahepatic ducts
malignant atrophic papulosis
malignant B-cell syndrome
malignant biliary obstruction
malignant carcinoid syndrome
malignant cell
malignant change
malignant degeneration
malignant dysphagia
malignant edema
malignant fibrous histiocytoma
malignant gastrointestinal disorder
malignant glioma tumor
malignant hyperphenylalaninemia
malignant hypertension
malignant insulinoma

malignant jaundice
malignant lentigo
malignant lentigo melanoma
malignant lesion
malignant lymphoma
malignant melanoma
malignant melanoma in situ
malignant melanoma metastatic to heart
malignant mesenchymal tumor
malignant mesothelioma
malignant mole
malignant mucoid adenocarcinoma
malignant neoplasm
malignant nephrosclerosis
malignant neurilemmoma
malignant obstructive jaundice
malignant pheochromocytoma
malignant polyp
malignant teratoma of heart
malignant tertian malaria
malignant thymoma
malignant thyroid nodule
malignant tumor
malignant tumor of thymus gland
malignant ulcer
Malignant dysphagia
Malis angled-up bipolar forceps
Malis bipolar cautery forceps
Malis bipolar coagulation forceps
Malis brain retractor
Malis elevator
Malis irrigation forceps
Malis-Jensen microbipolar forceps
Malis jeweler bipolar forceps
Malis nerve hook
Malis neurological scissors
Malis tube
malleable aluminum shaft
malleable aluminum stylet
malleable blade
malleable hook
malleable metal finger splint bandage
malleable plate
malleable probe

malleable retractor
malleable ribbon retractor
malleable scoop
malleable stylet
mallet (see also *hammer*)
    Acufex
    Bergman
    bone
    boxwood
    cervical
    copper
    Cottle
    Crane
    Doyen bone
    Gerzog
    Gerzog bone
    Hajek
    Heath
    Henning
    Hibbs
    Kirk
    lead-filled
    Lucae
    Lucae bone
    Mead
    Meyerding
    Miltex
    Ombredanne
    Ralks
    Richards
    Rush
    slotted
    Steinbach
    Surgical No Bounce
    Swanson
    Williger bone
    Wolfe-Boehler
mallet deformity
mallet finger
mallet fracture
mallet toe
malleus nipper
Mallinckrodt Laser-Flex endotracheal
    tube

Mallinckrodt Medical tracheal tube
Mallory body
Mallory-Head rasp
Mallory hyaline body
Mallory-Weiss lesion
Mallory-Weiss mucosal rupture
Mallory-Weiss mucosal syndrome
Mallory-Weiss mucosal tear
Mallory-Weiss procedure
Mallory-Weiss rupture
Mallory-Weiss syndrome
Mallory-Weiss tear
Malmstrom cup
malnourished
malnourishment
malnutrition
   profound
   protein-calorie (PCM)
   protein-energy (PEM)
malodorous fluid
malodorous stools
Maloney bougie
Maloney endo-otoprobe laser
Maloney mercury-filled esophageal
   dilator
malpighian body
malrotation of intestine
malt worker's lung
Maltsupex (nondiastatic barley malt
   extract)
Maltz cartilage knife
Maltz rasp
Maly test
Mam drill
mamillary suture
mammaplasty (see *mammoplasty*)
mammary atrophy
mammary calculus
mammary duct obstruction
mammary ductal ectasia
mammary ductogram
mammary dysplasia
mammary galactogram
mammary gland

mammary milk line
mammary ptosis
mammastatin protein
Mammex TR computer-aided
   mammography system
mammogram, mammography
   annual
   baseline
   bilateral
   computed tomography laser
   computed tomography laser
      mammography (CTLM)
   contoured tilting compression
   CT laser (CTLM)
   CTLM
   ductographic
   Dynamic Optical Breast Imaging
      System (DOBI)
   Egan
   GE Senographe 20001 digital
   laser
   magnetic resonance mammography
      (MRM)
   Mammex TR
   Opdima digital
   Palpagraph
   prebiopsy
   repeat
   scintimammography
   Senographe 2000D digital
   SenoScan
   Softscan laser
   step-oblique
   TDMS (Trex digital mammography
      system)
   Trex digital mammography system
      (TDMS)
   xeromammogram
   XMG (x-ray mammogram)
mammogram-guided core biopsy
mammographer
mammographically guided needle local-
   ization
mammographic findings

mammographic view
mammography (see *mammogram*)
mammoplasty, mammaplasty
  augmentation
  axillary approach in augmentation
  axillary endoscopic reduction
  BAMBI (breast augmentation
    mammoplasty by injection)
  "belly button" augmentation
  central cone technique reduction
  "cleavoplasty" augmentation
  "cross-the-heart" augmentation
  en bloc augmentation
  endoscopic-assisted transumbilical
    augmentation
  endoscopic transaxillary augmenta-
    tion
  free nipple transposition technique
    reduction
  Goulian
  inferior central pedicle reduction
  inferior pedicle technique reduction
  inframammary approach in
    augmentation
  laser reduction
  LeJour technique of reduction
  "mega-pocket" augmentation
  nonrigid technique reduction
  owl incision technique reduction
  pedicle technique reduction
  periareolar augmentation
  reconstructive
  reduction
  short-scar tumescent reduction
  subglandular augmentation
  superior pedicle technique reduction
  superwet reduction
  transaxillary subpectoral
  transumbilical augmentation
  vertical bipedicle flap technique
    reduction
  vertical reduction
  videoendoscopic augmentation
  wet-technique reduction

mammoplasty *(cont.)*
  Wise areola mastopexy breast
    augmentation (WAMBA)
  Wise pattern for reduction
MammoSite RTS (radiation therapy
  system) catheter
Mammotest breast biopsy system
Mammotest Plus breast biopsy system
Mammotome minimally invasive breast
  biopsy
Mammotome probe
Mammotome ultrasound system
management, palliative pain
Mandibular Excursiometer
mandibular fracture
mandibular gland
mandril set
maneuver
  Colanis
  Duecollement
  Epley
  Heimlich
  Hoguet
  Ko-Airan maneuver
  Kocher
  Mattox
  Mendelsohn
  Mueller
  Pringle
  Valsalva
mangofodipir trisodium
manipulation, transgenic
Mann-Bollman fistula
Mann-Whitney U test (data analysis)
Mannitol
manofluorography (MFG)
manometric assessment
manometric pattern
manometric study
manometry
  anal
  aneroid
  anorectal
  balloon reflex

manometry *(cont.)*
  biliary
  ERCP
  esophageal
  point of respiratory reversal
    on esophageal
  preoperative esophageal
  rectal
  rectosigmoid
  sphincter of Oddi
Mansfield balloon
M antibody
manual morcellator
manual resuscitator bag
MAO (monoamine oxidase) inhibitor
Maox 42 (magnesium oxide)
MAP (mean arterial pressure)
MAP–CVP/CO (mean arterial
  pressure–central venous pressure/
  cardiac output = systemic vascular
  resistance)
maple leaf flap
mapping
  anal
  functional anatomical
  intragastric pH
mapping marker
mapping pen
Maquet endoscopy table
marantic clot
marasmus protein-energy under-
  nutrition
Marathon guiding catheter
Marberger hilar retractor
marble bone pin
Marblen
Marburg virus
M.A.R.C. clip
Marcaine HCl (bupivacaine HCl)
Marcus grading scale for avascular
  necrosis
Marechal-Rosen test
Marezine

marfanoid body habitus
margin
  clear
  negative
  right costal
marginal artery of Drummond
marginal ulcer
marginal zone of the spleen
margination of white blood cells
marijuana usage
marimastat
Marinol (dronabinol)
Marino transsphenoidal hook
Marin reamer
Marjolin ulcer
marked afterload increase
marked stridor
marked thrombocytosis
marker (see also *genetic marker, tumor
  marker*)
  CA 15-3 RIA (radioimmunoassay)
    serum tumor
  Castroviejo
  CEA (carcinoembryonic antigen)
  Freeman cookie cutter areola
  genetic
  hepatitis serologic
  mapping
  methylene blue
  preoperative placement of radiologic
  radioactive-labeled
  radiopaque
  serum
  Sitzmarks radiopaque
  Skinmate
  tumor
marker transit study
Markham-Meyerding hemilaminectomy
  retractor
markings
  haustral (on x-ray)
  red wale (RWM)
Markov simulation model
Mark II Chandler retractor

Mark II distal femur retractor
Mark II Kodros radiolucent awl
Mark II PCL retractor
Mark II S retractor
Mark II Z knee retractor
Mark IV Moss decompression-feeding
    catheter
Markwalder bone rongeur
Markwalder rib forceps
Marlen double-faced adhesive disc
Marlen Gas Relief drainage pouch
Marlen Neoprene All-Flexible faceplate
Marlen Odor-Ban ileostomy pouch
Marlen Solo ileostomy pouch
Marlen Zip Klosed pouch
Marlex band
Marlex graft
Marlex hernia repair
Marlex mesh
Marlex mesh abdominal rectopexy
Marlex mesh rectopexy
Marlex PerFix plug
Marlex plug technique
Marlex polypropylene mesh
Marlex synthetic graft material
Marlow laparoscope
Marlow Primus instrument collection
Marlow rigid laparoscope
Marlow videolaparoscope
Marlow videoscope
Marmine (dimenhydrinate)
maroon-colored stools
Marquardt bone rongeur
marrow purging ex vivo pretransplant
Marseille classification of pancreatitis
MARSpo2 Tech pulse oximeter
Marsupial adjustable belt with
    attachable pouch
marsupial pouch
marsupialization of sublingual salivary
    cyst (ranula)
Martel clamp
Martin anoplasty
Martin cartilage chisel

Martin cartilage clamp
Martin cartilage forceps
Martin cartilage scissors
Martin cutting needle
Martin-Davis rectal speculum
Martin laryngectomy tube
Martin meniscus clamp
Martin muscle clamp
Martin needle
Martin nerve root retractor
Martin pelvimeter
Martin rectal hook
Martin scissors
Martin sheet rubber bandage
Martin stitch scissors
Martin tissue forceps
Martius flap and fascial sling
Martius graft
Martius labial fat pad flap
Martorell hypertensive ulcer
Maryland dissecting forceps, double-
    action
Maryland dissector
MAS (minimal access surgery)
Masimo SET (signal extraction
    technology) pulse oximeter
mask anesthesia
mask phenomenon
Mason abdominotranssphincteric
    resection
Mason Colly Seel Disc for ostomy skin
Mason gastroplasty
Mason suction tube
Mason vascular clamp
Mason vertical-banded gastroplasty
Mason-Judd suprapubic retractor
mason's lung
mass
    abdominal
    abdominopelvic
    appendiceal
    apperceptive
    apple-core configuration of
    body cell

mass *(cont.)*
  breast
  brittle
  colon
  concentrically laminated
  conical
  cystic
  discrete
  dominant
  dominant breast
  elongated
  encapsulated
  epigastric
  exophytic
  expansile abdominal
  fecal
  firm
  fleecy
  fluctuant
  fluid-filled
  friable
  fungating
  glistening
  groin
  hard fixed (in the thyroid)
  injection
  inner cell
  intra-abdominal
  intramural bowel
  ipsilateral brain
  irregular
  lean body
  liver
  lobulated
  lung
  molar
  molecular
  multilocular
  multinodular
  nodular
  nonthyroidal neck
  painless breast
  palpable
  palpable epigastric

mass *(cont.)*
  palpable retroareolar
  pearly white
  periumbilical
  phlegmonous
  pituitary
  polypoid
  pulsatile abdominal
  recanalization reducible
  rectal submucosal
  red cell
  reddish-brown tumor
  relative molecular
  retroareolar
  retroperitoneal
  right-sided
  right upper quadrant
  sex chromatin
  shiny
  slow-growing skin
  slowly enlarging
  soft tissue
  solid
  spiculated
  stellate
  stonelike
  tigroid
mass effect
Masset test for bile pigment in urine
Massie driver
Massie extractor
Massie II nail
Massie nail assembly
Massie plate
Massie sliding graft
Massie sliding nail
mass infection
massive acid secretion
massive bleeding
massive blood transfusion
massive coagulation
massive deposits of glycogen in muscle
massive embolism
massive fluid resuscitation

massive genital prolapse
massive hemorrhage
massive hemothorax
massive hepatic necrosis
massive ischemic necrosis
massive lower GI bleeding
massive pneumonia
massive pulmonary embolus
massive pulmonary hemorrhagic edema
massive splenic trauma
mass lesion
mass of congealed blood
Masson needle holder
Masson needle holder with tungsten
   carbide inlays
mastalgia
mast cell
mastectomy (pl. mastectomies)
   Auchincloss modified radical
   axillary node dissection
   bilateral
   breast-sparing
   complete
   Halsted radical
   lumpectomy
   McWhirter simple
   modified radical
   partial
   Patey modified radical
   preventive
   prophylactic
   quadrantectomy
   radical
   "scarless"
   segmental
   simple
   skin-sparing
   subcutaneous
   total
   two-stage technique of
   Willy Meyer incision for
mastectomy for gynecomastia
master duodenoscope
Masters intestinal clamp

Masters-Schwartz liver clamp
masticator space
Mastin muscle clamp
mastitis
   acute
   benign
   chronic
   chronic cystic
   cystic
   Dahl-Iverson
   diffuse cystic
   granulomatous
   parenchymatous
   periductal
   plasma cell
   postpartum
   puerperal
   tuberculous
mastocytosis, systemic
mastodynia
mastoid retractor
mastopathia chronica cystica
mastopexy
   anchor
   areolar
   augmentation
   Benelli
   Benelli lollipop
   Biesenberger technique of
   breast-lift
   central technique of
   circumareolar
   concentric
   crescent
   donut, doughnut
   double skin
   endoscopic-assisted
   full
   keyhole
   Keystone
   LeJour
   lollipop
   Louis
   modified

mastopexy *(cont.)*
  periareolar
  "purse-string"
  reduction
  Regnault type B
  "round block" technique of
  SAMBA (simultaneous areolar
    mastopexy and breast augmenta-
    tion)
  short-scar technique of
  simple
  vertical
  Wise
mastotomy with abscess drainage
MAST trousers
Masuka staging system, modified,
  for thymic carcinoma
matchstick graft
material
  amorphous
  "anchovy paste" (in hepatic abscess)
  base
  breadlike
  calcareous
  Cellolite patty
  coffee-grounds (CGM)
  collagen hemostatic
  colloid
  contrast
  cross-reacting (CRM)
  Curaderm hydrocolloid dressing
  Cutinova Cavity wound filling
  Cymetra tissue replacement
  cytoplasmic
  Dacron synthetic ligament
  DermAssist hydrocolloid dressing
  DermAssist wound filling
  Dermatell hydrocolloid dressing
  dried out
  Enteryx biopolymer
  eosinophilic
  extracellular (ECM)
  ExuDerm hydrocolloid dressing
  fecal

material *(cont.)*
  fluid
  foamy
  foreign
  functional
  gelatinous
  gel-like
  genetic
  globoid
  gritty
  grumous
  Healos bone-grafting
  Hedrocel bone substitute
  hemorrhagic
  hemostatic
  homogeneous
  inspissated
  jelly-like
  Kaltostat wound packing
  liquid
  lumpy
  Marlex synthetic graft
  mesh graft
  mucoid
  Multidex wound filling
  myxoid
  necrotic "anchovy paste"
  noncellular
  nonfibrous
  NuDerm hydrocolloid dressing
  polyglactin absorbable suture
  polyglyconate absorbable suture
  PolyWic wound filling
  Prolene suture
  purulent
  radiopaque contrast
  refractile
  RepliCare hydrocolloid dressing
  residual calculous
  Reston hydrocolloid dressing
  sandy
  sarcoplasmic
  semisolid
  SignaDress hydrocolloid dressing

material *(cont.)*
  suture
  thickened
  tissue equivalent
Mathews hand drill
Mathews rectal speculum
Mathieu forceps
Mathieu needle
Mathieu needle holder
Mathieu needle holder with tungsten
  carbide inlay
Mathieu rasp
Mathieu rectal speculum
Mathieu retractor
Mathieu-TC needle holder
Mathieu trivalve rectal speculum
Matritech NMP22 test kit
matrix, extracellular
MATRIX assay
Matson-Alexander elevator
Matson rib elevator
Matson rib stripper
matted lymph node
Matthew cross-leg clamp
Mattox aorta clamp
Mattox maneuver
mattress suture
mattress-type suture
mature T-tube tract
maturing the stoma
maturity-onset diabetes mellitus
  (MODM) (now classified as type 2)
maturity-onset diabetes of the young
  (MODY)
Maunsell-Weir operation
Max FiberScan laser
Max Fine tying forceps
Max Force balloon catheter
Max Force catheter
Maxamine (aldesleukin)
MaxCast tape
Maxidone
maxillary impression
maxillofacial tube

Maxima Forté blood oxygenator
maximal O_2
maximum anal resting pressure
  (MARP)
Maxolon (metoclopramide)
Maxon polyglyconate monofilament
  suture
Maxon suture
Maxorb alginate wound dressing
Maxxim Medical
Mayaro virus
Mayfield forceps
Mayfield incision
Mayfield miniature clip applier
Mayfield neurosurgical skull clamp
Mayfield rongeur
Mayfield skull clamp pin
Mayfield temporary aneurysm clip
  applier
Mayfield three-pin skull clamp
Maylard incision
Mayo abdominal clamp
Mayo abdominal retractor
Mayo-Adams abdominal retractor
Mayo-Adams appendectomy catheter
Mayo-Adams appendectomy retractor
Mayo-Adams spreader
Mayo-Blake gallstone forceps
Mayo clamp
Mayo Clinic system for primary biliary
  cirrhosis
Mayo-Collins retractor
Mayo common duct probe
Mayo common duct scoop
Mayo common duct spoon
Mayo curved dissecting scissors
Mayo dissecting scissors
Mayo dressing scissors
Mayo external vein stripper
Mayo gall duct probe
Mayo gallstone scoop
Mayo-Guyon kidney pedicle clamp
Mayo-Harrington scissors
Mayo-Hegar needle

Mayo-Hegar needle holder with tungsten carbide inlay
Mayo hemostat
Mayo iliac/femoral cannula
Mayo-Lexer scissors
Mayo needle
Mayo-Noble scissors
Mayo-Ochsner suction trocar cannula
Mayo-Péan forceps
Mayo-Robson clamp
Mayo-Robson forceps
Mayo-Robson intestinal forceps
Mayo-Robson position
Mayo-Russian tissue forceps
Mayo scissors
Mayo stand
Mayo sterilizing pin
Mayo-Stille scissors
Mayo straight dissecting scissors
Mayo subclavian cannula
Mayo towel forceps
Mayo trocar-point needle
Mazzariello-Caprini forceps
MB (methylene blue)
MBTS (modified Blalock-Taussig shunt)
MCAD (medium-chain acyl-CoA dehydrogenase) deficiency
MCAD deficiency
MCAG (multiple colloid adenomatous goiter)
MCAS (modular clip application system)
MCAT (modular coded aperture technology) collimator
McBride pin
McBride plate
McBurney appendectomy
McBurney incision
McBurney point
McBurney sign
MCC (mutated in colorectal carcinoma) gene
McCabe canal knife
McCabe-Farrior rasp
McCabe flap knife dissector
McCabe perforation rasp
McCain TMJ cannula
McCain TMJ forceps
McCain TMJ probe
McCain TMJ scissors
McCleery-Miller intestinal clamp
McClintock forceps
McCormick dissector
McCort sign (on x-ray)
McCraw gracilis myocutaneous flap
McCulloch long suction tube
McDonald dissector
McDougal clamp
McDougal prostatectomy clamp
M cell genesis
MCFA (medium chain fatty acids)
McFarland bone graft
McGaw volumetric pump
McGee-Priest wire forceps
McGee wire-crimping forceps
McGhan breast implant
McGhan saline-filled prosthesis
McGill forceps
McGivney grasping forceps
McGivney hemorroidal ligator
McGivney hemorrhoid forceps
McGlamry elevator
MCH (mean corpuscular hemoglobin)
MCHC (mean corpuscular hemoglobin concentration)
McHugh facial nerve knife
McHugh flap knife
McIndoe bone rongeur
McIndoe diathermy forceps
McIndoe dressing forceps
McIndoe rongeur forceps
McIndoe scissors
McIntosh laryngoscope blade
McIvor blades
McIvor mouth gag
McKee tri-fin nail
McKeever cartilage knife
McKenty rasp

McKenzie brain clip forceps
McKenzie clip-applying forceps
McKenzie clip-bending forceps
McKenzie clip-introducing forceps
McKenzie clip rack
McKenzie perforating twist drill
McKernan-Adson forceps
McKernan-Potts forceps
McKinley EpM analgesic infusion
  pump
McLaughlin intertrochanteric plate
McLaughlin modification of Bunnell
  pullout
McLaughlin nail
McLean pile clamp
McLean-Tucker obstetrical forceps
McMaster bone graft
McNealey-Glassman-Mixter forceps
McNemar test (for ascites)
McPherson forceps
MCS (Magnetic Controlled Suturing)
MCS (mesocaval shunt)
MCT (medium chain triglycerides)
MCTD (mixed connective tissue
  disease)
MCT oil
MCV (mean corpuscular volume)
McVay classification of groin hernias
  (types 1-4)
McVay herniorrhaphy
McVay inguinal hernia repair
McWhirter simple mastectomy
M.D. Anderson clamp
M.D. Paramedic Bag
MD-Gastroview (diatrozoate meglu-
  mine; diatrozoate sodium)
MDI deliver device
MD-111 bone allograft
MD-60 radiopaque contrast medium
MDR (multidrug resistance) 3 gene
MEA (multiple endocrine adenoma-
  tosis) syndrome
MEA type I (Wermer syndrome)
MEA type II or IIa (Sipple syndrome)

MEA type IIB or III (mucosal neuroma
  syndrome)
Mead bone rongeur
Mead mallet
Meadox Microvel arterial graft
Mead periosteal elevator
Mead rongeur
meal
  barium
  Boyden test
  butter
  double contrast barium
  Ewald test
  fatty
  isotope
  liver
  Lundh
  motor test
  opaque
  pain related to
  retention
  small bowel
  test
mean arterial pressure
mean corpuscular hemoglobin (MCH)
mean corpuscular hemoglobin concen-
  tration (MCHC)
mean corpuscular volume (MCV)
mean end-expiratory pressure
mean operative time
mean transit time
meandering artery of Gonzalez
Mears sacroiliac plate
measles virus
measurement test
meat wrapper's lung
meaty appearance
meaty texture
Mebadin (dehydroemetine)
mebendazole
mebrofenin hepatobiliary function test
mecasermin (insulin-like growth
  factor-1, recombinant human
  [rhIGF])

mechanical biliary obstruction
mechanical bowel obstruction
mechanical compression of viscera
   by tumor
mechanical dead space
mechanical diarrhea
mechanical duct obstruction
mechanical extrahepatic obstruction
mechanical ileus
mechanical intestinal obstruction
mechanical jaundice
mechanical lithotripsy for bile duct
   stone
mechanically defective sphincter
mechanical obstruction
mechanical small bowel obstruction
mechanical ventilation
mechanism
   antireflux
   deflecting
   deglutition
   feedback
   flap-valve
   Frank-Starling
   host defense
   humeral
   immune
   impaired cellular defense
   pinchcock
   sphincteric
   swallowing
mechanism of injury
mecholyl study
Meckel band
Meckel diverticulectomy
Meckel diverticulitis
Meckel diverticulum
Meckel ligament
Meckel rod
Meckel scan
Meckel space
meclizine HCl
meconium ileus
meconium plug syndrome

meconium-stained amniotic fluid
MECT (multipolar electrocoagulation
   therapy)
Mectizan (ivermectin)
Mectra Tissue Sample Retainer
medications (including pharmaceuticals,
      natural substances, imaging
      agents, and prescription and
      over-the-counter drugs)
   abarelix
   Abbokinase (urokinase)
   acarbose
   Accuprep HPF powder
   Accuzyme enzymatic debriding
      agent
   Accuzyme ointment
   Accuzyme topical enzyme
   Acephen analgesic suppositories
   Aceta (acetaminophen)
   Aceta with Codeine (codeine
      phosphate; acetaminophen)
   acetohexamide
   Acidulin (glutamic acid hydro-
      chloride)
   Aciphex (rabeprazole sodium)
   ACTH
   Actidose Aqua (activated charcoal)
   Actidose with Sorbital (activated
      charcoal; sorbital)
   Actigall (ursodiol-ursodeoxycholic
      acid)
   Actimmune (interferon gamma-1b)
   Actiprep skin preparation
   Actiq (oral transmucosal fentanyl
      citrate) ("lollipop")
   activated attapulgite
   activated charcoal
   Actos (pioglitazone hydrochloride)
   Actron (ketoprofen) pain reliever
   Acutrim
   Adcon-A
   Adcon-C
   Adcon-I
   Adcon-L gel

medications *(cont.)*
  Adcon-P solution
  Adcon-T/N gel
  adefovir dipovoxil
  ADEKs multivitamin supplement
  ADEKs pediatric drops
  Adept (icodextrin)
  Adipex-P (phentermine HCl)
  Adriamycin (doxorubicin)
  Adrucil (fluorouracil)
  AERx (morphine sulfate)
  AERx electronic inhaler (morphine
    sulfate)
  agalsidase beta
  Agoral (mineral; phenolphthalein)
  ALA (alpha lipoic acid)
  Alamag (aluminum hydroxide;
    magnesium hydroxide)
  Alamag Plus (aluminum hydroxide;
    magnesium hydroxide;
    simethicone)
  albendazole
  Albenza Tiltab (albendazole)
  Aldactone (spironolactone)
  aldesleukin
  Aldurazyme
  Alferon N (interferon alfa-n3)
  Algicon
  alglucerase
  Alibra (alprostadil/prazosin HCl)
  Aliminase
  AlitraQ formula
  alitretinoin
  Alka-Mints (calcium carbonate)
  Alka-Seltzer (sodium bicarbonate;
    citric acid; aspirin; phenyl-
    alanine)
  Alka Seltzer Extra Strength
  Alka Seltzer Gold
  Alkets (calcium carbonate)
  Allovectin-7 (DNA/lipid complex)
  Almacone (aluminum hydroxide;
    magnesium hydroxide;
    simethicone)
  Aloe Vesta protective ointment

medications *(cont.)*
  Alond (zopolrestat)
  alosetron HCl
  alpha-D-galactosidase enzyme
  alpha-galactosidase
  alpha lipoic acid (ALA)
  AlphaNine
  alprostadil
  Alprox-TD (alprostadil)
  Alramucil (psyllium hydrophilic
    mucilloid)
  ALRT1550 capsules
  ALternaGEL (aluminum hydroxide
    gel)
  Altracin (bacitracin)
  Alu-Cap (aluminum hydroxide gel)
  Aludrox (aluminum hydroxide;
    magnesium hydroxide;
    simethicone)
  aluminum carbonate gel, basic
  aluminum hydroxide gel
  aluminum sulfate
  Alu-Tab (aluminum hydroxide gel)
  ALX-0600
  Amaryl (glimepiride) tablets
  amber touch-and-heal (St. John's
    wort)
  amifostine
  aminoglutethimide
  aminosalicylic acid
  aminosidine
  aminosterol
  Aminosyn
  Aminosyn M
  Aminosyn II
  Amitone (calcium carbonate)
  Amphojel (aluminum hydroxide gel)
  amphotericin B
  Ampligen
  anakinra
  Analpram-HC (hydrocortisone
    acetate; pramoxine)
  ananain
  Anaspaz (hyoscyamine sulfate)

medications *(cont.)*
   anastrozole
   Ancef
   Andractim (dihydrotestosterone gel)
   Androderm testosterone transdermal
     patch
   Androgel (testosterone)
   Androsorb
   Angiocidin
   AngioMark contrast agent
   Angiozyme
   anisotropine methylbromide
   annamycin
   Anogesic (nitroglycerin ointment)
   antacid
   anthraquinone of cascara
   anti-IL-2 receptor antibody
   antibiotic
   anticholinergic drug
   Anticort
   antiemetic
   Antiminth (pyrantel pamoate)
   antiprostaglandin
   Antispas (dicyclomine HCl)
   Antivert (meclizine)
   Antrenyl
   Antrocol
   Anucort HC (hydrocortisone acetate)
   Anumed (bismuth subgallate;
     bismuth resorcin compound;
     benzyl benzoate; zinc oxide;
     Peruvian balsam)
   Anusol (pramoxine HCl; zinc oxide)
   Anusol-HC (hydrocortisone acetate)
   Anvirzel
   Anzemet (dolasetron mesylate)
   Apo-Domperidone (domperidone
     maleate)
   Apomate radiopharmaceutical
     imaging agent
   apomorphine
   Apra (CT-2584 mesylate)
   Aptosyn (exisulind)
   arbaprostil

medications *(cont.)*
   Arco-Lase (amylase; protease;
     lipase; cellulase)
   Arco-Lase Plus (amylase; protease;
     lipase; cellulase; hyoscyamine
     sulfate; atropine sulfate; pheno-
     barbital)
   Arilvax yellow fever vaccine
   Arimidex (anastrozole) tablets
   Aromasin (exemestane) tablets
   aromatic cascara fluidextract
   aromatic cascara sagrada
   Aroplatin
   arsenic trioxide (ATO)
   Arthrotec (diclofenac sodium;
     misoprostol)
   Asacol (mesalamine) delayed-release
     tablets
   ASAP antimicrobial solution
   Ascriptin A/D
   A-Spas S/L (hyoscyamine sulfate)
   Atabrine
   Atgam (lymphocyte immune
     globulin; antithymocyte)
   ATO (arsenic trioxide; As2O3)
   atorvastatin calcium
   atovaquone/proguanil
   Atrisol aerosol
   Atrocholin
   atropine sulfate
   attapulgite
   Avakine (infliximab)
   Avandia (rosiglitazone maleate)
   Avelox (moxifloxacin)
   Avicidin
   Avicine
   Avitene Hemostat (microfibrillar
     collagen hemostat)
   Axid; Axid AR (nizatidine)
   Axokine (ciliary neurotrophic factor
     [CNTF])
   azathioprine
   Azulfidine EN-tabs (sulfasalazine)
   BA-EDTA (bile acid-EDTA) solution

medications *(cont.)*
   bacitracin
   Bactrim
   BalAsa (balsalazide disodium) (now
     Colazal)
   balm of Gilead
   balmony
   Balneol
   balsalazide disodium
   Banalg
   Banthine (methantheline bromide)
   barberry (*Berberis vulgaris*)
   Barbidonna #2 (atropine sulfate;
     scopolamine hydrobromide;
     hyoscyamine hydrobromide;
     phenobarbital)
   Basaljel (aluminum carbonate gel,
     basic)
   Beano (alpha-D-galactosidase
     enzyme)
   becaplermin
   Bellacane (atropine sulfate; scopol-
     amine hydrobromide; hyoscya-
     mine sulfate; phenobarbital)
   Bellacane SR (belladonna alkaloids;
     phenobarbital; ergotamine
     tartrate)
   Belladenal
   belladonna alkaloid
   belladonna extract
   Bellafoline
   Bell/ans (sodium bicarbonate)
   Bellatal (phenobarbital)
   Bellergal-S (belladonna extract;
     phenobarbital; ergotamine
     tartrate)
   Bel-Phen-Ergot SR (belladonna
     alkaloids; phenobarbital; ergota-
     mine tartrate)
   BeneFin shark cartilage powder
   BeneFix (coagulation factor IX
     [recombinant])
   bentiromide
   Bentyl (dicyclomine HCl)

medications *(cont.)*
   benzocaine
   benzquinamide
   benztropine; benztropine mesylate
   Beta LT (beta-alethine)
   Betadine (povidone-iodine)
   Betadine gel
   Betathine (beta-alethine; Beta LT)
   bethanechol
   Bexxar (^{131}I tositumomab)
   Biaxin XL (clarithromycin)
     extended-release tablets
   Bicarbolyte
   bichloroacetid acid
   bile acid sequestrants
   bile salts
   bimoclomal
   Biofreeze with Ilex analgesic
     ointment
   BioGlue
   Bio-Hep-B
   biphasic insulin
   biphasic isophane insulin
   biricodar dicitrate
   bisacodyl tannex
   Bisco-Lax (bisacodyl)
   bismuth subcarbonate
   bismuth subgallate
   bismuth subsalicylate
   bisoxatin; bisoxatin acetate
   bithionol
   Bitin (bithionol)
   Black-Draught syrup (casanthranol;
     senna extract)
   Black-Draught tablets (senna
     concentrate)
   blood mononuclear cells, allogenic
     peripheral
   Blue Goo (Iamin hydrating gel)
   Bonine
   botulinum toxin
   Bouin solution
   bovine immunoglobulin concentrate
   BrachySeed iodine-125 (^{125}I)

medications *(cont.)*
BrevaRex
bromelain
Bromo-Seltzer (sodium bicarbonate;
  citric acid; acetaminophen)
bromocriptine mesylate
Brompton's Cocktail
Brompton's Mixture (oral narcotic
  alcohol solution)
broxuridine
Bucladin-S
buclizine HCl
bucrylate
budesonide
Buffets II (acetaminophen; aspirin;
  caffeine; aluminum hydroxide)
Bumex (bumetanide)
bupivacaine HCl
Buro-Sol (aluminum sulfate)
Burow solution
Buscopan
busulfan
Busulfanex (busulfan) for injection
  (now Busulfex)
Busulfex (busulfan)
butenafine
Butibel (belladonna extract;
  butabarbital sodium)
butyrylcholinesterase
C242-DM1
CA 72–4 gastric cancer antigen
  tumor marker
cA2 monoclonal antibody
cabergoline
calcifediol
Calcijex (cacitriol)
calcitriol
calcium carbonate
calcium polycarbophil
Calderol (calcifediol)
Calm-X (dimenhydrinate)
Camalox
cambendezole
Camptosar (irinotecan hydro-
  chloride) injection

medications *(cont.)*
Campyvax vaccine
Cancidas (caspofungin acetate)
Candistat-G
Candistroy
cannabinol
canstatin
Cantil (mepenzolate bromide)
capecitabine
capsaicin
Carafate (sucralfate)
carbantel lauryl sulfate
carbonyl iron
Cariel gel
CARN 750 (now CarraVex
  injectable)
Caroid
CarraVex injectable (formerly
  CARN 750)
casanthranol
Casec
caspofungin acetate
castor oil
cathartic
Cavilon barrier ointment
CDA (chenodeoxycholic acid)
CDCA (chenodeoxycholic acid)
Cd-texaphyrin photosensitizing agent
CEA-Cide
Cedax (ceftibuten)
cefadroxil
cefazolin
cefdinir
ceftibuten
Ceftin (cefuroxime)
cefuroxime
celandine (*Chelidonium majus*)
Celebra (celecoxib) (now Celebrex)
Celebrex (celecoxib)
CellCept (mycophenolate mofetil
  [MMF])
CellCept (mycophenolate mofetil)
Celsior organ preservation solution
Centara (priliximab)

medications *(cont.)*
   Ceo-Two (sodium bicarbonate;
      potassium bitartrate)
   cephalosporin
   Cephulac
   Ceredase (alglucerase)
   Cerezyme (imiglucerase)
   Certican (everolimus)
   Certiva vaccine
   Cetacaine
   cetraxate HCl
   cetuximab
   CharcoAid 2000 (activated charcoal)
   charcoal, activated
   Charcoal Plus (activated charcoal)
   CharcoCaps (charcoal)
   Charcodote
   Chardonna-2 (belladonna extract;
      phenobarbital)
   Chenix (chenodiol)
   chenodeoxycholic acid (CDCA)
   chenodiol
   Chenofalk
   Chirocaine (bupivacaine; levobupi-
      vacaine)
   chitosan
   ChloraPrep One-Step
   Chloresium (chlorophyllin copper
      complex)
   chlormethazine
   chlorophyllin copper complex
      (PALS tablets)
   cholagogue
   cholecystokinin
   Cholestagel (now Welchol)
   cholestyramine resin
   Choletec (^{99m}Tc mebrofenin)
      imaging agent
   choline chloride
   Cholografin Meglumine (iodipamide
      meglumine)
   Chooz (calcium carbonate)
   chromium (Cr)
   chromium picolinate

medications *(cont.)*
   chromium polynicotinate
   Chronulac (lactulose)
   Chrysalin
   Chymex (bentiromide)
   Cidex OPA
   cilansetron
   ciliary neurotrophic factor (CNTF)
   cimetidine HCl
   Cipro (ciprofloxacin)
   ciprofloxacin
   cisplatin/epinephrine gel
   Citra pH (sodium citrate)
   Citralax (magnesium citrate;
      magnesium sulfate)
   citrate of magnesia
   Citrocarbonate (sodium bicarbonate;
      sodium citrate)
   Citrotein
   Citrucel (methylcellulose)
   Citrucel Sugar Free (methylcellu-
      lose; phenylalanine)
   CLA (conjugated linoleic acid)
   clarithromycin
   clenoliximab (IDEC-151/SB-
      217969)
   clidinium
   clidinium bromide
   Clinimix E (amino acid with elec-
      trolytes in dextrose with calcium)
   Clinitest
   Clinoril (sulindac)
   Clomycin (polymyxin B sulfate;
      bacitracin; neomycin sulfate;
      lidocaine)
   clonidine gel
   clonidine hydrochloride injection
   clorsulon
   clortermine HCl
   closantel
   Clostridium botulinum toxin
   Clysodrast (bisacodyl tannex)
   CMV-IGIV (cytomegalovirus
      immune globulin, intravenous)

medications *(cont.)*

CNTF (ciliary neurotrophic factor)
coagulation factor IX recombinant
Coblation technology
Colace (docusate sodium)
Co-Lav (polyethylene glycol electrolyte solution; electrolytes)
Colax (phenolphthalein; docusate sodium)
Colazal (balsalazide disodium)
Colazide (balsalazide disodium)
colesevelam HCl
Colestid (colestipol)
colestipol
colistimethate
colistin
Collins solution
colloidal bismuth subcitrate
COLO-Vax
Colocort (hydrocortisone enema)
Cologel
Colomed
Colovage (polyethylene glycol-electrolyte solution)
Coly-Mycin M
Coly-Mycin S
Colyte (polyethylene glycol-electrolyte solution)
Combidex imaging agent
combretastatin
comosain
Compazine suppositories (prochlorperazine)
Compleat Modified Formula
Comply
Compro (prochlorperazine)
Comvax (*Haemophilus* b purified capsular polysaccharide; *Neisseria meningitidis* OMPC) (hepatitis B virus vaccine)
conjugated linoleic acid (CLA)
Constilac (lactulose)
Constulose (lactulose)
ConTE-Pak-4 (multiple trace elements)

medications *(cont.)*

Converspaz
Converzyme
ConXn (recombinant human relaxin, H_2)
Cope (aspirin; caffeine; magnesium hydroxide; aluminum hydroxide)
Cordox
coriander
Correctol (bisacodyl)
Correctol Extra Gentle (docusate sodium)
Cortenema (hydrocortisone)
Cortenema retention enema
Corticaine
corticorelin ovine triflutate
corticosteroid
Cortifoam (hydrocortisone acetate)
Cotara
Cotazym; Cotazym-S (lipase; protease; amylase)
Coumadin (warfarin sodium)
counterirritant
COX-2 inhibitor
Cr (chromium)
Creon
Crestor (rosuvastatin)
Cro-Man-Zin (chromium; manganese; zinc)
Cryptosporidium parvum bovine colostrum IgG concentrate
CT-2584 mesylate
CTLA4-Ig monoclonal antibody
CTP-37 theraccine
CTP37 vaccine
CY-1899
cyclizine
cyclophilin
cyclophosphamide
cycloserine (L-cycloserine)
cyclosporin A
CyPat
Cytadren (aminoglutethimide)
cytarabine liposomal

medications *(cont.)*
  CytoGam (cytomegalovirus immune globulin)
  CytoImplant (blood mononuclear cells, allogenic peripheral)
  Cytolex (pexiganan acetate) (now Locilex)
  Cytolex cream (pexiganan acetate)
  cytomegalovirus immune globulin, human
  cytomegalovirus immune globulin, solvent/detergent treated
  Cytomel (liothyronine sodium)
  cytoprotective agent
  Cytotec (misoprostol)
  Cytovene (oral ganciclovir)
  Cytoxan (cyclophosphamide)
  dacliximab monoclonal antibody
  daclizumab
  Dairy Ease (lactase enzyme)
  DairyCare
  Dakin solution
  dalanated insulin
  dalteparin sodium
  danaparoid sodium
  danthron
  daptomycin for injection
  Darbid (isopropamide)
  Daricon PB (oxyphencyclimine)
  darifenacin
  Darvocet-N 100
  dazopride; dazopride fumarate
  DC softgels (docusate calcium)
  DDAVP (desmopressin acetate)
  DDS-Acidophilus
  Debrisan (dextranomer)
  Decholin (dehydrocholic acid)
  decitabine
  Definity (perflutren)
  Degas (simethicone)
  DEHOP (diethylhomospermine)
  dehydrocholic acid
  dehydroemetine
  dehydroepiandrosterone (DHEA)

medications *(cont.)*
  Deliver 2.0 formula
  Demerol
  DENSPM (diethylnorspermine)
  deoxyspergualin
  DepoCyt (cytarabine liposomal)
  DepoMorphine (morphine sulfate)
  Derifil (chlorophyllin)
  DermaFreeze
  Dermol HC (hydrocortisone)
  Dermoplast (benzocaine; menthol)
  Dermuspray (trypsin; Peruvian balsam)
  desmopressin acetate (DDAVP)
  Devrom (bismuth gallate)
  dexamethasone sodium phosphate
  dexanabinol
  Dexatrim
  dexfenfluramine
  dexmedetomidine
  Dexol 300
  dexpanthenol
  dextran 40
  dextranomer
  DHEA (dehydroepiandrosterone)
  DHEA sulfate (DHEAS)
  DiaBeta (or Diaßeta)
  Diacol
  Dialose (docusate sodium)
  Dialose Plus (yellow phenol phthalein; docusate sodium)
  Dialume (aluminum hydroxide gel)
  Diapid (lypressin)
  Diar-Aid (loperamide)
  Diasorb (activated attapulgite)
  diazepam
  Dibent (dicyclomine)
  dibucaine
  diclofenac sodium
  dicyclomine hydrochloride
  diethylpropion
  diethylcarbamazine; diethylcarbamazine citrate
  diethylhomospermine (DEHOP; DEHSPM)

medications *(cont.)*
    diethylnorspermine (DENSPM)
    difenoximide HCl
    difenoxin; difenoxin HCl
    DiffGAM
    Diffistat-G
    Di-Gel (aluminum hydroxide; magnesium hydroxide; simethicone)
    Di-Gel Advanced Formula (magnesium hydroxide calcium carbonate; simethicone)
    Digepepsin (pancreatin; pepsin; bile salts)
    digestant
    Digestozyme (pancreatin; pepsin; dehydrocholic acid)
    Digibar 190 (barium sulfate for suspension)
    Digibar 190 imaging agent
    diloxanide furoate
    dimenhydrinate
    Dinate (dimenhydrinate)
    Diocto-C (docusate, casanthranol)
    Diocto-K (docusate potassium)
    Diocto-K Plus (casanthranol; docusate potassium)
    Dioctolose Plus (casanthranol; docusate potassium)
    Dioeze (docusate sodium)
    Dipentum (olsalazine sodium)
    diphenoxylate HCl
    Diprivan (propofol)
    Diquinol (iodoquinol)
    Dirame (propiram)
    disaccharide tripeptic glycerol dipalmitoyl
    disaccharide tripeptide glycerol tripalmitoyl
    Disanthrol (casanthranol)
    disodium cromoglycate (DSC; DSCG)
    Disolan (phenolphthalein; docusate sodium)

medications *(cont.)*
    Disolan Forte (casanthranol; carboxymethylcellulose sodium; docusate sodium)
    Disonate (docusate sodium)
    Disoplex (carboxymethylcellulose sodium; docusate sodium)
    Di-Spaz (dicyclomine)
    Dizmiss (meclizine HCl)
    DMP 504
    docetaxel
    docusate calcium
    docusate potassium
    docusate sodium
    DOK (docusate sodium)
    dolasetron mesylate
    Domeboro powder, tablets (aluminum sulfate; calcium acetate)
    domperidone
    Donna-Sed (atropine sulfate; scopolamine hydrobromide; hyoscyamine hydrobromide; phenobarbital)
    Donnagel (attapulgite)
    Donnagel-PG
    Donnatal No. 2 (atropine sulfate; scopolamine hydrobromide; hyoscyamine sulfate; pheno-barbital)
    Donnazyme (pancreatic lipase; protease; amylase)
    Donphen
    dopamine
    Dorbane
    Dorbantyl Forte
    DOS softgels (docusate sodium)
    Dosalax (senna concentrate; alcohol)
    Dostinex (cabergoline)
    Doxidan (phenolphthalein; docusate calcium)
    Doxil (doxorubicin hydrochloride liposome injection)
    Doxinate

medications *(cont.)*
   doxorubicin hydrochloride liposome injection
   D-penicillamine
   Dramamine II (meclizine HCl)
   Dramanate (dimenhydrinate)
   Dramilin (dimenhydrinate)
   Dr. Caldwell Senna Laxative (senna concentrate)
   Dr. Dermi-Heal (allantoin; zinc oxide; Peruvian balsam)
   droloxifene
   dronabinol
   droperidol
   DSC; DSCG (disodium cromoglycate)
   DSMC Plus (casanthranol; docusate potassium)
   D-S-S (docusate sodium)
   D-thyroxine
   D-xylose
   Dulcagen (bisacodyl)
   Dulcolax (bisacodyl)
   Dulcolax Bowel Prep Kit (bisacodyl)
   DuoDerm Hydroactive (hydrocolloid gel)
   Duphalac (lactulose)
   Duraclon (clonidine hydrochloride injection)
   Duragesic-100 (fentanyl) transdermal patches
   Duralone-80 (methylprednisolone acetate)
   Duramorph (morphine sulfate)
   Duranest MPF (etidocaine; epinephrine)
   Dyclone (dyclonine HCl)
   dyclonine HCl
   dymanthine HCl
   dimantine HCl
   Dymelor (acetohexamide)
   Dymenate (dimenhydrinate)
   EchoGen (perflenapent)
   Ecotrin

medications *(cont.)*
   edrophonium
   Effer-Syllium
   eflornithine
   8-methoxycarbonyloctyl oligosaccharides
   Elase (fibrinolysin; desoxyribonuclease)
   Eldisine (vindesine sulfate)
   Ellence (epirubicin hydrochloride)
   Elliott B solution
   Eloxatin (oxaliplatin)
   Elta wound cleanser
   Eltroxin (levothyroxine sodium)
   Emdogain
   Emete-con
   Emetrol (fructose, dextrose, and phosphoric acid)
   Emitasol (metoclopramide) nasal spray
   emitefur
   emulsified perflubron blood substitute
   Emulsoil
   Endocet (oxycodone/acetaminophen)
   Endocodone (oxycodone hydrochloride)
   Endodan (oxycodone/oxycodone terephthalate/aspirin)
   Endo-Flo irrigation
   Endostatin protein
   Engerix-B (hepatitis B vaccine [recombinant])
   Eno
   enprostil
   Entero Vu (barium sulfate for suspension)
   Entocort (budesonide)
   Entocort CR (budesonide)
   Entolase
   Entozyme
   EPC
   epinephrine & cisplatin injectable gel

medications *(cont.)*
   epirubicin hydrochloride
   Epivir (lamivudine)
   Epivir-HBV (lamivudine)
   epoetin alfa
   Equalactin (calcium polycarbophil)
   Equilet (calcium carbonate)
   Ergamisol (levamisole HCl)
   Ergoset (bromocriptine mesylate)
   ergotamine tartrate
   Esberitox
   esomeprazole magnesium
   esterified estrogens
   Estinyl (ethinyl estradiol)
   Estrace (estradiol)
   estradiol
   Estratab (esterified estrogens)
   estrone
   Estrone Aqueous (estrone)
   Ethamolin (ethanolamine oleate)
   ethanolamine oleate
   ethinyl estradiol
   Ethyol (amifostine)
   etidocaine
   etoformin HCl
   etomoxir
   etoposide injection
   Euglucon (glyburide)
   Evac-Q-Kwik (bisacodyl)
   Evac-Q-Mag (magnesium citrate; citric acid; potassium citrate)
   Evac-Q-Sert (sodium bicarbonate; potassium bitartrate)
   Evac-Q-Tabs (phenolphthalein)
   Evac-U-Gen
   Evac-U-Lac
   Evalose (lactulose)
   everolimus
   Ex-Lax
   Ex-Lax Extra Gentle
   Ex-Lax Gentle Nature
   Ex-Lax Maximum Relief
   Ex-Lax Stool Softener
   exemestane

medications *(cont.)*
   exisulind
   extended insulin human zinc (rDNA)
   extended insulin zinc
   FABRase (alpha-galactosidase)
   Fabrazyme (agalsidase beta)
   FAC (ferric ammonium citrate)
   factor VIII SQ, recombinant
   famotidine
   Fareston (toremifene citrate)
   Faslodex (fulvestrant)
   fedotozine
   Feen-A-Mint
   fenfluramine
   fenoctimine; fenoctimine sulfate
   fentanyl citrate (Actiq "lollipop")
   Fentanyl Oralet (fentanyl)
   fentanyl transdermal patches
   Feridex I.V. (ferumoxides injectable solution)
   ferric ammonium citrate (FAC)
   FerriSeltz (ferric ammonium citrate [FAC])
   Festalan (atropine)
   Festal II
   Fiberall (calcium polycarbophil)
   FiberCon (calcium polycarbophil)
   Fiber-Lax (calcium polycarbophil)
   Fiber-Norm (calcium polycarbophil)
   Fibrillex (NC-503)
   5-aminosalicylic acid
   5-ASA
   5-FU (fluorouracil)
   50% Dextrose with Electrolyte Pattern A (or N)
   Flagyl (metronidazole)
   Flatulex (simethicone)
   Fleet Babylax (glycerin)
   Fleet enema
   Fleet Bisacodyl enema
   Fleet Laxative (bisacodyl)
   Fleet Mineral Oil enema

medications *(cont.)*
    Fleet Phospho-Soda (monobasic sodium phosphate; dibasic sodium phosphate)
    Fletcher's Castoria (senna concentrate)
    Flocor (poloxamer 188)
    Florinef Acetate (fludrocortisone acetate)
    Floxin (ofloxacin)
    floxuridine (FUDR; FUdR [5-fluorouracil deoxyribonucleoside])
    fludrocortisone acetate
    flumecinol
    FluMist vaccine
    fluoropyrimidine
    fluorouracil & leucovorin
    fluorouracil (5-FU)
    fluoxymesterone
    Foamicon (aluminum hydroxide; magnesium trisilicate)
    Folergot-DF (belladonna alkaloids; phenobarbital; ergotamine tartrate)
    folinic acid
    Foloxatine (oxaliplatin)
    Foscan
    fotemustine (S 10036)
    Fourneau 309 (suramin sodium)
    Fragmin (dalteparin sodium injection)
    FRED (fog reduction elimination device) solution
    FRED Lite alcohol-free solution
    FUDR; FUdR (floxuridine)
    Furamide (diloxanide furoate)
    furazolidone
    furodazole
    G.B.S.
    gadodiamide
    Gadolite oral suspension
    Galzin (zinc acetate)
    gamma globulin

medications *(cont.)*
    Gantrisin
    Gardrin (enprostil)
    Gas Relief (simethicone)
    Gas-Ban (calcium carbonate; simethicone)
    Gas-X (simethicone)
    Gastrimmune (gemcitabine)
    Gastrimmune vaccine
    Gastrografin (meglumine diatrizoate)
    GastroMARK imaging agent (ferumoxsil)
    Gastrosed (hyoscyamine sulfate)
    Gastrozepine (pirenzepine HCl)
    Gaviscon (aluminum hydroxide; magnesium carbonate)
    Gaviscon-2
    Gelfoam soaked in sodium tetradecyl sulfate
    Gelusil (aluminum hydroxide; magnesium hydroxide; simethicone)
    Gelusil-M
    Gelusil-II
    gemcitabine HCl
    Gemzar (gemcitabine HCl)
    Genasense
    Genasoft Plus (casanthronate; docusate sodium)
    Genaton
    Genaton Extra Strength (aluminum hydroxide; magnesium carbonate)
    Gengraf (cyclosporine)
    Genotropin (somatropin lyophilized powder)
    Genotropin MiniQuick
    Genotropin Pen 5
    Genotropin Pen 12
    Gentlax (senna concentrate)
    Geref (sermorelin acetate)
    Geriplex-FS
    Germanin (suramin sodium)
    glimepiride tablets

medications *(cont.)*
  glipizide
  glitazone classification of diabetes
    drugs
  globin zinc insulin
  globulin, hepatitis B hyperimmune
  GlucaGen (glucagon)
  glucagon
  Gluco-Pro nutritional supplement
  Glucophage (metformin HCl)
  Glucophage XR (metformin HCl
    extended-release)
  glucose
  Glucotrol
  Glucotrol XL (glipizide)
  Glucovance (glyburide; metformin
    HCl)
  glutamic acid
  glutamine & somatropin
  Glutose
  glyburide
  glyburide/metformin hydrochloride
  glycerin
  glycerol
  glycerol monoctanoate (GMOC)
    solution
  glycopyrrolate
  glycopyrronium bromide
  Glynase Pres Tab (glyburide)
  Glypressin (terlipressin)
  Glyset (miglitol)
  GMOC (glycerol monoctanoate)
    solution
  Go-Evac (polyethylene glycol-
    electrolyte solution electrolytes)
  gold-198 (^{198}Au)
  GoLYTELY (polyethylene glycol-
    electrolyte solution)
  Gonadimmune
  gosereline acetate
  granisetron HCl
  Granocyte (lenograstim)
  Granulderm (trypsin; Peruvian
    balsam)

medications *(cont.)*
  Granulex (trypsin; Peruvian balsam)
  GranuMed (trypsin; Peruvian
    balsam)
  GVAX pancreatic vaccine
  Haley's M-O (magnesium hydrox-
    ide; mineral oil) (new name
    Phillips' M-O)
  halofuginone
  Halotestin (fluoxymesterone)
  Hanks balanced salt solution
    (HBSS)
  Havrix (hepatitis A vaccine,
    inactivated)
  H-BIG (hepatitis B immunoglobulin)
  H$_2$ blocker
  H$_2$ receptor blocker
  Hectorol (doxercalciferol)
  Helicide
  Helicosol (synthetic ^{13}C-urea)
    lyophilized powder
  Helidac (bismuth subsalicylate,
    metronidazole, and tetracycline)
  Helidac dose-pack (bismuth
    subsalicylate; metronidazole;
    tetracycline HCl)
  HemAssist blood substitute (hemo-
    globin crosfumaril)
  Hemocor HPH
  hemoglobin crosfumaril
  Hemopad (microfibrillar collagen
    hemostat)
  Hemorid for Women (pramoxine
    HCl; phenylephrine HCl)
  Hemorrhoidal HC (hydrocortisone
    acetate)
  Hemotene (microfibrillar collagen
    hemostat)
  Hem-Prep (phenylephrine HCl; zinc
    oxide)
  Hemril Uniserts (bismuth subga-1
    late; bismuth resorcin compound;
    benzyl benzoate; Peruvian
    balsam; zinc oxide)

medications *(cont.)*
  Hep-B-Gammagee
  Hep-Lock, Hep-Lock U/P (heparin
    sodium)
  Hepagene (hepatitis B vaccine)
  heparin sodium
  Heparin Lock Flush (heparin
    sodium)
  HepatAmine nutrient solution
  hepatitis B immune globulin
  Heptalac (lactulose)
  Heptavax-B
  Heptazyme
  Heptodin (lamivudine)
  Heptovir (lamivudine)
  Herceptin (trastuzumab) monoclonal
    antibody
  Herplex Liquifilm (idoxuridine)
  Herzyme
  Hespan (hetastarch)
  hetastarch
  Hetrazan (diethylcarbamazine
    citrate)
  hexocyclium
  Hextend
  Hirulog (bivalirudin)
  Histerone 100 (testosterone)
  Hi-Vegi-Lip
  Humalog (insulin lispro, human
    [rDNA])
  Humalog Mix 75/25
  Humalog Pen
  human insulin (recombinant)
  human insulin zinc
  Humatrope (somatropin)
  Humicade
  Humulin 30/70 (insulin; isophane
    insulin)
  Humulin 50/50 (isophane human
    insulin [rDNA]; human insulin
    [rDNA])
  Humulin 70/30 (isophane human
    insulin [rDNA]; human insulin
    [rDNA])

medications *(cont.)*
  Humulin L
  Humulin Pen
  Humulin R (human insulin [recom-
    binant])
  Humulin U (extended insulin zinc)
  Humulin U Ultralente (extended
    insulin human zinc [rDNA])
  hyaluronidase
  hydralazine
  Hydrate (dimenhydrinate)
  hydrazine sulfate
  hydrochloric acid
  Hydrocil Instant (psyllium
    hydrophilic mucilloid)
  hydrocortisone
  hydrocortisone acetate
  hydrocortisone enema
  hydrocortisone foam
  hydroxymethylacyfulvene [HMAF]
  hydroxyurea tablet
  HylaSine gel
  hyoscyamine
  hyoscyamine sulfate
  Hyosophen (atropine sulfate; scopol-
    amine hydrobromide;
    hyoscyamine hydrobromide;
    phenobarbital)
  HyperHep (hepatitis B immune
    globulin)
  I-Flow nerve block infusion kit
  Iamin hydrating gel (Blue Goo)
  Iamin-IB solution (prezatide copper
    acetate [PCA])
  Icar (carbonyl iron)
  icodextrin
  idoxifene
  Ilopan
  Ilopan-Choline (dexpanthenol;
    choline bitartrate)
  Ilozyme
  imiglucerase
  ImmTher (disaccharide tripeptide
    glycerol tripalmitoyl)

medications *(cont.)*
    Imodium A-D
    Imodium, Imodium A-D
      (loperamide)
    impromidine HCl
    ImuLyme vaccine
    Imuran (azathioprine)
    Inactivin
    Inapsine (droperidol)
    Incel (biricodar dicitrate)
    Indiclor (indium ^{111}In radioimaging
      agent)
    Infanrix vaccine
    Infergen (interferon alfacon-1)
    infliximab monoclonal antibody
    Innofem (estradiol)
    Innohep (tinzaparin sodium)
    [111]In satumomab pendetide
    insulin argine
    insulin aspart
    insulin defalan
    insulin glargine
    insulin human, isophane
    insulin human zinc, extended
    insulin lispro, human [rDNA])
    insulin zinc
    insulin zinc protamine
    insulin zinc suspension (amorphous)
    insulin zinc suspension (crystalline)
    insulin zinc [pork]
    Insulin Reaction (glucose)
    interferon alfa-2a
    interferon alfa-2b
    interferon alfa-2b recombinant
    interferon alfa-n1
    interferon alfa-n3
    interferon alfacon-1
    interferon beta
    interferon beta-1a
    interferon gamma-1b
    Intergel adhesion prevention solution
    interleukin-4 receptor (IL-4R)
    IntraDose (cisplatin/epinephrine) gel
    IntraSite (graft T starch copolymer)

medications *(cont.)*
    IntraSite gel
    Intron A (interferon alfa-2b,
      recombinant
    iodipamide meglumine
    iodixanol
    iodophor
    iodoquinol
    Iodosorb wound gel
    IoGen
    iohexol
    IontoDex (dexamethasone sodium
      phosphate)
    ipecac syrup
    Iressa
    irinotecan HCl injection
    irofulven
    ISG (immune serum globulin)
    ISIS 2302
    Isocaine HCl (mepivacaine HCl)
    isofylline
    Isopan (magaldrate)
    Isopan Plus (magaldrate;
      simethicone)
    isophane human insulin (rDNA)
    isosorbide mononitrate
    itraconazole
    ivermectin
    JTT-501
    Juven nutritional supplement
    Kaletra (lopinavir/ritonavir)
    Kanulase
    Kaodene Non-Narcotic (kaolin;
      pectin; bismuth subsalicylate)
    Kao Lectrolyte
    kaolin
    Kaopectate (attapulgite)
    Kao-Spen (kaolin; pectin)
    Kapectolin (kaolin; pectin)
    Kasof (docusate potassium)
    Kayexalate
    K-C (kaolin; pectin; bismuth
      subcarbonate)
    Kefzol (cefazolin)

medications *(cont.)*
   Kestrone 5 (estrone)
   Ketek (telithromycin)
   ketoconazole
   ketoprofen
   ketorolac tromethamine
   Kindercal supplement
   Kinesed
   Kinevac (sincalide)
   Kolantyl
   Konsyl (psyllium)
   Konsyl-D, Konsyl Orange (psyllium hydrophilic mucilloid)
   Konsyl Fiber (calcium polycarbophil)
   K-Pek (attapulgite)
   Kutrase (amylase; protease; lipase; cellulase; hyoscyamine sulfate; phenyltoloxamine citrate) digestive enzymes
   Ku-Zyme, Ku-Zyme HP (amylase; protease; lipase; cellulase) digestive enzymes
   Kytril (granisetron hydrochloride)
   Lactaid
   lactase enzyme
   Lactinex
   lactose enzyme
   Lactrase
   lactulose solution
   lamivudine
   lansoprazole
   Lantus (insulin glargine)
   lavoltidine, lavoltidine succinate
   laxative
   LDP-02
   lenercept
   Lente Iletin II (insulin zinc [pork])
   Lente L (insulin zinc [pork])
   letrazuril
   letrozole
   leucovorin
   leucovorin & fluorouracil
   Leukine (sargramostim)

medications *(cont.)*
   LeuTech radiolabeled imaging agent
   leuvectin
   levamisole HCl
   Levaquin (levofloxacin)
   Levbid (hyoscyamine sulfate)
   levobupivacaine
   levofloxacin
   Levo-T (levothyroxine sodium)
   Levothroid (levothyroxine sodium)
   levothyroxine sodium
   levothyroxine sodium & tiratricol
   Levoxyl (levothyroxine sodium)
   Levsin
   Levsin-PB drops (hyoscyamine sulfate; phenobarbital; alcohol)
   Levsin/SL (hyoscyamine sulfate)
   Levsin with Phenobarbital (hyoscyamine sulfate; phenobarbital)
   Levsinex Timecaps (hyoscyamine sulfate)
   lexipafant
   Lexirin
   liarozole fumarate
   Liazal (liarozole fumarate)
   Librax (clidinium; chlordiazepoxide)
   lidocaine
   lidocaine HCl
   lidocaine topical anesthetic
   Lidoject-2 (lidocaine HCl)
   lignocaine
   Limitrol-DM
   linezolid
   liothyronine sodium
   liotrix
   lipancreatin
   Lipitor (atorvastatin calcium)
   liposome encapsulated doxorubicin citrate complex
   LiquiBand topical wound closure glue
   Liqui-Char (activated charcoal)
   Liqui-Doss (mineral oil)
   lobucavir

medications *(cont.)*
   LoCholest
   LoCholest Light (cholestyramine
     resin)
   Locilex (pexiganan acetate)
   Lomanate (diphenoxylate HCl;
     atropine sulfate)
   Lomotil (diphenoxylate HCl;
     atropine sulfate)
   Lonox (diphenoxylate HCl; atropine
     sulfate)
   loperamide
   lopinavir/ritonavir
   Losec (omeprazole)
   Lotronex (alosetron HCl)
   Lovenox (enoxaparin)
   Lowsium Plus
   L-thyroxine
   Lu-Tex
   LYMErix vaccine
   lymph node-revealing solution
     (LNRS)
   Lymphazurin dye (isosulfan blue)
   lymphoblastoid interferon, human
     (L-IFN)
   lymphocyte immune globulin,
     antithymocyte (rabbit)
   lypressin
   Maalox (aluminum hydroxide;
     magnesium hydroxide)
   Maalox Plus
   Maalox TC (therapeutic concentrate)
   Maalox Whip
   Macrokine (WF10)
   mafenide acetate
   magaldrate
   Magaldrate Plus
   Magalox Plus (aluminum hydroxide;
     magnesium hydroxide;
     simethicone)
   Magnalox (aluminum hydroxide;
     magnesium hydroxide) (Canada)
   magnesium citrate
   magnesium oxide

medications *(cont.)*
   magnesium sulfate
   magnesium trisilicate
   Magnox (aluminum hydroxide;
     magnesium hydroxide)
   maladrate
   Malarone (atovaquone/proguanil)
   Maltsupex (nondiastatic barley malt
     extract)
   Mannitol
   Maox 42 (magnesium oxide)
   Marblen
   Marcaine HCl (bupivacaine HCl)
   Marezine
   marimastat
   Marinol (dronabinol)
   Maxamine (aldesleukin)
   Maxidone
   Maxolon (metoclopromide)
   MCT (medium chain triglycerides)
   MD-Gastroview (diatrozoate
     meglumine; diatrozoate sodium)
   Mebadin (dehydroemetine)
   mebendazole
   meclizine HCl
   Mectizan (ivermectin)
   Medicone (benzocaine)
   Medifil
   Mefoxin
   Megace (megestrol acetate)
   Megnatril
   Menest (esterified estrogens)
   Meni-D (meclizine HCl)
   mepenzolate bromide
   meperidine
   mepivacaine HCl
   Meridia (sibutramine HCl)
   meropenem
   Merrem (meropenem)
   mesalamine delayed-release tablets
   mesalazine
   Metamucil (psyllium hydrophilic
     mucilloid; sodium bicarbonate;
     potassium bicarbonate)

medications *(cont.)*
    metformin extended-release
    metformin HCl
    methantheline bromide
    methoxamine
    methoxyflurane
    methscopolamine bromide
    methylcellulose
    methylprednisolone acetate
    methylprednisolone sodium
        succinate
    methyl tertiary butyl ether (MTBE)
    methyltestosterone
    metoclopramide nasal spray
    metocurine iodide
    metrizamide
    metrizoate sodium
    Metro I.V. (metronidazole)
    metronidazole
    Metryl 500
    Metubine Iodide (metocurine iodide)
    MetXia
    microfibrillar collagen hemostat
    Micronase (glyburide)
    Micronized Glyburide (glyburide)
    midazolam HCl
    miglitol
    milk of magnesia (MOM)
    Milk of Magnesia–Cascara,
        Concentrated
    Milkinol (mineral oil)
    minalrestat
    mineral oil
    Mintezol (thiabendazole)
    Mintox (aluminum hydroxide;
        magnesium hydroxide)
    MiraLax (polyethylene glycol 3350)
    Miraluma (technetium ^{99m}Tc
        sestamibi)
    misoprostol
    MitoExtra
    mitomycin
    Mitrolan (calcium polycarbophil)
    Mivacron (mivacurium chloride)

medications *(cont.)*
    Moctanin (monoctanoin)
    Modane Bulk, Plus, and Soft
    Modane Plus
    Modane Soft
    Modane Versabran
    MOM (milk of magnesia)
    monooctanoin
    morantel, morantel tartrate
    Morphelan (oral morphine)
    MorphiDex
    morphine HCl
    morphine sulfate
    morrhuate
    Motilium (domperidone maleate)
    Motofen (difenoxin HCl; atropine
        sulfate)
    moxifloxacin
    MPI 5020
    MTBE (methyl tertiary butyl ether)
    Mucomyst
    MulTE-Pak-5 (multiple trace
        elements [metals])
    Multikine
    Multilyte-40 (combined electrolyte
        solution)
    Mutamycin (mitomycin)
    mycophenolate mofetil (MMF)
    Mycostatin
    Mylagen, Mylagen II
    Mylanta Natural Fiber Supplement
        (psyllium hydrophilic mucilloid)
    Mylanta-II
    Mylicon (simethicone)
    Myocet (liposome encapsulated
        doxorubicin citrate complex)
    Nabi-Altastaph vaccine
    Nabi-HB (hepatitis B immune
        globulin [human])
    Nabi-NicVAX vaccine
    Nabi-StaphVAX vaccine
    Naganol (suramin sodium)
    nandrolone phenpropionate
    Naphuride (suramin sodium)

medications *(cont.)*
    Naropin (ropivacaine)
    Nashville Rabbit Antithymocyte
      Serum (lymphocyte immune
      globulin, antithymocyte [rabbit])
    nateglinide
    Natural Vegetable (psyllium
      hydrophilic mucilloid)
    Nature's Remedy (cascara sagrada)
    Nausea Relief (phosphorated carbo-
      hydrate solution)
    Nausetrol (phosphorated carbohy-
      drate solution)
    NC-503 (Fibrillex)
    Neo-Cultol (mineral oil)
    Neo-Diaral (loperamide)
    Neocate One +
    Neoloid
    Neomark (broxuridine)
    neomycin sulfate
    Neoral (cyclosporine; alcohol)
    Neotrace-4 (multiple trace elements)
    Neovastat
    NE-0080
    Nephrox (aluminum hydroxide;
      mineral oil)
    Neuprex
    neutral insulin
    neutral protamine Hagedorn (NPH)
      insulin
    Nexium (esomeprazole magnesium)
    niacin
    Niaspan (niacin)
    nicotinamide
    Nilstat
    9-nitro-20-(S)-camptothecin (9-NC)
    nitrofural
    nitrofurazone
    nitroglycerin
    nitroglycerin ointment
    Nitrolan
    nitrous oxide
    nizatidine
    Nizoral

medications *(cont.)*
    No Pain-HP (capsaicin)
    nolinium bromide
    Nolvadex (tamoxifen citrate)
    Norco (hydrocodone bitartrate;
      acetaminophen)
    Normal Stool Formula
    Normal Stool Formula-IB (NSF-IB)
    Normosol-M and 5% Dextrose
    Normosol-R and 5% Dextrose
    Normosol-R pH 7.4 (combined
      electrolyte solution)
    Novamine 15% (amino acids)
    Novo-Domperidone (domperidone
      maleate)
    Novocain (procaine HCl)
    Novolin L (insulin)
    Novolin N PenFill
    Novolin N Prefilled (insulin)
    Novolin R PenFill
    Novolin R Prefilled (insulin)
    Novolin 70/30 PenFill
    Novolin 70/30 Prefilled
    Novolin 85/15 PenFill (insulin)
    NovoLog (insulin aspart)
    Novopaque (barium sulfate)
    NovoRapid (insulin)
    NPH (neutral protamine Hagedorn)
      insulin
    NPH Iletin II insulin
    NPH-N insulin
    NSF-IB (Normal Stool Formula-IB)
    NuLytely (polyethylene glycol-
      electrolyte solution)
    Numorphan (oxymorphone HCl)
    Nupercainal
    Nutraloric
    Nutren 1.0, 1.5, 2.0
    Nutrilan
    Nutrilyte II (combined electrolyte
      solution)
    Nutropin (somatropin)
    Nutropin Depot (somatropin)
    nystatin suspension

medications *(cont.)*
  Nystex
  OCL (polyethylene glycol electrolyte
    solution)
  Octamide PFS (metoclopramide)
  Octastatin (vapreotide)
  octatropine methylbromide
  Octocaine HCl (lidocaine HCl;
    epinephrine)
  OctreoScan imaging agent
  octreotide, octreotide acetate
  oestradiol (estradiol)
  oestrone (estrone)
  ofloxacin, Floxin
  OGT-918
  OKT3
  olsalazine sodium
  omega-3 fatty acid
  omeprazole sodium
  omeprazole plus amoxicillin
  Omnicef (cefdinir)
  Omnipaque iohexol)
  Omniscan (gadodiamide)
  Onco TCS
  Onconase (p30 protein)
  Oncophage vaccine
  OncoScint CR/OV ([111]In
    satumomab pendetide)
  OncoScint CR103 (colorectal)
    imaging agent
  OncoVax-P
  Oncovin (vincristine sulfate)
  ondansetron HCl
  Operand (povidone; iodine)
  opium tincture
  OptiMARK (gadoversetamide
    injection)
  Optison contrast medium
  Oralgen
  Orgaran (danaparoid sodium)
  orlistat
  Orzel (UFT/leucovorin calcium)
  Ostavir vaccine
  OvaRex

medications *(cont.)*
  ox bile extract
  oxaliplatin
  oxamniquine
  Oxandrin (oxandrolone)
  oxidized bile acids
  Oxiplex
  oxybuprocaine
  oxycodone and acetaminophen
  oxycodone HCl
  oxycodone terephthalate/aspirin
  OxyContin (oxycodone HCl)
  oxymorphone HCl
  oxyphencyclimine HCl
  oxyphenisatin, oxyphenisatin acetate
  oxyphenonium
  p10 protein
  p30 protein
  paclitaxel
  Pafase
  palmoxirate sodium
  palmoxiric acid
  palonosetron HCl
  PALS tablets (chlorophyllin copper
    complex)
  pamidronate disodium
  Pamine (methscopolamine bromide)
  Pamisyl (aminosalicylic acid)
  Pan-HER
  Panafil enzymatic debriding agent
  Panafil White ointment
  pancopride
  Pancrease, Pancrease MT 4,
    Pancrease MT 10, Pancrease MT
    16, Pancrease MT 20 (lipase;
    protease; amylase)
  pancreatic enzyme therapy
  Pancreatin 8X (pancreatin; lipase;
    protease; amylase)
  Pancrecarb MS-8 (lipase; protease;
    amylase; pancrelipase)
  pancrelipase
  Pancrex

medications *(cont.)*

Pancrezyme 4X (pancreatin; lipase; protease; amylase)
pancuronium bromide
Panretin (alitretinoin)
Pantoloc (pantoprazole)
pantoprazole
Pantozol (pantoprazole)
papain
Papaya Enzyme (papain; amylase)
paregoric (PG)
Parepectolin (attapulgite)
paricalcitol
paromomycin sulfate
Pathibamate-200
Pathilon (tridihexethyl chloride)
Pavulon (pancuronium bromide)
Paxene (paclitaxel)
Pazo Hemorrhoid (ephedrine sulfate; zinc oxide)
PCA (prezatide copper acetate)
pectin
Pedialyte (sodium, potassium, and chloride electrolytes)
PedTE-Pak-4 (multiple trace elements)
Pedtrace-4 (multiple trace elements)
PEG (polyethylene glycol)
PEG-interferon alfa-2a
PEG-interferon alfa-2b
PEG-Intron (PEG-interferon alfa-2b)
PEG-Intron A (interferon alfa 2b in a polyethylene glycol carrier)
Pegasys (PEG-interferon alfa-2a)
pegvisomant
pegylated interferon
Pentacea
pentagastrin
Pentasa (mesalamine)
Pepcid AC
Pepcid Complete
Pepcid RPD (famotidine)
Peptavlon (pentagastrin)

medications *(cont.)*

Pepto-Bismol (bismuth subsalicylate)
Pepto Diarrhea Control (loperamide)
Perdiem (psyllium husks; senna extract)
perflenapent
perflutren
Peri-Colace (casanthranol; docusate sodium)
Peri-Dos (casanthranol; docusate sodium)
Peruvian balsam
pexiganan acetate
PG (paregoric)
PG-TXL (polyglutamic acid paclitaxel)
PGG glucan
Phazyme (simethicone)
Phazyme-125
Phazyme-PB
Phenergan Fortis (promethazine HCl)
phenobarbital
Phenolax (phenolphthalein)
phenolphthalein
phentermine
Phillips' Milk of Magnesia (M-O) (magnesium hydroxide)
Phosphaljel
Photofrin (porfimer)
pimagedine HCl
Pink Bismuth (bismuth subsalicylate)
Pin-Rid (pyrantel pamoate)
Pin-X (pyrantel pamoate)
pioglitazone HCl
piperamide, piperamide maleate
piperazine, piperazine calcium edetate, piperazine edetate calcium
pirenzepine HCl
piritrexim
pirogliride, pirogliride tartrate
Pitressin
Pitressin Synthetic (vasopressin)

medications *(cont.)*

Pivanex
podophyllum
polidocanol
Polocaine (mepivacaine)
poloxamer 188
polyethylene glycol (PEG)
polyethylene glycol-electrolyte
   solution
polyethylene glycol 3350
polyglutamic acid paclitaxel
Pondimin (fenfluramine)
porcine islet preparation, encapsu-
   lated
porfimer sodium
Portagen
potassium iodide
PPMA (polymethylmethacrylate-
   copolymer) beads
pramlintide acetate
Pramoxine HC (hydrocortisone
   acetate; pramoxine)
Prandase (acarbose)
Prandin (repaglinide)
praziquantel
Precedex (dexmedetomidine)
Precose (acarbose)
prednisolone
prednisone
Premarin (conjugated estrogens)
Preparation H anorectal cream
Preparation H cleansing tissues
Preparation H Cooling Gel
Preparation H rectal suppositories
Prepodyne solution
Prevacid (lansoprazole)
Prevacid triple therapy
Prevalite (cholestyramine resin)
Prevatac (exisulind)
Prevenzyme
Prevpac (lansoprazole; clarithro-
   mycin; amoxicillin)
priliximab
Prilosec (omeprazole)

medications *(cont.)*

Pro-Banthine (propantheline
   bromide)
Pro-Cal-Sof (docusate sodium)
prochlorperazine
Proctocort (hydrocortisone)
ProctoCream HC (hydrocortisone
   acetate)
Procto-Esthesia
ProctoFoam NS (pramoxine HCl)
Proderm Topical (castor oil;
   Peruvian balsam)
profiromycin
Prograf (tacrolimus)
Proleukin (aldesleukin)
promethazine HCl
Promycin (porfiromycin)
propantheline bromide
Prophyllin (sodium propionate;
   chlorophyll derivatives)
Propimex-2
propiram
propofol
ProSol 20% (amino acids)
prostaglandin E1
ProstaScint (CYT-356 radiolabeled
   with ^{111}In indium chloride)
   imaging agent
Prostigmin
protamine zinc insulin
protease digestive enzyme
ProTec (isofylline)
protein pump inhibitor
Protenate (plasma protein fraction)
Prothecan
protirelin
Protonix (pantoprazole)
Protostat
Provir
Prulet (white phenolphthalein)
psyllium hydrophilic mucilloid
psyllium seed husks
Purge (castor oil)
Pylorid (ranitidine bismuth citrate)

medications *(cont.)*
>pyrantel pamoate
>Pyridium
>PZI (protamine zinc insulin)
>Quarzan (clidinium bromide)
>quassia (amargo; amara)
>Questran (cholestyramine)
>quiflapon sodium
>Quilimmune-M
>quinacrine HCl
>quinupristin/dalfopristin
>rabeprazole sodium
>raltitrexed
>ramoplanin
>ranitidine
>ranitidine bismuth citrate
>rapacuronium bromide
>Rapamune (sirolimus)
>rapamycin
>Rebetol (ribavirin)
>Rebetron (interferon alfa-2b injection)
>Rebetron (ribavirin and interferon alfa-2b)
>Reclomide (metoclopramide HCl)
>Recombivax HB
>Rectacort (hydrocortisone acetate)
>Rectagene (live yeast cell derivative; shark liver oil)
>Rectolax (bisacodyl)
>Reducin (somatostatin)
>Redux (dexfenfluramine)
>Reese's Pinworm (pyrantel pamoate)
>ReFacto (factor VIII SQ, recombinant)
>Reglan (metoclopramide HCl)
>Regranex (becaplermin)
>Regranex gel (becaplermin)
>Regulace (docusate sodium)
>Regular Iletin II (insulin)
>Regular Iletin II U-500 (concentrated insulin)
>Regular Purified Pork Insulin
>Regulax SS (docusate sodium)

medications *(cont.)*
>Reguloid (psyllium hydrophilic mucilloid)
>Regutol
>Rehydralyte (electrolyte solution)
>Remegel
>Remicade (infliximab)
>remifentanil
>Renacidin
>repaglinide
>Resol
>retinoid
>Rezipas (aminosalicylic acid)
>Rezulin (troglitazone)
>Rezyme
>Rheaban (activated attapulgite)
>Rheomacrodex (dextran 40)
>rhesus rotavirus-tetravalent vaccine (RRV-TV)
>ribavirin
>ribavirin and interferon alfa-2b
>rifaximin
>Riopan (magaldrate)
>Riopan Plus 2
>Ro-Bile
>Robinul Forte (glycopyrrolate)
>Rocaltrol (calcitriol)
>rofecoxib
>Rolaids, Calcium Rich
>ropivacaine
>rosiglitazone maleate
>rosuvastatin
>RotaShield vaccine
>Rowasa (mesalamine)
>roxatidine, roxatidine acetate HCl
>Roxicodone (oxycodone)
>Roxin (roxatidine acetate HCl)
>RRV-TV (rhesus rotavirus-tetravalent) vaccine
>rubitecan
>RuLox (aluminum hydroxide; magnesium hydroxide)
>sacrosidase
>salazosulfapyridine

medications *(cont.)*
  Salofalk (mesalamine)
  Sal-Tropine (atropine sulfate)
  Sandimmune (cyclosporine)
  Sandostatin
  Sandostatin LAR Depot
    (octreotide acetate)
  SangCya (cyclosporine; alcohol)
  Sani-Supp (glycerin)
  Saratoga (zinc oxide; boric acid;
    eucalyptol)
  sargramostim
  Satietrol Complete
  Satric-500
  satumomab pendetide
  SCCS (simethicone-coated cellulose
    suspension)
  Scleromate
  sclerosant
  Sclerosol
  scopolamine
  seabuckthorn seed oil
  secretin
  Secretin Ferring (secretin)
  SelCID (selective cytokine inhibitory
    drug)
  selenium-75 (^{75}Se) radioisotope
  Senexon (senna concentrate)
  senna concentrate
  Senna-Gen (senosides)
  Senokot (senna concentrate)
  Senokot-S
  Senokot X-prep
  Senokotxtra (senna concentrate)
  senosides
  Sensorcaine MPF (bupivacaine)
  Sepracoat coating solution
  Sepragel bioresorbable gel
  Septopal beads
  Septra
  sermorelin acetate
  Serutan
  shark cartilage
  shark liver oil

medications *(cont.)*
  short chain fatty acids
  sibutramine HCl
  Silace-C (docusate sodium)
  Silvadene (silver sulfadiazine)
  silver sulfadiazine (SSD, SSD AF)
  Simaal Gel 2 (aluminum hydroxide;
    magnesium hydroxide;
    simethicone)
  simaldrate
  Simeco
  simethicone
  simethicone-coated cellulose
    suspension (SCCS)
  Simulect (baxiliximab)
  sincalide
  sirolimus
  6-mercaptopurine (6-MP)
  SMX-TMP (sulfamethoxazole and
    trimethoprim)
  sodium bicarbonate
  sodium citrate
  sodium morrhuate
  sodium oxybate
  sodium perborate
  sodium phosphate
    dibasic
    monobasic
  sodium stibogluconate
  sodium tetradecyl (STD) sulfate
  sodium tetradecyl sulfate (sclerosant)
  sodium tyropanoate
  SomatoKine (IGF-BP3 complex)
  somatostatin
  somatropin
  somatropin & glutamine
  somatropin lyophilized powder
  Somavert (pegvisomant)
  SonoRx (simethicone-coated cellu-
    lose suspension)
  Sotradecol (sodium tetradecyl
    sulfate)
  Sparkles (sodium bicarbonate; citric
    acid; simethicone)

medications *(cont.)*
  Spasmolin (atropine sulfate;
    scopolamine hydrobromide;
    hyoscyamine hydrobromide;
    phenobarbital)
  Spasmophen
  Spastosed (calcium carbonate;
    magnesium carbonate)
  Spexil (trospectomycin)
  spironolactone
  Sporanox (itraconazole)
  Sporidin-G (bovine immunoglobulin
    concentrate)
  Sporidin-G (*Cryptosporidium
    parvum* bovine colostrum IgG
    concentrate)
  S-P-T (thyroid, desiccated porcine)
  squalamine (shark cartilage powder)
  SS (somatostatin)
  SSD, SSD AF (silver suladiazine)
  St. John's wort (amber; amber
    touch-and-heal)
  St. Joseph Anti-Diarrheal for
    Children (attapulgite)
  stannous sulfur colloid
  Starlix (nateglinide)
  steroid
  stillingia
  stool softener
  streptozocin
  Stresstein (multiple branched-chain
    amino acids)
  Stromagen
  Stromectol (ivermectin)
  Strong Iodine (iodine; potassium
    iodide)
  SU-5416
  sucralfate
  Sulfalax Calcium (docusate sodium)
  Sulfamylon (mafenide acetate)
  sulfasalazine
  sulfonylurea
  SuperChar
  suppository

medications *(cont.)*
  suramin sodium
  SureLac (lactose enzyme)
  Surfak (docusate calcium)
  Surgi–Prep (Betadine, povidone-
    iodine)
  sutilains
  Syllact
  Symlin (pramlintide acetate)
  Synercid (quinupristin/dalfopristin)
  Synsorb Cd
  Synsorb-PK
  synthetic ^{13}C urea lyophilized
    powder
  Synthroid (levothyroxine sodium)
  syrup of ipecac
  tacrolimus
  Tagamet, Tagamet HB (cimetidine)
  tamoxifen citrate
  taurolidine
  Taxol (paclitaxel)
  Taxotere (docetaxel)
  Tazocin
  tazofelone
  TBZ (thiabendazole)
  Tebamide (trimethobenzamide HCl)
  technetium macroaggregated albu-
    min (^{99m}Tc MAA)
  technetium ^{99m}Tc pertechnetate
  technetium sulfur colloid (^{99m}Tc-SC)
  tegaserod
  Telepaque (topanoic acid)
  telithromycin
  Tempo (aluminum hydroxide;
    magnesium hydroxide; calcium
    carbonate; simethicone)
  Ten-K
  Tensilon
  Tenuate
  Tepanil
  terlipressin
  Tesamone (testosterone)
  Teslac (testolactone)
  testosterone

medications *(cont.)*
Testred (methyltestosterone)
tetracaine, tetracaine HCl
tetradecyl sulfate
tetrahydrocannabinol (THC)
T-Gen (trimethobenzamide)
thalidomide
Thalomid (thalidomide)
theraccine
Theragyn
Theralax
Theratope-STn
Theratope vaccine
Therevac-Plus (docusate sodium; benzocaine)
Thermazene (silver sulfadiazine)
thiabendazole (TBZ)
thiazolidinedione
thiethylperazine
Thioplex (thiotepa)
thiosalan
thiotepa
Thrombin-JMI (thrombin)
thrombin-Keflin-sotredechol
Thrombogen (thrombin)
Thrombostat (thrombin)
thymalfasin
Thymitaq (nolatrexed dihydro-chloride)
thymosin alpha 1
Thypinone (protirelin)
Thyrar (thyroid, desiccated bovine)
Thyrel-TRH (protirelin)
Thyro-Block (potassium iodide)
Thyrogen (thyrotropin alfa)
thyroglobulin
thyroid
thyroid-stimulating hormone
Thyrolar (liotrix)
thyromedan HCl
thyrotrophic hormone
thyrotropin alfa
thyrotropin-releasing hormone (TRH)

medications *(cont.)*
thyroxine
Thytropar (thyrotropin)
tiabendazole
Ticlid (ticlopidine)
ticlopidine
Ticon (trimethobenzamide HCl)
Tigan (trimethobenzamide HCl)
tincture of benzoin
tincture of opium
tinzaparin sodium
tirolimus
Titralac
tolazamide
tolbutamide sodium
Tolinase (tolazamide)
tolrestat
Tomudex (raltitrexed)
Tonalin (conjugated linoleic acid)
topical bovine thrombin
Torecan
toremifene citrate
tositumomab
Transderm Scop (scopolamine hydrobromide)
transmucosal fentanyl citrate oral
Transplatin (oxaliplatin)
trastuzumab
Travasol in Dextrose
Travasol with electrolytes
Triacana (tiratricol; levothyroxine sodium)
Triban (trimethobenzamide HCl; benzocaine)
tridihexethyl chloride
Trimazide (trimethobenzamide HCl)
trimethobenzamide
trimethoprim-sulfamethoxazole
Triptone (dimenhydrinate)
Tritec (ranitidine bismuth citrate)
Trizivir
Trizyme (amylase; protease; cellulase)
troglitazone

medications *(cont.)*

Tronolane (pramoxine HCl)
tropisetron
trospectomycin
trovafloxacin
Trovan (trovafloxacin)
Trovax
troxacitabine
Tru-Scint AD imaging agent
trypsin
Tucks ointment
Tums
Twinrix vaccine
Tylenol No. 3
UDCA (ursodeoxycholic acid)
UFT (uracil plus tegafur)
Unilax (phenolphthalein; docusate
  sodium)
Unithroid (levothyroxine sodium)
uracil plus tegafur (UFT)
Urso (ursodiol)
ursodeoxycholic acid (UDCA)
ursodiol
V-Lax (psyllium hydrophilic
  mucilloid)
Valium (diazepam)
Valpin 50
Vansil (oxamniquine)
vapreotide
Vaqta (hepatitis A vaccine, inacti-
  vated) vaccine
vasoactive intestinal polypeptide
  (VIP)
vasopressin
vasopressin with nitroglycerin
Velban (vinblastine sulfate)
Velosulin Human BR (insulin)
Verluma (nofetumobab)
Vermox (mebendazole)
Versabran
Versed (midazolam HCl)
Vianain (ananain; comosain;
  bromelains)
Vicodin

medications *(cont.)*

VIMRxyn (synthetic hypericin)
vinblastine sulfate
Viokase
Vioxx (rofecoxib)
Virilon (methyltestosterone)
Virulizin
viscous lidocaine
viscous Xylocaine gargle
Visicol bowel prep
Vistaril
Vita-PMS, Vita-PMS Plus
vitamin K
VX-497
warfarin potassium
warfarin sodium
Welchol (formerly Cholestagel)
Wellferon (interferon alfa-n1)
wetting agents
white phenolphthalein
WinGel
Wyanoids Relief Factor (cocoa
  butter; shark liver oil)
Xcytrin (motexafin gadolinium)
Xeloda (capecitabine)
Xenical (orlistat) capsules
X-Prep
Xylocaine (lidocaine)
Xylocaine topical anesthetic
Xylo-Pfan (xylose)
xylose
yellow phenolphthalein
Zacutex (lexipafant)
zamifenacin
Zanosar (streptozocin)
Zantac, Zantac 75 (ranitidine)
Zantac EFFERdose
Zantac GELdose
Zeffix (lamivudine)
Zelmac (tegaserod)
Zemplar (paricalcitol)
Zenapax (daclizumab)
zinc acetate
Zixoryn (flumecinol)

medications *(cont.)*
   Zofran (ondansetron HCl)
   Zofran ODT (ondansetron)
   Zoladex (goserelin acetate)
   zoledronic acid
   Zometa (zoledronic acid)
   zopolrestat
   Zosyn (piperacillin sodium;
     tazobactam sodium)
   Zydone (hydrocodone bitartrate/
     acetaminophen)
   Zypan
   Zyvox (linezolid)
MedCam Pro Plus video camera
Medco Adson tissue forceps
Medco Allis tissue forceps
Medco Babcock forceps
Medco Bozeman uterine forceps
Medco Brown Adson forceps
Medco Carmalt splinter forceps
Medco Crile forceps
Medco eye dressing forceps
Medco Foerster sponge forceps
Medco forceps
Medco Halstead mosquito forceps
Medco Lister bandage scissors
Medco Schroder tenaculum forceps
Medco splinter forceps
Medco thumb dressing forceps
Medco tissue thumb forceps
Medebar Plus (barium sulfate)
Med-E-Jet inoculator injector
MED endoscope
Medescan (barium sulfate)
Medex Protégé 3010 syringe infusion
   pump
Medfusion 2001 syringe infusion pump
media (pl. of medium), contrast
medial cystic necrosis
medial genicular position
medial incision
medial parapatellar incision
medial pectoral nerve
medial thoracic nerve

medial to pectoral minor muscle
medial umbilical fold
median arcuate ligament
median incision
median length of survival
median lobe of prostate
median lymph node dissection
median parapatellar incision
mediastinal crunch
mediastinal cyst
mediastinal emphysema
mediastinal lymphadenectomy
mediastinal lymphatic and fibrofatty
   tissue
mediastinal lymphatics
mediastinal thickening
mediastinitis
mediastinodiaphragmatic pleural
   reflection
mediastinoscope
mediastinoscopy aspirating needle
mediastinum
mediated by gastrin
medical adhesive
medical blockade
medical therapy
medical vagotomy
medicated urethral system for erection
   (MUSE)
Medicina percutaneous button
Medicone (benzocaine)
Medicon-Jackson rectal forceps
Medicut catheter
Medicut shears
Medifil dressing
Mediflex-Gazayerli retractor
Mediflex video camera system
Medi-Ject needle-free insulin injection
   system
Medi-Jector Choice needle-free insulin
   injection system
Medilas laparoscope
Medina ileostomy catheter
mediolateral oblique view

medionodular cirrhosis
Medi plaster scissors
Medipore Dress-it surgical dressing
Mediskin hemostatic sponge
Medi-Tech bipolar probe
Medi-Tech catheter
Mediterranean fever
Mediterranean lymphoma
Medi-therm II Freon free unit
medium chain acyl-CoA dehydrogenase
   (MCAD) deficiency
medium chain fatty acids (MCFA)
medium chain triglycerides (MCT)
medium pressure catheter
medium pressure shunt
medius, scalenus
Medi-Vac bulk tubing
Medi-Vac CRD suction liner
Medi-Vac critical measurement unit
Medi-Vac Flex Advantage suction liner
Medi-Vac Flexi-Clear suction handle
Medi-Vac Yankauer suction handle
Medi-Vu endoscope
Medix anoscope
Medoc-Celestin endoprosthesis
Medoc-Celestin pulsion tube
Medoff sliding plate
MedPulser device
Medrad Mrinnervu (also MRinnervu)
   endorectal colon probe
Medstone STS lithotriptor
Medstone STS-T transportable litho-
   tripsy system
MedSystem III infusion pump
Med-Tech Teflon dilator
Medtronic Previa
Meduck anesthesia monitor
medulla (pl. medullas, medullae)
   adrenal
   dusky
   lymphatic
   ovarian
   renal
   spinal

medulla oblongata
medulla of bone
medulla of kidney
medulla of lymph node
medulla of thymus
medullary artery
medullary bone
medullary bone graft
medullary canal
medullary canal reamer
medullary carcinoma
medullary carcinoma of the thyroid
   (MTC)
medullary cavity
medullary cord
medullary nail
medullary ray
medullary sarcoma
medullary sinus
medullary sponge kidney
medullary substance
medullary thyroid cancer (MTC)
medullary thyroid carcinoma
medullary zone
medullated corneal nerve fibers
medulloadrenal hyperfunction
medulloblastoma
medusae, caput
Meeker forceps
Meeker gallbladder clamp
Meeker intestinal forceps
Mefoxin
Megace (megestrol acetate)
megacolon
   acquired
   congenital
   idiopathic
   toxic
megacystis-microcolon-intestinal
   hypoperistalsis syndrome
megaduodenum
MegaDyne all-in-one hand control
megaesophagus
megakaryocyte

Megalink biliary stent
"mega-pocket" augmentation mammo-
    plasty
megarectum
megestrol acetate
meglumine diatrizoate contrast medium
meglumine iocarmate
meglumine iothalamate
meglumine iotroxate contrast medium
meglumine ioxaglate
Meigs syndrome
melanocytes
melanoma
    acral-lentiginous
    amelanotic
    anorectal
    benign juvenile
    benign uveal
    desmoplastic malignant
    halo
    intraocular
    juvenile
    lentigo maligna
    malignant
    malignant lentigo
    minimal deviation
    mucosal
    nodular
    ocular
    staging of malignant
    subungual
    superficial spreading
    uveal
melanomatosis
melanophage
melanoplakia-intestinal polyposis
melanosis
melanosis coli
melanotic cancer
melanotic carcinoma
melanotic pigmentation
MELAS (mitochondrial encephalo-
    myopathy, lactic acidosis, and
    stroke-like episodes)

melena
melenic stool (*not* melanotic)
    basement
    peritoneal
    phrenoesophageal
    pleuroperitoneal
    TefGen guided tissue
membrane lipid composition
membrane phospholipid
membrane-puncturing forceps
membranous colitis
Memotherm colorectal stent
Memotherm endoscopic biliary stent
Memotherm Flexx biliary stent
Memotherm nitinol self-expanding stent
MEN (multiple endocrine neoplasia)
    syndrome
MEN 1 (multiple endocrine neoplasia,
    type 1) syndrome
MEN 2 (multiple endocrine neoplasia,
    type 2b or IIB, syndrome
menarche, early
Mendelsohn maneuver
Menest (esterified estrogens)
Menetrier disease
Menghini "one second" technique
Menghini liver biopsy needle
Menghini percutaneous liver biopsy
    technique
menginococcal septicemia
Meni-D (meclizine HCl)
meningeal adhesion
meningeal carcinoma
meningioma of the cribriform plate
meningitis
meningococcus
MENIN tumor
meniscal trimmer blade
meniscectomy blade
meniscectomy scissors
meniscotomy chisel
meniscotomy knife
meniscus clamp
meniscus forceps

meniscus hook
meniscus knife
meniscus retractor
meniscus scissors
meniscus sign
meniscutome
Menkes disease (kinky hair syndrome)
menopausal syndrome
menopause, early or late
mental status changes
Mentor breast implant
mentor tubing
Mentor wet-field electrocautery
mepenzolate bromide
meperidine
Mepiform
Mepilex self-adherent foam dressing
Mepitel contact-layer wound dressing
mepivacaine HCl
Mepore absorptive dressing
mercaptans
Mercator atrial high-density array
   catheter
Mercedes Benz sign, reversed
Mercedes cannula
Mercedes microtip
Mercedes One Piece cannula
Mercedes tip cannula
Mercedes Toomey syringe cannula
Merchant view
mercury-containing balloon
mercury-filled bougie
mercury-filled dilator
mercury-weighted dilator
mercury-weighted tube
Meriam dissecting forceps
Meridia (sibutramine HCl)
Merindino operation
Meritene liquid feeding
Merkel cell carcinoma
Merogel nasal dressing and stent
meropenem
Merrem (meropenem)
Mersilene braided nonabsorbable suture

Mersilene polyester fiber mesh
Mersilene polyester fiber suture
Mersilene suture
Mersilene tape
Mersilk braided silk suture
merycism
mesalamine delayed-release tablets
mesalamine enema
mesalazine
Mesalt ribbon dressing
mesenchymal tumor
mesenchyme
mesenteric abscess
mesenteric adenitis
mesenteric angina
mesenteric apoplexy
mesenteric artery syndrome
mesenteric attachment of colon
mesenteric cyst
mesenteric embolism
mesenteric fat creeping onto the
   antimesenteric border
mesenteric fat stranding (on CT scan)
mesenteric fistula
mesenteric gland
mesenteric infarction
mesenteric infiltration
mesenteric ischemia
mesenteric lymph node
mesenteric lymphadenitis
mesentericoparietal fossa
mesenteric rupture
mesenteric stranding
mesenteric tear
mesenteric thrombosis
mesenteric triangle
mesenteric vascular insufficiency
mesenteric vascular lesion
mesenteric vessel rupture
mesenteritis, retractile
mesenteropexy
mesentery
   appendiceal
   ileal

mesentery *(cont.)*
    jejunal
    plication of
    small bowel
    small intestine (SIM)
mesentery is divided
mesentery of appendix
mesentery of ileum
mesentery of jejunum
mesentery of small bowel
mesh
    Altex polypropylene
    Bard Composix
    Bard Sperma-Tex preshaped
    Bard Visilex
    bilayer polypropylene
    BioMesh
    Brennen biosynthetic surgical
    Composix
    Dacron
    Dexon polyglycolic acid
    freeform prosthetic
    Gore-Tex DualMesh Plus
    Gore-Tex MycroMesh Plus
    Guidor
    Hermesh-3
    Herniamesh surgical
    Hertra-2
    Marlex
    Marlex propylene
    Mersilene
    Mersilene polyester fiber
    monofilament microporous
    Omniderm
    Parietex composite
    Paritene
    PerFix Plus Plug
    polyglactin
    polyglycolic acid
    polypropylene
    preformed prosthetic
    Prolene polypropylene hernia
    prosthetic
    Resolut

mesh *(cont.)*
    Sepramesh Biosurgical Composite
    Sepramesh prosthetic surgical
    Sperma-Tex preshaped
    Surgipro
    SurgiSis sling
    synthetic
    Tramex
    Trelex
    Trelex mesh
    Vicryl knitted
    Vicryl woven polyglactin
    Visilex polypropylene
mesh plug hernioplasty
mesoappendicitis
mesoappendix
mesoatrial shunt
mesocaval anastomosis
mesocaval H-graft shunt
mesocaval interposition shunt
mesocaval shunt
mesocolic band
mesocolic gland
mesocolic shelf
mesocolic window
mesocolonic vessel
mesocolon, transverse
mesodermal cell
mesodermal cortex
mesoenteric vein
mesogastric fossa
mesophilic bacteria
mesorectum
mesosigmoid colon
mesosigmoiditis
mesothelioma, peritoneal
messenger RNA (mRNA)
MET-Rx
metabolic acidosis, intractable
metabolic alkalosis
metabolic calculus
metabolic cirrhosis
metabolic decompensation
metabolic deficiency

metabolic derangement
metabolic derangement from vomiting
metabolic encephalopathy
metabolic energy production
metabolic pathway
metabolic process
metabolic stone
metabolic waste
metabolism
   acid-base
   bacterial (in intestines)
   bilirubin
   calcium
   defect of
   drug
   estrogen
   fat
   fatty-acid
   glucose
   impaired fat
   liver
   nitrogen
   pyrrole
metabolite
metabolite level
metabolize
metacarpal retractor
metacarpal saw
metal clamp
Metalite+A4270
metallic clamp
metallic clip
metallic pin
metallic staple
metallic stent placement
metal needle
metal olive
metal prosthetic graft
metal-weighted Silastic feeding tube
metamass
Metamucil (psyllium hydrophilic mucil-
   loid; sodium bicarbonate; potassium
   bicarbonate)
metanephrine

metaphyseal abscess
metaplasia
   apocrine
   columnar
   intestinal
   myeloid
   specialized intestinal
   squamous
metaplastic polyp
metastasis (pl. metastases)
   advanced
   bone
   brain
   breast skin satellite
   distal lymph node
   distant
   extrahepatic (EHM)
   far-away
   focus of
   liver
   lung
   lymph node
   nodal
   nonskeletal
   peritoneal
   pleural
   port-site
   positive nodal
   satellite
   shunt-related
   skeletal
metastasis to liver
metastatic abscess
metastatic carcinoid syndrome
metastatic carcinoma
metastatic cascade
metastatic colorectal cancer
metastatic disease
metastatic gastric cancer
metastatic malignancy
metastatic polyp
metastatic septicopyemia
metastatic trophoblastic disease (MTD)
metastatic tumor

metatarsal head extractor
metatypical carcinoma
METAVIR classification of chronic
   hepatitis C (0–4)
meteorism
meter (see *blood glucose monitor*)
metformin HCl
methanethiol
methantheline
methantheline bromide
methicillin-resistant *Staphylococcus*
   aureus (MRSA, pronounced
   "mer-sah")
methimazole
method
   Benedict-Talbot body surface area
   Brown dietary (for colon prepara-
      tion)
   Cherry-Crandall (for testing serum
      lipase)
   dye scattering
   EMR (endoscopic mucosal
      resection) suction cap
   Gallego
   leading cord (of colonofibroscopy)
   modified Papanicolaou
   Morison
   Papanicolaou
   Parker-Kerr closed (of end-to-end
      enteroenterostomy)
   Siffert
   staging
   strip biopsy
   suction cap
methohexital sodium
methotrexate
methoxamine
methoxyflurane
methscopolamine bromide
methylcellulose
methylene blue dye
methylene blue enema
methylene blue instillation
methylene blue stain

methylmethacrylate adhesive
methylprednisolone acetate
methylprednisolone sodium succinate
methyl red test
methyl tertiary butyl ether (MTBE)
methyltestosterone
methyltestosterone-induced cholestasis
meticulous apposition
meticulous hemostasis
metoclopramide nasal spray
metocurine iodide
metopic cranial suture
MetraGrasp ligament grasper
MetraPass suture passer
MetraTie knot pusher
metrizamide
metrizoate sodium
Metro I.V. (metronidazole)
metronidazole
Metryl 500
mets (metastases)
Metubine Iodide (metocurine iodide)
MetXia
"Metz" or "Mets" (slang for
   Metzenbaum scissors)
Metzenbaum chisel
Metzenbaum dissecting scissors
Metzenbaum gouge
Metzenbaum scissors, curved, double-
   action
Metzenbaum-TC scissors
Meurig Williams plate
Mewi-5 sidehole infusion catheter
Meyerding chisel
Meyerding curved gouge
Meyerding finger retractor
Meyerding laminectomy blade
Meyerding laminectomy retractor
Meyerding mallet
Meyerding-Scoville blade
Meyerding self-retaining retractor
Meyer vein stripper
MFG (manofluorography)
Mg (magnesium)

MGB (mini-gastric banding)
MgSO$_4$ (magnesium sulfate)
M.G.H. needle holder
M.H.G. elevator
MH needle
MHV (middle hepatic vein)
MIBB breast biopsy system
MIC gastroenteric tube
MIC jejunostomy tube
MIC-Key G gastrostomy tube
MIC-Key J gastrostomy tube
MIC Thermal Option disposable biopsy
    forceps
MIC-TJ transgastric jejunal tube
micelle formation
Michel aortic clamp
Michel applying and removing forceps
Michel clip
Michel clip-removing forceps
Michele vertebral biopsy
Michel wound clip
Micral chemstrip urine test
Micral urine dipstick test
Micrins microsurgical suture
microabscess
microadhesiolysis
MicroAire blade
MicroAire drill
MicroAire oscillating saw
MicroAire power-assisted lipoplasty
    device
MicroAire reamer
micro artery forceps (see *forceps*)
micro balloon probe
Microban drape
micro bipolar forceps (see *forceps*)
Microblater ArthroWand
microbubble contrast agent
microcalcifications, clustered
microchromoendoscopy
microclip or micro clip (see *clip*)
micro cross-action bulldog clamp
microcyst formation
microcyst, lymphatic

microcytic anemia
Microdermabrader
Micro Diamond-Point microsurgery
    instruments
Micro dissecting forceps, fenestrated,
    double-action
microdissection of the cervical lymph
    node compartments
micro dissector or microdissector
Microdot technique for precision suture
    placement
micro dural hook
Microelectrode MI-506 small-caliber
    pH electrode
microerosion
microfibrillar collagen hemostat
microfixation plate
MicroFlow needle
MicroFlow phacoemulsification needle
Microfoam dressing
Microfoam surgical tape
micro forceps or microforceps (see
    forceps)
Microgyn resectoscope sheath
micro Halsted mosquito forceps
micro hook or microhook (see *hook*)
micro instruments, surgical
microinvasive carcinoma
micro irrigating cannula (see *cannula*)
Micro Jaw rotatable dissecting forceps
micro jaw rotatable Kelly (Metzenbaum,
    grasping, etc.) dissecting forceps
Micro-Kerrison rongeur
MicroKlenz wound cleanser
Microknit vascular graft
micro laminectomy rongeur (see
    rongeur)
MicroLap and Microlap Gold micro-
    laparoscopy system
micro laryngeal instruments
Microlase transpupillary diode laser
Microlet Vaculance
Microlight 830 laser
microlithiasis

microlobular cirrhosis
MicroMark clip
MicroMark tissue marker
micromelena
micrometastatic disease
MicroMewi multi-sidehole infusion
    catheter
MicroMite suture anchor
Micronase (glyburide)
Micron needle holder
micro needle or microneedle (see
    needle)
micro nerve hook (see *hook*)
micro neurosurgical scissors (see
    scissors)
Micronized Glyburide (glyburide)
micronodular cirrhosis of liver
micronodular fibrotic pattern
Micro-One dissecting forceps
Micro-One hook
Micro-One needle holder
Micro-One scissors
Micro-optical forceps
micro oscillating saw
micropapillary carcinoma
microperforation
micro pin or micropin (see *pin*)
micro plate or microplate
    C-shaped
    H-shaped
    half-circle
    Howmedica
    Leibinger
    L-shaped
    Luhr
    Microfixation cranial
    Storz Microsystem
    Synthes Microsystems
    T-shaped
    X-shaped
    Y-shaped
micropoint-reverse cutting
micropoint spatula
microport or micro port

Microprobe laser
Micro-Probe microdissection tip
micro probe or microprobe (see *probe*)
Micro QuickAnchor
Micropuncture Peel-Away introducer
microradiograph
micro rasp or microrasp (see *rasp*)
Micro-Retractor
microreamer or micro reamer
micro sagittal saw
microsatellite instability (MSI)
microsaw or micro saw (see *saw*)
micro scissors or microscissors (see
    scissors)
microscope
    darkfield
    double binocular operating
    electron
    Grenoble-Paris-Rennes (GPR) robot
    Leica Aristoplan laser-scanning
    light
    monocular
    Olympus OME-8000 dual stereo
        surgical
    operating
    phase-contrast
    robot neurosurgical
    stereotactic (or stereotaxic)
        operating
    Zeiss operating
    Zeiss OPMI surgical
microscopic blood in stool
microscopic colitis
microscopic diagnosis
microscopic dissecting needle
microscopic extension of tumor cells
microscopic hemorrhage of ligament
microscopic multicentric lesion
microscopic multifocal medullary
    carcinoma
microscopic scissors (see *scissors*)
microscopy
    darkfield
    electron

microscopy *(cont.)*
electronic
endoscopic confocal
immune electron
immunofluoresence
light
polarized light
scanning electron
microscopy of gastric biopsy
microscrew (see *screw*)
Microscribe 3DX digitizer
Micro Series wire driver
microsphere
Microspike approximator clamp
microstaple or micro staple (see *staple*)
microsurgery
computer-assisted
guided
stereotactic laser
transanal endoscopic (TEM)
video-endoscope-assisted
microsurgery drill (see *drill*)
microsurgery forceps (see *forceps*)
microsurgery or microsurgical scissors
microsurgical decompression
microsurgical dissection
microsurgical DREZ-otomy
microsurgical epididymovasostomy
(MSEV)
microsurgical free flap
microsurgical free tissue transfer
microsurgical technique
microsuture or micro suture (see *suture*)
Microtainer lancet
micro tear
Microtek Medical
microtelangiectasia
MicroTeq portable belt
Micro-Three microsurgery instruments
microthrombus
microtome object disc
microtrabecular hepatocellular
carcinoma
Micro-Two forceps

Micro-Two needle holder
Micro-Two scissors
microvascular anastomosis
microvascular clamp
microvascular decompression
microvascular disease
microvascular flap transfer
microvascular forceps
microvascular hemodynamics
microvascular knife
microvascular scissors
microvascular transfer
microvasculature
microvasculopathy
microvasive endoscopic balloon
Microvasive Glidewire
Microvasive Mini Button low-profile
balloon
Microvasive Rigiflex TTS balloon
Microvasive sclerotherapy needle
Microvasive stiff piano wire guidewire
MicroVent Resuscitator
microvesicular fat
microvilli of intestine
microvillus (pl. microvilli)
midabdominal transverse incision
midabdominal wall
Midas Rex craniotomy saw
Midas Rex knife
Midas Rex rongeur
midaxillary line
midaxillary line incision
midazolam HCl
midcolon
Middeldorpf retractor
middle colic artery
middle extrahepatic bile duct
middle hemorrhoidal artery
middle thyroid vein
midepigastric area
midepigastrium
midesophagus
midgut volvulus
midgut volvulus with malrotation

Mills vascular scissors
Miltex diagnostic instruments
Miltex ear loop
Miltex edge scissors sharpener
Miltex forceps
Miltex instrument guard
Miltex-Kerrison cervical rongeur
Miltex mallet
Miltex needle holder
Miltex punch
Miltex scissors
Miltex speculum
Miltex tendon-pulling forceps
Miltex tissue twist hook
minalrestat
mineral oil
mineralocorticoid
miner's lung
Ming classification of gastric carcinoma
mini applier
miniature stomach
Mini-CABG instrument set
Mini Crown stent
mini fragment plate
mini gastric bypass (MGB)
Mini GLS anchor
mini Hohmann podiatric retractor
minilap (minilaparotomy)
mini laparoscope, Storz
minilaparotomy incision
mini-Lexer gouge
minimal deviation melanoma
minimally invasive esophagectomy
minimally invasive surgery (MIS)
minimal urine output
MiniMed insulin pump
Minimedicut
mini meniscus blade
mini Metzenbaum scissors
mini papillotome or minipapillotome
Mini QuickAnchor anchor
Mini-Revo Screw suture anchor
mini Roux retractor
mini Ruskin rongeur

MiniSite laparoscope
MINI 6600 C-arm
Mini Virobac filter
Minnesota tube, modified
minor crossmatch
minor duodenal papilla
Mintezol (thiabendazole)
Mintox, Mintox Plus
minute bleeding mucosal ulcer
minute papule
minute ventilation
Mira cautery
Mirage ostomy appliance
MiraLax (polyethylene glycol 3350)
Miralene suture
Miraluma (technetium ^{99m}Tc sestamibi
    kit)
Miraluma nuclear breast imaging
Mira Mark III cranial drill
Mira reamer
Mirizzi syndrome
mirror
    Bramber head
    laryngeal
    Ziegler head
mirror image breast biopsy
MIS (minimally invasive surgery)
MIS Source colonoscope
MIS Source duodenoscope
MIS Source flexible endoscope
MIS Source gastroscope
MIS Source sigmoidoscope
Miskimon cerebellar retractor
misoprostol
missed accessory spleen
missile track abscess
MIST insufflator
MIST video camera system
Mitek bone anchor
Mitek GII suture anchor
Mitek knotless suture anchor
Mitek Mini GII suture
Mitek staple
Mitek Superanchor suture anchor

Mitek suture
Mitek suture anchor
Mitek Vapor probe
Mitek VAPR system
Mitek VAPRTM T thermal electrode
mitochondrial antibody
mitochondrial oxidative
    phosphorylation
MitoExtra
mitogen-activated protein kinase
    (MAPK) cascade
mitomycin
Mitraflex dressing
Mitraflex Plus dressing
Mitraflex SC dressing
Mitraflex SC sacral dressing
mitral orifice
mitral stenosis
mitral valve homograft
Mitrofanoff appendicovesicotomy
Mitrofanoff neourethra procedure
Mitrolan (calcium polycarbophil)
Mitscherlich test
Mittelman nasal cartilage graft kit
mittelschmerz
Mitutoyo digital calipers
Mivacron (mivacurium chloride)
mivacurium chloride
mixed cell Hodgkin disease
mixed cell sarcoma
mixed cell thymoma
mixed cell tumor
mixed-cholesterol gallstone
mixed elemental-fat diet
mixed growth on culture
mixed hemorrhoids
mixed hepatocholangiocellular
    carcinoma
mixed hiatal hernia
mixed infection
mixed lesion
mixed neuropathic picture
mixed protein-fat diet
mixed venous blood

Mixter artery forceps
Mixter clamp
Mixter dilating probe
Mixter dissecting forceps, 90° angle,
    double-action
Mixter-O'Shaughnessy artery forceps
Mixter right-angle clamp
Mixter thoracic forceps
Mixter ventricular needle
Mladick concave cannula
Mladick convex cannula
Mladick liposuction cannula
MLT microlaryngeal tracheal tube
MMC (migrating motor complex)
MMF (mycophenolate mofetil)
MMMP (mucosal neuroma, medullary
    thyroid carcinoma, marfanoid body
    habitus, pheochromocytoma)
mmol/L (millimole per liter)
MM virus
MoAb monoclonal antibody
Mobetron electron accelerator
mobile axillary node
mobile gallbladder
mobile suction cart
mobilization of breast
mobilization of cecum
mobilization of gastric fundus
mobilization of small intestine through
    the mesocolon
mobilization of upper pole of thyroid
mobilize the duodenum and pancreas
mobilizer, Derlacki
MOC (metronidazole, omeprazole,
    clarithromycin)
Moctanin (monoctanoin)
Modane Bulk
Modane Plus
Modane Soft
Modane Versabran
model
    Claus breast cancer
    Gail breast cancer
    Markov simulation

moderate ductal hyperplasia
moderately differentiated adenoma
moderately well-differentiated
  carcinoma
moderate-size polymorphic inflamma-
  tory cell infiltrate
modified Allis grasping forceps,
  double-action
modified barium swallow
modified Bassini inguinal hernia repair
modified Delphi technique
modified dorsal lithotomy position
modified double Allis grasping forceps,
  double-action
modified Dukes staging (A-D)
modified Kessler suture
modified lithotomy position
modified Minnesota tube
modified neck dissection
modified Papanicolaou method
modified radical mastectomy
modified Robert Jones dressing
modified Shouldice hernioplasty
modified TAPP hernioplasty
modified tumescent technique
modified Whitehead hemorrhoidectomy
MODM (maturity-onset diabetes
  mellitus)
Modny pin
MODS (multiorgan [multiple organ]
  dysfunction syndrome)
Modudose A4398 unit dose saline vial
Modulap probe
Modulith SL 20 lithotriptor
MODY (maturity-onset diabetes of the
  young)
Moe distraction rod
Moe gouge
Moe intertrochanteric plate
Moe-modified Harrington rod
Moe spinal hook
Moe square-ended hook
MOF (multiple organ failure)
Mogen circumcision clamp

Mohr test
Mohs fresh tissue chemosurgery
moist sponge on ring forceps
molar mass
molar pregnancy (hydatidiform mole)
molecular death
molecular lesion
molecular marker
molecular mass
molecule
  antibody
  filtered
  middle
  PEG (polyethylene glycol)
  RNA
  secreted
moleskin dressing
moleskin scissors
moleskin strips dressing
Mollelast bandage
Mollison retractor
molluscum contagiosum
molluscum contagiosum virus
MOLLY bipolar forceps
Molt mouth gag
Molt periosteal elevator
Molypen (ammonium molybdate
  tetrahydrate)
MOM (milk of magnesia)
Mon-a-therm esophageal stethoscope
  temperature sensor
Mon-a-therm Foley catheter
Mon-a-therm skin temperature sensor
Mondor disease
mongolian spot-like lesion
monilial infection
monitor, monitoring (see also *blood
  glucose monitor*)
  Biotrack coagulation
  Cardiocap 5
  chronicle implantable hemodynamic
  Diasensor 1000 glucose
  Digital Response (DRx)
  DRx (Digital Response)

monitor *(cont.)*
    Duet glucose control
    esophageal pH
    FastTake blood glucose
    gastric pH
    Glycosal diabetes
    Health Buddy
    HealthCheck
    hemodynamic
    HemoMatic
    HERMES surgery
    Hewlett Packard temperature
    high-resolution video
    HomMed Sentry/Observer
    incuTemp
    IVAC
    Laserflo blood perfusion (BPM)
    Licox
    LifeShirt
    Lifestream Personal Cholesterol
        Monitor
    Meduck anesthesia
    Optical Sensors blood gas
    Prestige Smart System (PSS)
        glucose
    PSA 4000 anesthesia
    SureStep glucose
    TD Glucose
    24-hour ambulatory esophageal pH
monitored anesthesia care (MAC)
monitoring lumen
monocautery cable
monoclonal antibody (see *medication*)
    altumomab (^{111}In altumobab
        pentetate)
    altumomab pentetate (^{111}In
        altumobab pentetate)
    anti-HER2
    anti-HER2 humanized
    basiliximab
    B43.13 (BrevaRex) vaccine for solid
        tumors
    BTI-322
    cA2

monoclonal *(cont.)*
    Campath
    CB-45RB
    CEA-Cide
    cedelizumab
    Cotara
    CTLA4-Ig
    dacliximab (daclizumab)
    Ha1A
    Herceptin (trastuzumab) anti-HER2
    IgG 2A
    Immurait (IgG 2A)
    ^{111}In altumomab pentetate
    infliximab
    MAb
    MAb-170
    MoAb
    murine
    muromonab-CD3
    Orthoclone OKT3
    Ostavir (tuvirumab)
    satumomab pendetide
    Simulect (baxiliximab)
    technetium ^{99m}Tc solesomab
    Therex (huHMFG1)
    trastuzumab
monoclonal antibody to CEA,
    humanized
monoclonal antibody to hepatitis B
    virus, human
monoclonal B cell proliferation
    Muromonab-CD3
Monocryl (poliglecaprone 25) suture
monoctanoin
monocular microscope
monocytes
monofilament absorbable suture
monofilament microporous mesh
monofilament nylon drain
monofilament nylon suture
monofilament polypropylene suture
monofilament stainless steel suture
Monojector fingerstick device
monojet Toomey syringe

mosquito forceps
mosquito hemostat
Moss decompression feeding catheter
Mosse syndrome
Moss gastrostomy tube (G-tube)
Moss G-tube PEG kit
Moss hook
Moss nasal tube, Mark IV
Moss rod
Moss Suction Buster tube
Moss T-anchor needle introducer gun
moth-eaten appearance (on imaging)
mother cyst
mother/daughter endoscope
Mother Jones (modified Robert Jones)
  dressing
motility
  colonic
  cornflake esophageal
  esophageal
  gastrin-stimulated intestinal
  GI
  intestinal
  primary esophageal
motility disorder
  esophageal
  gastric
  intestinal
  nonspecific esophageal motility
    (NEMD)
  smooth-muscle
  primary esophageal
Motilium (domperidone maleate)
motion pain
motion sickness
Motofen (difenoxin HCl; atropine
  sulfate)
motorized gouge
motor meal barium GI series
motor oil peritoneal fluid
motor test meal
mottled appearance
moulage for breast implant
moulage for custom breast implant

moulage sign
Mount laminectomy rongeur
Mouradian rod
mouse, peritoneal
Mousseaux-Barbin intraluminal tube
Mousseaux-Barbin prosthetic tube
mouth gag
  Ackland
  Crowe-Davis
  Davis
  Denhardt
  Dingman
  Doyen-Jensen
  Jennings
  McIvor
  Molt
mouth guard
mouth to anus
movable kidney
movement, bowel (BM)
moxifloxacin
Moynihan artery forceps
Moynihan bile duct probe
Moynihan forceps
Moynihan gall duct forceps
Moynihan gallstone probe
Moynihan gallstone scoop
Moynihan test
Moynihan towel clamp
MPC scissors
MPD (main pancreatic duct) stent
MPEC (multipolar electrocoagulation)
MPH (medullary thyroid carcinoma,
    pheochromocytoma, hyperpara-
    thyroidism)
MPI 5020
MPM hydrogel dressing
MPT (multiple parameter telemetry)
MRC (magnetic resonance cholangi-
    ography)
MRCP (magnetic resonance cholangio-
    pancreatography)
MRCP using HASTE with a phased
    array coil

MRI (magnetic resonance imaging)
MRM (magnetic resonance mammography)
MRN (magnetic resonance neurography)
MRP (magnetic resonance pancreatography)
MR peritoneography
MRSA (pronounced "mer-sah") (methicillin-resistant *Staphylococcus aureus*)
MS Classique balloon dilatation catheter
MSA (microsomal antibody)
MSEV (microsurgical epididymovasostomy)
MSI (microsatellite instability)
MSOF (multisystem organ failure)
MS-1 hepatitis
MS-2 hepatitis
MS-325 imaging agent
MTBE (methyl tertiary butyl ether)
mtDNA (mitochondrial DNA)
M2A Swallowable Imaging Capsule
M-25 virus
mucin clot formation
mucin clot test
mucin, gastric
mucinoid degeneration
mucinosis
    follicular
    papular
mucinous adenocarcinoma
mucinous adenoma
mucinous carcinoma
mucinous cystadenocarcinoma
mucinous degeneration
mucinous nest
mucocele, appendiceal
mucocele of gallbladder
mucocutaneous hemorrhoids
mucocutaneous junction
mucocutaneous line

mucocutaneous pigmentation of Peutz-Jeghers syndrome
mucoepidermal carcinoma
mucoepidermoid carcinoma
mucoid material
mucoid secretion
mucoid stool
Mucomyst
Mucopolysaccharidoses
mucopurulent drainage
mucormycosis
mucosa
    alimentary
    alveolar
    anorectal
    antral
    auditory
    Barrett
    blanching of
    bronchial
    buccal
    bulging of
    burned out (on x-ray)
    cardiac (of stomach)
    cobblestone
    cobblestoning of
    colorectal
    denuded
    discolored
    ectopic gastric
    edematous
    endocervical
    esophageal
    foveolar gastric
    foveolosulciolar gastric
    friable
    fundic
    gallbladder
    gastric antral
    gastrointestinal
    gingival
    hemorrhagic
    honeycomb

mucosa *(cont.)*
  hyperemic
  hyperplastic
  hypertrophied
  intestinal
  irregular
  Neisseria
  normal-appearing
  outpouching of
  oxyntic
  polyp of hypertrophied
  protrusion of the
  pyloric
  rectal
  sloughing of
  small bowel
  spiraling of rectal
  sulciolar gastric
  thumbprinting of
  tracheobronchial
  urinary
  vaginal
mucosal abnormality
mucosal advancement
mucosal atrophy
mucosal bridge
mucosal disease virus
mucosal folds
mucosal guideline pattern
mucosal hyperemia
mucosal hyperplasia
mucosal ileal diaphragms
mucosal immune system
mucosal injection
mucosal involvement
mucosal island (on x-ray)
mucosal junction, squamocolumnar
mucosal melanoma
mucosal necrosis
mucosal neuroma syndrome (MEA
  type III)
mucosal neuromas
mucosal patch
mucosal pattern

mucosal proctectomy
mucosal ring, esophageal
mucosal sleeve resection
mucosal surface
mucosal suspensory ligament
mucosal ulcer
mucosal ulceration
mucosal view
mucosal zone
mucosanguineous discharge
mucosectomy, rectal
mucoserous cell
mucositis
  candida
  cytolomegalovirus
  herpes
mucous (adj.)
mucous carcinoma
mucous cell
mucous colic
mucous colitis
mucous cyst
mucous degeneration
mucous diarrhea
mucous fistula
mucous gland of duodenum
mucous lake of stomach
mucous membrane
mucous neck cell
mucous plug
mucous polyp
mucous salivary gland
mucous shred
mucous stool
mucous strand
mucous surface
mucoviscidosis
mucus (noun); mucous (adj.)
mucus per rectum
mucus plug
mucus plugging
mucus-secreting cell
mucus-secreting gland
mud, biliary

Mueller (Müller)
Mueller compression blade plate
Mueller maneuver
Mueller rongeur
Mueller saw
Mueller 0° 5 mm rigid laparoscope
"muffs" bandage
Muir hemorrhoid forceps
mulberry calculus
mulberry gallstone
mule-spinner's cancer
Mulholland sphincterotomy
Muller pediatric clamp
Müller (see *Mueller*)
Mullins catheter introducer
MultAport cannula
MultApplier device
MultApump device
MultAvalue laparoscopic device
MulTE-Pak-4: MulTE-Pak-5 (multiple
　　trace elements [metals])
multi-agent therapy
Multibite biopsy forceps
multicellular organism
multicentric lesion
multicentric thyroid
multicentricity
Multiclip ligating clip device
Multidex hydrophilic powder dressing
Multidex wound-filling material
multidisciplinary transplant team
multidrug resistant (MDR)
multidrug systemic chemotherapy
multifactorial etiopathogenesis
multifilament suture
Multifire Endo GIA stapler
Multifire Endo Hernia clip applicator
Multifire Endo Hernia stapler
Multifire GIA surgical stapler
Multifire TA surgical stapler
Multifire VersaTack stapler
multiflanged Portnoy (for hydrocephalus
　　shunt) catheter
Multi-Flex stent

multifocal lesion
multifocal tumor
multifunction port
Multikine
Multikuf sphygmomanometer
Multi-Link Tetra coronary stent system
multilobular cirrhosis
multilocular mass
multiloculated tumor
multilumen probe
Multilyte-40 (combined electrolyte
　　solution)
multimodal therapy
multinodular gland
multinodular goiter
multinodular mass
Multi-Operatory Dentalaser (MOD)
　　laser
multiorgan dysfunction syndrome
　　(MODS)
multiorgan failure
multiplanar fluoroscopic stress view
multiple abscess formation
multiple colloid adenomatous goiter
　　(MCAG)
multiple cysts
multiple dysplastic nevi
multiple endocrine adenomatosis
　　(MEA) syndrome, type 2
multiple endocrine deficiency
　　syndrome, type 2
multiple endocrine neoplasia, type 2B
multiple familial polyposis
multiple hamartoma syndrome
multiple hamartomatous polyps
multiple idiopathic hemorrhagic
　　sarcoma
multiple inert gas elimination
　　techniques (MIGET)
multiple infarcts
multiple inflammatory fibrous
　　thickenings
multiple intestinal polyposis
multiple myeloma

multiple myositis
multiple neuritis
multiple nodules
multiple organ dysfunction
multiple organ dysfunction syndrome
    (MODS)
multiple organ failure (MOF)
multiple organ failure syndrome
    (MOFS)
multiple organ involvement
multiple pain afferents
multiple parameter telemetry (MPT)
multiple polyp
multiple previous surgical procedures
multiple proinflammatory cytokines
multiple sclerosis
multiple-strand suture
multiple thyroid nodules
multiple transfusions
multipolar coagulation
multipolar electrocautery
multipolar electrocoagulation (MPEC)
    therapy (MECT)
Multipurpose-SM catheter
multiseptate gallbladder
multisized reamer
multistep carcinogenesis
multistrand
multisystem disease
multisystem organ failure (MOM)
Multitak SS suture anchor
multivariate analysis
multiverrucous friable lesion
multivisceral transplantation
mumps hepatitis
mumps pancreatitis
mumps virus
Munchausen syndrome
Munro point
mural kidney
mural thickening
MUR (multiuse reposable) clip applier
murine leukemia virus
murine monoclonal antibody

Murless fetal head extractor
muromonab-CD3 monoclonal antibody
Murphy common duct dilator
Murphy eye
Murphy gallbladder retractor
Murphy gouge
Murphy-Lane bone skid
Murphy retractor
Murphy sign
Murphy tip
Murray Valley encephalitis virus
muscle biopsy
muscle biopsy clamp
muscle carnitine deficiency
muscle fasciculation
muscle guarding
muscle hook
muscle necrosis
muscle pedicle
muscle-splitting incision
muscle-to-bone suture
muscle wasting
muscular propria
muscular ring, esophageal
muscularis
musculature, intra-abdominal wall
musculoaponeurotic band
musculoaponeurotic sheath tumor
MUSE (medicated urethral system
    for erection)
mushroom catheter
mushroom gastrostomy tube
mushroom-shaped mass
mushy stools
musical bowel sounds
Mustang steerable guidewire
Mutamycin (mitomycin)
mutation
    BRCA
    gene
    P53
MVR blade
Mya hook
myalgia

myasthenia gravis
mycobacterial antibody
mycobacterial spheroplast
Mycobacterium avium-intracellulare
 (MAI) complex
Mycobacterium gordonae
Mycobacterium tuberculosis
mycophenolate mofetil (MMF)
Mycoplasma pneumoniae
mycosis, gastric
Mycostatin
mycotoxin aflatoxin
MycroMesh biomaterial graft
myelin kidney
myelogenic sarcoma
myelogenous leukemia
myeloid metaplasia
myeloid sarcoma
myeloma kidney
myelophthisic splenomegaly
myeloproliferative disorder
myelosuppression
myelotomy knife
myenteric plexus
Myers-Fine test
Myers knee retractor
Mylagen, Mylagen II (aluminum
 hydroxide; magnesium hydroxide;
 simethicone)
Mylanta (calcium carbonate; magne-
 sium hydroxide; simethicone)
Mylanta Natural Fiber Supplement
 (psyllium hydrophilic mucilloid)
Mylanta-II
Mylar patch
Mylicon (simethicone)
Mylius test
myoblastoma, granular cell
myocardial necrosis
Myocet (liposome encapsulated doxoru-
 bicin citrate complex)
myocutaneous flap
myocutaneous graft

myodesis suture
myoelectric dysrhythmia
myofibroblast
myofibroma
myolysis
myoma
myomatous polyp
myomectomy, anorectal
myoneural junction
myoneural necrosis
myopathic carnitine deficiency
myopathic electromyography
myopathy
 infantile mitochondrial
 inflammatory
 ipecac-induced
 myxedema
 steroid
 thyrotoxic
 toxic
myopectineal opening of Fruchaud
myopectineal orifice (MPO)
myotomy
 circular
 cricoid
 cricopharyngeal
 esophageal
 extramucosal
 Heller
 laparoscopic
 longitudinal
myotonic dystrophy
myxedema ascites
myxedema coma
myxedema madness
myxedema myopathy
myxedema, pretibial
myxofibroma
myxoid material
myxomatous tumor
myxorrhea gastrica
myxovirus

N, n

N (nitrogen)
NA (Narcotics Anonymous)
Na (sodium)
Nabi-Altastaph vaccine
Nabi-HB (hepatitis B immune globulin
    [human])
Nabi NicVAX vaccine
Nabi-StaphVAX vaccine
nabothian gland
NABS (normoactive bowel sounds)
N-acetylcysteine (NAC)
NaCl (sodium chloride)
Nadler coaptation bipolar forceps
Naganol (suramin sodium)
nagging pain
nail
    adjustable
    Ainsworth modification of Massie
    antegrade femoral
    AO slotted medullary
    AP
    Augustine boat
    Bailey-Dubow
    Barr
    Bickel intramedullary
    Bionx SmartNail
    blind medullary
    boat

nail *(cont.)*
    Brooker femoral
    Brooker-Wills
    cannulated
    Chick
    Christensen interlocking
    closed
    closed Küntscher (Kuentscher)
    closed unlocked
    cloverleaf intramedullary
    cloverleaf Küntscher (Kuentscher)
    condylocephalic
    crutch-and-belt femoral closed
    Curry hip
    Derby
    Deyerle pin
    diamond-shaped medullary
    Dooley
    double-ended
    double-hollow
    dynamic locking
    elastic stable intramedullary (ESIN)
    Ender
    Ender flexible medullary
    Engel-May
    extension
    femoral neck
    fixator-augmented

nail *(cont.)*
    fluted titanium
    four-flanged
    gamma locking
    Grosse-Kempf interlocking
      medullary
    Hagie pin
    Hahn bone
    half-and-half
    hallux
    Hansen-Street
    Harris condylocephalic
    Harris hip
    Harris medullary
    Holt
    hooked intramedullary
    hooked medullary
    Huckstep
    ingrown (onychocryptosis)
    INRO surgical
    interlocking
    interlocking intramedullary
    intramedullary (IM)
    Inyo
    Jewett
    Johannson hip
    Kaessmann
    Ken
    Ken sliding
    Knowles
    Küntscher (Kuentscher) medullary
    left-sided
    Lewis
    locked intramedullary
    locking
    Lottes triflanged medullary
    Massie II
    Massie sliding
    McKee tri-fin
    McLaughlin
    medullary
    Moore
    nailing
    nested

nail *(cont.)*
    Neufeld
    noncannulated
    Nylok self-locking
    open
    OrthoSorb pin
    Palmer bone
    PGP
    Pidcock
    pre-bent
    Pugh sliding
    reconstruction
    retrograde femoral
    Richards reconstruction
    right-sided
    Rush flexible medullary
    Rush pin
    Russell-Taylor (R-T) interlocking
      medullary
    Rydell
    Sage triangular
    Sampson medullary
    Sarmiento
    Schneider medullary
    Seidel humeral locking
    self-broaching
    self-locking
    Slocum
    SmartNail
    Smillie
    Smith-Petersen femoral neck
    Smith-Petersen transarticular
    spring-loaded
    static locking
    Steinmann extension
    Street
    Sven-Johansson femoral neck
    telescoping
    Temple University
    Terry
    Thatcher
    Thornton
    Tiemann
    titanium

nail *(cont.)*
    triangular medullary
    triflange
    triflanged Lottes
    Uniflex intramedullary
    Venable-Stuck
    Vesely-Street split
    Vitallium Küntscher (Kuentscher)
    V-medullary
    Watson-Jones
    Webb
    Z fixation
    Zickel intramedullary
    Zickel subtrochanteric
    Zickel supracondylar medullary
nail assembly, Massie
nail atrophy
nail bed
nail driver
nail-extracting hook
nail nipper
nail plate
nail-pulling forceps
nail rotational guide
nail scissors
nail splitter
nail-splitting scissors
Nakao snare I and II
Nakayama test
Namalwa cell
NANB (non-A, non-B) hepatitis (now hepatitis C)
nandrolone phenpropionate
N&V (nausea and vomiting)
NAP hepatitis B virus (HBV) quantitative panel
Naphuride (suramin sodium)
napkin-ring annular lesion
Narco esophageal motility machine
narcotic addiction
Narcotics Anonymous (NA)
Nardi test (morphine-prostigmine)
Naropin (ropivacaine)
narrow blade retractor

narrow neck mini Hohmann retractor
narrowing of thoracic aorta
nasal dressing sponge
nasal elevator
nasal instrumentation
nasal intubation
nasal olives glass
nasal polyp
Nasal RAE uncuffed tube
nasal septal hematoma
nasal smear
nasal sponge
nasal suction/irrigator with sheath
NASH (nonalcoholic steatohepatitis)
Nashold biopsy needle
Nashville Rabbit Antithymocyte Serum (lymphocyte immune globulin, antithymocyte [rabbit])
nasobiliary catheter
nasobiliary drain
nasobiliary drainage
nasobiliary drainage catheter
nasobiliary drainage tube
nasoduodenal feeding tube
nasoendoscopy
nasogastric (NG)
nasogastric feeding tube
nasogastric suction
nasogastric aspirate
nasogastric drainage
nasogastric intubation
nasogastric tube
nasogastric tube suction
nasojejunal (NJ) feeding tube
nasolabial fistula
nasolaryngopharyngoscope
nasopancreatic drainage
nasopancreatic drainage tube
nasopancreatic tube
nasopharyngeal carcinoma
nasopharyngeal hemorrhage
nasopharyngeal reflux
nasopharynx
nasotracheal intubation

nasotracheal tube
nateglinide
National Cancer Institute (NCI)
National Diabetes Data Group (NDDG)
National Digestive Diseases
 Information Clearinghouse
 (NDDIC)
National Donor Family Council
 (NDFC)
National Hospital percussor
National Institute of Diabetes and
 Digestive and Kidney Diseases
 (NIDDK)
National Kidney Foundation
National Organization for Rare
 Disorders, Inc.
native vasculature
Native American heritage
native tissue Harmonic imaging (NTHI)
natural body fluid
natural death
natural killer (NK) antigen
natural killer cell
natural resin, propolis
Natural Vegetable (psyllium hydrophilic
 mucilloid)
Nature's Remedy (cascara sagrada)
Naunton Morgan proctoscope
Naunton Morgan rectal speculum
nausea and vomiting (N/V, N&V)
nausea, postprandial
Nausea Relief (phosphorated carbo-
 hydrate solution)
nauseous
Nausetrol (phosphorated carbohydrate
 solution)
NAVEL (nerve, artery, vein, extra-
 lymphatic material, lymphatics)
navicular shoe cookie (pad)
navicular view
Navigator flexible endoscope
Navigator system for lymph node detec-
 tion
Naviguide introducer

Navion BioNavigation system
Naviport catheter
Naviport deflectable tip-guiding catheter
Navi-Star catheter
Navitrack system
Navratil retractor
NBT (nitroblue tetrazolium)
NBT-PABA test
NCCH (National Cancer Center
 Hospital)
NCI (National Cancer Institute)
NCPF (noncirrhotic portal fibrosis)
NDDG (National Diabetes Data Group)
NDDIC (National Digestive Diseases
 Information Clearinghouse)
NDFC (National Donor Family Council)
Nd:YAG (neodymium:yttrium-
 aluminum-garnet) laser
Neal fallopian cannula
near-anatomic position
near-far suture
near-infrared spectroscopy (NIRS)
Nearly Me breast prosthesis
near-syncopal episode
near-syncope
near-total esophagectomy
near-total pancreatectomy
near-total removal
near-total thyroidectomy
nebulizer
 handheld
 large-volume
 ultrasonic
NEC (necrotizing enterocolitis)
Necator americanus
neck crepitus
neck exploration
neck hematoma
neck irradiation
neck masses
neck of gallbladder
neck of pancreas
necrosectomy

necrosis
    acute sclerosing hyaline (ASHN)
    acute tubular
    aseptic
    avascular (AVN)
    bacillary
    Balser fatty
    bilateral cortical
    biliary piecemeal
    blood vessel
    bloodless zone of
    bone
    bony
    bowel
    bridging
    caseous
    central
    centrilobular
    cerebral radiation (CRN)
    cheesy
    coagulation
    colliquative
    colonic
    contraction band
    cortical
    cystic medial
    diffuse
    dry
    embolic
    epiphyseal ischemic
    Erdheim cystic medial
    exanthematous
    extensive pancreatic
    fat
    fatty
    femoral head
    fibrinoid
    fibrosing piecemeal
    focal
    focal hepatic
    frank
    gallbladder
    gangrenous
    gangrenous pulp

necrosis *(cont.)*
    hemorrhagic
    hemorrhoidal
    hepatic
    hepatocellular
    hyaline
    indurative
    infected
    infectious pancreatic
    intestinal
    liquefaction
    liver
    localized
    malarial
    Marcus grading scale for avascular
    massive hepatic
    massive ischemic
    medial cystic
    midzonal
    mucosal
    muscle
    myocardial
    myoneural
    neuronal
    Paget quiet
    pancreatic
    papillary
    peripheral
    peripheral hepatic
    phosphorus
    piecemeal
    postpartum pituitary
    postreduction ischemic
    pressure
    progressive emphysematous
    radiation
    renal tubular
    segmental
    septic
    skin
    small bowel
    soft tissue
    sterile pancreatic
    stomal

necrosis *(cont.)*
   strangulation
   stromal
   subacute
   subacute hepatic
   subcutaneous fat
   submassive
   submassive hepatic
   superficial
   syphilitic
   thermal
   tissue
   total
   tracheobronchial mucosal
   tumor
   Zenker
   zonal
necrosis and perforation
necrosis of bladder epithelium
necrosis of bladder mucosa
necrosis of ductal epithelium
necrosis of gallbladder wall
necrosis of hepatocyte
necrosis of muscle
necrosis of muscle cells
necrosis of small bowel mucosa
necrosis of tissue
necrotic abscess
necrotic "anchovy paste" material
necrotic bone
necrotic bowel
necrotic debris
necrotic fibroid
necrotic hemorrhoids
necrotic inflammation
necrotic lesion
necrotic segment
necrotic tissue
necrotic tumor
necrotic ulceration
necrotizing arteriolitis in kidney
necrotizing arteritis
necrotizing arteritis associated
   with hepatitis B infection

necrotizing enterocolitis (NE, NEC)
necrotizing fasciitis
necrotizing gastritis
necrotizing gingivitis
necrotizing glomerulonephritis
necrotizing granulomatous lymph-
   adenitis
necrotizing migratory erythema
necrotizing nephrosis
necrotizing pancreatitis
necrotizing papillitis
necrotizing pneumonia
necrotizing vasculitis of bowel
NED (no evidence of disease)
needle
   Abrams
   Abrams biopsy
   Accucore II core biopsy
   Adson aneurysm
   Adson scalp
   Ailee
   Aldrete
   AMC
   aneurysm
   aortic root perfusion
   Arruga
   Arthrotek RC
   aspirating
   aspiration
   aspiration injection
   Atraloc surgical
   Backlund biopsy
   band circling
   Barraquer
   B-D spinal
   B-D Weiss epidural with fixed wings
   Becton Dickinson Teflon-sheathed
   Bengash-type
   beveled thin-walled
   Beyer paracentesis
   Bier lumbar puncture
   Bierman
   BiLAP bipolar needle electrode

needle *(cont.)*
    biopsy
    Biopty cut
    bone biopsy
    bone round
    Bonney
    bore
    Bouge
    Boynton
    BRK series transseptal
    Brockenbrough transseptal
    Bunnell tendon
    butterfly
    BV-2
    BV130-5
    cardioplegic
    Cardiopoint
    Castroviejo
    Castroviejo-Mayo
    cataract
    Charles flute
    Chiba
    Chiba aspiration biopsy
    Chiba cholangiography
    Cibis ski
    CIF-4
    coaxial sheath cut-biopsy
    Cobb-Ragde
    Colapinto curved
    Colapinto transjugular liver biopsy
    Colorado microdissection
    cone biopsy
    cone ventricular
    Control-Release pop-off
    conventional cutting-sternum
    Cook aspiration biopsy
    Cook endoscopic curved
    Cope biopsy
    core biopsy
    Core aspiration/injection
    Core CO_2 insufflation
    Core laparoscopic aspiration/
      injection
    Cournand arteriogram

needle *(cont.)*
    Cournand-Grino arteriogram
    Craig biopsy
    Crawford
    Crile-Wood
    C-type acupuncture
    culposuspension
    Cushing ventricular
    cut-biopsy
    cutting
    cutting biopsy
    cyst aspiration
    Dandy ventricular
    DeBakey
    Derf
    Derf-TC
    D'Errico ventricular
    Deschamps
    Deschamps ligature
    Dieckmann intraosseous
    discission
    DLP cardioplegic
    docking
    Dos Santos
    double-pointed
    D-TACH removable
    dural
    Echo-Coat ultrasound biopsy
    electrode
    EMG (electromyogram)
    Endoknot suture
    Endopath Ultra Veress
    Estridge biopsy
    Ethalloy TruTaper cardiovascular
    Ethibond
    ExtreSafe
    eye
    Feild-Lee brain biopsy
    fine
    Finochietto
    fistula
    Framer tendon-passing
    Franklin-Silverman liver biopsy
    Franseen stereotactic

needle *(cont.)*
    Frazier ventricular
    French-eye
    Gabriel hemorrhoidal
    Gallie
    gastrointestinal
    Gillies
    GraNee
    Greene biopsy
    Gripper
    Gynex extended-reach
    Hagedorn
    Halsy
    Hariri-Heifetz
    Hawkeye suture
    Hawkins
    Hegar-Baumgartner
    Hemo-Drain
    Hoen ventricular
    hollow
    House
    House-Barbara shattering
    House-Rosen
    Howell biopsy aspiration
    hubbed
    Huber
    hypodermic
    insufflation
    Intracath
    J
    Jamshidi liver biopsy
    Jelco
    Jordan
    Kalt
    Keith
    Keith abdominal
    Klatskin liver biopsy
    Klima-Schleicher biopsy
    Knight needle
    Kobak pudendal block
    Koch nucleus hydrolysis
    Kopans breast lesion localization
    Kronecker aneurysm
    laparoscopy

needle *(cont.)*
    large bore
    large-bore slotted aspirating
    Lee cutting biopsy
    Lewis Pair-Pak
    Lewy-Holinger Teflon injection
    Lewy-Rubin Teflon glycerine
        mixture injection
    Lichtenberg
    ligature
    liver and peritoneum biopsy
    liver biopsy
    lumbar puncture
    Maciol laparoscopic suture
    Madayag biopsy
    MAGneedle controller
    Maho-Hegar
    Martin
    Martin cutting
    Mathieu
    Mayo Hegar
    Mayo noncutting
    Mayo trocar-point
    mediastinoscopy aspirating needle
    Menghini liver biopsy
    metal
    MH
    micro
    MicroFlow
    microscopic dissecting
    Microvasive sclerotherapy
    milliner's
    Mixter ventricular
    Nashold biopsy
    Neivert
    nonferromagnetic
    Nordenstrom biopsy
    Nottingham
    olive-tipped
    Olsen-Hegar
    OmniTip laser
    Optivis
    Pace ventricular
    Paparella straight

needle *(cont.)*
    Parhad-Poppen arteriogram
    Parham band-circling
    PC-7
    P.D. Access
    Pencan spinal
    Penfine
    PercuCut cut-biopsy
    percutaneous cutting
    Pereyra
    pericardiocentesis
    peritoneal biopsy
    P-4
    phacoemulsification
    Pitkin spinal
    pleural biopsy
    Plum-Blossom
    PMT biopsy
    Pneu-Stick abdominal
    pneumoinsufflation
    pneumoperitoneum
    Poppen ventricular
    port closure
    postmortem
        double-curve cutting-edge
        half-curved cutting-edge
    Potts-Cournand
    pressure (teishein)
    Protect Point
    Punctur-Guard
    Quincke lumbar puncture
    Quincke spinal
    Redon wound drainage
    Reichert-Mundinger biopsy
    Retter aneurysm
    Reverdin suture
    Rhoton
    Riza-Ribe grasper
    root
    Rosch-Uchida transjugular liver
        access needle-catheter
    Rosen
    Rosenthal
    Rotex cutting biopsy

needle *(cont.)*
    Rotex II biopsy
    Ruskin antrum trocar
    Ryder
    Sabreloc spatula
    SafeTap tapered spinal
    Safetrak epidural
    Safety AV fistula
    Sahli biopsy and aspiration needle
    SampleMaster biopsy needle
    Sarot
    scalp
    sclerotherapy
    SC-1
    Scoville ventricular
    Seldinger
    Seldinger gastrostomy
    self-aspirating cut-biopsy
    Sensi-Touch anesthesia
    Shambaugh palpating
    Shaw aneurysm
    Sheldon-Spatz vertebral arteriogram
    side-aspirating biopsy
    side-cutting spatulated
    Sieman irrigation injection
    Silverman
    Silverman-Boeker
    Simcoe
    skinny
    skinny Chiba
    slotted
    SmallPort
    SmartNeedle
    Smiley-Williams arteriogram
    Solitaire
    spatulated half-circle
    spinal
    Spinell biopsy
    spinocan spinal
    Sprotte
    Stamey
    steel-winged butterfly
    Steis
    stereotactic biopsy

needle *(cont.)*
    Stifcore aspiration
    straight cutting
    Stratte
    Sureshot metal sheathed injection
    Surgalloy
    Surgineedle pneumoperitoneum
    suture
    SutureLoop
    suture-release
    swaged
    swaged-on
    Swedish
    Syme aneurysm
    Szabo-Berci needle driver
    tapered
    taper point
    teasing
    Teflon-coated hollow-bore
    teishein
    tendon-passing
    Terry-Mayo
    THI
    Thomas
    thoracentesis
    transjugular access
    transseptal
    Troutman
    Tru-Cut biopsy
    Tru-Cut cutting biopsy
    Tru-Cut liver biopsy
    Tru-Cut/Vim Silverman
    Tuohy epidural
    Tuohy lumbar puncture
    Tuohy point
    Tuohy thin-wall
    Turner biopsy
    ultrasound biopsy
    UMI
    Unimar J-Needle
    venting aortic Bengash-type
    ventricular
    ventriculostomy
    Verbrugge

needle *(cont.)*
    Veress (not Verres)
    Vim-Silverman
    Visi-Black surgical
    Voorhees (do not confuse with
        Veress)
    Wangensteen
    Waterfield
    Webster
    Westcott cutting biopsy
    Westerman-Jensen
    Whitacre spinal
    wire circling
    Wright
    Yankauer
NeedleAid device
needle and spud
needle aspiration, fine-
needle aspiration for culture
needle biopsy (see *biopsy*)
    confirmatory
    core
    CT-directed
    CT-scan directed
    fine-
    guided
    random
    stereotactic core needle (SCNB)
    transthoresis (TNB)
    ultrasound-guided
    Vim/Silverman
needle case
needle catheter jejunostomy
needle core biopsy
needle drainage
needle driver, Zsabo-Berei
needle electro probe
needle EMG
needle guide
    Iowa trumpet
    Site ~ Rite
needle holder
    Adson dural
    Ayers

needle holder *(cont.)*
   Barraquer
   Baumgartner-TC
   Berry sternal
   boomerang
   Boynton
   Bozeman Thomas Walker
   Brown
   Castroviejo
   Castroviejo-Mayo
   Castroviejo-TC
   Castroviejo-TC spring
   Collier
   Converse-TC
   Crile-Wood
   DeBakey-TC
   Derf, Derf-TC
   Diethrich-TC
   Donaghy angled suture
   Dubecq-Princeteau angulating
   Foster-TC
   Fukushima-Giannotta
   Gillies
   Gillies-Finochietto
   Halsey-TC
   Heaney
   Jacobson microvascular
   Jacobson-TC
   Kalman
   Kilner-TC
   Lichtenberg-Ryder
   Masson
   Mathieu-TC
   Mayo-Hegar
   M.G.H.
   Micro-One
   Micron
   Miltex
   Neivert-TC
   New Orleans
   Olsen-Hegar-TC
   Olsen-Mathieu-TC
   Parell-TC
   Parks-TC

needle holder *(cont.)*
   ratchet-on-demand
   Ryder-TC
   Ryder micro
   Sarot-TC
   Stevens
   Stratte-TC
   TC (tungsten carbide)
   Thomson
   Thomson Walker-TC
   titanium microsurgical
   Twisk
   Vantage
   Vickers
   Vital Cooley microvascular
   Vital Ryder microvascular
   Wangensteen
   Ward
   Webster
   Webster-TC
   Wright
   Young-Millin boomerang holder
needle holder+A4654 with tungsten
   carbide (TC) inlays
needle hub
needle inserted under fluoroscopic
   control
needle introducer
needle knife
needle-knife sphincterotome
needle lavage
needle localization, mammographically
   guided
needle localization of breast lesion
needle manometer technique
needle-nose dissecting forceps,
   double-action
needle-nose pliers
needlepoint electrocautery
needle-pulling forceps
needle puncture
needle puncture wound
needle raiser
needlescope
needlescopic TAPP hernia repair

needle sprotte
needlestick exposure
needle thoracostomy
needle-tip electrocautery
needle with Hustead wing
needle with tungsten carbide (TC)
  inserts, double-action
Neer lateral view
Neer transscapular view
Neff meniscus knife
negative antibody screen
negative appendectomy
negative breast biopsy
negative feedback
negative inotropic effect
negative inspiratory pressure
negative margin
negative pleural space pressure
negligible blood loss
Negus rigid esophagoscope
Neisseria
Neivert needle
Neivert polyp hook
Neivert-TC needle holder
Nélaton fold
Nélaton rubber tube drain
Nélaton sphincter
Nelson cannula
Nelson forceps
Nelson rib retractor
Nelson scissors
Nelson syndrome
Nelson thoracic trocar
Nelson tissue forceps
Nelson trocar
NEMD (nonspecific esophageal
  motility disorder)
neobladder construction following total
  cystectomy
Neocate One +
neocholangiole
Neo-Cultol (mineral oil)
NeoCure Cryoablation System
NeoDerm

Neo-Diaral (loperamide)
neodymium-YAG laser
neodymium:yttrium-aluminum-garnet
  (Nd:YAG) laser
Neoflex bendable knife
Neoflex bendable-knife electrocautery
Neoloid
Neomark (broxuridine)
Neomark-BU (broxuridine) test
Neo-Med cautery unit
Ne-Osteo bone morphogenic protein
  (BMP)
Neo-Sert umbilical vessel catheter
neotherm probe
Neo tracheal tube
neomycin sulfate
neonatal diabetes mellitus
neonatal diagnosis
neonatal diaphragmatic hernia
neonatal hepatitis
neonatal hyperbilirubinemia
neonatal hypoglycemia
neonatal hypoparathyroidism
neonatal intestinal obstruction
neonatal jaundice
neonatal lupus
neonatal lymphedema
neonatal thyrotoxicosis
neoplasia, anal epithelial
neoplasm (see also *tumor*)
  benign
  breast
  encapsulated
  firm
  functioning
  gonadal
  grading
  hormone-dependent
  Hürthle cell
  invasive
  islet cell
  lethal
  malignant
  ovarian

neoplasm *(cont.)*
  periampullary
  premalignant
  spherical
  staging
  thyroid
  well-circumscribed
neoplastic disease
neoplastic disorder
neoplastic extension
neoplastic polyp
Neoprobe 100 gamma-detection probe
Neoral (cyclosporine; alcohol)
neorectum
neostigmine
NeoTect disease-specific imaging agent
NeoTect kit
Neotrace-4 (multiple trace elements)
neovagina, rectal
Neovastat
nephritic calculus
nephritic colic
nephritis, interstitial
nephrogenic ascites
nephrogenic diabetes insipidus
nephroscope, Pentax ECN-1530 chole-
  dochonephroscope
nephrostomy-type catheter
nephrotic syndrome
nephrotoxic agent
Nephrox (aluminum hyroxide; mineral
  oil)
NERD (nonerosive reflux disease)
nerve biopsy
nerve block anesthesia
Nerve Block Infusion Kit
nerve block, percutaneous celiac
nerve graft
nerve hook
nerve hook plain
nerve of Latarjet
nerve root retractor
nerve suture
nervous gut

nervous vomiting
Nesacaine MPF (chloroprocaine)
nesidioblastosis
nested nail
Neufeld nail
Neufeld plate
Neukomm test
Neupogen (filgrastim) recombinant
  G-CSF
Neuprex
neural cell adhesion molecule (NCAM)
  expression
neural tube
neuralgia
neurinoma
neuroblockage
NeuroCol sponge
NeuroDrape surgical drape
neuroectoderm
neuroectodermal dysplasia
neuroendocrine C cells of the thyroid
neuroendocrine carcinoma of skin
neuroendocrine malignancy
neurofibroma, gastrointestinal
neurofibromatosis
neurogastroenterology
neurogenic arthropathy
neurogenic dysphagia
neurogenic intestinal obstruction
neurogenic sarcoma
neurohypophysis
neuroimmune dysfunction
neurolimmoma, malignant
neurologic gut dysfunction
neurological hammer
neurological insulin
neurological or neurosurgical scissors
neurolytic drug
neuroma, mucosal
Neuromeet nerve approximator
neuromuscular actions of
  catecholamines
neuromuscular irritability
neuromuscular transmission

neuronal necrosis
neuronoma, VIP-secreting
neuropathy
  alcoholic
  angiopathic
  ascending
  Dejerine-Sottas
  Denny Browne (Denis Browne)
  descending
  diabetic
  entrapment
  familial visceral
  peripheral
  peripheral autonomic
  postherniorrhaphy
  postoperative
  somatic
  visceral
Neuro-Patties sponge
neuroplasty fat graft
neuroplexus block
neurosurgical chisel
neurosurgical needle holder with
  tungsten carbide (TC) inlay
Neurotone multipurpose instrument
neurotransmitter
Neurotrend probe
neurovascular bundle
neurovascular island graft
neurovascular stent
NeuroVasx (Sub-Microinfusion)
  catheter
neutral and load drill guide
neutral calcaneal stance position
neutral drill guide
neutral hip position
neutral protamine Hagedorn (NPH)
  insulin
neutral spine position
neutralization plate
neutropenia
neutrophil activation
neutrophilic infiltration
Neville-Barnes forceps

nevus (pl. nevi), spider
Nevyas drape retractor
newborn hepatitis
newborn jaundice
newborn pneumonitis virus
Newcastle disease virus
New Eder Corporation trocar
Newman anoscope
Newman plate
Newman proctoscope
new-onset constipation
New Orleans needle holder
NEW Speaking Tube
New York Glass suction tube
new variable stiffness (VS) colonoscope
Nexium (esomeprazole magnesium)
NexStent carotid stent
Nexus 2 linear ablation catheter
Nezhat-Dorsey Trumpet Valve
NFkB-dependent gene activation
NG (nasogastric)
NG aspirate
NG feeding tube
NG suction as needed
NG tube decompression
NGT (nasogastric tube)
NGT aspiration
NGT suction
N High Sensitivity CRP (C-reactive
  protein) assay
niacin
Niaspan (niacin)
Nibbler device for dissection, morcella-
  tion, suction, and irrigation
Nibblit laparoscopic device
Nibs mapping pen
NIC (Nursing Interventions
  Classification)
nick, nicking (of fascia)
Nicola forceps
Nicola pituitary rongeur
Nicola rasp
Nicola scissors
Nicoll cancellous bone graft

Nicoll extractor
Nicoll graft
Nicoll plate
Nicoll rasp
nicotinamide
NIDDK (National Institute of Diabetes and Digestive and Kidney Diseases)
NIDDM (non-insulin-dependent diabetes mellitus)
Nidek EC-5000 excimer laser
nidus of inflamed tissue
nidus of necrotic tissue
nidus of stone formation
Niedner anastomosis clamp
Niemann-Pick disease
Niemeier classification of gallbladder perforation
Niemeier gallbladder perforation
night sweats, chills, and fever
Nigro protocol
NIH mitral valve forceps
Nilstat
Niopam contrast medium
nipple (pl. nipples)
   accessory
   cracked
   everted
   inverted
   level of
   slough of
   supernumerary breast
   ulcer of
nipple-areola complex
nipple change
nipple discharge
   bloody
   guaiac-positive
   milky
   persistent
   spontaneous
nippled stoma
nipple eversion
nipple exploration with excision
nipple-flap duct resection

nipple inversion
nipple lesion
nipple level
nipple rash
nipple reconstruction
nipple retraction
nipple valve
Niro bone-cutting forceps
NIR ON Ranger premounted stent system
NIR Primo Monorail stent system
Niro wire-twisting forceps
Niroyal Elite Monorail stent
NIRS (near-infrared spectroscopy)
Nissen antireflux operation
Nissen fundoplasty
Nissen fundoplication wrap
Nissen gall duct forceps
Nissen laparoscopic fundoplication
Nissen technique and partial posterior hemifundoplication (Toupet and Lind techniques)
Nissen 360° wrap fundoplication
Nissen wrap
nitinol mesh-covered frame
nitinol stent
nitrazoxanide
nitric oxide (NO)
nitrofural
nitrofurazone
nitrogen (N)
nitrogen balance
   negative
   positive
nitrogen partition test
nitroglycerin (NTG)
nitroglycerin I.V. (IV) drip
nitroglycerin ointment
Nitrolan
nitroprusside
nitrosamine
nitrous oxide
nitrous oxide insufflator
nizatidine

nodule *(cont.)*
  cold
  ectopic thyroid
  encapsulated
  fibroadenomatous
  freely movable
  HCC
  hot
  infiltration of
  lymphoid tissue
  malignant thyroid
  Morgagni
  multiple thyroid
  nondiscrete
  palpable
  regenerative cirrhotic
  rubbery
  satellite
  solitary thyroid
  subcutaneous
  thyroid
nodule uptake of intravenous ^{131}I or ^{99m}Tc
no evidence of disease (NED)
nolinium bromide
Nolvadex (tamoxifen citrate)
NOMSI (nonoperative management of splenic injury)
nonabsorbable blue monofilament suture
nonabsorbable dark blue braided stainless steel suture
nonabsorbable green and white braided suture
nonabsorbable green braided Ethibond suture
nonabsorbable steroid
nonabsorbable surgical suture
nonabsorbable white braided suture
nonadherent gauze dressing
nonadhesive bandage
nonadhesive dressing
nonadrenal tumor

nonalcoholic cirrhosis
nonalcoholic patient
nonalcoholic steatohepatitis
non-alpha, non-beta pancreatic islet cell
nonan malaria
non-A, non-B hepatitis (now hepatitis C)
nonbacterial gastroenteritis
nonbilious vomiting
nonbeta islet cell tumor of the pancreas
nonbloody stools
noncalcified stone
noncannulated nail
noncaseating tubercle-like granuloma
noncellular material
noncholecystokinin substance
noncirrhotic hepatitis C
noncirrhotic liver
noncirrhotic portal fibrosis (NCPF)
noncirrhotic portal hypertension
nonclinical diabetes
noncompliant patient
noncompliant ventricle
nonconductive tubing
noncontrast-enhanced CT scan
noncrushing bowel clamp
noncrushing vascular clamp
noncutaneous region
noncyclic pain
nondiabetic gastroparesis
nondiabetic insulin coma
nondiscrete nodule
nondistended abdomen
nondistensible
nondysenteric colitis
nonepithelial wall
nonerosive nonspecific gastritis
nonerosive reflux disease (NERD)
noneverting suture
nonfamilial intestinal pseudo-obstruction
nonferromagnetic needle
nonfibrous material
nonfilling gallbladder

nonfunctioning adrenal mass
nonfusion of cranial suture
nonhealing ulcer
non-heart-beating donor
nonhemolytic jaundice
nonhemolytic strep (streptococcus)
non-Hodgkin lymphoma
noniatrogenic cause
nonicteric sclerae
nonicteric skin
noninfectious colitis
noninfectious hepatitis
noninfective endocardial lesion
noninfiltrating lobular carcinoma
non-insulin-dependent diabetes mellitus (NIDDM)
non-Lynch syndrome
nonmedullary thyroid cancer
noninvasive carcinoma
noninvasive exploration of biliary tract
noninvasive imaging study
noninvasive localization study
nonionic contrast media
nonislet cell tumor
nonketotic coma
nonketotic hyperglycemic-hyperosmolar coma (NKHHC)
nonketotic hypoglycemia and carnitine deficiency due to MCAD deficiency
nonmalodorous fluid
nonmucosal hemorrhoidectomy
nonmutagenic surgical suture
nonobstructive hepatic parenchymal disease
nonobstructive ileus
nonocclusive intestinal infarction
nonocclusive mesenteric thrombosis
nonopaque stone
nonoperative management of splenic injury (NOMSI)
nonoperative therapy
nonoptical rigid bronchoscope
nonorganic dyspepsia
nonoxygenated blood

nonpalpable mass on mammogram
nonpalpable parathyroid
nonpathogenic organism
nonpenetrating wound
nonperforated appendicitis
nonperforated appendix
nonpliable
nonpuerperal breast abscess
nonrebreathing anesthesia
nonreducible mass
nonreflux esophagitis
nonrigid technique reduction mammo-plasty
nonskeletal metastases
non-small cell lung cancer
nonspecific colitis
nonspecific enteritis
nonspecific esophageal motility disorder (NEMD)
nonspecific gas pattern
nonspecific ulcerative proctitis
nonstanding lateral oblique view
Nonsterile Guedel Airways
nonsteroidal anti-inflammatory drug (NSAID)
Non-Stix sponge
nonsuppurative cholangitis
nonsuppurative thyroiditis
nontender gallbladder
nonthyroidal neck mass
nontoxic diffuse goiter
nontoxic nodular goiter
nontraumatic hernia
nontropical sprue
nontubed closed distant flap graft
nontubed open distant flap graft
nonulcer dyspepsia (NUD)
nonventilated patient
nonviable bowel
nonviable tissue
nonvisualization of gallbladder
nonweightbearing view
Noon AV fistula clamp
No Pain-HP (capsaicin)

no peritoneal signs
NoProfile balloon catheter
Norco (hydrocodone bitartrate; aceta-
    minophen)
Nordenstrom (Rotex II) biopsy needle
Nordt knot tightener
norepinephrine (NE)
norepinephrine analog
norepinephrine level
Norfolk-Norwich retractor
normal active bowel sounds
normal adrenal physiology
normal anatomic position
normal appendix
normal bile duct
normal calcitonin concentration
normal caliber duct
normal carrier hepatitis
normal colonic epithelium
normal flora
normal gas exchange in lung
normal gastric slow wave
normal hepatocyte
normal intestinal microflora
normal negative feedback loop
normal rectal exam
normal saline
normal saline drip
normal saline solution
Normal Stool Formula-IB (NSF-IB)
normal-appearing mucosa
normally apposed parietal and visceral
    pleura
normetanephrine
Normigel hydrogel dressing
normoactive bowel sounds
normochloremic metabolic acidosis
normochlorhydria
normocytic
normoglycemia, absolute
Normosol-M and 5% Dextrose
Normosol-R and 5% Dextrose
Normosol R pH 7.4 (combined
    electrolyte solution)

Northbent stitch scissors
North-South retractor
Norton ball reamer
Norwalk agent
Norwalk gastroenteritis
Norwalk virus
Norwood rectal snare
nosocomial infection
No Sting Barrier Film
not amenable to percutaneous drainage
notchplasty blade
notch, suprasternal
notch view
"no-trocar" zone (in path of epigastric
    arteries or immediately under costal
    margins)
Nottingham colposuspension needle
Nottingham introducer, semirigid
Nottingham Key-Med introducing
    device
NovaCath multi-lumen infusion catheter
Novafil suture
NovaGold breast implant
Novak suction curette
NovaLine Litho-S DUV excimer laser
Novamine 15% (amino acids)
NovaPulse CO_2 laser
NovaSaline inflatable saline breast
    implant
NovaSaline pre-filled breast implant
Novocain (procaine HCl)
Novo-Domperidone (domperidone
    maleate)
Novofil suture
Novolin L (insulin)
Novolin N PenFill
Novolin N Prefilled (insulin)
NovolinPen insulin device
Novolin R PenFill
Novolin R Prefilled (insulin)
Novolin 70/30 PenFill
Novolin 70/30 Prefilled (insulin)
Novolin 85/15 PenFill (insulin)
NovoLog (insulin aspart)

O, o

O_2 (oxygen)
O&P (ova and parasites) test
Oasis One Action stent introducer
Oasis wound dressing
oat cell carcinoma of lung
oat cell tumor of lung
O'Beirne sphincter
O'Brien rib hook
O'Brien staple
Oberhill laminectomy retractor
obesity
    adult-onset
    alimentary
    endogenous
    exogenous
    hyperinsulinar
    hyperinterrenal
    hyperplasmic
    hyperplastic
    hyperplastic-hypertrophic
    hypertrophic
    hypogonad
    hypoplasmic
    hypothyroid
    lifelong
    morbid
    simple
    truncal

obesity-associated diabetes
obesity hypoventilation syndrome
    (OHS)
obesity index
oblique course
oblique film
oblique hernia
oblique incision
oblique view
obliterated umbilical vein
obliteration of diverticulum
obliteration, percutaneous transhepatic
oblong-shaped onlay component
OBL RC5 soft tissue anchor
O_2 (oxygen) Boot
O'Brien scissors
Obrinsky syndrome
observation
obstipation
obstructed shunt tube
obstruction
    adynamic intestinal
    airway
    appendiceal lumen
    arterial
    bilateral ureteral (BUO)
    bile duct
    biliary

obturator *(cont.)*
   Frazier suction tube
   LaparoSAC single-use
   Soft Thoracoport
   Versaport
obturator canal
obturator fossa
obturator hernia
obturator node
obturator sign
obturator test
occipital suture
occipital view
occipitoanterior position
occipitocervical plate
occipitomastoid suture
occipitoparietal suture
occipitoposterior position
occipitosphenoid suture
occipitotransverse position
occluding clamp
occlusion
   balloon
   blood outflow line
   hepatic vein
   rectal
   splenic vein
occlusion clamp
occlusive dressing
occlusive ileus
occlusive lesion
occult blood
occult blood in stool
occult blood in urine
occult blood, positive test for
occult cancer
occult hepatitis
occult lesion
OCG (oral cholecystogram)
Ochsner artery forceps
Ochsner flexible spiral gallstone probe
Ochsner gall duct probe
Ochsner gallbladder probe
Ochsner gallbladder trocar

Ochsner hemostat
Ochsner ribbon retractor
Ochsner ring
OCL (polyethylene glycol electrolyte
   solution) bowel prep
o'clock (position, i.e., 9 o'clock
   position)
OCP (oral contraceptive pills)
ocrylate tissue adhesive (also ocrilate)
Ocrilon
OCT (optical coherence tomography)
   surgical imaging probe
Octamide PFS (metoclopramide)
Octastatin (vapreotide)
octatropine methylbromide
Octocaine HCl (lidocaine HCl;
   epinephrine)
Octopus tissue stabilizer
OctreoScan 111 (^{111}In pentetreotide)
octreotide
octreotide acetate
octreotide scan
ocular infection
ocular melanoma
ocular myasthenia
OcuLight SL diode laser
oculopharyngeal muscular dystrophy
OD (overdose)
Oddi sphincter
Oder-Weber-Rendu telangiectasia
O'Donoghue dressing
odontoid view
odynophagia
Oehler tissue and needle-pulling forceps
oestradiol (estradiol)
oestrone (estrone)
Oettingen abdominal retractor
Officer sigmoidoscope biopsy forceps
Officer tissue forceps
ofloxacin
OFS (organ failure score)
O'GAWA two-way cataract aspirating
   cannulas
Ogden anchor

Ogden plate
Ogilvie obstruction
Ogilvie pseudo-obstruction
Ogilvie syndrome (pseudo-obstruction
  of colon)
OGT (oral gastric tube)
OGT-918
Ogura tissue and cartilage forceps
O'Hanlon intestinal clamp
Ohio air
OHS (obesity hypoventilation
  syndrome)
oil
  castor
  evening primrose
  MCT (medium chain triglyceride)
  mineral
  oil-red-O
  peppermint
  rice bran
  seabuckthorn seed
  shark liver
oil enema
oil-red-O stain
oil retention enema
oily stools
OKT3 antibody
Okuda staging classification
Okuda transhepatic obliteration
  of varices
Oldberg brain retractor
Oldberg intervertebral disk rongeur
Oldberg pituitary forceps
Oldberg pituitary rongeur
Oldfield syndrome
Olds pin
O'Leary gastroplasty
O'Leary lesser curvature gastroplasty
Olerud PSF rod
oligomerization
Oligon catheter
olive (instrument)
  Eder-Puestow
  expandable

olive *(cont.)*
  metal
  palpable pyloric
Olivecrona clip-applying and removing
  forceps
Olivecrona dissector
Olivecrona dural scissors
Olivecrona-Gigli saw
Olivecrona rasp
Olivecrona rongeur
Olivecrona-Toennis clip-applying
  forceps
Olivecrona trigeminal knife
Olivecrona trigeminal scissors
olive over guidewire
olive-tipped needle
Olivier retractor
Ollier incision
Ollier rake retractor
Ollier thick split free graft
Ollier-Thiersch skin graft
OLM (ophthalmic laser micro-
  endoscope)
olsalazine sodium
Olsen cholangiogram clamp
Olsen-Hegar needle
Olsen-Hegar needle holder with
  tungsten carbide (TC) inlays
Olsen-Mathieu-TC needle holder
OLT (orthotopic liver transplant or
  transplantation)
Olympus (see *endoscope*)
Olympus clip applier
Olympus heat probe
Olympus hot biopsy forceps
Olympus hysteroscope
Olympus laparoscope
Olympus ligator
Olympus lithotriptor
Olympus monopolar cannula
Olympus needle-knife papillotome
Olympus OME-8000 dual stereo
  surgical microscope
Olympus One-Step Button gastrostomy
  tube

Olympus reusable hot biopsy forceps
Olympus rotatable clip applicator
Olympus rectal probe
Olympus SonoSurg ultrasonic cutting
    and coagulation
Olympus sphincterotome
Ombredanne forceps
Ombredanne mallet
Omed bulldog vascular clamp
omega-shaped incision
omega sign
omega-3 fatty acid
omental abscess
omental adhesion
omental band
omental bursa
omental cyst
omental flap
omental pack
omental patch (Graham closure)
omental pedicle
omental studding
omental wrapping
omentectomy
omentopexy
omentum
    colic
    gastric
    gastrocolic
    gastrohepatic
    gastrosplenic
    greater (omentum majus)
    incarcerated
    lesser (omentum minus)
    pancreaticosplenic
    splenogastric
    viable
omeprazole, omeprazole sodium
omeprazole plus amoxicillin
Omiderm dressing
Omiderm plain and mesh occlusive
    dressing
Omiderm transparent adhesive film
    dressing

Ommaya ventriculoperitoneal shunt
Omnican Piston syringe
OmniCath atherectomy catheter
Omnicef (cefdinir)
OmniFilter
Omni-Lift retractor
Omnipaque (iohexol)
OmniPulse holmium pulsed laser
OmniPulse-MAX holmium laser
Omni retractor
Omniscan (gadodiamide)
OmniStent
OmniTip laser needle
Omni-Tract adjustable wishbone
    retractor
omphalectomy
omphalocele
omphalomesenteric duct
Omsk hemorrhagic fever virus
Onchocerca volvulus
OncoChek immunoassay
oncogene
    Bc1-2
    c-erb B-2
    c-fos
    HER2/neu
oncogenesis
oncogenic virus
On-Command (male and female)
    catheter
Onconase (p30 protein)
Oncophage vaccine
OncoScint CR/OV (^{111}In satumomab
    pendetide)
OncoScint CR103 (colorectal) imaging
    agent
OncoScint OV103 imaging agent
oncosuppressor gene
Onco TCS
OncoVax-P
Oncovin (vincristine sulfate)
oncovirus
OnCyte assay
ondansetron HCl

one-chip camera
one-hour glucose tolerance test
O'Neill clamp
one-piece ostomy pouch
One Piece cannula
one-piece shunt
one-quadrant hemorrhoidectomy
One Touch Basic blood glucose monitor
One Touch FastTake blood glucose
    monitor
One Touch Profile blood glucose
    monitor
One Touch II blood glucose monitor
One Touch Ultra blood glucose monitor
On-Q anesthesia delivery system
On-Q postoperative pain management
    system
One-Shot anastomotic instrument
One Shot vascular clip applier
one-stage enterolithotomy and cholecys-
    tectomy
one-stage operation
One Touch Basic blood glucose monitor
One Touch blood glucose monitor
One Touch FastTake blood glucose
    monitor
One Touch Profile glucose monitor
One Touch reagent strips
One Touch II blood glucose monitor
One Touch II glucose monitor
one-tube cuff
onion bulb changes (on biopsy)
onion peel appearance
onion scale lesion
onion-shaped dilatation (of the
    duodenum)
onionskin appearance
onionskin lesion
onlay cancellous iliac graft
onlay mesh graft
onset of pain
OnSite stainless steel instrument
    repair
oophoropexy

ooze
oozing (of blood or fluid)
oozing, venous
opacification
    complete
    incomplete
    poor
Opal R.F. tissue ablation device
opaque calculi
opaque meal
Opdima digital mammography system`
open anesthesia
open biopsy
open brain biopsy
open diathermy-excision hemorrhoidec-
    tomy
open drainage
open drop anesthesia
opened in direction of its fibers
open-end ostomy pouch
open esophagectomy
open gastric banding procedure
opening of ampulla of Vater
open investing peritoneum over the
    internal inguinal ring
open laparoscopy cannula adapter
open laparotomy
open liver biopsy
open loop reflex
open mesh-plug hernioplasty
open-mouth odontoid view
open nail
open periprosthetic capsulotomy, breast
open pin
open pneumothorax
open posterior approach
open procedure
Open Sky MRI
open weave mesh graft
open wedge biopsy of the liver
open wound
Operand (povidone; iodine)
operating laparoscope
operating microscope

operating scissors (see *scissors*)
operating thorascope
operation or procedure (quick-reference
    list of diagnostic procedures and
    studies, and surgical procedures,
    approaches, maneuvers, methods,
    techniques, and therapies)
    Abbe
    Abbott esophagogastrostomy
    abdominal colectomy
    abdominal exploration
    abdominal pull-through
    abdominal-sacral colpoperineopexy
    abdominoperineal or abdominal-
      perineal resection (APR)
    Acucise retrograde procedure for
      incision of ureteral stricture and
      ureteropelvic junction obstruction
    afferent jejunostomy
    Albert-Lembert gastroplasty
    Alden loop gastric bypass
    Allison gastroesophageal reflux
    Alliston GE reflux correction
    Altemeier repair of rectal prolapse
    ampullectomy
    Amussat
    anal anastomosis
    anal stretch
    antireflux
    argon plasma coagulation
    anoplasty
      Martin
      posterior sagittal and 3-flap
    anorectoplasty, Laird-McMahon
    anorectovaginoplasty
    antecolic anastomosis
    anterior colon resection
    antiperistaltic
    antireflux
    antrectomy
    antrostomy
    antrotomy
    appendectomy
    appendicovesicotomy

operation *(cont.)*
    APR (abdominoperineal resection)
    Aries-Pitanguy correction of
      mammary ptosis
    Auchincloss modified radical
      mastectomy
    augmentation mammoplasty
    autologous bone marrow transplanta-
      tion
    autotransplantation of parathyroid to
      forearm
    axillary approach in augmentation
      mammoplasty
    axillary dissection
    axillary endoscopic reduction
    Aylett
    Baldy-Webster operation
    Ball operation for treatment of
      pruritus ani
    balloon tamponade
    BAMBI (breast augmentation
      mammoplasty by injection)
    banding (hemorrhoidal)
    band ligation of esophageal varices
    band sigmoidopexy
    band-snare technique
    bariatric
    Barron hemorrhoidal banding
      technique
    Bassini hernia repair
    Bassini herniorrhaphy
    Battle
    "belly button" augmentation
      mammoplasty
    Belsey antireflux Mark IV
    Belsey IV fundoplasty
    Belsey Mark IV 240° fundoplication
    Belsey two-thirds wrap fundoplica-
      tion
    Benelli mastopexy
    bilateral inguinofemoral
      lymphadenectomy
    bilayer patch hernia repair
    biliary enteric anastomosis

operation *(cont.)*
    biliary sphincterotomy and stent placement
    biliointestinal bypass (BIB)
    biliopancreatic bypass (BPB)
    Billroth gastroenterostomy
    Billroth I (truncal vagotomy, antrectomy, gastroduodenostomy)
    Billroth II (truncal vagotomy, antrectomy, gastrojejunostomy)
    Billroth II-type gastrectomy
    Bishop-Koop ileostomy
    blind esophageal brushing (BEB)
    Bloch-Paul-Mikulicz
    Blumgart technique for hepaticojejunostomy
    blunt dissection
    Boerema anterior gastropexy
    Boerema hernia repair
    Brackin ureterointestinal anastomosis
    Braun anastomosis
    Braun-Jaboulay gastroenterostomy
    breast augmentation mammoplasty by injection (BAMBI)
    breast reconstruction during mastectomy
    breast reconstruction with latissimus dorsi flap
    breast reduction
    Bricker ureteroileostomy
    Brooke ileostomy
    Brunschwig
    Burch colposuspension
    Burch iliopectineal ligament urethrovesical suspension
    Burch laparoscopic procedure
    Burhenne biliary duct stone extraction
    buttonhole puncture technique for hemodialysis needle insertion
    buttonpexy fixation for stomal prolapse
    CAGEIN (catheter-guided endoscopic intubation)

operation *(cont.)*
    Camey ileocystoplasty
    capsulectomy of breast
    cardiomyotomy (stomach)
    CASH (classic abdominal Semm hysterectomy)
    catheter balloon valvuloplasty
    catheter-directed thrombolysis and endovascular stent placement
    cecopexy
    cecorrhaphy
    cecostomy
    central cone technique reduction mammoplasty
    cervical esophagotomy
    Child pancreaticoduodenostomy
    Childs-Phillips bowel plication
    cholecystectomy, three-trocar technique
    cholecystoduodenostomy
    cholecystoenterostomy
    cholecystojejunostomy
    choledochoduodenostomy
    choledochoenterostomy
    choledochojejunostomy
    choledochostomy
    choledochotomy
    cholelithotripsy
    Clagett-Barrett esophagogastrostomy
    "cleavoplasty" augmentation mammoplasty
    Coblation-Channeling
    Coffey ureterointestinal anastomosis
    colectomy, total abdominal (TAC)
    Collis antireflux
    Collis gastroplasty
    Collis-Nissen fundoplication
    Collis-Nissen gastroplasty
    coloanal anastomosis
    colocolostomy
    colopexy
    coloplasty procedure
    coloproctostomy

operation *(cont.)*
  colorrhaphy
  colosigmoid resection
  colostomy
  combined Collis gastroplasty-
    fundoplication for scleroderma
    reflux esophagitis
  combined liver and intestinal
    transplantation
  Commando glossectomy
  common bile duct exploration
  complete wrap Nissen
  composite
  conductive keratoplasty (CK)
  continent ileostomy
  contralateral subtotal thyroid
    lobectomy
  Cooper ligament repair
  Cordonnier ureteroileal loop
  corner mouth lift
  Courvoisier gastroenterostomy
  cricopharyngeal myotomy
  "cross-the-heart" augmentation
    mammoplasty
  cryptectomy
  CT cholangiography
  CT PEG (CT-guided percutaneous
    endoscopic gastrostomy)
  culdolaparoscopy
  curative
  cut-back
  cystogastrostomy
  cystojejunostomy
  cystopericystectomy
  decompression
  defatting of panniculus
  Delorme rectal prolapse
  Dennis-Brooke ileostomy
  Dennis-Varco pancreaticoduo-
    denostomy
  Depage-Janeway gastrostomy
  Devine
  DGHAL (Doppler-guided hemor-
    rhoidal artery ligation)

operation *(cont.)*
  diagnostic laparoscopy
  dilatation of stenotic hepatico-
    jejunostomy
  distal gastrectomy with excision
    of ulcer
  distal near-total pancreatectomy
  distal pancreatectomy
  distal Roux-en-Y gastric
  distal subtotal pancreatectomy
  diverticulectomy
  donut mastopexy
  Doppler-guided HAL (hemorrhoid
    artery ligation) (DGHAL)
  Doubilet sphincterotomy
  double seton modified surgical
    approach to transsphincteric anal
    fistula repair
  double-wrap graciloplasty
  Douglas procedure
  Douglas suture of tongue
    for micrognathia
  drainage
  duct-to-duct anastomosis
  Duecollement hemicolectomy
  Duhamel laparoscopic pull-through
  duodenal diversion
  duodenal seromyectomy
  duodenoenterostomy
  duodenoileal bypass (DIB)
  duodenojejunostomy
  duodenotomy
  Duval distal (caudal) pancreatico-
    jejunostomy
  Duval pancreaticojejunostomy
  dynamic graciloplasty
  Eckhout gastroplasty
  Eckhout vertical gastroplasty
  elective shunt procedure
  elective sigmoid resection
  electrohydraulic lithotripsy for bile
    duct stone
  emergency
  emergency laparotomy

operation *(cont.)*
- emergency tracheostomy
- en bloc augmentation mammoplasty
- en bloc distal pancreatectomy
- en bloc resection
- en bloc vein resection
- Endo Lumenal gastroplication procedure (ELGP)
- endorectal ileal pull-through
- endoscopic antireflux procedure
- endoscopic-assisted transumbilical augmentation mammoplasty
- endoscopic cryoablation
- endoscopic cryotherapy
- endoscopic cystogastrostomy
- endoscopic gastroplasty
- endoscopic injection
- endoscopic laser cholecystectomy
- endoscopic mucosal ablation
- endoscopic mucosal resection (EMR)
- endoscopic mucosectomy
- endoscopic papillectomy (EP)
- endoscopic papillotomy
- endoscopic resection
- endoscopic retrograde balloon dilation
- endoscopic retrograde cholangiography (ERC)
- endoscopic retrograde cholangiopancreatogram (ERCP)
- endoscopic sphincterotomy (ES)
- endoscopic stent placement
- endoscopic transpapillary catheterization of the gallbladder (ETCG)
- endoscopic Zenker diverticulectomy
- endoscopy with tumor ablation
- enteroenterostomy
- enterolithotomy
- enterotomy
- end-to-back bowel anastomosis
- end-to-end anastomosis
- end-to-end jejunoileal bypass
- end-to-side anastomosis

operation *(cont.)*
- end-to-side choledochojejunostomy
- end-to-side jejunoileal bypass
- epiploectomy
- esophageal-jejunal anastomosis
- esophageal sling procedure
- esophageal transection with para-esophagogastric devascularization
- esophagectomy
- esophagoduodenostomy
- esophagoenterostomy
- esophagogastrectomy
- esophagogastric anastomosis
- esophagogastric fundoplasty with fundic patch (Thal-Nissen procedure)
- esophagogastric tamponade
- esophagogastrostomy
- esophagojejunostomy
- esophagomyotomy (Heller type)
- esophagostomy
- EUS-guided fine-needle aspiration
- exclusion bypass
- explantation of breast implant
- exploratory celiotomy
- exploratory laparotomy
- extended right hepatectomy
- extended right hepatic lobectomy
- external fistulization of intestine
- extracorporeal shock-wave lithotripsy
- extramucosal myotomy
- failed shunt surgery
- femoral hernia repair
- Finney pyloroplasty
- fissurectomy
- fistulectomy
- fistulotomy
- floppy Nissen fundoplication
- Fobi pouch
- formal laparotomy
- Fredet-Ramstedt pyloromyotomy
- free nipple transposition technique reduction mammoplasty

operation *(cont.)*
  frenoplasty
  fundic mobilization in Nissen
    fundoplication
  fundoplasty
  fundoplication
  gasless laparoscopic-assisted
    colostomy
  gastrectomy
  gastric bypass (GBP)
  gastric loop-type bypass
  gastric neobladder procedure
  gastric partitioning
  gastric resection
  gastric restrictive procedure
  gastric stapling
  gastroduodenopancreatectomy
  gastroduodenostomy
  gastroenterostomy
  gastrogastrostomy
  gastrojejunal anastomosis
  gastrojejunostomy
  gastropexy
  gastroplasty
  gastrorrhaphy
  gastrostomy
  Gauderer-Ponsky PEG
  Gauderer-Ponsky-Izant PEG
  gift-wrap suture technique
  glossectomy
  Goligher ileostomy
  Gomez fundoplasty
  Gomez gastroplasty
  Gore-Tex banding of sigmoid colon
    to abdominal wall
  Goulian mammoplasty
  gracilis muscle transposition
  graciloplasty
  Greenville gastric bypass
  Griffen Roux-en-Y bypass
  groin dissection
  Grondahl-Finney esophagogastro-
    plasty
  Gross

operation *(cont.)*
  HAL (hemorrhoid arterial ligation),
    Doppler-guided
  HALS (hand-assisted laparoscopic
    surgery)
  Halsted-Bassini herniorrhaphy
  Halsted inguinal herniorrhaphy
  hand-assisted laparoscopic
    colectomy
  hand-assisted laparoscopic gastrec-
    tomy
  hand-assisted laparoscopy
  hand-assisted sigmoidectomy
  Harrington esophageal diverticu-
    lectomy
  Hartmann pouch
  Hartmann resection of bowel
  Hasson technique
  Heineke-Mikulicz gastroenterostomy
  Heineke-Mikulicz pyloroplasty
  Heller-Belsey operation for achalasia
    of esophagus
  Heller cardiomyotomy
  Heller-Dor operation for achalasia
    of esophagus
  Heller esophagomyotomy
  Heller myotomy
  hemicolectomy
  hemigastrectomy
  hemorrhoid arterial ligation (HAL)
  hemorrhoidal banding
  hemorrhoid cryotherapy
  hemorrhoid infrared photo-
    coagulation
  hemorrhoid laser excision
  hemorrhoid sclerotherapy
  hemorrhoid vaporization
  hemorrhoidectomy
  hepatectomy
  hepatic lobectomy
  hepatic resection
  hepatic segmentectomy
  hepaticojejunostomy with cutaneous
    stoma

operation *(cont.)*
   hepatopancreatoduodenectomy
   hepatoportoenterostomy
   hepatorrhaphy
   hepatotomy
   herniorrhaphy
   Higgins technique for uretero-
      intestinal anastomosis
   highly selective vagotomy
   Hill antireflux
   Hill cluster harvest technique
   Hill fundoplasty
   Hill gastropexy
   Hill hiatus hernia
   Hill median arcuate repair
   Hill repair for esophageal reflux
   Hofmeister anastomosis
   Hofmeister gastroenterostomy
   Horsley anastomosis
   Horsley gastrectomy
   Hunt-Lawrence pouch
   hydrocelectomy
   hypophysectomy
   ileal pouch-anal anastomosis
   ileal pull-through
   ileal resection
   ileectomy
   ileoanal anastomosis
   ileoanal endorectal pull-through
   ileocolectomy
   ileocolic resection
   ileocolostomy
   ileocystoplasty
   ileogastrostomy
   ileo-ileal anastomosis
   ileoproctostomy
   ileorectal anastomosis (IRA)
   ileorectostomy
   ileostomy
   Indiana pouch
   inferior central pedicle reduction
      mammoplasty
   inferior pedicle technique reduction
      mammoplasty

operation *(cont.)*
   infrahepatic caval anastomosis
   inframammary approach in augmen-
      tation mammoplasty
   inguinal exploration
   inguinal lymphadenectomy
   intestinal anastomosis
   intestinal bypass
   intestinal transplantation
   intracorporeal shock-wave lithotripsy
      (ISWL)
   intrahepatic cholangioenterostomy
   intrahepatic transjugular porto-
      systemic shunt
   intraoperative cholangiography
      (IOC)
   intraperitoneal onlay mesh (IPOM)
      hernia repair
   inversion-ligation appendectomy
   inverted U-pouch ileal reservoir
   IPAA (ileal pouch-anal anastomosis)
   ipsilateral thyroid lobectomy
   isoperistaltic anastomosis
   isthmusectomy
   Ivalon rectopexy
   Ivalon sponge-wrap
   Ivor Lewis esophagectomy
   Ivor Lewis esophagogastrectomy
   Jaboulay gastroduodenostomy
   Jaboulay pyloroplasty
   Janeway procedure
   jejunoileal bypass
   jejunoileostomy
   jejunojejunostomy
   jejunostomy
   Jenckel cholecystoduodenostomy
   Johnson esophagogastrostomy
   Judd ventral hernia repair
   Kader gastrostomy
   Karydakis pilonidal cyst excision
   Kasai portoenterostomy
   Kiricuta breast reconstruction
   Kocher anastomosis
   Kocher pylorectomy

operation *(cont.)*
    Kocher pyloromyotomy
    Kock ("coke") ileostomy
    Kock pouch modified procedure
    Kugel hernia repair
    Kugel patch
    Kuzmak gastric banding
    Kuzmak gastroplasty
    Ladd correction of malrotation
      of the bowel
    Lane
    laparoscopic adrenalectomy
    laparoscopically assisted colorectal
      resection
    laparoscopically assisted sigmoid
      resection
    laparoscopic anterior fundoplication
    laparoscopic antireflux surgery
    laparoscopic appendectomy
      ("lap appy")
    laparoscopic approach
    laparoscopic-assisted procedure
    laparoscopic-assisted vaginal
      hysterectomy
    laparoscopic bile duct exploration
    laparoscopic biopsy of liver
    laparoscopic bladder neck suture
      suspension procedure
    laparoscopic bowel resection
    laparoscopic Burch procedure
    laparoscopic cholecystectomy
      ("lap chole")
    laparoscopic colectomy
    laparoscopic common bile duct
      exploration
    laparoscopic dissection
    laparoscopic distal pancreatectomy
    laparoscopic duct exploration
    laparoscopic esophagogastroplasty
      with Nissen fundoplication
    laparoscopic exploration of common
      bile duct
    laparoscopic fundoplication
    laparoscopic Heller myotomy

operation *(cont.)*
    laparoscopic hernia repair
    laparoscopic herniorrhaphy
    laparoscopic Kittner
    laparoscopic laser cholecystectomy
      (LLC)
    laparoscopic liver biopsy
    laparoscopic lysis of adhesions
    laparoscopic micro scissors
    laparoscopic monopolar scissors
    laparoscopic Nissen and Toupet
      fundoplication
    laparoscopic Nissen fundoplication
    laparoscopic Nissen fundoplication
      with esophageal lengthening
    laparoscopic paraesophageal hernia
      repair (LPHR)
    laparoscopic placement of peritoneal
      dialysis catheter
    laparoscopic pneumodissection
    laparoscopic posterior hemi-
      fundoplication
    laparoscopic radical prostatectomy
    laparoscopic repair of para-
      esophageal hernia (LRPH)
    laparoscopic retroperitoneal
      lymphadenectomy
    laparoscopic Roux-en-Y gastric
      bypass procedure (LRYGBP)
    laparoscopic supracervical
      hysterectomy (LASH)
    laparoscopic surgery for peptic ulcer
      disease
    laparoscopic Toupet fundoplication
    laparoscopic transcystic duct
      exploration
    laparoscopic transcystic papillotomy
    laparoscopic tubal ligation
    laparoscopic urinary diversion
    laparotomy
    laparotomy with splenectomy
    laparotomy with splenorrhaphy
    Lap-Band adjustable gastric banding
      (LAGB)

operation *(cont.)*
    "lap chole" (laparoscopic cholecystectomy)
    lap Nissen (laparoscopic Nissen fundoplication)
    LAP-TAPP (laparoscopic transabdominal preperitoneal) hernioplasty
    LAR/CAA (low anterior resection in combination with coloanal anastomosis)
    large-volume paracentesis
    LARS (laparoscopic antireflux surgery)
    laryngopharyngectomy
    laser ablation
    laser-assisted spinal endoscopy (LASE)
    laser-assisted tissue welding technique
    laser-assisted uvulopalatoplasty (LAUP)
    laser biomicroscopy
    "Laser Bra" (see *L.I.F.T.*)
    laser correlational spectroscopy (LCS)
    laser Doppler flowmetry (LDF)
    laser hemorrhoidectomy
    laser image custom arthroplasty (LICA)
    laser-induced thermotherapy (LITT)
    laser lithotripsy
    laser myringotomy
    laser nucleotomy
    laser photoablation
    laser reduction mammoplasty
    laser thermal keratoplasty (LTK)
    laser trabeculodissection (LTD)
    laser uterosacral nerve ablation (LUNA)
    LASH (laparoscopic supracervical hysterectomy)
    lateral cervical lymphadenectomy
    lateral cervical node dissection

operation *(cont.)*
    lateral crural steal (LCS)
    Latzko vesicovaginal fistula repair
    LAUP (laser-assisted uvulopalatoplasty)
    LAVH (laparoscopically assisted vaginal hysterectomy)
    Laws gastroplasty
    Lazaro da Silva continent perineal colostomy creation technique
    Lazarus-Nelson pneumoperitoneum technique
    Leadbetter-Politano ureterovesicoplasty
    LeDuc anastomosis
    LeDuc-Camey ileocolostomy
    LeDuc-Camey ileocystoplasty
    LEEP (loop electrosurgical excision procedure)
    LeFort urethral sound
    left hepatic lobectomy
    left-to-right subtotal pancreatectomy
    LeJour technique of reduction mammoplasty
    LeJour-type breast reduction
    LESA (lower esophageal sphincter augmentation)
    Lester Martin modification of Duhamel procedure
    levator muscle imbrication
    Lewis-Tanner subtotal esophagectomy and reconstruction
    Lich-Gregoire kidney transplant surgery
    Lichtenstein herniorrhaphy
    Lich ureteral implantation in transplantation surgery
    L.I.F.T. (laser-assisted internal fabrication) of breast
    ligamentum teres cardiopexy
    lip lift
    Lipostructure technique
    LLETZ (large loop excision of the transformation zone)

operation *(cont.)*
   lobectomy
   long limb gastric bypass
   Longmire-Gutgemann gastric
     reconstruction
   Longo hemorrhoidectomy
   loop choledochojejunostomy
   loop-end ileostomy
   Lord hemorrhoidectomy
   Lortat-Jacob hepatic resection
   low anterior resection
   low-intensity laser therapy (LILT)
   LRYGBP (laparoscopic Roux-en-Y
     gastric bypass procedure)
   LULA (laparoscopy under local
     anesthesia)
   lumpectomy of breast
   LUNA (laparoscopic uterine nerve
     ablation)
   lung tumor resection
   lung volume reduction surgery
     (LVRS)
   lymph node dissection
   Macewen herniorrhaphy
   Madden herniorrhaphy
   Madden repair of incisional hernia
   Madigan prostatectomy
   Magerl screw placement in lower
     cervical spine
   magnetic resonance cholangiography
     (MRC)
   magnetic resonance cholangiography
     with HASTE
   magnetic resonance cholangio-
     pancreatography (MRCP)
   magnetic resonance mammography
     (MRM)
   MAGPI (meatal advancement,
     glanuloplasty, penoscrotal
     junction meatotomy)
   Maki pylorus-preserving gastrec-
     tomy
   Mallory-Weiss procedure
   Marlex mesh rectopexy

operation *(cont.)*
   Martin anoplasty
   Mason abdominotranssphincteric
     resection
   Mason vertical-banded gastroplasty
   mastotomy
   Maunsell-Weir
   Mayo
   McBurney
   McVay herniorrhaphy
   mechanical lithotripsy for bile duct
     stone
   Meckel diverticulectomy
   mediastinal lymphadenectomy
   "mega-pocket" augmentation
     mammoplasty
   Menthini "one second" technique
   Merindino
   mesenteropexy
   mesh plug hernioplasty
   mesocaval anastomosis
   Miles abdominoperineal resection
   minilaparotomy
   minimally invasive esophagectomy
   mirror-image breast biopsy
   Mitrofanoff appendicovesicotomy
   Mitrofanoff neourethra procedure
   modified Bassini inguinal hernia
     repair
   modified radical mastectomy
   Mohs fresh tissue chemosurgery
   Morinaga hemorrhoidectomy
   MR peritoneography
   mucosal sleeve resection
   mucosectomy
   Mulholland sphincterotomy
   multipolar electrocoagulation
     therapy (MECT)
   multivisceral transplantation
   necrosectomy
   needle biopsy
   needle catheter jejunostomy
   needlescopic TAPP hernia repair
   Newman procedure

operation *(cont.)*
    nipple-flap duct resection
    Nissen antireflux
    Nissen fundoplasty
    Nissen fundoplication
    Nissen laparoscopic fundoplication
    Noble bowel plication
    noninvasive exploration of the biliary tract
    nonrigid technique reduction mammoplasty
    O'Leary gastroplasty
    omentectomy
    omentopexy
    omphalectomy
    open diverticulectomy
    open esophagectomy
    open gastric banding procedure
    open mesh-plug hernioplasty
    open wedge biopsy of the liver
    one-stage
    optical coherence tomography
    Oriental V-Y flap technique
    Orr-Loygue transabdominal proctopexy
    Orr rectal prolapse repair
    Owl incision technique reduction mammoplasty
    palliative resection
    palliative surgical
    pancreas after kidney (PAK) transplantation
    pancreas-preserving total gastrectomy
    pancreas transplantation
    pancreatectomy
    pancreatic islet cell transplantation
    pancreaticobiliary
    pancreaticocystostomy
    pancreaticoduodenectomy
    pancreaticoduodenostomy
    pancreaticogastrostomy
    pancreaticojejunal anastomosis
    pancreaticojejunostomy
    pancreatoduodenectomy

operation *(cont.)*
    pancreatoscopy
    percutaneous endoscopic gastro-jejunostomy
    percutaneous transhepatic cholangiography (PTC)
    plication of mesentery (mesenteropexy)
    proctocolectomy
    pancreas-preserving total gastrectomy
    pancreatorrhaphy
    pancreatotomy
    panproctocolectomy
    pants-over-vest hernia repair
    papillectomy
    papillotomy transection of the sphincter of Oddi
    paracentesis
    paraesophageal hernia, type 2
    parietal cell vagotomy
    Parker-Kerr enteroenterostomy
    Parks fistulotomy
    Parks ileoanal anastomosis
    Parks posterior anal repair
    Parks sphincterotomy
    Parks transanal anastomosis
    partial distal gastrectomy
    partial ileal bypass
    partial pancreatectomy
    Partipilo gastrostomy
    Paul-Mikulicz resection
    Payne-DeWind jejunoileal bypass
    PCTCL (percutaneous transhepatic cholecystolithotomy)
    pedicle technique reduction mammoplasty
    PEG (percutaneous endoscopic gastrostomy)
    PEJ (percutaneous endoscopic jejunostomy)
    per anum intersphincteric rectal dissection and coloanal anastomosis

operation *(cont.)*
   percutaneous catheter cecostomy
   percutaneous cholecystostomy
   percutaneous choledochoscopy
   percutaneous deflation of sigmoid loop
   percutaneous endoscopic gastro-jejunostomy
   percutaneous endoscopic gastrostomy (PEG)
   percutaneous endoscopic jejunostomy (PEJ)
   percutaneous gastroenterostomy (PGE)
   percutaneous gastrostomy (PG)
   percutaneous nephrostolithotomy (PCNL)
   percutaneous stone dissolution
   percutaneous transfemoral dilatation
   percutaneous transhepatic cholangiogram (PTC)
   percutaneous transhepatic cholangiography (PTC)
   percutaneous transhepatic cholangi-oscopy (PTCS) tube stenting
   percutaneous transhepatic cholangi-oscopy and lithotripsy for complicated hepatolithiasis
   percutaneous transhepatic cholangi-oscopy tube stenting through a mature T-tube tract
   percutaneous transhepatic chole-dochoscopic electrohydraulic lithotripsy (PTCS-EHL)
   periareolar augmentation mammo-plasty
   periprosthetic capsulectomy of breast
   peritoneocentesis
   pharyngoesophageal repair
   pharyngogastrostomy
   pharyngostomy (fistulization of pharynx)
   plication of bowel

operation *(cont.)*
   plug-and-patch hernia repair
   Polya gastrectomy
   polypectomy
   polyvalent pneumococcal vaccine postsplenectomy
   Ponka herniorrhaphy
   portacaval anastomosis
   portal systemic anastomosis
   portoenterostomy
   portoportal anastomosis
   portosystemic anastomosis
   posterior diaphragmatic gastropexy
   posterior repair of the diaphragmatic hiatus
   posterior sagittal and 3-flap anoplas-ty
   PPPD (pylorus-preserving pancreatoduodenectomy)
   precut sphincterotomy
   preperitoneal approach
   preperitoneal hernioplasty
   preperitoneal prosthetic mesh repair of hernia via laparoscopy
   Pringle maneuver for clamping the hepatic pedicle
   proctectomy, mucosal
   proctocolectomy
   proctopexy
   Prolene Hernia System (PHS) bilayer patch repair
   prophylactic cholecystectomy
   prophylactic gastrojejunostomy
   proximal duct excision
   proximal gastric vagotomy
   proximal subtotal pancreatectomy
   Puestow pancreaticojejunostomy
   Puestow-Gillesby
   pull-through
   push enteroscopy
   pyeloileocutaneous anastomosis
   pylorectomy
   pyloromyotomy
   pyloroplasty

operation *(cont.)*

pylorotomy
pylorus-preserving modification
pylorus-preserving pancreato-
    duodenectomy (PPPD)
pylorus-preserving resection
pylorus-preserving Whipple
pylorus-sparing Whipple procedure
radical mastectomy
radioguided parathyroidectomy
radioiodide ablation
Ramstedt-Fredet pyloromyotomy
Ramstedt pyloroplasty
rapid pull-through (RPT)
reconstructive mammoplasty
rectal mucosectomy
rectal prolapse repair
rectal sleeve advancement
rectopexy
rectosigmoidectomy
rectovaginopexy
reduction mammoplasty
Rehne-Delorme plication
resection and primary anastomosis
    of bowel
resection with Roux-en-Y hepatico-
    jejunostomy
retrocolic choledochojejunostomy
retropharyngeal approach
retropubic prostatectomy
right colectomy with ileostomy
right hepatic lobectomy
Ripstein rectal prolapse repair
Ripstein rectopexy
robot-assisted
Rodney Smith biliary stricture
Roux-en-Y anastomosis
Roux-en-Y chimney surgical
    technique
Roux-en-Y choledochojejunostomy
Roux-en-Y cystojejunostomy
Roux-en-Y esophagojejunostomy
    reconstruction
Roux-en-Y gastric bypass
Roux-en-Y gastrojejunostomy

operation *(cont.)*

Roux-en-Y hepaticojejunostomy
Roux-en-Y jejunoileostomy
Roux-en-Y pancreaticojejunostomy
Roux-en-Y reconstruction
Roux-Y (see *Roux-en-Y*)
rubber band hemorrhoid ligation
Russell percutaneous endoscopic
    gastrostomy
Rutkow sutureless plug and patch
    repair for inguinal hernia
sacroabdominoperineal pull-through
sacrofixation
sacrospinous
SBE (small bowel enteroscopy)
Schoemaker anastomosis
Schwartz-Pregenzer urethropexy
Scopinaro pancreaticobiliary bypass
Scott jejunoileal bypass
second-look laparotomy
segmental bowel transplantation
segmental colon resection
segmental mastectomy
segmental reduction and split-graft
    techniques
segmental resection of bowel
segmentectomy
SEPS (subfascial endoscopic
    perforator surgery)
serosal patch repair
shoelace technique for delayed
    primary closure of fasciotomy
short-scar procedure in breast
    reduction
short-scar tumescent reduction
    mammoplasty
Shouldice hernia repair
Shouldice herniorrhaphy
sialodochoplasty
sialolithotomy
side-to-side anastomosis
sigmoid colectomy
sigmoid colostomy
sigmoidoscopic decompression
    of volvulus

operation *(cont.)*
  sigmoidoscopic reduction of
    volvulus
  Simonsen technique for large
    rectovaginal fistula repair
  simple mastectomy
  Sistrunk procedure
  small bowel resection
  snare resection (band and snare)
  Soave abdominal pull-through
  Soave endorectal pull-through
  solid organ transplantation
  sphincterotomy of papilla
  sphincterotomy with stone extraction
  sphincter-saving procedure
  Stretta
  splenectomy
  splenorrhaphy
  Ssabanejew-Frank gastrostomy
  staging
  staging laparotomy
  Stamm gastrostomy
  standard Whipple pancreatico-
    duodenectomy
  stapler-facilitated rectal eversion
  stapling esophago-diverticulostomy
    by endoscopy
  stapling off of small gastric pouch
  State end-to-end anastomosis
  station pull-through
  stereotactic transsphenoidal
    hypophysectomy
  stereotaxic core needle biopsy
  Stoppa posterior approach
  Stoppa-Rives giant prosthetic repair
    of the visceral sac
  stricturoplasty
  subcutaneous mastectomy
  subfascial endoscopic perforator
    surgery (SEPS)
  subglandular augmentation mammo-
    plasty
  submucosal tunnel technique
  subserosal needle catheter
    jejunostomy

operation *(cont.)*
  subtotal colectomy
  subtotal pancreatectomy
  subtotal thyroidectomy
  suction-assisted lipectomy (SAL)
  Sugiura esophageal varices
    procedure
  superior pedicle technique reduction
    mammoplasty
  superwet reduction mammoplasty
  suprahyoid neck
  sutureless plug and patch repair
    for inguinal hernia
  Swenson abdominal pull-through
  Tanner
  TAPP (transabdominal preperi-
    toneal) hernia repair
  TAPP (transabdominal preperi-
    toneal) laparoscopic hernioplasty
  Teflon sling repair
  temporary colostomy
  temporary ostomy
  tension-eliminating repair
  tension-free anastomosis
  tension-free hernia repair
  tension-free prosthetic repair
  TEP (totally extraperitoneal) laparo-
    scopic hernioplasty
  T-fastener gastropexy
  Thal esophageal stricture repair
  Thal esophagogastrostomy
  Thal stricturoplasty
  Thal-Nissen fundoplasty
  Thiersch anal incontinence proce-
    dure
  thoracoabdominal esophagectomy
  thoracophrenolaparotomy
  thoracoscopic esophagomyotomy
  thorascopic esophagomyotomy
  three-trocar technique of cholecys-
    tectomy
  thymectomy
  TIPS (transjugular intrahepatic
    portal shunt procedure)

operation *(cont.)*
    total abdominal colectomy (TAC)
    total abdominal evisceration (TAE)
    total colectomy
    total esophagectomy
    total fundic wrap (Nissen-Rossetti)
    total gastrectomy
    total hepatectomy
    total lobectomy
    totally (or total) extraperitoneal laparoscopic hernioplasty
    total mastectomy
    total mesorectal excision (TME)
    total pancreatectomy
    total parathyroidectomy
    total protocolectomy and ileostomy
    total sac excision
    total thoracic esophagectomy
    total thyroidectomy
    Toupet (partial posterior) fundoplication
    Toupet fundoplasty
    Toupet fundoplication
    transabdominal preperitoneal laparoscopic hernioplasty
    transabdominal repair
    transabdominal retroperitoneal lymph node dissection
    transanal deflation of sigmoid volvulus
    transanal endoscopic microsurgery (TEM)
    transanal pouch advancement
    transaxillary subpectoral mammoplasty
    transcystic common bile duct exploration
    transcystic duct/common bile duct exploration (TCD/CBDE)
    transduodenal sphincterotomy
    transected vertical gastric bypass with Silastic ring band and gastrostomy
    transection of esophagus
    transectomy of vagus nerves

operation *(cont.)*
    transhiatal esophagectomy
    transhiatal pyloroplasty
    transjugular intrahepatic porto-systemic shunt procedure (TIPS)
    transomental posterior gastro-enterostomy
    transpapillary endoscopic cholecystotomy
    transthoracic Nissen fundoplication
    transumbilical augmentation mammoplasty
    transumbilical breast augmentation (TUBA)
    transurethral balloon Laserthermia prostatectomy
    transurethral laser-induced prostatectomy (TULIP)
    transverse colectomy
    transverse wedge
    transversostomy
    Traverso-Longmire technique
    T-tack gastropexy
    TUBA (transumbilical breast augmentation)
    tube duodenostomy with feeding jejunostomy
    tumescent liposuction technique
    Turbinger gastric reconstruction
    Turnbull multiple ostomy
    typhlorrhaphy
    umbilectomy
    unilateral adrenalectomy
    unilateral groin dissection
    UPPP (uvulopalatopharyngoplasty)
    Urban
    ureteral reimplantation
    ureteroileocutaneous anastomosis
    ureteroileostomy
    uvulopalatopharyngoplasty (UPPP)
    vaginal lengthening
    vagotomy
    venovenous bypass
    vermilionectomy
    vertical-banded gastroplasty (VBG)

operation *(cont.)*
  vertical bipedicle flap technique
    reduction mammoplasty
  vertical reduction mammoplasty
  vest-over-pants hernia repair
  V-excision
  video-assisted thoracic surgery
    (VATS)
  videoendoscopic augmentation
    mammoplasty
  videoscopic fundoplication
  Von Haberer-Finney anastomosis
  Von Haberer gastroenterostomy
  WAMBA (Wise areola mastopexy
    breast augmentation)
  Waugh Clagett pancreatico-
    duodenostomy
  wedge resection
  weight reduction
  Weinberg pyloroplasty
  Wells rectopexy
  wet-technique breast reduction
    with liposuction
  Wheeless surgical construction
    of J rectal pouch
  Whipple pancreaticoduodenectomy
  Whitehead hemorrhoidectomy
  Wise pattern for reduction mammo-
    plasty
  Witzel duodenostomy
  Witzel gastrostomy
  Witzel jejunostomy
  Womack procedure
  xanthogranulomatous cholecystitis
  Y-V anoplasty
  Y-V plasty
  zipper sphincterotomy
operative biliary bypass
operative cholangiogram
operative cholangiogram catheter
operative debridement and placement
  of drain
operative diagnosis
operative drainage

operative field
operative laparoscope
operative stone removal
operculectomy
OpEX instrument service
ophthalmic retractor
opiates
Opisthorchis sinensis
opisthotonic position
Opmi microscope drape
Opmilas 144 Plus laser
Opmilas CO_2 multipurpose laser
OP-1 implant graft
opportunistic infection
Opraflex incise drape
OpSite dressing
OpSite Flexigrid transparent adhesive
  film dressing
OpSite occlusive dressing
opsonin production
Opteform 100HT bone graft
Op-Temp cautery
optical biopsy
optical biopsy forceps
optical biopsy instruments
Optical Biopsy system
optical bronchoscopes
optical coherence tomography (OCT)
optical forceps
optical retractor
Optical Sensors blood gas monitor
Optical Tracking System (OTS)
Optik rigid laparoscope
Optima fabric
optimal tracheal seal
OptiMARK (gadoversetamide injection)
optimized serum pancreolauryl test
option, therapeutic
OptiPen insulin delivery pen
OptiPen Pro insulin delivery pen
Optipore sponge dressing
Optipore wound-cleaning sponge
Opti-Port right-angle, double-swivel
  connector

OptiQue sensing catheter
Optiray 350 (ioversal)
OptiSet insulin delivery pen
Optison contrast agent
Opti-Sorb reinforcement
Optistar MR contrast delivery system
Optistat power injector
Optiva I.V. catheter
Optivis needle
Oracle Focus catheter
Oracle Megasonics catheter
Oracle Micro catheter
Oracle Micro Plus catheter
Oragrafin contrast medium
Oragrafin Sodium (ipodate sodium)
oral airway
oral calcium
oral cholecystogram (OCG)
oral contraceptive
oral gastric calibration tube
oral gastric tube (OGT)
oral hypoglycemic agent
   biguanide
   sulfonylurea
oral intubation
oral papilloma
oral propanolol
oral purge
oral sepsis
oral smear
oral transmission
oral ulcer
Oral RAE uncuffed tube
Oralgen oral aerosol insulin
orange peel appearance (peau d'orange)
Oratec electrocautery probe
orbital plate
orbital reducer seal
orbital retractor
orbital rim dissector
Oreopoulos-Zellerman catheter
Oretorp arthroscopy knife
organ
   ancestral
   cadaveric

organ *(cont.)*
   distant
   donor
   extraperitoneal
   failure of
   glandular
   harvesting of
   inadequate perfusion of
   recipient of
   reticuloendothelial
   retroperitoneal
   target
   Zuckerkandl
organ donation
organ donor registry
organ harvesting
organic acids
organic lesion
organism
   acid-fast
   blood-borne
   gram-negative
   intracellular
   multicellular
   nonpathogenic
   pathogenic
      bacterium
      fungus
      parasite
      rickettsia
      virus
   pleuropneumonia-like (PPLO)
   pyogenic
   unicellular
   urease-producing
   virulent
Organización Nacional de Transplantes
   (Spain)
organized clot
organized thrombus
organoaxial gastric volvulus
organomegaly
organ procurement agency
organ recipient
organ recovery

organ-sparing surgery
Orgaran (danaparoid sodium)
ORI electronic endoscopy system
Oriental cholangiohepatitis
Oriental V-Y flap technique
orienting reflex
orienting suture
orifice
    anal
    aortic
    appendiceal
    atrioventricular
    cardiac
    esophagogastric
    external urethral
    gastroduodenal
    golf-hole ureteral
    hernial
    ileocecal
    internal urethral
    mitral
    myopectineal (MPO)
    pharyngeal
    pulmonary
    pyloric
    tricuspid
    ureteral or ureteric
    urethral
    vaginal
orifice of appendix
Origin balloon
Origin distention balloon system
Origin Medsystems trocar
Origin Tacker laparoscopic tacking
    device
Origin trocar
Oris pin
orlistat
Ormond disease
Ormon rectal scissors
oroendotracheal tube
orofacial fistula
orofacial herpes
orogastric tube

OR1 electronic endoscopy system
oropharyngeal anesthesia
oropharyngeal cancer
oropharyngeal dysphagia
    from esophageal dysphagia
oropharyngeal hemorrhage
oropharyngeal tumor
orotracheal intubation
Orozco cervical plate
orphan virus
Orr gall duct forceps
Orr-Loygue transabdominal proctopexy
Orr rectal prolapse repair
Orthair oscillating saw
Orthoairtome wire driver
Orthoclone OKT3 monoclonal antibody
orthogonal view
Ortholav stand
orthopedic mallet
orthosis, Gillette joint
OrthoSorb absorbable fixation pin
OrthoSorb pin nail
orthostasis
orthostatic blood pressure
orthostatic change
orthostatic hypotension
Orthotec handpiece and tubing
Orthotec pulsed irrigation
orthotic plate
orthotopic liver transplant (transplanta-
    tion) (OLT)
Ortho-Trac adhesive bandage
Ortho-Vent nonadhesive bandage
Orzel (UFT/leucovorin calcium)
O_2 (oxygen) saturation
Osborne plate
oscillating blade
oscillating gouge
oscillating microsaw
oscillating saw
oscillating sternotomy saw
Oscillo III plaster saw
O'Shaughnessy artery forceps
OSI Extremity elevator

Osler-Weber-Rendu disease
Osler-Weber-Rendu syndrome
Osler-Weber-Rendu telangiectasia
OsmoCyte Island wound dressing
OsmoCyte PCA pillow wound dressing
OsmoCyte pillow
osmolality equilibration
osmolality, fecal
osmolarity
Osmolite HN enteral feeding
osmotic agent
osmotically active particles
osmotic diarrhea
osmotic edema
osmotic fragility of red cells
osmotic laxative
osmotic pressure
osseous polyp
osseous tuberosity
Ossoff-Karlan microlaryngeal suction
    tube
Ostavir (tuvirumab) monoclonal
    antibody
osteoarticular graft
OsteoBiologics, Inc.
osteoblastic bony metastasis
osteocartilaginous graft
osteochondral graft
osteoclastic activity
osteoclast tension staple
osteogenic sarcoma
osteoid carcinoma
osteolytic activity
osteoma
Osteomark monoclonal antibody-based
    agent
Osteomark test
osteomyelitis
Osteone air drill
osteoperiosteal graft
osteophyte elevator
osteophyte nipper rongeur
osteophytes and skeletal abnormalities
osteoporosis

Osteoset bone graft substitute graft
osteotome
OST-577 human antihepatitis B
    antibody
ostial lesion
ostiomeatal stent
ostomate
ostomy (pl. ostomies) (see *colostomy;*
    pouch; operation)
ostomy appliance
ostomy bag
O'Sullivan-O'Connor abdominal
    retractor
O'Sullivan scoring system for dysphagia
OTC (over-the-counter) medications
otic obstruction
Otis urethrotome
OtoLam laser
OtoLam laser therapy
otologic drill
otorrhea, clear
O_2 (oxygen) toxicity
OTW (over the wire)
outer capsule
outer crossbar
outflow cannula
outflow, pancreatic duct
out-in-out technique suture
outlet constipation
outlet delay
outlet disorder of anorectum
outlet view
outpatient anesthesia
outpatient percutaneous liver biopsy
outpouching of mucosa
outpouching of testicular tissue
oval cherry-red raised lesion
oval-cup jaws
oval dissector
ovale malaria
oval-form colonic groove
OvaRex MAb
ovarian cancer
ovarian cyst

ovarian medulla
ovarian neoplasm
ovarian torsion
ovarian tumor
over-and-over suture
over-and-over whip suture
over-the-counter (OTC) medications
over-the-top position
overactivity, acquired benign adrenal
    androgenic
overbed table
overdistention of hollow viscus
overexpression, P53 protein
overhead film
overhead oblique view
overhead view
Overholt artery forceps
Overholt clip-applying forceps
Overholt thoracic forceps
overlap syndrome (connective tissue
    disease)
overlapping suture
overlay plate
overload, circulatory
overlying skin erythema
overlying structures
overnight basal acid output (BAO)
overnight dexamethasone suppression
    test
overnutrition
overproduction of normal adrenal
    hormones
oversewn, oversewing
overt colonic polyposis
Overton dowel graft
overventilation
overwhelming postsplenectomy sepsis
    (OPSS)
ovolactovegetarian diet
Ovum curette
Owen gauze
Owen gauze dressing
Owen silk suture
Owestry staple

owl incision technique reduction
    mammoplasty
oxaliplatin
oxaluria, enteric
oxamniquine
Oxandrin (oxandrolone)
oxandrolone
ox bile extract
Oxequip air
oxidation
oxidative stress
oxide radical
oxidized bile acid
Oximax pulse oximeter
oximeter
    MARSpo2 Tech pulse
    Masimo SET pulse
    Oximax pulse
    Oxi-Reader
    pulse
oximetry
Oxiplex
Oxi-Reader pulse oximeter
Oxo kitchen scissors
oxybuprocaine
Oxycel (oxidized cellulose) pad
Oxycel (oxidized cellulose) pledget
Oxycel (oxidized cellulose) strip
oxycodone HCl
oxycodone/oxycodone terephthalate/
    aspirin
OxyContin (oxycodone HCl)
oxygen bound to hemoglobin
oxygen-carrying capacity of blood
oxygen saturation
Oxygen Sensors (fuel cells)
oxygenated blood
oxygenation
oxygenator, Maxima Forté blood
Oxygent (emulsified perflubron) blood
    substitute
oxymetric data
oxymorphone HCl
oxyntic cell

oxyntic gland
oxyntic mucosa
oxyphenisatin, oxyphenisatin acetate

oxyphenonium
oxyphil cell hyperplasia

P, p

PA (posteroanterior) film
PA (posteroanterior) view
PA (pulmonary artery pressure)
PABA (p-aminobenzoic acid) test
Pace bipolar pacing catheter
pacemaker
    Enterra gastrointestinal
    gastric
    transvenous
pacemaker (gastric) cell
pacemaker (stomach) cell
pacemaker region, gastric
Pacesetter introducer
Pace ventricular needle
Pacifico-type suction tube
pack, packing (see also *bandage*)
    Adaptic
    Aquacel Hydrofiber
    Barrier
    ENTaxis nasal
    gauze
    iodoform gauze
    Kaltostat wound
    moist lap (laparotomy)
    Nu-Brede
    omental
    Pedi-Boro Soak Packs
    perihepatic

pack *(cont.)*
    petrolatum gauze
    Silverlon wound
    Sorbsan
    Tilley
    wound
packed cells, transfusion of (measured
    in units)
packed red blood cells
paclitaxel
PaCO$_2$
pad (see also *dressing*)
    abdominal (ABD)
    abdominal fat
    abdominal lap (laparotomy)
    ABS
    acetone prep
    alcohol prep
    Alpha Protech
    Alpha Protech Unreal Lambskin
        Soft Touch
    Aluma foam
    antimesenteric fat
    arch cookie
    axillary fat
    B-D Sensability Breast Self-
        Examination Aid
    calcium alginate

pain *(cont.)*
  epicritic
  epigastric
  esophageal
  exacerbation of
  exquisite
  flank
  functional
  gallbladder
  gastrointestinal
  gnawing
  gynecologic
  headache
  hunger
  incapacitating
  intermittent
  intractable
  jaw
  knifelike
  lancinating
  left flank
  left lower quadrant
  left upper quadrant
  localized
  loin
  midline
  migrating
  motion
  musculoskeletal
  nagging
  nocturnal
  noncyclical
  onset of
  parietal (somatic)
  perirectal
  phantom breast
  phantom rectal
  pleuritic chest
  point of maximal
  poorly localized
  postlaparoscopic shoulder
  postoperative
  postprandial
  postural

pain *(cont.)*
  prolonged
  protopathic
  psychogenic
  radiating
  rebound
  rectal
  recurrent
  recurring
  referred
  referred periumbilical
  referred right subscapular
  refractory
  remission of
  retrosternal chest
  right flank
  right lower quadrant
  right-sided abdominal
  right upper quadrant
  severe
  sharp
  shoulder
  small of back
  somatic
  steady
  stomach
  subscapular
  substernal
  sudden onset of
  suprapubic
  tearing
  terrifying
  testicular
  unexplained abdominal
  unrelenting
  unrelieved
  unremitting
  vaginal
  visceral
  vise-like
pain abolished by breath-holding
pain accompanied by abdominal
  fullness
pain accompanied by nausea

pain accompanied by palpitation
pain accompanied by sensation of gas
pain accompanied by shortness
   of breath
pain accompanied by sweating
pain accompanied by weakness
pain aggravated by coughing
pain aggravated by deep breathing
pain aggravated by deep inspiration
pain and tenderness
PainBuster infusion pain management
   kit
pain continued unabated
pain control (see *anesthesia*)
pain following heavy meal
painful anesthesia
painful hepatomegaly
painful palpable gallbladder
painful swollen thyroid
pain in sternal articulations
pain indistinguishable from angina
pain induced with methacholine
painless breast mass
painless edema
painless indurated ulcer
painless jaundice
painless, large thyroid
painless lower GI bleeding
painless mammogram
painless pancreatitis
painless rectal bleeding
painless thyroiditis
pain "like being crushed under a heavy
   load"
pain "like being caught in a vise"
pain "like someone sitting on my chest"
pain migration
pain of gastrointestinal origin
pain of musculoskeletal origin
pain of psychogenic origin
pain on drinking cold liquid
pain on exposure to cold
pain on strong emotion
pain on swallowing

pain precipitated by emotional upset
pain precipitated by exertion
pain precipitated by strong emotion
pain radiating to back
pain radiating to epigastrium
pain radiating to jaw
pain radiating to left arm
pain radiating to neck
pain radiating to right arm
pain radiating to throat
pain rapidly extinguished by withdrawal
   of stimulus
pain relieved by antacids
pain relieved by belching
pain relieved by bowel movement
pain relieved by carotid massage
pain relieved by cimetidine
pain relieved by eating
pain relieved by food intake
pain relieved by leaning forward
pain relieved by passage of flatus
pain relieved by rest
pain reproduced by palpation
pain reproducible with moderate
   exercise
Painter colic
pain unaffected by position
pain unrelated to meals
pain unrelieved by nitroglycerin
pain when angry
pain when excited
pain with defecation
pair of pliers
PAIS (Psychosocial Adjustment
   to Illness Scale)
PAK (percutaneous access kit)
PAL (probe for aspiration and lavage)
Palacos cement adhesive
palate
palatopharyngeal fold
palatopharyngoplasty
palatoplasty
Palco EM-100 Oxylato
pale cell

pale skin
palliation of pain
palliation, surgical
palliation therapy
palliative care
palliative chemotherapy
palliative hepatojejunostomy
palliative operative procedure
palliative pain management
palliative resection
palliative surgery
palliative surgical procedure
palliative therapy
pallor
palmar erythema
palmar incision
palmar plate
Palmaz balloon-expandable stent
Palmaz Corinthian biliary stent
Palmaz Corinthian transhepatic biliary
    stent and delivery system
Palmaz-Schatz balloon-expandable stent
Palmaz-Schatz Crown balloon-expand-
    able stent
Palmaz-Schatz Mini Crown stent
Palmaz-Schatz stent (PSS)
Palmer bone nail
palmitin test
palmoxirate sodium
palmoxiric acid
palm-to-axilla dressing
Palomar E2000 ruby laser
palonosetron hydrochloride
palpable adenopathy
palpable epigastric mass
palpable gallbladder
palpable mass
palpable mass after aspiration
palpable nodule
palpable, nontender, distended
    gallbladder
palpable pulse
palpable pyloric olive
palpable retroareolar mass

palpably enlarged gallbladder
Palpagraph breast tissue examination
    device
Palpagraph mammography device
palpation
palpitation
PALS tablets (chlorophyllin copper
    complex)
pamidronate disodium
Pamine (methscopolamine bromide)
P-aminosalicylic acid (PAS) hypothy-
    roidism
Pamisyl (aminosalicylic acid)
pampiniform plexus
Panacryl absorbable suture
Panacryl braided synthetic absorbable
    suture
Panafil (papain; urea; chlorophyllin
    copper complex)
Panafil enzymatic debriding agent
Panafil White (papain; urea) ointment
Panalok RC absorbable soft tissue
    anchor
Panalok RC QuickAnchor Plus
Panalok suture anchor
pancake kidney
pancolitis
pancolonoscopy
pancopride
pancreas
    aberrant
    accessory
    anlage
    annular
    anterior surface of
    Aselli
    beta cells of the
    biopsy of
    blunt injury to
    body of
    burned-out
    cancer of
    Christmas tree appearance of
    congenital lipomatosis of

pancreas *(cont.)*
   degeneration of
   dorsal
   endocrine
   exocrine
   fibrofatty infiltration of
   head of
   heterotopic
   inferior surface of
   inflammation of
   lesser
   longitudinal filleting of the
   lower border of the
   neck of
   posterior surface of
   tail of
   uncinate process of
   ventral
   Willis
   Winslow
pancreas acinar cell growth
pancreas after kidney (PAK) trans-
   plantation
pancreas divisum
pancreas encircling the duodenum
pancreas transplant
Pancrease MT 20 (lipase; protease;
   amylase)
pancreatectomy (see *operation*)
   distal
   distal laparoscopic
   distal near-total
   distal subtotal
   donor
   en bloc distal
   laparoscopic distal
   left-to-right subtotal
   limited
   near-total
   partial
   proximal subtotal
   subtotal
   total
   transduodenal
   Whipple

pancreatic abscess
pancreatic acinar cells
pancreatic acinus atrophy
pancreatic adenoma
pancreatic allograft
pancreatic alpha$_2$ islet cell tumor
pancreatic amylase (P-type)
pancreatic ascites
pancreatic bed
pancreatic bud
pancreatic calculus
pancreatic cancer, exocrine
pancreatic carcinoma
pancreatic cholera
pancreatic cholera syndrome
pancreatic colic
pancreatic cutaneous fistula
pancreatic cyst
pancreatic cystic disease
pancreatic D cells
pancreatic diabetes
pancreatic divisum
pancreatic duct
   accessory
   duodenal end of dorsal
   duodenal end of main
   genu of
   main
   obstruction of
   proximal part of dorsal
pancreatic ductal adenocarcinoma
pancreatic ductal carcinoma
   iatrogenic
   traumatic
pancreatic duct disruption
pancreatic duct obstruction
pancreatic duct outflow
pancreatic duct sphincter (PDS)
pancreatic duct stent
pancreatic endocrine insufficiency
pancreatic endocrine tumor (PET) cell
pancreatic endoscopy
pancreatic endotherapy
pancreatic enteric fistula
pancreatic enzyme

pancreatic enzyme replacement
pancreatic enzyme therapy
pancreatic exocrine insufficiency
pancreatic exocrine secretions
pancreatic fibrosis
pancreatic fistula
pancreatic fluid
pancreatic function test (testing)
pancreatic gastrinoma (Zollinger-Ellison syndrome)
pancreatic gastrinoma and peptic ulcer disease
pancreatic glucagonoma tumor
pancreatic hamartoma
pancreatic head
pancreatic hormone
pancreatic infantilism
pancreatic insufficiency
pancreatic insulinoma
pancreatic islet
pancreatic islet cell
pancreatic islet cell markers
pancreatic islet cell transplantation
pancreatic islet cell tumor
pancreatic juice
pancreatic leak
pancreatic lipase
pancreatic malignancy
pancreatic necrosis
pancreatic non-beta islet cell tumor
pancreaticobiliary common channel
pancreaticobiliary diversion
pancreaticobiliary ductal junction
pancreaticobiliary sphincter
pancreaticobiliary tract
pancreatic obstruction
pancreaticocutaneous fistula
pancreaticocystostomy
pancreaticoduodenal artery
pancreaticoduodenectomy, Whipple
pancreaticoduodenostomy (see also *operation*)
  Child
  Dennis-Varco

pancreaticoduodenostomy *(cont.)*
  Waugh-Clagett
  Whipple
pancreaticogastrostomy
pancreaticohepatic syndrome
pancreaticojejunal anastomosis
pancreaticojejunostomy or pancreato-jejunostomy (see also *operation*)
  Cattell-Warren
  caudal
  distal
  ductal
  duct-to-mucosa
  DuVal or Duval
  end-to-end intussuscepted
  end-to-end inverting
  end-to-side
  Frey
  invagination technique of
  isolated
  laparoscopic
  lateral
  longitudinal
  modified dunking
  Partington-Rochelle
  Puestow
  retrocolic end-to-end
  Roux-en-Y
  Roux loop
  side-to-side
  two-layer end-to-side
pancreaticolienal lymph node
pancreatic oncofetal antigen (POA) test
pancreaticopleural fistula
pancreaticosplenic gland
pancreaticosplenic lymph node
pancreaticosplenic omentum
pancreatic phlegmon
pancreatic pleural effusion
pancreatic polypeptide (PP)
pancreatic pseudocyst
pancreatic rest
pancreatic sepsis in acute pancreatitis
pancreatic steatorrhea

Papanicolaou smear
Papanicolaou test
Paparella angled ring curette
Paparella canal knife
Paparella drum elevator knife
Paparella duckbill elevator
Paparella fenestrometer
Paparella incudostapedial knife
Paparella mastoid curette
Paparella pick
Paparella retractor
Paparella sickle knife
Paparella straight needle
Paparella tissue press
papaya enzyme
PA–PCWP/CO x 80 (mean pulmonary
   artery pressure – pulmonary capil-
   lary wedge pressure/cardiac output x
   80 = pulmonary vascular resistance)
paper drape
papilla (pl. papillae)
   acoustic
   anal
   bile
   circumvallate
   clavate
   conical
   dentinal
   dermal
   disinsertion of
   duodenal
   filiform
   foliate
   fungiform
   hypertrophic
   lingual
   major duodenal
   minor duodenal
   renal
   urethral
papilla of Vater
papillary adenocarcinoma
papillary adenoma
papillary carcinoma of thyroid gland

papillary cluster of cells
papillary cystadenocarcinoma
papillary cystic adenoma
papillary dermis
papillary gastric carcinoma
papillary hyperplasia of follicles
papillary hypertrophy of conjunctiva
papillary layer of dermis
papillary lesion
papillary muscle
papillary necrosis
papillary proliferation
papillary stenosis
papillary tumor
papillated surface
papillation
papillectomy
papillitis
   necrotizing
   necrotizing renal
papilloadenocystoma
papillocarcinoma
papilloma
   basal cell
   benign squamous
   choroid plexus
   cockscomb (also coxcomb)
   cutaneous
   duct
   fibroepithelial
   friable
   Hopmann
   intracanalicular
   intracystic
   intraductal
   inverted
   inverted ductal
   oral
   soft
   squamous
   transitional cell
   villous
   vocal cord
   warty

papilloma lactiferous duct
papilloma of bladder
papilloma of vocal cord
papillomavirus (also, papilloma virus)
papillomatosis
papillomatous benign tumor
papillotome
    Accuratome
    Apollo3 triple-lumen
    Bard high-flow
    bowed
    Cape Town steerable
    Classen-Demling
    Danish pattern
    double-lumen
    endoscopic
    Erlangen
    guidewire
    Howell rotatable
    Huibregtse
    Huibregtse-Katon
    Olympus needle-knife
    piggyback needle-knife
    precut
    ProForma
    shark fin
    single-lumen
    triple-lumen
    two-lumen
    Wilson-Cook
    Zimmon
papillotomy, endoscopic (EPT)
papillotomy transection of the sphincter
   of Oddi
Papineau graft
papovavirus
Pappenheimer body
Pap (Papanicolaou) smear
Pap test
papular lesion
papular mucinosis
papule
    fluid-filled
    Gottron

papule *(cont.)*
    lichenoid
    minute
    pearly penile
    pedunculated
    piezogenic
    pruritic urticarial (of pregnancy)
    rust-colored
    sessile
    split
    transitory
papulonecrotic lesion
PAR (postanesthesia recovery)
para-aortic lymph node
para-aortic node biopsy
para-aortic region
paracecal appendix
paracentesis, abdominal
paracentesis needle
paracentesis tray
paracetamol hepatotoxicity
Parachute corkscrew suture anchor
paracolic abscess
paracolic gutter
paracolic lymph node
paracolon bacillus
paracolostomy hernia
paracrine regulation pattern
paracystic pouch
paracytic
paradoxic increase
paradoxical movement
paraductal adenopathy
paraduodenal fold
paraduodenal fossa
paraesophageal hernia
paraesophageal herniation
paraesophageal hiatus hernia
paraesophageal varices
paraesophagogastric devascularization
paraffin cancer
paraffin tumor
parafollicular C cell
paraganglia

Paragon Champion stent system
Paragon CO_2 laser system
Paragon coronary stent
paraileostomal hernia
parainfluenza 2 virus
parainfluenza 3 virus
parainfluenza 4 virus
parallel to the tracheoesophageal groove
paralytic colonic or intestinal
   obstruction
paralytic ileus
parajejunal fossa
Paramax angled driver
paramedial incision
paramedian incision
parameters
   clinical
   clotting
paraneoplastic syndrome
parapatellar incision
parapharyngeal approach
pararectal abscess
pararectal pouch
pararectus incision
pararenal pseudocyst
parasite
   Enamoeba histolytica
   Giardia
   intestinal
   Isospora
parasitemia
parasitic abscess
parasitic cyst
parasitic disease
parasitic infection
parasitic infestation
Parasmillie double-bladed knife
parasternal gunshot wound
parasternal long-axis view
parasternal short-axis view
parasternal stab wound
parastomal hernia
parasympathomimetic drugs
parathyroid autotransplantation to
   forearm

parathyroid carcinoma
parathyroidectomy
   endoscopic
   incidental
   minimally invasive
   minimally invasive video-assisted
     (MIVAP)
   radioguided
   subtotal
parathyroid gland
parathyroiditis
parathyroid gland
parathyroid hormone analysis
parathyroid-hormone-related protein
   (PTHrp)
parathyroid hormone test
parathyroid hyperplasia
parathyroid tetany
parathyroid tissue placed in forearm
   muscles
parathyroid tumor
parathyroprival tetany
paratracheal node
paratyphoidal cholangiolitis
paraumbilical hernia
paraumbilical region
paravariceal sclerotherapy
paravertebral anesthesia
paravesical fossa
paravesical pouch
parchment induration
paregoric (PG)
Parell needle holder
parenchyma
   breast
   destruction of
   hepatic
   hepatic lobular
   heterogenous
   liver
   lung
   renal
   splenic
   thyroid

parenchymal cell
parenchymal damage
parenchymal destruction
parenchymal hemorrhage
parenchymal jaundice
parenchymal liver disease
parenchymal tissue
parenchymatous degeneration
parenchymatous goiter
parenchymatous inflammation
parenchymatous mastitis
parenchymatous myocarditis
parenchymatous nephritis
parenchymatous neuritis
parenchymatous pneumonia
parenchymography, endoscopic
    retrograde (ERP)
parenchymous degeneration of liver
parenteral alimentation
parenteral antibiotic therapy
parenteral feeding
parenteral fluids
parenteral nutrition
Parepectolin (attapulgite)
paresis
paresthesias
Parfocal zoom
Parhad-Poppen arteriogram needle
Parham band circling needle
Parham-Martin fracture clamp
paricalcitol
parietal cell antibody
parietal cell index
parietal cell of fundus
parietal cell receptor
parietal cell vagotomy (PCV)
parietal fistula
parietal pain
parietal peritoneum
parietal (somatic) pain
parietal suture
Parietex composite mesh for hernia
    surgery
parietomastoid suture

parieto-occipital suture
Paritene mesh graft for hernia surgery
park bench position
Parker-Kerr closed method of
    end-to-end enteroenterostomy
Parker-Kerr enteroenterostomy
Parker-Kerr intestinal clamp
Parker knife
Parker retractor
Parkinson disease
Park posterior anal repair
Parks anal retractor
Parks anoscope
Parks fistulotomy
Parks hemorrhoidectomy
Parks ileal reservoir
Parks ileoanal anastomosis
Parks ileoanal reservoir
Parks ileostomy pouch
Parks partial sphincterotomy
Parks rectal retractor
Parks sphincterotomy retractor
Parks staged fistulotomy
Parks-TC needle holder
Parks transanal anastomosis
paromomycin sulfate
parotid abscess
parotid duct diversion, bilateral
    (Wilke procedure)
parotid enlargement
parotid gland
paroxysmal motor disease
paroxysmal nocturnal hemoglobinuria
parrot clamp
parrot's beak clamp
Parsonnet clamp
partial adrenalectomy
partial bowel obstruction
partial colectomy
partial-curve blade
partial esophagectomy
partial fundoplication procedure
partial gastrectomy
partial hepatectomy

partial ileal bypass
partial lesion
partial lobectomy of liver
partial mastectomy
partial occluding clamp
partial occlusion clamp
partial pancreatectomy
partial pressure of oxygen
partial shunt
partial small bowel obstruction
partial thromboplastin (PTT)
partial thromboplastin time coagulation
   panel
partial thymectomy
partial transplantation
partially intrahepatic gallbladder
partially occluding vascular clamp
partially threaded pin
partially threaded rod
particle, Dane
particulate graft
Partipilo gastrostomy
partition, gastric
partitioning, gastric
Partsch chisel
Partsch gouge
parumbilical abscess
parvovirus B19, human
Pascal principle
PAS (P-aminosalicylic acid) hypothy-
   roidism
PAS (periodic acid Schiff) stain
PAS (periodic acid Schiff) test
P.A.S. (peripheral access system)
P.A.S. Port catheter
P.A.S. Port Fluoro-Free catheter
passage
   biliary
   flatus
   hard stool
   stone
Passage catheter
passage of flatus per vagina
passage of gallstones

passage of perforated fluid
passage of stool
passage pressure
Passager introducing sheath
passive clot
passive congestion
passive congestion of stomach
passive congestive cirrhosis
passive cutaneous anaphylaxis
passive hyperemia
passive pneumonia
Passow chisel
patch
   Androderm testosterone transdermal
   bilayer
   BioGlue surgical
   Carrel
   circumferentially sutured onlay
   colic
   colonic
   Dacron
   Fluoropassiv
   fundic
   Graham
   Hemarrest
   Hemaseel HMN
   HRT (hormone replacement therapy)
   InterGard
   Kugel hernia
   Lichtenstein onlay
   Lyrelle
   mucosal
   Osteopatch
   Peyer
   pleural
   plug and
   preperitoneal
   RapiSeal
   Rutkow sutureless
   ScopeSeal endoscope
   seromuscular intestinal
   serosal
   vascularized gastric tissue
   white

patch and plug
patch-clamp
patch dressing
patch-reinforced mattress suture
patchy colonic ulceration
patchy intercellular edema
Patella disease (pyloric stenosis)
patellar clamp
patellar drill
patellar drill guide
patellar skyline view
patellar tendon graft
patency of common bile duct
patency, splenic vein
patent ductus arteriosus
patent ductus clamp
patent splenic and portal veins
Paterson-Brown-Kelly syndrome
Paterson-Kelly syndrome
Paterson rectal biopsy forceps
Patey modified radical mastectomy
Pathfinder catheter
Pathfinder irrigation device
Pathfinder microcatheter
Pathfinder mini microcatheter
Pathibamate
Pathilon (tridihexethyl chloride)
pathoanatomy
pathogenesis
pathogenic bacteria
pathogenic microorganism
pathogenic organism
    bacterium (pl. bacteria)
    fungus (pl. fungi)
    parasite (pl. parasites)
    virus (pl. viruses)
pathogenic pneumococci
pathognomic for hyperparathyroidism
pathognomonic feature
pathognomonic sign of a fistula
pathologic atrophy
pathologic diagnosis
pathologic fracture
pathologic nipple disease

pathologic reflux
pathological hypersecretory conditions
pathologist
pathology
    anatomic
    clinical
    forensic
    general
pathology report
pathophysiologic mechanism
pathophysiology
PathVysion HER-2 DNA probe kit
PATI (Penetrating Abdominal Trauma
    Index)
patient-controlled analgesia (PCA)
    pump
pattern
    abdominal wall venous
    adenoid
    airspace-filling
    airway
    alveolar
    anhaustral colonic gas
    ballerina-foot
    basket weave
    bowel gas
    branching
    breast reconstruction
    breathing
    butterfly
    cartwheel
    chromatin
    cobblestone
    cribriform
    elongate
    feathery
    fibrotic
    fleur de lis
    fold
    frondlike
    gas
    ground-glass
    haustral
    honeycomb

pattern *(cont.)*
  hourglass
  ineffective breathing
  interstitial
  irregular amputated mucosal
  juvenile
  lamellated
  layered
  lobular
  manometric
  micronodular fibrotic
  miliary
  mosaic
  mosaic duodenal mucosal
  mucosal
  mucosal guideline
  nonspecific gas
  nutmeg
  progestational
  proliferative
  railroad track
  rugal
  sawtooth
  signet ring
  speckled
  starry-sky
  stellate
  undifferentiated
  venous
  vesicular
  wax
  Wyse
Patterson trocar
patulous anus
patulous cardia
patulous hiatus
paucity of colon gas
paucity of fat
Paufique blade
Paufique knife
Paul-Miculicz resection
Paul-Mixter tube
Paulson knee retractor
Paulus plate

Pavlik bandage
Pavlov stomach
Pavulon (pancuronium bromide)
Paxene (paclitaxel)
Payne-DeWind jejunoileal bypass
Payr director
Payr forceps
Payr pyloric clamp
Pazo Hemorrhoid (ephedrine sulfate; zinc oxide)
PBC (primary biliary cirrhosis)
PBC-associated antibody
PBN catheter
PBTE (percutaneous transhepatic liver biopsy with tract embolization)
p.c. (L. *post cibum*, after meals)
PCA (prezatide copper acetate)
PCA cutting guide
PCA medullary guide
PCA (patient-controlled analgesia) pump
PCC (peripheral cholangiocarcinoma)
PCCL (percutaneous cholecysto-lithotomy)
PCI (pneumatosis cystoides intestinalis)
PCL (posterior collateral ligament) retractor
PCNA (proliferating cell nuclear antigen)
PCNL (percutaneous nephrosto-lithotomy)
pCO_2
PC Polygraf HR
PCPS (peroral cholangiopancrea-toscopy)
PCR (polymerase chain reaction)
PCS (postcholecystectomy syndrome)
PCT (porphyria cutanea tarda)
PCTCL (percutaneous transhepatic cholecystolithotomy)
PCV (parietal cell vagotomy)
PCWP (pulmonary capillary wedge pressure)
PDB (preperitoneal distention balloon)

PDB laparoscopic balloon system
PDC (peritoneal dialysis catheter)
PDS (pancreatic duct sphincter)
PDS (polydioxanone suture) pin
PDS (polydioxanone suture) II
 Endoloop suture
PDS Vicryl suture
PDT (photodynamic therapy) laser
PE (portal embolization)
peak and trough levels
PEAK channeled plate
peaked T waves
peak flow meter
peak inspiration
peak plasma concentration
peak pressure
peaks and troughs
peaks and valleys
peak secretory flow rate (PSFR)
Péan clamp
Péan forceps
peanut (small dissecting sponge)
peapod intervertebral disk forceps
peapod intervertebral disk rongeur
pearly white mass
Pease bone drill
pea soup stool
peau d'orange
PeBA C 4-mm anchor
PeBA RCR 5-mm anchor
PeBA S 2.8-mm anchor
PeBA suture anchor
PEBB (percutaneous excisional breast
 biopsy)
Peck-Joseph dissecting scissors
pectin
pectinate line
pectineal ridge
pectineus fascia
pectineus muscle
pectoral fascia
pectoral minor muscle
pectoral muscle
pectoralis fascia

pectoralis major muscle
pectoralis minor muscle
pedal edema, trace
pedal lymphangiography
Pederson vaginal speculum
Pedialyte (sodium, potassium, and
 chloride electrolytes) solution
Pedialyte RS (rehydrating solution)
 electrolyte solution
pediatric bulldog clamp
Pediatric Crohn's & Colitis
 Association, Inc.
pediatric Deaver retractor
pediatric endoscope
pediatric esophagoscope
pediatric Foley catheter
pediatric gastroscope
pediatric hernia
pediatric nasogastric feeding tube
pediatric ribbon retractor
pediatric scopes and instrumentation
pediatric vascular clamp
pediatric video optical intubation stylet
pediatric Y tube
Pedi-Boro Soak Packs (modified Burow
 solution)
pedicle
 inferior
 long splenic
 muscle
 omental
 vascular
 vertical
pedicle bone graft
pedicle clamp
pedicle graft
pedicle hook
pedicle plate
pedicle probe
pedicle technique reduction mammo-
 plasty
pedicular rod
Pedi PEG tube
PediPort trocar

PedTE-Pak-4 (multiple trace elements)
Pedtrace-4 (multiple trace elements)
pedunculated mass of polyp
pedunculated papule
pedunculated polyp
pedunculation
peel-away introducer
PEEP (positive end-expiratory pressure)
Peers towel forceps
Peet splinter forceps
PEG (percutaneous endoscopic
    gastrostomy)
  PEG balloon
  PEG catheter
  PEG tube
PEG (polyethylene glycol)
  PEG-interferon alfa-2a
  PEG-interferon alfa-2b
  PEG-Intron (PEG-interferon
    alfa-2b)
  PEG-Intron A (interferon alfa-2b
    in polyethylene glycol carrier)
  PEG lavage
  PEG molecule
Pegasus Nd:YAG surgical laser
Pegasys (PEG-interferon alfa-2a)
peg-base plate
peg graft
pegvisomant
pegylated interferon
pegylated protein
pegylation
Peiper-Beyer laminectomy rongeur
PEJ (percutaneous endoscopic jejunos-
    tomy)
peliosis hepatis
pellegra skin changes
pelleted stools
pellet, radiopaque
Pelosi Illuminator device
Pelosi manipulator set
pelvic abscess
pelvic adhesion
pelvic brim

pelvic colon
pelvic exenteration
pelvic floor dysfunction
pelvic floor electromyography
pelvic floor function study
pelvic hematoma
pelvic infection
pelvic inflammatory disease (PID)
pelvic kidney
pelvic lymph node
pelvic peritoneum
pelvic plexus
pelvic sidewall
pelvimeter, Martin
pelvirectal abscess
pelvirectal achalasia
pelviscopy instrumentation
PEM (protein-energy malnutrition)
Pemberton sigmoid clamp
Pemberton spur-crushing clamp
pen
    Disetronic Insulin Pen
    Eckhoff mapping
    Humulin Pen
    Humulin R Pen
    Humalog Pen
    mapping
    Nibs mapping
    Novolin Pen
    Securline skin-marking
    Skin-Scribe skin-marking
pencil
    cautery
    electrocautery
    electrosurgical
pencil-like stool
PenduLaser 115 surgical laser system
pendulous pouch
penetrating abdominal trauma
Penetrating Abdominal Trauma Index
    (PATI)
penetrating atherosclerotic aortic ulcer
penetrating drill
penetrating injury

penetrating injury through the platysma
penetrating stab injury
penetrating trauma
penetrating ulcer
penetrating wound
Penfield dissector
Penfield elevator
Penfield retractor
Penfine needle
Penn fingernail drill
Pennington clamp
Pennington grasping forceps
Pennington rectal speculum
Pennington tissue forceps
Penn pouch for continent urinary
    diversion
Penn umbilical scissors
Penn wire-cutting scissors
Penrose drain
Penrose seton
pentagastrin gastric secretory test
pentagastrin infusion test
pentagastrin provocative test
pentagastrin-stimulated analysis test
pentagastrin-stimulated calcitonin
    concentration
pentagastrin stimulation
pentagastrin test
pentamidine-induced pancreatitis
Pentasa (mesalamine)
Pentax ECN-1530 choledochonephro-
    scope
Pentax EC videoendoscope
Pentax EC-3430F videocolonoscope
Pentax EC-3430L videocolonoscope
Pentax EC-3440F videocolonoscope
Pentax EC-3440L videocolonoscope
Pentax EC-3830 videocolonoscope
Pentax EC-3830L videocolonoscope
Pentax EC-3830TL video colonoscope
Pentax EC-3840L videocolonoscope
Pentax EC-3840T videocolonoscope
Pentax ED-3430T videoduodenoscope
Pentax ED-3440T videoduodenoscope

Pentax EG videoendoscope
Pentax EG-1840 videogastroscope
Pentax EG-2530 gastroscope
Pentax EG-2540 videogastroscope
Pentax EG-2731 gastroscope
Pentax EG-2901 flexible gastroscope
Pentax EG-2930 gastroscope
Pentax EG-2940 videogastroscope
Pentax EG-3430 videogastroscope
Pentax EG-3440 videogastroscope
Pentax EG-3830T videogastroscope
Pentax EG-3840T videogastroscope
Pentax EndoNet endoscope
Pentax endoscopic camera
Pentax ES-3830 videosigmoidoscope
Pentax ES-3840 videosigmoidoscope
Pentax EUP-FC124 ultrasound
    gastroscope
Pentax FC endoscope
Pentax FC-38LV fiberoptic colonoscope
Pentax FC-38LX flexible colonoscope
Pentax FC-38LX flexible gastroscope
Pentax FC-38MV fiberoptic colono-
    scope
Pentax FCN-15H flexible choledocho-
    scope
Pentax FD-32A side-viewing endoscope
Pentax FD-34V fiberoptic duodeno-
    scope
Pentax FG-24V fiberoptic gastroscope
Pentax FG-29H flexible gastroscope
Pentax FG-29V fiberoptic gastroscope
Pentax FG-29X flexible gastroscope
Pentax FG-36UX echoendoscope
Pentax fiberoptic sigmoidoscope
Pentax flexible sigmoidoscope
Pentax FS-34A flexible sigmoidoscope
Pentax FS-34V fiberoptic sigmoido-
    scope
Pentax FS-38H flexible sigmoidoscope
Pentax-Hitachi FG32UA endosono-
    graphic system
Pentax side-viewing endoscope

Pentax SIG-E2 fiberoptic sigmoido-
scope
Pentax videoendoscope
Pentax VSB-P2900 pediatric colono-
scope
Pentax W fiberoptic endoscope
Pepcid AC (famotidine)
Pepcid RPD (famotidine)
PEPCK (phosphoenolpyruvate
carboxykinase) deficiency
Pepgen test
peppermint oil
pepsin
pepsinogen
Peptamen liquid diet
Peptavlon (pentagastrin)
peptic cell
peptic esophagitis
peptic stricture
peptic ulcer
peptic ulcer disease (PUD)
peptic ulceration
peptid bond hydrolysis
peptide bonds
peptide hormone
peptide, regulatory
Pepto-Bismol (bismuth subsalicylate)
Pepto Diarrhea Control (loperamide)
per anum intersphincteric rectal dissec-
tion and coloanal anastomosis
per os (p.o.)
per primam healing
per rectum
Perative formula
Perception 5000 PC-based ultrasound
scanner
Percival gastric balloon
Perclose suture device
Percor DL-II (dual-lumen) intra-aortic
balloon
Percor-Stat intra-aortic balloon
PercScope percutaneous diskectomy
endoscope
PercuCut cut-biopsy needle

Percuflex Plus biliary stent
PercuGuide
PercuPump disposable syringe and
injector
percussion hammer
percussion note
percussion tenderness
percutaneous ablation
percutaneous abscess and fluid drainage
(PAFD)
percutaneous access kit (PAK)
percutaneous appendectomy
percutaneous aspiration
percutaneous aspiration and drainage
percutaneous autogenous dowel bone
graft
percutaneous balloon dilation
percutaneous biopsy
percutaneous catheter
percutaneous catheter cecostomy
percutaneous catheterization (of the
portal vein)
percutaneous celiac nerve block
percutaneous cholecystolithotomy
(PCCL)
percutaneous cholecystostomy
percutaneous choledochoscopy
percutaneous closed-catheter drain
percutaneous cutting needle
percutaneous deflation of cecum
percutaneous deflation of sigmoid loop
percutaneous drain placement
percutaneous drainage
percutaneous drainage catheter
percutaneous drainage with CT
guidance
percutaneous drainage with ultrasound
guidance
percutaneous endoscopic gastrostomy
(PEG) tube
percutaneous endoscopic jejunostomy
(PEJ)
percutaneous ethanol injection (PEI)
percutaneous ethanol tumor injection

percutaneous excisional breast biopsy
(PEBB)
percutaneous fibrin glue
percutaneous fine-needle biopsy
percutaneous gastroenterostomy (PGE)
percutaneous gastrostomy (PG) tube
percutaneous hepatic vein angioplasty
(PHVA)
percutaneous jejunostomy tube
percutaneous lead introducer
percutaneous liver biopsy
percutaneous needle muscle biopsy
percutaneous nephrostolithotomy
(PCNL)
percutaneous pin
percutaneous resection
percutaneous stent
percutaneous stone dissolution
percutaneous transfemoral dilatation
percutaneous transhepatic catheteriza-
tion
percutaneous transhepatic biliary
drainage (PTBD) catheter
percutaneous transhepatic cholangio-
gram (PTC)
percutaneous transhepatic cholangi-
ography (PTC)
percutaneous transhepatic cholangi-
oscopy (PTCS) tube stenting
percutaneous transhepatic cholangi-
oscopy and lithotripsy for compli-
cated hepatolithiasis
percutaneous transhepatic cholangi-
oscopy tube stenting through a
mature T-tube tract
percutaneous transhepatic cholecysto-
lithotomy (PCTCL)
percutaneous transhepatic choledocho-
scopic electrohydraulic lithotripsy
(PTCS-EHL) of common bile duct
stones
percutaneous transhepatic decompres-
sion

percutaneous transhepatic liver biopsy
with tract embolization (PTBE)
percutaneous transhepatic obliteration
percutaneous transhepatic pigtail
catheter
Percy amputating saw
Percy amputation retractor
Percy intestinal forceps
Percy-Wolfson gallbladder retractor
perendoscopic biopsy specimen
Pereyra improved ligature cannula
PerFix Marlex mesh plug
PerFix plug and patch repair
PerFix Plus Plug polypropylene mesh
perflenapent
Perflex stainless steel stent and delivery
system
perflisopent
perflubron
perflutren
perforate
perforated acid peptic ulcer
perforated acute appendicitis
perforated appendicitis
perforated appendix
perforated carcinoma
perforated cholecystitis
perforated colon
perforated gallbladder
perforated, Smillie
perforated ulcer
perforated viscus
perforating abscess
perforating aneurysm
perforating forceps
perforating injuries
perforating twist drill
perforating ulcer
perforating vessel
perforating wound
perforation
   bowel
   closure of
   colonic

perforation *(cont.)*
   duodenal
   endoscopic intraperitoneal
   extraperitoneal
   frank
   free
   gallbladder
   gastric
   gastrointestinal
   GI tract
   intestinal
   small bowel
   stomach
   subacute
   traumatic
   ulcer
   uterine
   vesiculocolic
perforation of bowel
perforation of diverticulum
perforation of stomach
perforator
perfusion
   altered tissue
   inadequate
   intraperitoneal hyperthermic (IPHP)
   peripheral
   portal venous liver
   remote access (RAP)
perfusion cannula
perfusion defect
periadrenal tissue
periampullary carcinoma
periampullary neoplasm
periampullary region
periampullary tumor
perianal abscess
perianal Bowen disease
perianal condyloma
perianal drainage
perianal hematoma
perianal hygiene
perianal reflex
perianal region

perianal skin
perianal skin tag
perianal soak
perianal wart
periaortic node
periappendiceal abscess
periappendiceal fluid
periappendiceal gas
periareolar augmentation mammoplasty
periareolar incision
pericardial effusion
pericardial effusion fluid
pericardial fluid
pericardial sac
pericardiocentesis
pericardiocentesis needle
pericardiophrenic artery
pericarditis
pericecal abscess
pericholangiolitic biliary cirrhosis
pericholangitis
pericholecystic abscess
pericholecystic adhesion
pericholecystic collection
pericholecystic edema
pericholecystic fluid
pericholedochal lymph node
perichondritis, auricular
Peri-Colace (casanthranol; docusate
   sodium)
pericolic abscess
pericolic membrane syndrome
pericolic phlegmon
pericolitis
pericolonic abscess
pericolonic fat
pericolostomy area
pericoronal tissues
pericostal suture
peridiverticular tissue
Peri-Dos (casanthranol; docusate
   sodium)
periductal fibrosis
peridural anesthesia

periesophageal abscess
periesophageal inflammation
Periflow peripheral balloon catheter
perihepatic abscess
perihepatic packing
perihepatic peritoneum
perihepatitis (Fitz-Hugh–Curtis
    syndrome)
perihepatitis, gonococcal
perihepatitis syndrome
peri-ileal periampullary duodenal tumor
perilobar pancreatitis
perilobular duct
perimolysis
perimylolysis
perineal descent
perineal ecchymosis
perineal nerve terminal motor latency
perineal rectosigmoidectomy
perineal sinus
perineovaginal fistula
perinephric tissue
perineural anesthesia
periodic abdominalgia
periodic acid Schiff (PAS) test
periodic familial peritonitis
periodic liver biopsy
periodic peritonitis syndrome
periodic vomiting
periodontal anesthesia
periodontal mucosal grafting
PerioGlas bone graft material graft
PerioLase laser
perioperative antibiotic
perioperative muscle strength
perioperative steroid replacement
perioperative vomiting
perioral numbness
perioral tingling
periorbital edema
periosteal elevator
periosteal release double-edge knife
periosteal sarcoma
peripancreatic area

peripancreatic drain
peripancreatic space
peripancreatic tumor
periperitoneal fat stripe
peripheral alimentation
peripheral autonomic neuropathy
peripheral blood
peripheral blood smear
peripheral cyanosis
peripheral edema
peripheral embolism
peripheral hepatic necrosis
peripheral intravenous access
peripheral intravenous alimentation
peripheral lesion
peripheral necrosis
peripheral neurologic disorder
peripheral neuropathy
peripheral perfusion
peripheral smear
peripheral wasting
periportal area
periportal cirrhosis
periportal fibrosis of liver
periportal hepatocyte
periportal sinusoidal dilatation
periprosthetic capsulectomy, breast
perirectal abscess
perirectal cellulitis
perirectal injection
perirectal lymph node
perirectal pain
perirenal tissue
perisigmoid colon
perisinusoidal fibrosis
perisinusoidal space
peristalsis
    absent
    decreased
    equivocal primary
    gastrointestinal
    impaired esophageal
    visible
peristaltic activity

peristaltic contraction
peristaltic dysfunction
peristaltic reflex
peristaltic rush
peristaltic wave
peristomal area
peristomal skin
Peri-Strips Dry surgical staple-line
    reinforcement
Peri-Strips Dry wound sealant
peritoneal adhesion
peritoneal abscess
peritoneal-atrial shunt
peritoneal attachment
peritoneal band
peritoneal biopsy needle
peritoneal catheter
peritoneal cavity
peritoneal contamination from bowel
    perforation
peritoneal cytology
peritoneal dialysis
peritoneal dialysis catheter (PDC)
peritoneal drain
peritoneal edge
peritoneal effusion
peritoneal effusion fluid
peritoneal exudation
peritoneal flap
peritoneal fluid
peritoneal fold
peritoneal friction rub
peritoneal hernia
peritoneal implant
peritoneal irritation
peritonealization
peritonealize
peritoneal lavage
peritoneal metastasis
peritoneal mouse
peritoneal reflection
peritoneal rupture
peritoneal sac
peritoneal scarring

peritoneal seeding
peritoneal sign
peritoneal soilage
peritoneal soiling
peritoneal space
peritoneal studding
peritoneal tap
peritoneal toilet
peritoneal traverse by missile
peritoneal trocar
peritoneal-venous shunt (PVS)
peritoneal washings
peritoneocaval shunt
peritoneocentesis
peritoneography
peritoneointestinal reflex
peritoneoscope
peritoneoscopy
peritoneovenous shunt (PVS)
peritoneum
    abdominal
    parietal
    pelvic
    perihepatic
    posterior parietal
    visceral
peritoneum identified with hemostats
peritoneum was reapproximated
peritonism
peritonitis
    bacterial
    benign paroxysmal
    bile
    biliary
    chemical
    chronic proliferative
    diffuse
    exudative
    fecal
    full-blown bacterial
    generalized
    gonococcal
    periodic familial
    pneumococcal

peritonitis *(cont.)*
  primary
  proliferative
  puerperal
  sclerosing encapsulated
  spontaneous
  spontaneous bacterial (SBP)
  starch
  subacute nonspecific
  suppurative
  syphilitic
  tuberculous
peritonize
periumbilical abscess
periumbilical lymph node
periumbilical mass
periumbilical region
periumbilical vein engorgement
perivascular goiter
perivenular fibrosis
perivenular or pericellular fibrosis
Perkins left retractor
Perkins otologic retractor
Perkins right retractor
PermaClip endoscopic clip applier
Perma-Flow coronary bypass graft
Perma-Hand braided silk suture
Perma-Hand silk suture
Perma-Hand suture
PermaMesh graft
PermaMesh suture
Perman cartilage forceps
permanent colostomy
permanent end colostomy
permanent hypoparathyroidism
permanent lead introducer
permanent loop ileostomy
permanent section
permanent stoma
permanent tracheostomy
Perma-Seal dialysis access graft
PermCath double-lumen ventricular
  access catheter
permeability, intestinal

Perneczky aneurysm clamp
pernicious anemia
pernicious malaria
pernicious vomiting of pregnancy
peroneus brevis graft
peroral bougienage
peroxidase oxidation of iodide
peroxidase stain
peroxisome
Perras breast prosthesis
Perras-Papillon breast prosthesis
Perry ileostomy bag
PerryMeter anal EMG sensor
persistence, viral
persistent acidosis
persistent bacteremia
persistent breast abnormality
persistent hyperparathyroidism
persistent loop of distended small bowel
persistent mass after aspiration
persistent nipple discharge
persistent oligoanuria
persistent pylorospasm
persistent viral hepatitis (PVH)
persistent viral hepatitis C (PVH-C)
persistent viral hepatitis non-A, non B
  (PVH-NAB)
persistently raised E2-antimitochondrial
  antibody (AMA)
persisting fibrosis and nodule formation
personality changes
Perthes reamer
Peruvian balsam
pes cavus
pes planum
pessary, vaginal
pesticide, hepatocarcinogenic
PET (positron emission tomography)
PET balloon
petechia (pl. petechiae)
petechial angioma
petelin dissector
Petit hernia
Petit triangle

petrobasilar suture
petrosal ACTH
petrosphenobasilar suture
petrospheno-occipital suture
petrosquamous suture
Pettenkofer test
Petz clamp
Peutz-Jeghers gastrointestinal polyposis
Peutz-Jeghers polyp
Peutz-Jeghers syndrome (PJS)
Peutz-Jeghers syndrome of familial
    gastrointestinal polyposis
Peutz-Touraine syndrome
pexiganan acetate
Peyer gland
Peyer patch
Pezzer catheter
Pezzer drain
Pfannenstiel incision
p53 adenoviral gene
p53 mutation
p53 protein overexpression
PFGE (pulsed-field gel electrophoresis)
PFR95 filter
PFTE (polyfluorotetraethylene) graft
PG (paregoric)
PG (percutaneous gastrostomy)
PGA synthetic absorbable suture
PGA II (polyglandular autoimmune
    syndrome, type 2)
PGC (proximal gastric vagotomy)
PGE (percutaneous gastroenterostomy)
PGG glucan
PGP nail
PgR (progesterone receptor)
PG-TXL (polyglutamic acid paclitaxel)
PGV (proximal gastric vagotomy)
pH probe
    esophageal
    intraesophageal
phagocytic stellate cell
phagocytosis
Phalen position
Phaneuf artery forceps

phantom breast pain
phantom breast sensation
Phantom 5 Plus balloon catheter
phantom rectal pain
pharyngeal flap
pharmacomechanical coupling
pharmacotherapy
Pharmasealt tray
pharyngeal constrictor muscle
pharyngeal manometry
pharyngeal musculature
pharyngeal orifice
pharyngeal pouch
pharyngeal pouch syndrome
pharyngeal swallow reflex
pharyngoconjunctival fever virus
pharyngoesophageal function
pharyngoesophageal repair
pharyngoesophageal segment
pharyngoesophageal sphincter
pharyngogastrostomy
pharyngoglottal adduction reflex
pharyngoscope
pharyngostomy (fistulization of
    pharynx)
pharyngo-UES (upper esophageal
    sphincter) contractile reflex
pharynx
phase
    convalescent, of hepatitis
    gastric, of acid secretion
    icteric, of hepatitis
    intestinal, of acid secretion
    intradeglutitive, of swallowing
    postdeglutitive, of swallowing
    posticteric, of hepatitis
    preicteric
    venous
phase-contrast microscope
phasic contractions
Phazyme (simethicone)
Phemister elevator
Phemister onlay bone graft
Phemister rasp

Phenergan Fortis (promethazine HCl)
phenobarbital
Phenolax (phenolphthalein)
phenolphthalein
phenoltetrachlorophthalein test
phenomenon
    common cavity
    dawn
    Jod-Basedow
    mask
    satellite
    yo-yo weight fluctuation
phenoxybenzamine therapy
phentermine
phenylbutazone-induced hypothy-
    roidism
phenylethanolamine-N-methyltrans-
    ferase
pheochromocytoma
    bladder
    disseminated
    extra-adrenal
    malignant
    remote
PHG (portal hypertensive gastropathy)
Phillips LaxCaps
Phillips' Milk of Magnesia (magnesium
    hydroxide)
Phillips' M-O
pHisoHex scrub
phlebitis of thoracoepigastric vein
phlegmon formation
phlegmonous change
phlegmonous colitis
phlegmonous gastritis
phlegmonous mass
phlegmon, subhepatic
Phoenix cranial drill
Phoenix ventriculostomy catheter
phosphasoda cathartic
phosphate-binding antacid
phosphate buffered saline
phosphate depletion
phosphate enema

phosphatidyl choline (PC)
phosphoenolpyruvate carboxykinase
    (PEPCK) deficiency
phospholipase A
phospholipid, serum
phospholipid signal pathway
phosphoric acid
phosphorus necrosis
phosphorylase deficiency glycogen
    storage disease
phosphorylase, liver
phosphosoda enema
photocoagulation
    hemorrhoid
    infrared
    laser
photodynamic therapy (PDT)
photodynamic therapy, Foscan
    (temoporfin, mTHPC)
Photofrin (porfimer)
photometer, reflectant spectral
photon-deficient lesion
Photon Radiosurgery System (PRS)
photon scan
PhotoPoint laser
PhotoPoint light-activated technique
photosensitivity
photosensitizer
photothermal laser ablation of Barrett
    esophagus
phrenicocolic ligament
phrenicoesophageal ligament
phrenoesophageal ligament
phrenoesophageal membrane
phrenofundal reflection
phrenogastric ligament
phrygian cap deformity
physic (noun)
physical diagnosis
Physick pouch
physiograph for esophageal manometry
physiological gut-loop herniation
physiological irrigating solution
physiologic dead space

physiologic jaundice
physiologic reflux test (PRT)
physiological irrigating solution
phytobezoar
pica
PIC (peripherally inserted) catheter
PICC (peripherally inserted central
   catheter)
Piccolo blood analyzer
Pichinde virus
Pick cell
Pick chisel
picket fence guide
pickup
   DeBakey
   rat-tooth
pickup forceps
picornavirus
Pico-ST II catheter
Pidcock check pin
Pidcock nail
piecemeal necrosis
piecemeal swallowing
Pierse micro dissecting forceps
Pierse tip forceps
Piezolith-EPL (extracorporeal piezo-
   electric lithotriptor)
pigeon-breeder's lung
piggybacking of I.V.
pigmentary cirrhosis
pigment cirrhosis
pigmented gallstone
pigmented liver
pigmented satellite lesion
pigment stone
pigskin graft
pigtail catheter
pigtail connector
pigtail stent
pile, sentinel
piles (hemorrhoids)
Piliel gel (hair regrowth) dressing
pill esophagitis
Pilling-Liston rongeur

Pilling rigid laparoscope
Pilling Weck Surgical
Pilling Weck Y-stent forceps
Pillo Pro dressing
pillow sign
pilonidal abscess
pilonidal cyst
pilonidal disease
pilonidal fistula
pilonidal sinus
Pilot drill
Pilot suture
Pilot suturing guide
pimagedine HCl
pin
   absorbable
   absorbable polyparadioxanone
   Acufex distractor
   alignment
   Allofix freeze-dried cortical bone
   Austin Moore
   ball guide
   ball-point guide
   ball-tip guide
   beaded hip
   beaded reamer guide
   Beath
   Bilos
   biodegradable
   Biofix system
   Böhler (Boehler)
   Bohlman
   breakaway
   Breck
   calcaneal
   calibrated
   Canakis
   Charnley
   clavicle
   closed
   collapsible
   Compere threaded
   Compton clavicle
   Conley

pin *(cont.)*
 Crego-McCarroll
 cross
 Crowe pilot point on Steinmann
 Davis
 Day
 Denham
 DePuy
 Deyerle II
 distractor
 drawing
 drill
 Ender
 Fahey-Compere
 femoral guide
 Fischer transfixing
 Fisher half
 fixation
 Gardner skull clamp
 Gingrass and Messer
 Gouffon hip
 guide
 Hagie
 half
 halo
 Hansen-Street
 Hare
 Hatcher
 Haynes
 Hessel-Nystrom
 hip
 hook
 hook-end intramedullary
 hydroxyapatite-coated
 in situ
 Intraflex intramedullary
 intramedullary
 Jones compression
 Knowles
 Krankendonk
 Küntscher (Kuentscher)
 LIH (Lars Ingvar Hansson) hook
 locating
 Lottes

pin *(cont.)*
 marble bone
 Mayfield skull clamp
 Mayo sterilizing
 McBride
 metallic
 Modny
 Moore
 Olds
 open
 Oris
 OrthoSorb absorbable fixation
 partially threaded
 PDS (poly-p-dioxanone)
 percutaneous
 Pidcock check
 poly-p-dioxanonc (PDS)
 polyparadioxanone, absorbable
 precurved ball-tipped guide
 Pritchard Mark II
 rasp
 resorbable
 Rhinelander
 Riordan
 Roger Anderson
 Rush
 Schanz
 Schneider
 Schweitzer
 self-broaching
 Serrato forearm
 Shriner
 skeletal traction
 skull
 Smith-Petersen
 smooth Steinmann
 socket
 Sofield
 Stader
 Steinmann
 Street medullary
 strut-type
 tapered
 threaded

pin *(cont.)*
    threaded Steinmann
    tibial drill
    titanium half
    traction
    transarticular
    transfixing
    transfixion
    Turner
    Tutofix cortical
    Varney
    Venable-Stuck
    Vom Saal
    Wagner closed
    wrench
    Zimmer
pinch-band forceps
pinchcock effect
pinchcock mechanism at esophago-
    gastric junction
pinch forceps
pin clamp
pin cutter
PI90 double-headed stapler
Pink Bismuth (bismuth subsalicylate)
pinked up (verb)
Pinn.ACL guide
pinpoint gastric mucosal defect
    bleeding
PinPoint stereotactic arm
pinpoint suction
pin-retained palatal prosthesis
pin retractor
Pin-Rid (pyrantel pamoate)
Pinto Cobra, The
Pinto loop underminer
pinworm (*Enterobius vermicularis*)
Pin-X (pyrantel pamoate)
pioglitazone hydrochloride
PIP (pressure inversion point)
    on esophageal manometry
pipe, food
pipestem cirrhosis
pipestem stool

Pipelle endometrial suction catheter
Piper obstetrical forceps
piperamide maleate
piperazine, piperazine calcium edetate,
    piperazine edetate calcium
PIPIDA scan
pi plate
pirenzepine HCl
piriform fossa
piriform sinus
piritrexim
pirogliride, pirogliride tartrate
PI surgical stapler
pit
    anal
    colonic
    gastric
    postanal
pitch worker's cancer
pitchfork retractor
Pitkin spinal needle
pit of stomach
Pitressin Synthetic (vasopressin)
pitting edema
Pittman IMA retractor
pituitary adenoma
pituitary cachexia
pituitary Cushing syndrome
pituitary dwarfism
pituitary enlargement
pituitary forceps
pituitary gland
pituitary hyperfunction
pituitary hypersecretion
pituitary insufficiency
pituitary irradiation
pituitary knife
pituitary mass
pituitary rongeur
pituitary scissors
pituitary secretion
pituitary suppression
pituitary tumor

pituitary tumor syndrome (acromegaly,
  galactorrhea, Cushing syndrome)
Pivanex
PIVKA-II levels
Pivotal coagulator
Pivotal dissector
Pivotal grasper
Pivotal scissors
Pixie fiberoptic scope
PiZZ alpha$_1$ antitrypsin deficiency
PJS (Peutz-Jeghers syndrome)
placement of intraperitoneal drain
placement of silastic ring band
placement, trocar
placental polyp
plain catgut suture
plain film of abdomen
plain gut
plain gut suture
plain pattern plate
plain splinter forceps
plain suture
plain tissue forceps
plain view
planar plate
planar view
plane (pl. planes)
  axial
  biparietal
  coronal
  fascial
  fat
  horizontal
  ischiorectal fossa
  pelvic
  sagittal
  subcostal
  subfascial
  supracrestal
  transumbilical
  transverse
  umbilical
  vertical

planing brush
planned pancreaticoduodenectomy
plantar axial view
plantar plate
plantar puncture wound
plantar flexion stress view
planus, lichen
plaquelike linear defect
Plasbumin-25 (human albumin)
plasma aldosterone
plasma assay coagulation panel
plasma basal and stimulated (with
  pentagastrin or calcium) calcitonin
  measurements
plasma carbon dioxide
plasma cell dyscrasia
plasma cell hepatitis
plasma cell mastitis
plasma clotting time
plasma coagulation time
plasma concentration
plasma electrolytes
plasma Endotoxin concentration
plasma expander
plasma, fresh frozen (FFP)
plasma gastrin level
plasma glucose level
plasma lipotropic hormone (LPH,
  lipotropin) concentration
Plasma-Lyte A pH 7.4
Plasma-Lyte 148 (combined electrolyte
  solution)
Plasmanate (plasma protein fraction)
plasma pH
plasmapheresis
Plasma-Plex (plasma protein fraction)
plasma pool
plasma protein fraction
plasma renin activity
Plasma Scalpel
Plasmatein (plasma protein fraction)
plasma total cortisol

plasma volume expander (see also
   medications)
  dextran 40 (10% LMD)
  dextran 40 (Rheomacrodex)
  Hespan (hetastarch)
  Hextend
  Rheomacrodex (dextran 40)
  10% LMD (dextran 40)
Plasmodium falciparum
Plasmodium malariae
plaster cast instruments
plaster knife
plaster of Paris (POP) bandage
plaster saw
plaster scissors
plaster shears
plastic clot
plastic drape
plastic nasopharyngeal airway
plastic-sheathed malleable aluminum
  stylet
plastic suture
plate
  acetabular reconstruction
  AcroMed VSP
  Aesculap ABC cervical
  alar
  anal
  anchor
  AO blade
  AO condylar blade
  AO contoured T
  AO hook
  AOI blade
  AO reconstruction
  AO semitubular
  AO small fragment
  Armstrong
  ASIF right-angle blade
  axial
  Badgley
  Bagby angled compression
  basal
  Batchelor

plate *(cont.)*
  biodegradable
  blade
  Blount blade
  bone
  bone flap fixation
  bony
  Bosworth spine
  Burns
  buttress
  Calandruccio side
  cap-and-anchor
  cartilaginous growth
  CASP (contoured anterior spinal)
  Caspar cervical
  cervical locking
  cloverleaf
  coaptation
  cobra-head
  Collison
  compression
  condylar
  conical tectal
  connecting
  Continuum total knee base
  contoured T-plate
  cortical
  cranial bone fixation
  cribriform
  C-shaped
  DCP (dynamic compression)
  deck
  DePuy
  Deyerle
  dorsal
  double-H
  Driessen hinged
  dual
  Duopress
  Dwyer-Hall
  dynamic compression (DCP)
  eccentric dynamic compression
    (EDCP)
  Eggers bone

plate *(cont.)*
    11-hole
    Elliott femoral condyle blade
    end
    epiphyseal cartilage
    ethmovomerine
    E-Z Flap cranial bone
    femoral
    fibrocartilaginous
    fiducial
    five-hole (5-hole)
    fixed-angle blade
    flat
    flexor palmar
    foot
    Forte distal radius
    four-hole (4-hole)
    frontal
    fusion
    gait
    Gallannaugh bone
    growth
    Hagie sliding nail
    Haid cervical
    half-circle
    Hansen-Street
    Harlow
    Harm posterior cervical
    Harris
    heavy-duty femur
    heavy side
    Hicks lugged
    hilar
    Hoen skull
    Holt nail
    Howmedica Microfixation cranial
    H-shaped
    Hubbard
    interfragmentary
    intertrochanteric
    I plate of Yuan
    Jergesen I-beam
    Jergesen tapered
    Jewett nail overlay

plate *(cont.)*
    Jones compression
    Kaneda
    Kessel
    Laing
    Lane
    Lawson-Thornton
    LC-DCP
    Leibinger Micro Plus
    Leibinger Micro System cranial
        fixation
    Leibinger 3-D
    Letournel
    limiting
    liver cell
    localization-compression grid
    Lorenz cranial
    Louis
    low contact dynamic compression
        (LC-DCP)
    L-shaped
    Luhr micro
    Luhr Microfixation cranial
    Luhr mini
    Luhr pan
    Lundholm
    Luque-Galveston
    Luque II
    malleable
    Massie
    McBride
    McLaughlin intertrochanteric
    Mears sacroiliac
    Medoff sliding
    meningioma of the cribriform
    Meurig Williams
    micro
    microfixation
    Milch
    mini
    minifragment
    Moe intertrochanteric
    Moore sliding nail
    Moreira

plate *(cont.)*
    Morscher cervical
    Müller (Mueller) compression blade
    nail
    Neufeld
    neutralization
    Newman
    Nicoll
    occipitocervical
    Ogden
    orbital
    Orozco cervical
    orthotic
    Osborne
    overlay
    palmar
    Paulus
    PEAK channeled
    pedicle
    peg-base
    pi
    plain pattern
    planar
    plantar
    pterygoid
    Pugh
    pylon attachment
    quadrangular positioning
    quadrigeminal
    reconstruction
    resorbable
    Richards-Hirschhorn
    Richards side
    roof
    Rotator Cuff Buttress (RCB)
    Roy-Camille cervical
    Roy-Camille occipitocervical
    Roy-Camille pedicle
    Schweitzer spring
    semitubular compression
    Senn
    serpentine
    seven-hole (7-hole)
    17-hole

plate *(cont.)*
    Sherman bone
    side
    Simmons
    six-hole (6-hole)
    skull
    slide
    slotted femur
    Smith-Petersen
    Smith-Petersen intertrochanteric
    SMO (supramalleolar orthosis)
    spoon
    stabilization
    stainless steel
    stainless steel preformed skull
    steel sole
    Steffee
    Steffee pedicle
    Steffee screw
    stem base
    Storz Microsystems cranial fixation
    subchondral bone
    supracondylar
    Synthes cervical
    Synthes dorsal distal radius
    Synthes Microsystems cranial
        fixation
    Synthes mini L-plate
    Syracuse I
    T
    tantalum preformed skull
    tarsal
    T buttress
    tectal
    Temple University
    tendon
    Thornton nail
    3-D (three-dimensional)
    three-hole (3-hole)
    titanium
    toe
    Townley tibial plateau
    Townsend-Gilfillan
    trial base

plate *(cont.)*
   T-shaped
   T-shaped AO
   tubular
   Tupman
   twisted
   two-hole (2-hole)
   UCP compression
   Uslenghi
   V blade
   Venable
   vertebral body
   Vitallium
   V nail
   volar
   VSP (variable screw placement)
   Wainwright
   Wenger
   Whitman
   Wilson
   wing
   Wright
   Wurzburg
   X-shaped
   Y bone
   Y-shaped
   Zimmer femoral condyle blade
   Zimmer side
   Zimmer Y
   Z-shaped
   Zuelzer hook
plate driver
plate-holding forceps
platelet activating factor (PAF)
platelet-activating factor acetylhydro-
   lase, recombinant (rPAF-AH)
platelet activity
platelet count
platelet count coagulation panel
platelet-derived growth factor
platelet dysfunction
platelet plug
platelet-poor blood (PPB)
platelet storage

platelet trapping
platysma
PLE (protein-losing enteropathy)
pleating of small bowel
Pleatman sac
pledget dressing
pledgeted Ethibond suture
pledgeted mattress suture
pledget, Oxycel
Plenk-Matson rasp
pleomorphic destructive cholangitis
Plester self-retaining retractor
Plester suction tube
pleural biopsy needle
pleural effusion
pleural fluid
pleural metastasis
pleural patch
pleural space
pleural space flow of fluid
pleural tube
Pleur-evac suction tube
pleuritic chest pain
pleuropericardial effusion
pleuroperitoneal canal
pleuroperitoneal membrane
pleuropneumonia-like (PPLO)
   organism
plexus
   abdominal aortic
   Auerbach mesenteric
   biliary
   brachial
   choroid
   colic
   colonic myenteric
   cystic
   esophageal
   gastric
   gastroesophageal variceal
   hemorrhoidal
   hepatic
   ileocolic
   muscularis

plexus *(cont.)*
  myenteric
  nerve
  pampiniform
  pelvic
  prostatic venous
  rectal
  submucosal venous
  testicular pampiniform venous
  venous
pliable stent
plica (pl. plicae)
plicae circulares
plicae gastropancreaticae
plicate, plicated
plicating
plication
  Childs-Phillips bowel
  fundal
  intestinal
  Noble bowel
  Rehne-Delorme
  suture
  transgastric
  transmesenteric
plication of bowel
plication of fascia
plication of mesentery (mesenteropexy)
plication suture
pliers
  Compaction
  double-action wire-extraction
  flat-nose
  Howmedica Microfixation System
  Leibinger Micro System
  locking
  Luhr Microfixation System
  mesh
  needle-nose
  needle-nose locking
  pair of
  polypropylene mesh
  PowerGrip
  slip joint

pliers *(cont.)*
  Storz Microsystems
  Synthes Microsystems
  taper-nose
  wire-cutting
plug
  bile
  bone
  decannulation
  Gilbert free-formed umbrella-shaped
  Herniamesh surgical mesh
  Marlex PerFix
  meconium
  mucus
  patch and
  PerFix Marlex mesh
  platelet
  R-Med
  Rutkow sutureless plug and patch
  sutureless
plug effect of connector
plug and patch
plug-and-patch hernia repair
plugged liver biopsy
plug of tissue
Plum drug delivery pump
plume
  laser
  smoke
Plummer disease
Plummer esophageal dilator
Plummer-Vinson syndrome
plunging goiter
Plus Reusable Silicone Resuscitator
PMC (pseudomembranous colitis)
PMMA (polymethylmethacrylate) rod
PMN (polymorphonuclear leukocyte)
PMT biopsy needle
pneumatic bag
pneumatic bag esophageal dilatation
pneumatic balloon catheter dilation
pneumatic balloon dilator
pneumatic compression boot
pneumatic drill

pneumatosis coli
pneumatosis cystoides intestinalis (PCI)
pneumatosis intestinalis
pneumatosis of the bowel
pneumaturia
pneumobilia
pneumococcal peritonitis
pneumococcus vaccine
pneumocolon
Pneumocystis carinii (PCP)
pneumogastric
pneumogastrography
pneumoinsufflation needle
Pneumo-Needle reusable instrument
pneumonia
pneumoperitoneum, carbon dioxide
pneumoperitoneum needle
pncumoscrotum, ipsilateral
Pneumo Sleeve laparoscopic airlock
pneumothorax
Pneu-Stick needle
PNTML (pudendal nerve terminal
    motor latency) test
pO$_2$
p.o. (L. *per os*, by mouth, orally)
p.o. antibiotic
POA (pancreatic oncofetal antigen) test
pocket aneroid
pocketed calculus
pocket
    breast reconstruction
    fluid
    pus
    subcutaneous
point
    acupressure
    Addison
    bleeding
    blunt
    Boas
    Chauffard
    Crowe pilot
    Desjardins
    dorsal

point *(cont.)*
    drill
    Ethiguard blunt
    Hartmann
    Lane
    Lanz
    Mackenzie
    McBurney
    Munro
    pressure inversion (PIP)
    Ramond
    respiratory inversion
    Robson
    Sudeck
pointed awl
pointed-nose grasper
point-in-space stereotactic biopsy
point of attachment
point of maximal pain
point of respiratory reversal
    on esophageal manometry
Poirier gland
poison, poisoning
    acetaminophen
    bacterial food
    carbon tetrachloride
    caustic acid
    caustic alkali
    chloroform
    ethylene glycol
    food
    halothane
    salicylate
    salmonella food
    staphylococcal food
    toxic mushroom
Poison Control Center
Polaris 1.32 Nd:YAG laser
Polaris RF catheter
polarographic P(ti)O$_2$ catheter probe
Polaroid camera
Polaroid endocamera EC-3
Polaroid SX-70 with ACMI adapter
Polhemus-Schafer-Ivemark syndrome

Policot II sponge
polidocanol sclerosant
poliglacaprone absorbable suture
  material
polio
poliomyelitis virus
poliovirus
pollen, bee
Pollock grasper
Polocaine (mepivacaine)
poloxamer 188 (Flocor)
Polya anastomosis
Polya gastrectomy
Polya technique
polyarteritis nodosa
polybutester suture
polycystic chronic esophagitis
polycystic kidney
polycystic liver
polycystic liver disease
polycythemia vera
Polydek suture
Polyderm foam wound dressing
Polyderm hydrophilic polyurethane
  foam dressing
polydioxanone suture (PDS)
polydipsia
polydrug therapy
polyester mesh (Mersilene)
polyester mesh + silicone with
  memory, pre-shaped
polyester suture
polyester tripled hamstring graft
polyester-reinforced Dacron tape
polyester-reinforced silicon sheeting
polyethylene cannula
polyethylene glycol (PEG)
polyethylene glycol electrolyte solution
polyethylene tube
PolyFlo peripherally inserted central
  catheter (PICC)
polyfluorotetraethylene (PTFE) plastic
  graft material
PolyGIA stapler

polyglacine suture
polyglactin mesh dural graft
polyglactin rod
polyglactin suture material
polyglactin 370, polyglactin 910
  absorbable suture material
polyglactin 910 mesh
polyglactin 910 suture
polyglandular autoimmune syndrome,
  type II (PGA II)
polyglandular deficiency syndrome,
  type II
polyglandular dysfunction
polyglutamic acid paclitaxel (PG-TXL)
polyglycolic acid mesh
polyglycolic acid suture material
polyglycolic suture
polyglycolide, self-reinforced rod
polyglyconate absorbable suture
  material
polyglyconate suture
PolyHeme (human hemoglobin cross-
  linked with glutaral) blood substitute
polylobar liver
PolyMem foam wound dressing
polymerase chain reaction (PCR)
polymerase technique
polymeric IgA antigen complex
polymethylmethacrylate-copolymer
  beads
polymicrobial bacteremia
polymorphic fungi
polymorphism
polymorphonuclear leukocyte (PMN)
polymorphonuclear leukocyte cell
polymyositis
polyneuropathy
  diabetic
  familial amyloid
polyoma virus
polyp
  adenomatous
  benign
  benign adenomatous

polyp *(cont.)*
  bleeding
  broad-based
  bronchial
  cardiac
  cellular
  cervical
  choanal
  colon
  colonic mucosubmucosal elongated
  colorectal
  cystic
  dental
  diffuse GI hamartoma
  duodenal
  endometrial
  fibrinous
  fibroepithelial
  fibrovascular
  gallbladder
  gastric
  gastrointestinal
  gelatinous
  hamartomatous gastric
  Hopmann
  hydatid
  hyperplastic gastric
  inflammatory fibroid
  juvenile
  laryngeal
  lipomatous
  lymphoid
  malignant
  metaplastic
  metastatic
  mucous
  multiple hamartomatous
  myomatous
  nasal
  neoplastic
  osseous
  pedunculated mass of
  Peutz-Jeghers
  placental

polyp *(cont.)*
  polypoid adenocarcinoma
  postinflammatory
  premalignant colonic
  pulp
  rectal
  regenerative
  retention
  sessile
  sigmoid
  single
  stalk of
  tubular
  tubulovillous
  uterine
  vascular
  villous
polyparadioxanone, absorbable pin
poly-p-dioxanone suture (PDS) pin
polypectomy
  colonoscopic
  electrosurgical snare
  endoscopic
polypectomy snare
polypectomy snare with banana plug
  connector
polypectomy snare with Olympus
  connector
polypeptide
  gastric inhibitory (GIP)
  glucose-dependent insulinotropic
    (GIP)
  islet amyloid (IAPP)
  pancreatic (PP)
  parathyroid-like
  vasoactive intestinal (VIP)
polypeptide antigen
polypeptide chain
polyp forceps
polyp grasper, four-pronged
polyp grasping forceps
polyphagia
polyp hook
polyphrenic gene

polyplastic cell
polypoid adenocarcinoma polyp
polypoidal tumor
polypoid carcinoma
polypoid lesion
polypoid lymphoid hyperplasia
polypoid lymphoma
polypoid mass
polypoid polyp
polypoid tissue
polyposis
   adenomatous
   diffuse mucosal
   familial
   familial adenomatous (FAP)
   familial colorectal
   familial gastrointestinal
   familial intestinal
   filiform
   gastric
   gastrointestinal
   hamartomatous intestinal
   hyperplastic
   intestinal
   juvenile
   melanoplakia-intestinal
   multiple familial
   multiple intestinal
   Peutz-Jeghers gastrointestinal
polyposis coli, familial
polypous gastritis
polypropylene mesh
polypropylene mesh/gelatin film graft
polypropylene mesh with memory
polypropylene suture
polyps and spots syndrome
polyps of hypertrophied mucosa
polyp snare technique
polyp stalk
polys (polymorphonuclear leukocytes)
Polyskin II dressing
Polysorb braided synthetic absorbable
   suture
polysplenia syndrome

Polystan catheter
polytetrafluoroethylene mesh graft
Polytrac Gomez retractor
polyurethane foam (PFD) dressing
polyvalent pneumococcal vaccine post-
   splenectomy
polyvinyl alcohol sponge
polyvinyl sponge graft
PolyWic wound filling material
Pondimin (fenfluramine)
Ponka anesthesia technique in herni-
   orrhaphy
Ponka classification of groin hernias
   (types 1–2)
Ponka herniorrhaphy
Ponka technique for local anesthesia
Ponsky Endo-Sock retrieval bag
Ponsky "Pull" gastrostomy feeding
   device
Pontén-type tubed pedicle
Pontocaine HCl (tetracaine HCl)
pool, pooling
   abdominal
   bile acid
   blood
   gastric
   plasma
   vallecular
Poole abdominal suction tube
pooled plasma
Poole instrument
Poole suction
Poole suction tube
Poole tip
poorly defined vascular space
poorly differentiated adenocarcinoma
poorly differentiated adenoma
poorly differentiated carcinoma
poorly localized pain
poorly opsonized pathogen
poor operative candidate
poor prognosis
poor tissue turgor
poor uptake

poor visualization
POP (plaster of Paris) bandage
popliteal pulse
pop-off needle
pop-off suture
pop-off valve
Poppen-Blalock carotid clamp
Poppen-Blalock-Salibi clamp
Poppen forceps
Poppen-Gelpi laminectomy retractor
Poppen Gigli saw guide
Poppen intervertebral disk rongeur
Poppen saw
Poppen ventricular needle
population, viral
porcelain gallbladder
porcine dermal collagen graft
porcine islet preparation, encapsulated
porcine transmissible gastroenteritis
porcine xenograft
porfimer sodium
porfiromycin
porous polyethylene graft
porphyria
   acute
   acute intermittent (AIP)
   congenital erythropoietic
   hepatic
   hepatoerythropoietic (HEP)
porphyria cutanea tarda (PCT)
port
   endoscopic
   Fastrac gastrostomy access
   Hasson
   Import vascular-access port
     with BioGlide
   Port-A-Cath
   suction
   two-way laparoscopic
portable blood irradiator
portable film
portable insulin infusion pump
portable view
Port-A-Cath

portacaval anastomosis
portacaval H graft
portacaval shunt
Portagen diet
Portagen formula
porta hepatic lymph node
porta hepatis
portal and splenic veins
portal and systemic endotoxemia
portal azygous collateral
portal canal
portal cannula
portal catheter
portal circulation
portal cirrhosis
portal decompression
portal embolization (PE)
portal endotoxin
portal fibrosis
portal fibrosis of liver
portal fissure
portal hypertension from liver cirrhosis
portal hypertension-induced variceal
   bleeding
portal hypertension with severe
   hypersplenism
portal hypertensive gastropathy (PHG)
portal lobule
portal pressure
portal pyemia
portal pylethrombophlebitis
portal space
portal spread
portal systemic anastomosis
portal-systemic anastomotic area
portal-systemic collateral blood flow
portal-systemic collateral circulation
portal-systemic encephalopathy (PSE)
portal-systemic (or portosystemic) shunt
portal system of veins
portal thrombophlebitis
portal-to-portal bridging
portal-to-portal fibrosis
portal triad

portal vascular bed
portal vein
portal vein (end) to IVC (side)
portal vein gas
portal vein resection
portal vein thrombosis
portal venous hypertension
portal venous liver perfusion
portal venous pressure (PVP)
portal venous system thrombosis
portal vessel rupture
portal zone
portal zone granuloma
port closure needle
Porter duodenal forceps
Portex blue line intubation
Portnoy ventricular cannula
Portnoy ventricular catheter
portocaval shunt
portocaval synthetic H-graft
portoenterostomy, Kasai
portogram
portography, percutaneous transhepatic
portoportal anastomosis
portopulmonary shunt
portosystemic (or portal-systemic)
portosystemic anastomosis
portosystemic encephalopathy
portosystemic gradient
portosystemic shunt
portosystemic shunting
port site
port-site metastasis
port-site recurrence of tumor
POSICAM system
position
    abdominal brace
    antero-oblique
    barber chair
    bayonet fracture
    beach chair
    Bonner
    Bozeman
    Brickner

position *(cont.)*
    Buie
    calcaneal stance
    conjugate forward gaze
    decubitus
    dorsal
    dorsal lithotomy (*not* dorso-
        lithotomy)
    dorsal recumbent
    dorsal supine
    dorsosacral
    figure-4
    Fowler
    frog-leg
    full lateral
    Gaynor-Hart
    hook-lying
    horizontal
    infraumbilical
    intrinsic plus
    jackknife
    jet pilot
    Jones
    jumper's knee
    knee-chest
    knee-elbow
    kneeling
    Kraske jackknife
    lateral decubitus
    lateral park bench
    leapfrog
    left decubitus
    left lateral decubitus
    lithotomy
    lotus
    Mayo-Robson
    medial genicular
    modified dorsal lithotomy
    modified lithotomy
    near-anatomic
    neutral calcaneal stance
    neutral hip
    neutral spine
    normal anatomic

position *(cont.)*
   occipitoanterior
   occipitoposterior
   occipitotransverse
   opisthotonic
   over-the-top
   park bench
   Phalen
   prayer
   prone
   proximal bow
   rectus
   resting calcaneal stance
   reverse Trendelenburg
   right antero-oblique
   right lateral decubitus
   Robson
   Rose
   scissor-leg
   semi-Fowler
   semi-sitting
   side-lying
   Sims
   sitting
   ski
   spinal fusion
   static
   stress tolerant
   supine
   three-quarters prone
   Trendelenburg
   W-sitting
positional stasis
positive bowel sounds
positive Chvostek sign
positive family history
positive inotropy
positive margin
positive Murphy sign
positive nodal metastasis
positive peritoneal space pressure
positive peritoneal tap
positive-pressure ventilation
positive surgical margins

positive test for occult blood
positive tetany
positive Trousseau sign
positron emission tomography (PET)
positron emission tomography with
   fluorodeoxyglucose
possible paracrine growth of adeno-
   carcinoma of the stomach
postablative hypopituitarism
postablative hypothyroidism
postadenoidectomy
postage stamp-type skin graft
postanal pit
postanal repair
postanesthesia recovery room
postaugmentation mammoplasty bra
postaural regurgitation
post balloon angioplasty restenosis
postbulbar duodenal ulcer
postcholecystectomy flatulent dyspepsia
postcholecystectomy syndrome (PCS)
postcibal symptoms
postcoital bleeding
postcolonoscopy distention syndrome
postcricoid area
postcricoid web
postdeglutitive phase of swallowing
postemesis longitudinal tear
postemetic esophageal rupture
postendoscopic cholangitis
post-ERCP-induced pancreatitis
posterior abdominal wall
posterior choanal atresia
posterior colporrhaphy
posterior diaphragm
posterior diaphragmatic gastropexy
posterior extension of the lateral thyroid
   lobe
posterior fixation
posterior fossa-atrial shunt
posterior fossa retractor
posterior hemifundoplication
posterior hiatoplasty
posterior horn of the spinal cord

posterior incision
posterior inferior pancreaticoduodenal
  artery
posterior midline
posterior perforated duodenal ulcer into
  the pancreas
posterior rectopexy
posterior rectus fascia
posterior rectus sheath
posterior repair of the diaphragmatic
  hiatus
posterior sagittal and 3-flap anoplasty
posterior superior pancreaticoduodenal
  artery
posterior surface of pancreas
posterior surface of prostate
posterior triangle of the neck
posterolateral
posteromedial aspect of the thyroid
  gland
postevacuation film
postevacuation view
postfundoplication dysphagia
postfundoplication syndrome
postgastrectomy
postgastrectomy stasis
postgastrectomy syndrome
postgastric surgery syndrome
posthepatic cirrhosis
postherniorrhaphy neuropathy
posticteric phase of hepatitis
postinflammatory polyp
postinjury immunologic defect
postlaparoscopic shoulder pain
postlymphangiography abdomen
postmastectomy radiation therapy
postmenopausal
postmortem clot
postmortem knife
postmortem needle
  double-curve cutting-edge
  half-curved cutting-edge
postmyotomy reflux
postnecrotic cirrhosis

postnecrotic scar
postop (postoperative)
postoperative chemotherapy
postoperative abscess
postoperative adhesion
postoperative anesthesia
postoperative antibiotic
postoperative atelectasis
postoperative complications
postoperative diagnosis
postoperative ductal dilation
postoperative dysphagia
postoperative esophagitis
postoperative feeding schedule
postoperative hematoma
postoperative hemorrhage
postoperative hernia
postoperative hydrocele
postoperative hypocalcemia
postoperative ileus
postoperative incentive spirometry
postoperative infection
postoperative neuropathy
postoperative pain
postoperative pancreatitis
postoperative paraesophageal hiatus
  hernia
postoperative regimen for oral early
  feeding (PROEF)
postoperative residual stone
postoperative seroma
postoperative serum calcitonin level
postoperative "settling" of breast
  following reduction
postoperative T-tube cholangiography
postoperative view
postoperative vomiting
postpancreatectomy hyperglycemia
postpartum constipation
postpartum mastitis
postpartum period
postpartum pituitary necrosis
postpolio syndrome
postpolypectomy coagulation syndrome

postprandial abdominal discomfort
postprandial abdominal distention
postprandial antral hypomotility
postprandial blood glucose level
postprandial discomfort
postprandial distention
postprandial fullness
postprandial hypoglycemia
postprandially
postprandial pain
postprandial rise in peripheral glucose
postprandial vomiting
postpyloric feeding tube
postpyloric ulcer
postreduction ischemic necrosis
post-retching hematemesis
post-retching longitudinal tear
post-secretin challenge gastric level
post-shunt encephalopathy
postsplenectomy complications
postsplenectomy sepsis
postsurgical abdomen
postsurgical gastric stasis
postsurgical hypoglycemia
postsurgical hypothyroidism
postsurgical muscular or neurogenic
postsurgical nonabsorption syndrome
postsurgical recurrent ulcer
postsurgical stricture
post-transfusion hepatitis
post-transplant diabetes mellitus
post-transplant lymphoproliferative
  disorder
post-transplantation lymphoproliferative
  disorder (PTLD)
post-tussive vomiting
postural response of aldosterone
postvagotomy diarrhea
postvagotomy dysphagia
postvagotomy gastroparesis
postvagotomy syndrome
potassium (K)
potassium iodide
potassium supplement

potassium-titanyl-phosphate (KTP)
  laser light therapy
potato liver
Pott abscess
Potter syndrome
Potts aortic clamp
Potts bronchus forceps
Potts bulldog forceps
Potts clamp
Potts-Cournand needle
Potts-DeMartel vascular scissors
Potts forceps
Potts needle
Potts-Nieder clamp
Potts patent ductus clamp
Potts rib shears
Potts right-angled scissors
Potts-Satinsky clamp
Potts 60° angled scissors
Potts-Smith aortic occlusion clamp
Potts-Smith dressing forceps
Potts-Smith tissue forceps
Potts-Smith vascular scissors
Potts tenotomy scissors
Potts thumb forceps
Potts tie suture
Potts vascular forceps
Potts-Yasargil scissors
pouch (see also *appliance; barrier;
    device*)
  antral
  apophyseal
  Bard Extra Ileo B
  Bard Integrale
  blind
  blind upper esophageal
  branchial
  Broca pudendal
  celomic
  closed-end ostomy
  Coloplast Flange
  coloplasty
  continent ileal
  ConvaTec Little One Sur-Fit

pouch *(cont.)*
    Cymed Micro Skin
    Dansac DuoSoft
    Dansac Karaya Seal
    Dansac Nova ostomy
    Dansac Standard Ileo
    deep perineal
    Denis Browne
    dilatation of the
    Douglas rectouterine
    drainable ostomy
    endodermal
    endorectal ileal
    esophageal
    fluid collection
    Fobi
    formation of intestinal
    fourth bronchial
    fourth pharyngeal
    gastric
    Graham omental
    Greez EZ Access drainage
    Hartmann
    haustral
    Heidenhain
    hepatorenal
    hernia
    Hollister First Choice
    Hollister Holligard
    Hollister Karaya 5 ostomy
    Hollister Karaya Seal
    Hollister Premium
    Hunt-Lawrence
    hypophysial
    ileal J
    ileal S
    ileal W
    ileoanal
    ileocecal
    Indiana
    jejunal
    J-shaped ileal
    Karaya ring ileostomy
    Kock ("coke")

pouch *(cont.)*
    lateral-lateral
    Mainz pouch urinary reservoir
    Marlen Gas Relief
    Marlen Odor-Ban
    Marlen Solo ileostomy
    Marlen Zip Klosed
    marsupial
    Morison
    Nu-Hope ileostomy
    Nu-Hope Nu-Self
    one-piece ostomy
    open-end ostomy
    ostomy
    Pagedas retrieval
    paracystic
    pararectal
    paravesical
    Parks ileostomy
    pendulous
    Penn
    pharyngeal
    Physick
    Prussak
    Rathke
    rectal
    rectouterine
    rectovaginal
    rectovaginouterine
    rectovesical
    Remedy
    renal
    Seessel (2 e's, 2 s's)
    S-shaped
    superficial inguinal
    superficial perineal
    Sur-Fit Mini
    terminal ileal
    third branchial
    third pharyngeal
    three-loop ileal
    two-loop J-shaped ileal
    two-piece ostomy
    UCLA

pouch *(cont.)*
 ultimobranchial
 United Bongort Lifestyle
 United Max-E
 United Surgical Bongort Lifestyle
 United Surgical Featherlite
  ileostomy
 United Surgical Shear Plus
 United Surgical Soft & Secure
 uterovesical
 vertical stapled small gastric
 vesicoureterine
 VPI nonadhesive
 water-filled
 Willis
 W-shaped
 Zenker
pouched ilcostomy
pouchitis
pouchlike
pouch of Douglas
pouchography, evacuation
Poupart ligament shelving edge
povidone-iodine impregnated drape
powder (see also *enteral nutrition;*
  feeding; medications)
 absorbable dusting
 Accuprep HPF
 Amin-Aid
 Domeboro
 Helicosol lyophilized
 Hepatic-Aid
 hyCURE protein
 hydrophilic
 karaya
 Lonalac
 Multidex hydrophilic
 Precision Isotein HN
 Precision Isotonic
 Precision LR
 Seidlitz
 Sween Micro Guard
 Travasorb HN
 Vivonex elemental
 Vivonex HN

powdered bone graft
powder-free Latex exam gloves
PowerCut drill blade
PowerCut gold surgical system
PowerCut pneumatic power system
power-driven reamer
power-driven saw
power driver
power-drive staple
PowerGrip pliers
PowerGrip stent delivery system
PowerLink endoluminal graft
power magnification
power-mode color Doppler imaging
power oscillating saw
PowerPro
power rasp
power reamer
PowerSculpt cosmetic surgery system
power setting (for laser)
PowerVision ultrasound system
PPAF (progressive perivenular
  alcoholic fibrosis)
PP (pancreatic polypeptide) cell
PP-CAP IgA enzyme immunoassay
PPI treatment
PPMA (polymethylmethacrylate-
  copolymer) beads
PPoma
PPP (pituitary, pancreas, parathyroid
  tumors)
PPPD (pylorus-preserving pancreato-
  duodenectomy)
Prader-Willi syndrome
pramlintide acetate
Pramoxine HC (hydrocortisone acetate;
  pramoxine)
Prandase (acarbose)
Prandin (repaglinide)
Pratt bivalve retractor
Pratt crypt hook
Pratt proctoscope
Pratt rectal forceps
Pratt rectal hook
Pratt rectal probe

Pratt rectal scissors
Pratt rectal speculum
Pratt scissors
Pratt speculum
Pratt tumor forceps
prayer position
praziquantel
prazosin
PRBC transfusion
preampullary portion of bile duct
Pre-Attain
pre-bent nail
prebiopsy mammogram
precancerous lesion
PreCare Conceive nutritional
    supplement
Precedex (dexmedetomidine)
precipitating factor
precirrhosis
Precision Dynamics Corp.
Precision High Nitrogen
Precision HN (high nitrogen) powdered
    feeding
Precision Isotein HN powdered feeding
Precision Isotonic powdered feeding
Precision LR powdered feeding
precision-point conventional cutting
precision-point reverse cutting
Precision QID blood glucose monitor
Precision Therapy
precore-core promoter mutant infection
Precose (acarbose)
precursor lesion
precurved ball-tipped guide pin
precut foam bandage
Precut intermediate Hi-Lo tracheal
    tube with stylet
precut sphincterotome
precut sphincterotomy
prediabetes (diet-controlled gestational
    diabetes)
predigested protein formula
predisposing factor
prednisolone enema

prednisone
pre-eclampsia
pre-esophageal dysphagia
preexisting condition
preexisting infection
Prefil nebulizer
preformed prosthetic mesh
Pregestimil (enzymatically hydrolyzed
    protein formula)
pregnancy, ectopic
prehepatic
prehyoid gland
preicteric phase
preileal appendix
preinvasive carcinoma
preinvasive lesion
preliminary diagnosis
preliminary film
preliminary view
preload
premalignant colonic polyp
premalignant neoplasm
premalignant skin lesion
premalignant state
Premarin (conjugated estrogens)
prematurely closed suture
premenstrual edema
Premidex-Aldehyde
Premier Platinum HpSA test
Premilene suture
Premium Americot sponge
Premium Barrier for ostomy skin
Premium CEEA circular stapler
Premium dissecting knife
Premium Plus CEEA disposable stapler
premium-point reverse cutting suture
premium-point spatula suture
prenatal diagnosis
prenatal genetic diagnosis
preneoplastic intraductal lesion
preoperative antibiotic
preoperative assessment
preoperative chemotherapy
preoperative diagnosis

preoperative endoscopic biliary stenting
preoperative endoscopic drainage
preoperative esophageal manometry
preoperative localization
preoperative placement of needle
 localization wire
preoperative placement of radiologic
 marker
preoperative plasmapheresis
preoperative view
prep (bowel prep) (see *bowel prep;
 enema*)
prepapillary bile duct
Preparation H anorectal cream
Preparation H cleansing tissues
Preparation H Cooling Gel
Preparation H rectal suppositories
preparation, islet cell
prepared and draped in a sterile fashion
Prepcat (barium sulfate)
preperitoneal approach
preperitoneal compartment
preperitoneal distention balloon (PDB)
preperitoneal fat
preperitoneal fat on the cord structures
preperitoneal hernioplasty
preperitoneal patch and plug hernia
 repair technique
preperitoneal prosthetic mesh repair
 of hernia via laparoscopy
preperitoneal space
preplaced suture
Prep Mitt surgical adhesive mitt
Prepodyne solution
prepped and draped in a sterile fashion
prepped and draped in the usual sterile
 manner
prepyloric antrum
prepyloric atresia
prepyloric gastric ulcer
prepyloric sphincter
prepyloric ulcer
prereduction view
prerenal FENa

presacral anesthesia
presacral drainage
presacral edema
presacral rectopexy
presacral space
presacral tumor
presbyesophagus
Presbyterian Hospital staphylorrhaphy
 elevator
Presbyterian Hospital tubing clamp
Presbyterian tube-occluding clamp
presence of bile
preservation of vagal innervation
preserved dural homograft
presinusoidal intrahepatic portal hyper-
 tension
pressor support
pressure
 anal sphincter squeeze
 atmospheres of
 backup of portal
 bile duct
 biliary-duodenal
 blood
 central venous (CVP)
 choledochal basal
 continuous positive airway (CPAP)
 decreased blood
 diastolic blood
 direct
 duodenobiliary
 elevated portal
 end-expiratory
 esophageal peristaltic
 free hepatic venous
 gastric
 gastrosphincteric
 hepatic venous
 hepatic wedge
 increased gastric
 increased intra-abdominal
 increased intracranial
 increased intraluminal
 increased portal

pressure *(cont.)*
   indirect hepatic vein wedge
   intra-abdominal
   intra-anal
   intracranial
   intraductal
   intraesophageal peristaltic
   intragastric
   intraluminal esophageal
   Koala intrauterine
   left ventricular end diastolic
     (LVEDP)
   LES (lower esophageal sphincter)
   lower esophageal sphincter
   low urethral (LUP)
   maximum anal resting (MARP)
   mean arterial (MAP)
   mean end-expiratory
   needle
   negative inspiratory
   negative pleural space
   orthostatic blood
   osmotic
   passage
   peak
   portal
   portal venous (PVP)
   positive end-expiratory (PEEP)
   positive peritoneal space
   pulmonary artery (PA)
   pulmonary capillary wedge (PCWP)
   resting anal sphincter
   sinusoidal
   splanchnic
   squeeze
   systemic
   systolic blood
   UOS tonic
   wedged hepatic venous (WHVP)
pressure anesthesia
pressure dressing
pressure gauge
pressure inversion point (PIP)
pressure measurement of sphincter
  of Oddi

pressure necrosis
pressure needle
pressure-sensitive valve in shunt tube
pressure sore
pressure support (ventilatory)
pressure symptoms
Pressure Ulcer Scale for Healing
   (PUSH) tool
pressurized pulsatile irrigation system
Prestige Smart System (PSS) glucose
   monitor
prestomal ileitis
Preston ligamentum flavum forceps
presumptive diagnosis
preternatural anus
pretibial edema
pretibial myxedema
pretransplant crossmatch
PRE 2 suture
Prevacid (lansoprazole)
Prevacid triple therapy
Prevail gel
Prevalite (cholestyramine resin)
Prevatac (exisulind)
Prevenzyme
prevertebral fascia
Prevpac (lansoprazole; clarithromycin;
   amoxicillin)
PreVue *B. burgdorferi* antibody
   detection assay
prezatide copper acetate
Pribham suction tube
Price muscle biopsy clamp
Price-Thomas bronchial forceps
prickle cell carcinoma
priliximab
Prilosec (omeprazole)
Prima laser
Primaderm semipermeable foam
   dressing
Primapore absorptive wound dressing
primary adrenocortical insufficiency
primary anastomosis
primary benign liver tumor

primary bile duct cancer
primary biliary cirrhosis (PBC)
primary carcinoma
primary (preoperative) chemotherapy
primary closure
primary contraction
primary diffuse malignant peritoneal
 mesothelioma
primary direct linear closure
primary esophageal motility
primary GI tract lymphoma
primary hepatic carcinoma
primary hyperaldosteronism
primary hyperparathyroidism
primary hypersplenism
primary ileal villous atrophy (PIVA)
primary intestinal lymphangiectasia
primary intraosseous carcinoma
primary lesion
primary liver cancer
primary malignancy
primary peristaltic wave
primary peritonitis
primary pituitary pathology
primary reanastomosis
primary sclerosing cholangitis (PSC)
primary suture
primary thyroid hyperplasia
primary thyroid malignancy
primary tumor
Primer compression dressing or wrap
principal diagnosis
Pringle maneuver for clamping
 the hepatic pedicle
Pritchard lipiodol syringe
Pritchard Mark II pin
Pritchard syringe
p.r.n. (L. *pro re nata*, as needed)
p.r.n. antacid
PRN bandage
Pro-Banthine (propantheline bromide)
probe
 Acculite Contour Tip
 AccuProbe 600 cryotherapy probe

probe *(cont.)*
 Acufex
 angled
 Arthrocare Wand
 arthroscopic
 Barr D/E fistula
 Barr fistula
 Beckman 39042 pH
 BiCAP electrocoagulation
 BiLAP bipolar cutting and
  coagulating
 biliary balloon
 biplane sector
 bipolar
 bipolar cautery (BiCAP)
 blunt
 Bowman
 broach
 Brodie
 Buie rectal
 Bunnell dissecting
 Bunnell forwarding
 buttonhole
 Cameron-Miller monopolar
 Circon-ACMI electrohydraulic
  lithotriptor
 continuously perfused
 core
 Core suction/irrigation
 Dandy
 Desjardins gallstone
 dissecting
 double ended
 Earle rectal
 8-channel cross-sectional anal
  sphincter
 electrohydraulic
 electromagnetic focusing field (EFF)
 endoesophageal
 Endo-Flo
 endoscopic BiCAP
 endoscopic heat
 Endotrac
 esophageal temperature

probe *(cont.)*
  Fenger gallbladder
  Fisch rectal
  fistula
  Fluhrer rectal
  Fogarty biliary
  forwarding
  Frigitronics
  gallstone
  galvanic
  heater
  hemispherical contact
  high-frequency
  high-frequency miniprobe
  Hydromer coated bipolar
    coagulation
  Hydro-Temp
  intraosseous
  Jacobson
  Jacobson micro
  Jannetta
  J-hook ElectroProbe
  Jobson Horne
  Klear-Temp
  lacrimal duct
  laparoscopic Doppler
  Larry rectal
  laser
  laser Doppler
  Laserflo Doppler
  LDF (laser-Doppler flowmetry)
  malleable
  Maloney endo-otoprobe
  Mammotome
  Mayo common duct
  Mayo gall duct
  McCain TMJ
  Medi-Tech bipolar
  Medrad Mrinnervu (also
    MRinnervu) endorectal colon
  micro
  microballoon
  Microelectrode MI-506 small-
    caliber

probe *(cont.)*
  Mitek Vapor
  Mixter dilating
  Modulap
  Moynihan bile duct
  Moynihan gallstone
  multilumen
  needle electroprobe
  neo-therm
  Neurotrend
  Nucleotome aspiration
  Nucleotome Flex II cutting
  Ochsner flexible spiral gallstone
  Ochsner gall duct
  OCT surgical imaging
  Olympus heat
  Olympus RU-12M-R1 rectal
  Olympus RU-75M-R1 rectal
  Olympus UM-1W endoscopic
  Oratec electrocautery
  PathVysion HER-2 DNA probe kit
  pedicle
  pH
  polarographic $P(ti)O_2$ catheter
  Pratt rectal
  radiofrequency
  Radiometer GK2803C pH
  Sandhill P32 pH antimony
  silver
  simple suction
  skin temperature monitoring
  SmokEvac electrosurgical
  spatula electroprobe
  spear-ended
  Steffee
  StrykeFlow electrocautery
  suction irrigation
  Surgical Dynamics aspiration
  Surgiflex
  tactile
  telomere-specific
  TEMPprobe
  thermal
  tulip

probe *(cont.)*
  24-hour pH
  ultrasonic
  Valleix
  Vanguard splinter
  Verbatim balloon
  water
  Watson-Cheyne
  wire-guided
  Wound Stick
  Yankauer
probe dilator
probe for aspiration and lavage (PAL)
probes/grooved director
probe with eye
probiotic agent
procaine HCl
Pro-Cal Sof (docusate sodium)
procedure (see *operation* for a quick-
  reference list of diagnostic,
  operative, and therapeutic
  procedures)
Proceed hemostatic surgical sealant
process (pl. processes)
  altered thought
  autoimmune
  AuTolo Cure Process
  chronic inflammatory
  energy-producing respiratory
  finger-like epithelial
  inflammatory
  metabolic
  Tutoplast
  uncinate
prochlorperazine
procidentia
  anal
  internal
  rectal
procidentia recti
Pro-Clude dressing
Pro-Clude transparent film wound
  dressing
procoagulants (PCA)

ProCross Rely over-the-wire balloon
  catheter
proctalgia fugax
proctectomy
  abdominoperineal
  intersphincteric
  Kraske transsacral
  laparoscopic
  mucosal
  partial
  perineal
  permanent
  radical
  restorative
  sphincter-preserving
  subtotal
  total
Procter-Livingstone endoprosthesis
proctitis
  acute
  diversion
  factitial
  gonorrheal
  nonspecific ulcerative
  radiation
  ulcerative
proctocolectomy
  laparoscopic total
  pan-
  primary
  restorative
  secondary stage
  single-stage total
  total
proctocolitis
  idiopathic
  radiation
  venereal
Proctocort (hydrocortisone)
ProctoCream-HC (hydrocortisone
  acetate)
Procto-Esthesia
ProctoFoam NS (pramoxine HCl)
proctogenous constipation

proctogram, proctography
  balloon
  evacuation
proctopexy, Orr-Loygue transabdominal
proctoplasty
proctorectoscopy
Proctor-Livingston tube
proctoscope (also *anoscope, endoscope, rectoscope, speculum*)
  ACMI
  Alan-Parks rectal speculum
  Arakawa
  Bensaude
  Blond
  Brinkerhoff
  disposable
  Enproct disposable
  Fansler
  Fansler-Ives anoscope
  front lifting hood rectoscope
  Gabriel
  Galencia disposable
  Heine
  Hirschman
  Jasan rigid
  Ives
  Ives-Fansler
  Karl Storz
  Kelly straight
  Kelly tapered
  KleenSpec disposable
  Medix
  Naunton Morgan
  Newman anoscope
  Pratt
  Ricord rectal speculum
  Romanoscope
  Roschke rectal speculum
  Sani-Scope
  Sapimed
  Sawyer rectal speculum
  Sklar
  slotted
  St. Mark's

proctoscope *(cont.)*
  Storz
  Strauss rectoscope
  Tuttle
  UniSpec disposable
  videorectoscope
  Welch anoscope
proctoscope and obturator
proctoscopy
proctosigmoiditis
proctosigmoidoscope
proctosigmoidoscopy
proctotomy
ProCyte transparent adhesive film dressing
Proderm Topical (castor oil; Peruvian balsam)
prodromal symptoms
prodrome
production
  catecholamine
  decreased pituitary
  digestion
  ectopic hormone
  endogenous inflammatory mediator
  exocrine
  excessive cortisol
  gastric acid
  gastrin-induced excessive gastric acid
  glucocorticoid
  increased gastric acid and pepsin
  metabolic energy
  pepsin
  suboptimal thyroid hormone
products of digestion
PROEF (postoperative regimen for oral early feeding)
proemial breast
Profiber enteral nutritional formula
profile
  adverse event
  ASTRA
  Contour Profile

profile *(cont.)*
  gut-hormone
  lipid
  liver function
  ultra-low
Pro-Flo XT catheter
Profore four-layer bandaging system
profound catabolic response
profound dehydration
profound malnutrition
profuse bleeding
profuse vomiting
progastrin
progeria
progestational pattern
progesterone-associated colitis
progesterone receptor (PgR)
progesterone-receptor analysis
progesterone-receptor-negative tumor
progesterone-receptor-positive tumor
progesterone-receptor status
prognosis
prognostic indicator
prognostic marker
Prognostic Nutritional Index (PNI)
prognostic value
Prograf (tacrolimus)
program, "Be In Charge" hepatitis
programmed cell death (apoptosis)
progressive abdominal distention
progressive ascites
progressive coagulopathy
progressive decline in mental status
progressive decompensation
progressive diet
progressive distention
progressive dysphagia
progressive emphysematous necrosis
progressive familial cirrhosis
progressive hypoxemia
progressively larger reamer
progressive obstruction
progressive perivenular alcoholic
  fibrosis

progressive suppurative cholangitis
progressive thinning of stool
PRO infusion catheter
proinsulin level
projectile vomiting
prokinetic agent
prokinetic drugs
prolactin deficiency
prolactin level
prolapse
  anal
  anorectal mucosal
  bladder
  hemorrhoidal
  intestinal
  massive genital
  rectal
  stomal
  uterine
  vaginal vault
prolapsed hemorrhoids
prolapsed stoma
prolapsed vaginal vault
prolapse gastropathy
prolapse with defecation
prolapsing internal hemorrhoids
ProLease drug delivery system
Prolene Hernia System (PHS) bilayer
  patch repair
Prolene mesh tape
Prolene polypropylene hernia mesh
Prolene polypropylene mesh
Prolene polypropylene suture
Prolene suture
Proleukin (aldesleukin)
proliferating cell nuclear antigen
  (PCNA)
proliferation
  bile duct
  cytotoxic lymphocytic
  ductal
  monoclonal B cell
  papillary
  vascular

proliferation of acini
proliferation signal inhibitor
proliferative hypertrophic gastritis
proliferative of undifferentiated cells
proliferative pattern
proliferative peritonitis
prolonged bleeding from wound
prolonged fasting
prolonged H_2-receptor blockade
prolonged ischemia
prolonged nausea or vomiting
prolonged pain
prolonged respiratory alkalosis
prolonged ventilatory support
prolonged vomiting
PROloop coagulator
PROloop electrosurgical device
promethazine HCl
Prometheus test
prominent thyroid nodule
promontory cartilage
promontory, sacral
Promycin (porfiromycin)
prone film
prone lateral view
prone position
prone view
pronounced leucocytosis
Pronova nonabsorbable suture
Pronova poly (hexafluoropropylene-
    VDF) suture
ProOsteon 500 bone graft substitute
ProOsteon 500 bone implant
propantheline bromide
Propel cannulated interference screw
properdin
properitoneal fat
properitoneal flank stripe (on x-ray)
properitoneal hernia
properitoneal space
prophylactic antibiotic
prophylactic cholecystectomy
prophylactic colectomy
prophylactic drain

prophylactic gastrojejunostomy
prophylactic intravenous antibiotic
prophylactic penicillin
prophylactic removal of uninvolved
    lymph node
prophylactic subcutaneous mastectomy
prophylactic thyroidectomy
prophylaxis
    antibiotic
    antimicrobial
    CMV
    long-term
Prophyllin (sodium propionate;
    chlorophyll derivatives)
Propimex-2
propiram
Proplast graft
propofol
propolis natural resin
Propper scalpel
propranolol
propylthiouracil (PTU)
Proscope
ProSobee liquid formula
ProSol 20% (amino acids) nutrition mix
Prosphyg sphygmomanometer
ProstaCoil self-expanding stent
prostaglandin E1 (PGE1)
prostaglandin E2 (PGE2)
Prostalase laser
Prostar percutaneous closure device
Prostar Plus percutaneous closure
    device
Prostar XL percutaneous closure
    device
ProstaScint (CYT-356 radiolabeled with
    [111]In) imaging agent
prostate
    adenocarcinoma of
    apex of
    ballotable
    high-riding
    inferolateral surfaces of
    lateral lobe of

prostate *(cont.)*
   lymph vessel of
   median lobe of
   posterior surface of
prostate cancer
prostate chip
prostatectomy
   laser
   Madigan
   perineal
   radical
   retropubic
   retropubic prevesical
   suprapubic prevesical
   transurethral
   transurethral balloon
   TULIP (transurethral laser-induced)
prostate enlargement
prostate gland
prostate-specific antigen (PSA)
prostatic abscess
prostatic acid phosphatase (PAP)
prostatic adenocarcinoma
prostatic calculus (pl. calculi)
prostatic capsule
prostatic carcinoma
prostatic concretion
prostatic cyst
prostatic duct
prostatic fluid
prostatic hyperplasia
prostatic malignancy
prostatic shaving
prostatic sinus
prostatic urethra
prostatic venous plexus
prostatitis
   acute
   acute bacterial
   allergic
   chronic
   chronic bacterial prostatitis (CBP)
   eosinophilic
   nonspecific granulomatous

prosthesis (see also *breast implant;*
     endoprosthesis; implant)
   Acticon neosphincter implantable
   Amoena breast
   Angelchik antireflux ring
   antireflux
   asymmetrical breast
   Becker breast
   Becker tissue expander/breast
   Belle-Amie breast
   bilioduodenal
   bladder neck support
   breast
   Charnley femoral
   CUI gel breast
   CUI saline breast
   delayed insertion of breast
   Discrene breast
   Dow Corning Silastic breast
   Dumon-Gilliard
   endoscopic
   endoscopic biliary endoprosthesis
   esophageal
   Gianturco expandable (self-expand-
     ing) metallic biliary
   GunSlinger shoulder orthosis
   Hartley breast
   HD II (or 2) total hip prosthesis
   Hemobahn endovascular
   iridium
   large-bore bile duct
   Leading Lady breast
   McGhan saline-filled
   Moore
   Nearly Me breast
   Perras breast
   Perras-Papillon breast
   pin-retained palatal
   Restore orthobiologic soft tissue
     implant
   silicone donut
   Spenco breast
   stent
   subpectoral breast

protocol
  chemotherapy
  Edmonton fresh islet
  Gerson therapy protocol
  Haemonetics red blood cell
    collection
  immunomodulatory
  immunosuppressive
  Nigro
  treatment
protocolectomy
Protocult stool sampling device
proton-density image
proton efflux rate
Protonix (pantoprazole)
proton magnetic resonance
  spectroscopy
proton permeability
proton pump inhibitor (PPI)
protopathic pain
protoporphyria, erythrohepatic
Protostat (metronidazole)
protozoal infection of bowel
Protractor retractor and wound
  protector
protruded gastric carcinoma
protruding fat
protrusion of mucosa
protuberant abdomen
proud graft
proudflesh
Providence Hospital artery forceps
Providencia alcalifaciens
Providencia rettgeri
Provir (sirirumab)
Provis cannula
provisional anatomic diagnosis
provocative test
proximal bile duct obstruction
proximal bow position
proximal clot
proximal diverting ostomy
proximal duct excision
proximal end of colon

proximal esophageal lumen
proximal esophagus
proximal gastrectomy
proximal gastric vagotomy (PGV)
proximal jejunum
proximal part of dorsal pancreatic duct
proximal saline injection
proximal splenorenal shunt
proximal to the ligament of Trietz
Proximate flexible linear stapler
Proximate ILS curved intraluminal
  stapler
Proximate linear cutter
Proximate skin staple
PRS (Photon Radiosurgery System)
PRT (physiologic reflux test)
Pruitt-Inahara shunt
Prulet (white phenolphthalein)
prune-belly abdomen
prune-belly syndrome
prune juice peritoneal fluid
pruning sign
pruritic urticarial papule
pruritus
pruritus ani
Prussak pouch
PSA 4000 anesthesia monitoring system
psammoma body
PSC (primary sclerosing cholangitis)
PSE (portal-systemic encephalopathy)
Pseudallescheria boydii
pseudoaneurysm
pseudobacillus
pseudobacterium
pseudocapsule of tumor
pseudochylous ascites
pseudocirrhosis, cholangiodysplastic
pseudocyst
  adrenal
  communicating
  pancreatic
  pararenal
  pulmonary
pseudocyst gastrostomy, pancreatic

pseudocyst of pancreas
pseudodiverticulum
pseudoductular transformation of
    hepatocyte
pseudohermaphroditism
pseudohyperparathyroidism
pseudohypoparathyroidism
pseudolymphoma, gastric
pseudomelanosis
pseudomembranous colitis (PMC)
pseudomembranous enterocolitis
pseudomembranous gastritis
pseudomembranous inflammation
pseudomembranous radiation gastritis
Pseudomonas-like bacteria
pseudomucinous cystadenocarcinoma
pseudomyxoma peritonei
pseudo-obstruction
    bowel
    chronic idiopathic intestinal (CIIP)
    chronic intestinal (CIP)
    colonic
    familial intestinal
    idiopathic intestinal
    intestinal
    nonfamilial intestinal
    Ogilvie
pseudo-obstructive syndrome
pseudopalisade formation
pseudopalisading
pseudoparenchyma
pseudopolyp
pseudopolyposis
pseudoprecocious puberty
pseudopseudohypoparathyroidism
pseudopyogenic granuloma
pseudorabies virus
pseudosac
pseudosacculation
pseudosarcoma
pseudostone
pseudoxanthoma elasticum
PSFR (peak secretory flow rate) test

p.s.i. or psi (pronounced "sigh")
    (pounds per square inch)
PSI-TEC aspirator
PSI-TEC system
PSI-TEC tubing
psoas abscess
psoas fascia
psoas gap
psoas hitch
psoas inflammation
psoas major muscle
psoas margin
psoas muscle
psoas muscle abscess
psoas shadow
psoas sign
psorelcosis
psorenteritis
PSS (Prestige Smart System) glucose
    monitor
PSS (progressive systemic sclerosis)
PST staging
psychogenic colic
psychogenic colitis
psychogenic vomiting
Psychosocial Adjustment to Illness
    Scale (PAIS)
psyllium hydrophilic mucilloid
PT (prothrombin time)
PTBD (percutaneous transhepatic
    biliary drainage) catheter
PTC (percutaneous transhepatic
    cholangiography)
PTCS tube
PTD (percutaneous transhepatic
    drainage)
p10 protein
pterygoid plate
PTFE (polytetrafluoroethylene) graft
PTH (parathyroid hormone) test
PTH assay
p30 protein
PTHrp (parathyroid-hormone-related
    protein)

PTLD (post-transplantation lympho-
    proliferative disorder)
ptosis, mammary
ptosis of breasts
ptosis of testicle
ptotic breasts
PT (prothrombin time)
PTT (partial thromboplastin time)
ptyocrinous cell
pubic hair line
pubic symphysis
pubic tubercle
pubocervical ligament`
pubococcygeal line
pubococcygeus muscle
puborectalis loop
puborectalis sling
PUD (peptic ulcer disease)
puddle sign
puddling on barium enema
Puddu view
pudendal anesthesia
pudendal artery
pudendal hernia
pudendal nerve terminal motor latency
    (PNTML) test
Pudenz peritoneal catheter
Pudenz shunt
puerperal breast abscess
puerperal peritonitis
puerperal sepsis
puerperium
Puestow-Gillesby operation
Puestow pancreaticojejunostomy
Pugh-Child grading system for bleeding
    esophageal varices
Pugh classification of Child liver
    criteria
Pugh sliding nail
Puka chisel
pullout suture
pullout wire suture
pull-through procedure
    abdominal
    continuous

pull-through procedure *(cont.)*
    Duhamel laparoscopic
    endorectal
    endorectal ileal
    ileal
    ileoanal
    rapid (RPT)
    sacroabdominoperineal
    Soave endorectal
    station (SPT)
    Swenson abdominal
Pull-thru Network
pulmonary autograft (PA)
pulmonary cirrhosis
pulmonary congestion
pulmonary consolidation
pulmonary edema
pulmonary embolism
pulmonary embolus
pulmonary emphysema
pulmonary function
pulmonary gas exchange
pulmonary gases
pulmonary hypertension
pulmonary infarct
pulmonary infection
pulmonary orifice
pulmonary pseudocyst
pulmonary segment
pulmonary stenosis
pulmonary tissue–blood barrier
pulmonary venous blood
pulpar cell
pulpiform nucleus forceps
pulp polyp
pulp, splenic
Pulsalith lithotriptor
Pulsar CO_2 laser system
pulsatile abdominal mass
pulsatile mass in the neck
pulsation balloon
Pulsavac III wound debridement system
pulse (pl. pulses)
    abdominal
    brachial

punch *(cont.)*
    Hartmann tonsil
    Hirsch hypophyseal
    Hunstad
    Inner Dyne single-action single-tooth biopsy
    Inner Dyne spoon biopsy
    intervertebral disk
    Kerrison
    Keyes cutaneous
    Keyes dermal
    laminectomy
    Miltex
    Raney laminectomy
    Rhoton sellar
    rotary basket
    Rowe glenoid
    Sauerbruch-Frey bone
    Schlesinger
    Schmeden tonsil
    sellar
    skull
    suture
    tibial
    tubular
    window
    Yankauer
punch biopsy
punch-drunk syndrome of boxers
punched-out ulcer
punch forceps
punctate area
punctate hemorrhage
punctate keratotic lesion
punctate ulcer
Punctur-Guard needle
puncture aspiration of cyst of breast
puncture incision
puncture site for laparoscopy
puncture wound
pupil, blown
pure respiratory acidosis
pure respiratory alkalosis
pure tissue hernia repair

purgative
Purge (castor oil)
purging, self-induced
Puri-Clens wound cleanser
purified factor VIII concentrations
Puritan oxyadaptor
purple striae
purpura
    adult chronic immune thrombo-cytopenic
    Henoch-Schönlein
    hyperglobulinemic
    idiopathic thrombocytopenic (ITP)
    thrombotic thrombocytopenic (TTP)
purpuric bleeding
purpuric lesion
pursestring ligature
pursestring or purse-string suture
pursestringed (verb)
pursestring ligature
Purstring device
Pursuer CBD (common bile duct) basket
Pursuer CBD Helical or Mini-Helical stone basket
Purtilo syndrome
purulent debris
purulent discharge
purulent lesion
purulent material
purulent pancreatitis
pus-forming bacteria
push enteroscope
push enteroscopy
pusher (small dissecting sponge)
pusher catheter
pusher tube
push-pull ankle stress view
push-pull hip view
PUSH (Pressure Ulcer Scale for Healing) tool
pus, frank
pus smear
pus under pressure

Putti bone rasp
Putti bone raspatory
putty kidney
PVH (persistent viral hepatitis)
PVH-B (persistent viral hepatitis,
    type B)
PVH-NAB (persistent viral hepatitis,
    non-A, non-B)
PVP (portal venous pressure)
PVP-I Solution Skin Prep Trays
PVR (pulmonary vascular resistance)
PVS (peritoneovenous shunt)
PWB (Puno-Winter-Byrd) rod
pyeloileocutaneous anastomosis
pyelonephritic kidney
pyemia, portal
pylephlebitis
pylethrombophlebitis
pylon attachment plate
pylorectomy
    Billroth
    Kocher
Pylori-Check test kit (also, Pylori-
    Chek)
pyloric antrum
pyloric antrum cardiacum
pyloric artery
pyloric canal
pyloric channel
pyloric channel obstruction
pyloric channel ulcer
pyloric exclusion with gastro-
    jejunostomy
pyloric gland
pyloric lymph node
pyloric mucosa
pyloric orifice
pyloric outlet obstruction
pyloric ring
pyloric sphincter
pyloric spreader
pyloric stenosis
pyloric stricture
pyloric string sign

Pylorid (ranitidine bismuth citrate)
PyloriProbe assay
Pyloriset
PyloriTek *Helicobacter pylori* test
pyloroduodenal junction
pyloroduodenal obstruction
pyloromyotomy
    circumumbilical
    extramucosal
    Fredet-Ramstedt
    Kocher
    laparoscopic
    Ramstedt-Fredet
    surface umbilical
    umbilical
pyloroplasty
    double
    Finney
    Heineke-Mikulicz
    Jaboulay
    laparoscopic
    Mikulicz
    Ramstedt
    reconstructive
    transhiatal
    vagotomy and
    Weinberg modification of
    Yu
pylorospasm
pylorostenosis
pylorotomy
pylorus (pl. pylori), hypertrophic
pylorus-preserving modification
pylorus-preserving pancreatoduo-
    denectomy (PPPD)
pylorus-preserving resection
pylorus-preserving Whipple procedure
pylorus-sparing Whipple procedure
Pynchon suction tube
pyoderma gangrenosum
pyogenic abscess
pyogenic bacteria
pyogenic cholangitis
pyogenic infection

pyogenic liver
pyogenic liver abscess
pyogenic organism
pyogenic thyroiditis
pyopneumocholecystitis
pyopneumohepatitis
pyopneumoperitoneum
pyopneumoperitonitis
pyopneumothorax, subphrenic
pyostomatitis vegetans
pyramid tip
pyramidal lobe
pyramidal tip trocar

pyramidal trocar
pyrantel pamoate
Pyridium
pyridostigmine
pyriform (see *piriform*)
pyrogen-free heparin
pyroglycolic acid suture
pyrosis (heartburn)
Pyrost graft
pyrrole metabolism
pyruvate kinase deficiency
PYtest (^{14}C urea)
PZI (protamine zinc insulin)

Q, q

QALY (quality-adjusted life-year)
QHS (quantitative hepatobiliary
  scintigraphy)
QLI (quality of life index)
QOL (quality of life)
QRS complex
Q-switched neodymium:YAG laser
Q-switched ruby laser
QT change
Quad-Lumen drain
quadrangular positioning plate
quadrant
  left lower (LLQ)
  left upper (LUQ)
  right lower (RLQ)
  right upper (RUQ)
quadrant of breast
  lower inner
  lower lateral
  lower medial
  lower outer
  upper inner
  upper lateral
  upper medial
  upper outer
quadrantectomy, axillary dissection, and
  radiotherapy (QUART) for breast
  cancer

quadrants, all four
quadrants of abdomen
  left lower
  left upper
  right lower
  right upper
quadrate lobe of liver
quadratus lumborum
quadrigeminal plate
Quadripolar cutting forceps
Quadripolar electrosurgical forceps
Quadripolarity
quadruple therapy (bismuth, ranitidine,
  amoxicillin, and metronidazole)
QualiCode test
quality-adjusted life-year (QALY)
quality of life (QOL)
quality of life index (QLI)
Quantison imaging agent
quantitative fecal fat test
quantitative hepatobiliary scintigraphy
  (QHS)
QUART (quadrantectomy, axillary
  dissection, and radiotherapy)
  for breast cancer
quartz rod and laser scalpel
Quarzan (clidinium bromide)
quasispecies distribution

queasiness
queasy
Quervain abdominal retractor
query
questionable calcifications
questionnaire, Rhodes Inventory
    of Nausea and Vomiting
Questran (cholestyramine)
Questran Light (cholestyramine resin)
Questus Leading Edge cutter
Questus Leading Edge grasper
Questus Leading Edge sheathed knife
Quick AC Enema Kit
Quick Bend flex clamp
QuickSilver hydrophilic-coated guide
    wire
Quick test
QuickVue one-step *H. pylori* test
QuickVue one-step influenza test

QuickVue UrinChek 10+ urine test
    strips
quiescent hepatitis
quiet bowel sounds
quiflapon sodium
Quilimmune-M vaccine
quilted suture
Quimby scissors
quinacrine HCl
Quincke edema
Quincke lumbar puncture needle
quinidine intoxication
Quinlan test
Quinton Mahurkar dual-lumen
    peritoneal catheter
Quinton suction biopsy instrument
Quinton tube
quotidian malaria

R, r

rabbit stools
rabeprazole sodium
rabies virus
Rabiner neurological hammer
Rabuteau test
raccoon eyes
race-track oval shaped polypropylene
mesh graft with pocket
Rachitome
Racobalamin-57 radioactive agent
racquet-shaped incision
RAD Airway laryngeal blade
radial groove
Radial Jaw single-use biopsy forceps
Radial Osteo Compression (ROC)
soft tissue anchor
radial scar
radial sclerosing lesion
radiating pain
radiation colitis
radiation enteritis
radiation esophagitis
radiation gastritis
radiation-induced colitis
radiation-induced ulceration
radiation, intestinal graft
radiation necrosis
radiation proctitis

radiation proctocolitis
radiation therapy
radical cholecystectomy
radical D2 gastrectomy
radical, free
radical mastectomy, including pectoral
muscles, axillary and internal
mammary lymph node (Urban
operation)
radical mediastinal dissection
radical neck dissection
radical surgery
radicle
biliary
intrahepatic
tertiary
radicular abscess
radioactive agent (see *imaging agent*)
radioactive-labeled marker
radioactive therapy
radiocholesterol analogue
radiocontrast agent
Radiofocus Glidewire
radiofrequency energy
radiofrequency probe
radiograph
radiographic imaging
radiographic procedure

radio-guided parathyroidectomy
radioimmunoassay (see *assay; test*)
radioimmunoluminography
radioiodine ablation
radioiodine-labeled metaiodobenzyl-
guanidine (MIBG)
radioiodine scan
radioiodine uptake
radioisotope (see *imaging agent;
medications*)
radioisotope bone scan
radioisotope scan
radioisotope scanning of the thyroid
radioisotope scintigraphy
radioisotope stent
radiolabeled peptide alpha-M2
radiolabeled RBC scan
radiologically proven arthritis
radiolucency
radiolucent filling defect
radiolucent gallstone
radiolucent stone
Radiometer GK2803C pH probe
radionuclide esophageal emptying time
radionuclide-labeled leukocytes
radionuclide-labeled platelets
radionuclide scan
radionuclide scanning
radionuclide uptake
radiopacity
radiopaque calculus
radiopaque contrast material
radiopaque density
radiopaque dye
radiopaque gallstone
radiopaque marker
radiopaque Ocrilon polyurethane
radiopaque stone
radiopaque suture
radiopaque Teflon biliary dilating
catheter
radiopharmaceutical
radioresistant tumor
radioscintigraphy

radiosensitizer
Broxine (broxuridine)
Neomark (broxuridine)
radiotherapy
adjuvant
extended-field (EFRT)
3-D conformal
radiotherapy-induced hypopituitarism
Radius coronary stent
Radius enteral feeding tube
radius of varices
Radolf forceps
RAE endotracheal tube
ragged red appearance
Ragnell-Davis retractor
Ragnell dissecting scissors
Ragnell handheld retractor
Ragnell retractor
railroad track pattern
railroad track scars
Raimondi hemostatic forceps
Raimondi peritoneal catheter
Raimondi scalp forceps
Raimondi spring catheter
Raimondi ventricular catheter
raised, slightly pigmented lesion
rake retractor
rake ulcer
Ralk hand drill
Ralks mallet
raltitrexed
Ramond point
ramoplanin
Rampley sponge-holding forceps
Ramsay tissue forceps
Ramstedt-Fredet pyloromyotomy
Ramstedt pyloroplasty
Randall stone forceps
Randall suction curette
randomized trial
random needle biopsy
random stool sample
Raney clamp
Raney clip

Raney clip-applying forceps
Raney coagulating forceps
Raney cranial drill
Raney hemostasis clip
Raney laminectomy punch
Raney laminectomy rongeur
Raney perforator drill
Raney rongeur forceps
Raney saw
Raney saw guide
Raney scalp clip-applying forceps
Ranfac cholangiographic catheter
Ranfac laparoscopic instruments
range, hepaptotoxic
ranitidine
Rankin clamp
Ranson criteria for acute pancreatitis
ranula
RAO (right anterior oblique) view
RAP (recurrent abdominal pain)
rapacuronium bromide
Rapamune (sirolimus)
rapamycin
raphe, anococcygeal
Rapicide disinfectant/sterilant
rapid-acting anesthetic
rapid emptying of dye
rapid enlargement
Rapide suture
Rapidgraft arterial vessel substitute graft
rapid premature sexual development
rapid pull-through (RPT) esophageal
    manometry technique
rapid relapse
rapid serum amylase test
rapid transit time
rapid uptake
rapid weight loss
RapiSeal patch
Raplon (rapacuronium bromide) anes-
    thesia
Rappaport classification of gastric
    lymphoma

rasp, raspatory
    Acufex
    Acufex convex
    Alexander
    Alexander-Farabeuf
    angled
    Aufricht glabellar
    Austin Moore
    Babcock
    Bacon
    Bardeleben
    Black
    Bristow
    Brown
    carbon-tungsten
    Charnley
    convex
    Coryllos
    costal
    Cottle-MacKenty
    DePuy
    diamond
    Doyen costal
    Doyen rib
    Endotrac
    Epstein bone
    Farabeuf bone
    Farabeuf-Collin
    Farabeuf-Lambotte
    Filtzer interbody
    Fisher
    Fomon
    Forman nasal
    Gallagher
    glabellar
    Good
    Herczel rib
    Hylin
    interbody
    intramedullary
    Israel
    Jansen
    Joseph nasal

rasp *(cont.)*
>Key
>Kirmission periosteal
>Kleinert-Kutz
>Koenig
>Lambotte
>Langenbeck
>Lewis periosteal
>Mallory-Head
>Maltz
>Mathieu
>McCabe-Farrior
>McCabe perforation
>McKenty
>micro
>Miller
>Nicola
>Nicoll
>Olivecrona
>Phemister
>Plenk-Matson
>power
>Putti bone
>rib
>Rubin
>Schneider
>Schneider-Sauerbruch
>Seawell
>Sedillot
>Semb rib
>sympathetic
>Thompson
>Yasargil micro
>Zoellner

rasp pin
ratchet on demand
Rathke pouch
Rathke pouch cyst
ratio
>amylase to creatinine clearance
>antigen-antibody
>basal maximal acid output
>>(BAO:MAO)

ratio *(cont.)*
>BCAA/AAA plasma
>effective thyroxine (ETR)
>Hybritech Tandem PSA (free PSA/
>>total PSA)
>insulin:glucose
>lactulose/rhamnose permeability
>>(L/R ratio)
>thyroid hormone-binding (THBR)
>thyroxine/TBG

Ratliff-Blake gallstone forceps
Ratliff-Mayo forceps
rat-tail appearance on pancreatogram
rat-tail sign
rat-tooth forceps
rat-tooth pickup
raw surface of liver bed
Ray-Cot sponge
rayon cotton ball
Raypaque sponge
Ray-Parsons-Sunday staphylorrhaphy
>elevator
Rayport dural dissector and knife
Rayport muscle biopsy clamp
Ray-Tec x-ray detectable sponge
Ray TFC device
Ray ventricular cannula
razor blade
RBC (red blood cell)
RBC casts
RBC smear
RCF (Ross carbohydrate-free) formula
RC Mini-Open lighted retractor
RCS (red color sign)
RCT (randomized controlled trials)
RDG (retrograde duodenogastroscopy)
RE (reflux esophagitis)
re-FRED the lens
Re-New forceps
Re-New laparoscopic scissors
Re-New laparoscopic surgical tip
Reabilan HN enteral nutritional therapy
reabsorbable suture

reabsorption of H_2O
reaction
   acute hypersensitivity
   antibody-mediated immune
     (type III)
   argentaffin
   cell-mediated immune
   delayed hypersensitivity
   glucose
   graft versus host
   hot-shot PCR (polymerase chain
     reaction)
   IgE-mediated immune (type I)
   intragraft PCR (polymerase chain
     reaction)
   insulin
   PCR (polymerase chain)
   reverse-transcriptase polymerase
     chain (RT-PCR)
   scar tissue
   Sgambati
   single and rapid polymerase chain
     reaction/restriction fragment
     length
   transfusion
reactive hypoglycemia
Read gouge
reagent strips
   Clinistix
   Diascan
   DiaScreen
   First Choice
   Glucofilm
   Glucometer Elite
   Glucometer Encore
   Glucostix
   One Touch
   Tes-Tape
Real coronary artery scissors
real-time electronic imager
real-time ultrasonography
reamer
   acetabular
   Anspach

reamer *(cont.)*
   Arthrex coring
   Aufranc
   Austin Moore
   ball
   barrel
   blunt tapered T-handled
   bone
   brace-type
   calcar
   Campbell
   cannulated Henderson
   chamfer
   Charnley
   Charnley deepening
   Charnley expanding
   Charnley taper
   Charnley trochanter
   Christmas tree
   congruous cup-shaped
   conical
   corrugated
   cup
   deepening
   DePuy
   expanding
   female
   femoral shaft
   fenestrated
   flexible medullary
   grater
   Gray
   grooving
   Hall Versipower
   handle-type
   Harris center-cutting acetabular
   hemispherical
   hollow mill
   Indiana
   Intracone intramedullary
   intramedullary
   Küntscher (Kuentscher) intra-
     medullary
   male

reamer *(cont.)*
 Marin
 medullary canal
 MicroAire
 Mira
 Moore bone
 multisized
 Norton ball
 Perthes
 power
 power-driven
 progressively larger
 Richards
 rigid
 Rotalink flexible-shaft
 Rush awl
 self-centering
 Smith-Petersen
 spherical
 spiral cortical
 spiral trochanteric
 square
 starting
 step-cut
 straight
 Swanson
 tapered
 tapered hand
 T-handled
 triangular bone
 trochanteric
 Wagner acetabular
reaming awl
reanastomosis
reapproximate
reapproximating
Rebar microcatheter
Rebetol (ribavirin)
Rebetron (ribavirin/interferon alfa-2b)
rebiopsy
rebleed
rebound hypocalcemia
rebound pain

rebound sign
rebound tenderness on palpation
rebreathing anesthesia
Recamier curette
recanalization
recanalization reducible mass
recently healed surgical incision
receptor, insulin
receptor protein
receptor status
recess
 azygoesophageal
 cecal
 duodenal
 duodenojejunal
 hepatorenal
 ileocecal
 inferior duodenal
 inferior omental
 intersigmoid
 paracolic
 paraduodenal
 retrocecal
 retroduodenal
 splenic
 splenorenal
 subphrenic
 superior azygoesophageal
 superior duodenal
 superior ileocecal
 superior omental
recipient hepatectomy
recipient, organ
recipient site
reciprocating saw
Reclomide (metoclopramide HCl)
recombinant human thyroid-stimulating
 hormone (rhTSH)
recombinant human thyroid-stimulating
 hormone, thyrotropin alfa
recombinant immunoblot assay (RIBA)
Recombivax HB (hepatitis B virus
 vaccine, recombinant)

reconstruction (see also *breast recon-
    struction; operation*)
    biliary
    breast
    free flap breast
    full-thickness
    Kiricuta breast
    lateral transverse thigh flap on breast
    Lewis-Tanner subtotal esophagec-
        tomy and
    Roux-en-Y esophagojejunostomy
    Rubens flap
    "saddle bags" breast
    transverse rectus abdominis myo-
        cutaneous flap
reconstruction nail
reconstruction plate
reconstructive mammoplasty
reconstructive pyloroplasty
recording, esophageal pressure
recovery, organ
Rectacort (hydrocortisone acetate)
Rectagene (live yeast cell derivative;
    shark liver oil)
rectal abscess
rectal akinesia
rectal alimentation
rectal ampulla
rectal-anal inhibitory reflex
rectal anesthesia
rectal artery
rectal balloon
rectal biopsy forceps
rectal biopsy punch
rectal bleeding
rectal cancer
rectal cellulitis
rectal contrast medium
rectal dilator
rectal distention
rectal endoscopic ultrasonography
    (REU)
rectal evacuatory disorder
rectal examination

rectal fissure
rectal fistula
rectal fold
    inferior transverse
    superior transverse
rectal granuloma
rectal incontinence
rectal inhibitory reflex
rectal instruments
rectal intussusception
rectal linitis plastica (RLP)
rectal manometry
rectal mucosa
rectal mucosectomy
rectal multiplane transducer
rectal muscle cuff
rectal neovagina
rectal nerve
rectal occlusion clamp
rectal plexus
rectal polyp
rectal pouch
rectal probe
rectal procidentia
rectal prolapse
rectal prolapse repair
rectal reflex
rectal shelf
rectal sleeve advancement
rectal snare
rectal speculum (see *speculum;
    proctoscope*)
rectal sphincter
rectal stenosis
rectal stricture
rectal stump
rectal submucosal mass
rectal submuscula fluctuance
rectal trauma
rectal tube
rectal valve
rectal varices
rectal vault
rectal vein

recurrent upper respiratory tract
   infection (RURTI)
recurrent volvulus
recurring acute pancreatitis
recurring hernia
recurring pain
red blood cell casts
red blood cells (RBCs), packed
red cell mass, increased
red cell membrane
red cell surface area
red color sign (RCS)
red light neon laser
red pulp of spleen
red Robinson catheter
red rubber catheter
red wale marking (RWM)
Reddick cystic duct cholangiogram
   catheter
Reddick grasper
Reddick Olsen forceps
Reddick-Saye screw
Reddick-Saye screw catheter
Reddick-Saye suture
Reddick-Saye suture grasper
reddish-brown tumor mass
reddish tumor
Redifurl TaperSeal IAB catheter
Redigrip pressure bandage
redness and inflammation
Redo intestinal clamp
Redon wound drainage needle
REDS (remote endoscopic digital
   spectroscopy)
reduced lactose diet
reduced liver transplant (RLT)
reduced-size liver transplant (RSLT)
reduce spontaneously
reduced transhepatic blood flow
reducer
   cannula
   Seal-Up II
   Versaport Plus

reducible hernia
Reducin (somatostatin)
reducing substances in stool
reducing substances test
reduction mammoplasty (see *mammo-*
   plasty)
reduction mastopexy (see *mastopexy*)
redundant hernia sac
redundant loop of bowel
redundant sac tissue
redundant sigmoid
redundant sigmoid loop
redundant tissue
Redux (dexfenfluramine)
reentry
Reese osteotomy guide
Reese's Pinworm (pyrantel pamoate)
Rees-Martel flap forceps
Rees scissors
reexploration
ReFacto (factor VIII SQ, recombinant)
referred epigastric discomfort
referred hip pain
referred pain
referred pain from CO_2 on the
   diaphragm
referred pain to the tip of the shoulder
referred periumbilical pain
referred right subscapular pain
reflectance spectroscopy
reflectant spectral photometer
reflected portion of Poupart ligament
reflecting edge of ligament
reflection
   costopleural
   hepatoduodenal
   hepatoduodenal-peritoneal
   hepatoduodenoperitoneal
   lateral pleural
   mediastinodiaphragmatic pleural
   peritoneal
   phrenofundal
   sternal pleural
   vertebral pleural

reflex (pl. reflexes)
  abdominal
  abdominocardiac
  absent gag
  accommodation
  acquired
  anal
  arc
  cardiac
  cremasteric
  crossed
  Cushing
  deep tendon (DTRs)
  deglutition
  emetic
  epigastric
  esophagoglottal closure
  esophagosalivary
  gag
  gastrocolic
  gastroileac
  gastroileal
  gastropancreatic
  ileogastric
  intestinointestinal
  open loop
  orienting
  perianal
  peristaltic
  peritoneointestinal
  pharyngeal swallow
  pharyngo-UES (upper esophageal
    sphincter) contractile
  pharyngoglottal adduction
  rectal
  rectal inhibitory
  rectal-anal inhibitory
  renointestinal
  Rogers
  somatointestinal
  vasovagal
Reflex ELC clip applier
ReFlex wand

reflux
  abdominojugular
  acid
  bile
  cholangiovenous
  duodenobiliary
  duodenogastric (DGR)
  duodenopancreatic
  endoscopy-negative
  esophageal
  free
  gastroesophageal (GER)
  hepatojugular (HJ)
  high-volume
  intrarenal
  long-term duodenobiliary
  nasopharyngeal
  nocturnal gastric
  pathologic
  postmyotomy
  silent
  vesicoureteral
reflux bile gastritis
reflux esophagitis (RE)
reflux gastritis
refluxant
refluxed gastric contents
reflux of gastric contents
refractile material
refractory ascites
refractory bile duct stone
refractory bleeding
refractory constipation
refractory gastroesophageal reflux
  disease
refractory hepatic hydrothorax
refractory hyperplasia
refractory pain
refractory pancreatic fistula
refractory to conservative treatment
refractory to medical management
refractory to medical therapy
refractory to medication
refrigeration anesthesia

Regan isoenzyme
Regen Biologics, Inc.
regenerating hepatic nodule
regeneration, liver
regenerative polyp
regimen
    antireflux
    chemotherapy
    diabetic
    empiric antibiotic
    medical
    postoperative
    Prevacid triple therapy
    treatment
region
    abdominal
    anal
    ankle
    axillary
    Beckwith-Wiedemann chromosome
    buccal
    calcaneal
    centrilobular
    choledochal
    colonic crypt
    cricopharyngeal
    deltoid
    epigastric
    femoral
    floor of inguinal
    frontal
    gastric pacemaker
    gluteal
    hypochondriac
    hypogastric
    hypopharyngeal
    inguinal
    long segment
    lumbar
    noncutaneous
    pacemaker
    para-aortic
    paraumbilical
    periampullary

region *(cont.)*
    perianal
    periumbilical
    retroperitoneal
    scapular
    subdiaphragmatic perirenal
    suprapubic
    umbilical
    urogenital
regional anesthesia
regional anesthetic
regional colitis
regional enteritis
regional enterocolitis
regional ileitis (Crohn disease)
regional ileocolitis
regional lymph node metastasis
regional lymphatic drainage
Regional Organ Procurement Agency
    (ROPA)
regional osteopenia in anorexia nervosa
regional spread of infection
regional thoracic lymphadenectomy
registry
        Autologous Bone Marrow Trans-
            plant Registry (ABMTR)
        bone marrow transplant
        International Islet Transplant
            Registry (ITR)
        International Pancreas Transplant
            Registry
        Laparoscopic Bowel Registry
        organ donor
        tumor
Reglan (metoclopramide HCl)
Regnault type B mastopexy
Regranex (becaplermin) gel
regression, sacral
Regulace (docusate sodium)
regular diet
Regular Iletin II (insulin)
Regular Iletin II U-500 (concentrated)
    (insulin)
Regular Purified Pork Insulin

regulatory peptide
Regulax SS (docusate sodium)
Reguloid (psyllium hydrophilic
    mucilloid)
regurgitant esophagitis
regurgitant fraction
regurgitation
    acid
    chronic
    nocturnal
    postural
Regutol
rehabilitation, nutritional
reherniation
Rehfuss test
Rehfuss tube
Rehne abdominal retractor
Rehne-Delorme plication
Rehydralyte (electrolyte solution)
Reichert fiberoptic sigmoidoscope
Reichert flexible sigmoidoscope
Reichert FPS-3 fiberoptic sigmoido-
    scope
Reichert MH-1 flexible sigmoidoscope
Reichert MS-1 flexible sigmoidoscope
Reichert-Mundinger biopsy needle
Reichert SC-48 flexible sigmoidoscope
Reichmann syndrome
Reich-Nechtow forceps
REI rigid laparoscope
Reimann syndrome
reimplantation of parathyroid glands
Reiner bone rongeur
Reiner plaster knife
Reiner rongeur
reinforced tracheal tube
reinforcing suture
Reinhoff clamp
reinsertion
reinsulate "U" style handle
reintubation
Reitman-Frankel test for SGOT
Reitman-Frankel test for SGPT

rejection
    cardiac transplant
    cellular xenograft
    chronic graft
    graft
    hyperacute
    irreversible
    kidney transplant
    organ
    transplant
rejection response
relaparotomy
relapsing appendicitis
relapsing febrile nodular nonsuppura-
    tive panniculitis
relapsing malaria
relapsing pancreatitis
relative
    first-degree
    second-degree
relative contraindications
relative molecular mass
relax the conjoint tendon
relaxation of pylorus
relaxation suture
relaxing incision
Release-NF catheter
release of ACTH
release of exocrine products
Reliance urinary control insert catheter
ReliaSeal skin barrier adhesive
Relia-Vac drain
ReliefBand NST
relief of symptoms
relieved with antacids
relieved with food
relieving incision
Remegel
Remicade (infliximab)
remifentanil
Remington Hobbs diathermy forceps
remission of pain
remittent malaria

remnant of the omphalomesenteric duct
remote access perfusion (RAP) cannula
catheter
remote endoscopic digital spectroscopy
(REDS)
remote pheochromocytoma
removal of ectopic tissue
removal of extrahepatic duct
removal of foreign body
removal of intact mammary implant
removal with clear margins
remove the appendix from abdomen
Renacidin Irrigation (bladder) solution
renal artery stenosis
renal calculus
renal cell carcinoma
renal dose dopamine
renal edema
renal failure of unknown cause
renal function parameters
renal impression
renal impression on liver
renal lithiasis
renal medulla
renal obstruction
renal papilla
renal parenchymal disease
renal pouch
renal stone
renal threshold for calcium
renal transplant patient
renal tubular acidosis
renal tubular necrosis
renal vasodilation
Rendu-Osler-Weber disease
renin-angiotensin system
renin serum level
Reno-M contrast medium
Reno-M-Dip
Renografin contrast medium
renointestinal reflex
renovascular hypertension
rent (a tear or rupture)
Renu enteral feeding

REO (respiratory enteric orphan) virus
reoperation
reovirus
repaglinide
repair (see *operation*)
repeat endoscopic sclerotherapy
repeat mammogram
repeat thoracentesis
Repel abdominal film
Repela surgical glove
Repel bioresorbable barrier film
Repel-CV abdominal film
reperfusion
reperfusion syndrome
reperitonealization
reperitonealize
repetitive nerve stimulation
replacement, pancreatic enzyme
replantation bandage
Replete enteral nutritional therapy
Replicare dressing
Replicare paste dressing
RepliCare hydrocolloid dressing
material
Repliderm collagen-based dressing
Repliderm wound dressing
Repliform graft
Replogle tube
reposable clip applier
reposable trumpet
Repose surgical system
repositionable
reprep
Res-Q-Vac hand-powered suction
rescue treatment
resectable
resected malignant breast tumor
resected segment
resected tissue
resection (see also *operation*)
abdominoperineal (APR)
anterior colon
band and
colosigmoid

resection *(cont.)*
    curative restorative
    distal
    distal pancreatic
    en bloc
    endometrial
    endoscopic mucosal (EMR)
    esophageal
    gastric
    Harmann
    hepatic
    ileal
    ileocolic
    interval (of redundant sigmoid)
    laparoscopic bowel
    liver
    localized
    Lortat-Jacob hepatic
    low anterior (LAR)
    lung
    lymph node
    Mason abdomino-transsphincteric
    Miles abdominoperineal
    mucosal sleeve
    nipple flap duct
    palliative
    Paul-Mikulicz
    percutaneous
    portal vein
    pylorus-preserving
    segmental colon
    sigmoid
    small bowel
    snare
    surgical
    transsphenoidal
    wedge
resection and colostomy
resection and primary anastomosis
    of bowel
resection knife
resection of involved segment
resection of lung tumor
resection of pancreatic tail

resection of pylorus
resection of tail of pancreas
resection with Roux-en-Y hepatico-
    jejunostomy
resective colostomy
resectoscope (see *endoscope*)
reservoir (see also *pouch*)
    Camey
    colonic
    continent ileal
    decreased gastric
    double-barrel
    double J-shaped
    fecal
    gastric
    ileal
    ileoanal
    ileoperistaltic
    intra-abdominal ileal
    J ileal
    J-shaped
    J-Vac suction
    Kock ileal
    lateral internal pelvic
    LeBag ileocolic urinary reservoir
    Mainz pouch urinary reservoir
    Parks ileal
    Parks ileoanal
    shunt
    S ileal
    sigmoid colon
    S-shaped
    W-stapled urinary
residual abscess
residual barium
residual calculous material
residual capacity
residual carcinoma
residual flaccid paralysis
residual locoregional differentiated
    thyroid cancer
residual postoperative hepatolithiasis
    and intrahepatic strictures
residual stone

residual stool
residual thrombus
residual tumor
resin, bile-salt binding
resistance to portal flow
Resol electrolyte solution
resolution, fluoroscopic
Resolut barrier
Resolut surgical mesh
resorbable pin
resorbable plate
resorbable rod
resorcinol-induced hypothyroidism
Resource enteral feeding
Resource Plus enteral nutritional
   therapy
respiratory acidosis
respiratory alkalosis
respiratory distress syndrome
respiratory embarrassment
respiratory-esophageal fistula
respiratory inversion point
respiratory obstruction
respiratory quotient
respiratory syncytial virus (RSV)
respiratory virus
response
   biochemical
   end-of-treatment
   end-organ
   fibroblastic tissue
   gag
   gastrocolonic
   inflammatory
   immune
   inflammatory
   postural
   profound catabolic
   rejection
   sustained
   vagal efferent tonic
   vasovagal
   virologic
Response electrophysiology catheter

rest
   bowel
   pancreatic
resting anal sphincter pressure
resting and residual lower esophageal
   sphincter pressures
resting calcaneal stance position
Reston foam wound dressing
Reston hydrocolloid dressing material
Restore (psyllium hydrophilic
   mucilloid)
Restore orthobiologic soft tissue
   implant
restrictive bandage
restrictive pulmonary disease
resuscitation, massive fluid
resuscitative measures
resuscitator
RET gene test for familial medullary
   thyroid carcinoma
RET proto-oncogene
retained antrum syndrome
retained barium
retained calculus
retained gallstone
retained gastric antrum following
   incomplete antrectomy
retained suture
retching
retching without emesis
retention
   barium
   chronic stool
   gastric (GR)
   stool
   suture
   water
retention cyst
retention enema
retention esophagitis
retention jaundice
retention meal
retention polyp
retention suture

rete pegs
Rethi incision
reticular network
reticulocyte
reticulocytosis
reticuloendothelial organ
  liver
  lymphatics
  spleen
reticuloendothelial system
reticulum cell sarcoma
reticulum, sarcoplasmic
retinal edema
retinal tumor
retinoblastoma hereditary human
  carcinoma
retinoids
retracted stoma
retraction of clot
retraction of nipples
retraction of skin of breast
retraction suture
retractor
  Adson-Anderson cerebellar
  Adson brain
  Adson cerebellar
  Adson hemilaminectomy
  Adson Zenker artery forceps
  Airlift balloon
  Alan-Parks rectal
  Allison lung
  Allport
  Alm self-retaining
  Alm wound
  amputation
  anal
  Anderson-Adson scalp
  angled
  Ankeney sternal
  appendiceal
  Army-Navy
  Aronson esophageal
  atrial
  Aufranc cobra

retractor *(cont.)*
  automatic skin
  baby Balfour
  baby Balfour abdominal
  baby Deaver
  baby Gelpi
  baby Harrington
  baby Mollison
  baby Roux
  Badgley laminectomy
  Bailey-Gibbon rib contractor
  Balfour abdominal
  Balfour self-retaining
  Ballantine hemilaminectomy
  Bankart shoulder
  Barr rectal
  Beardsley esophageal
  Beckman
  Beckman-Adson laminectomy
  Beckman-Eaton laminectomy
  Beckman thyroid
  Beckman-Weitlaner laminectomy
  B.E. Glass abdominal
  Bennett bone
  Bennett self-retaining
  Bennett tibia
  bent malleable
  bent-tine, forklike
  Berens esophageal
  Berkeley-Bonney self-retaining
    3-blade abdominal
  Billingham-Bookwalter
  Billroth
  blade
  Blount anvil
  Blount hip
  Blount knee
  Bodnar
  bone
  Bookwalter
  Boyes-Goodfellow
  brachial plexus root
  brain
  Breisky

retractor *(cont.)*
  Breisky-Navratil
  Brooke-Bookwalter retractor
  Buck-Gramcko
  Budde-Greenberg-Sugita
  Buie-Smith
  bunion
  Burford
  Burford-Finochietto
  Cairns
  Cairns ribbon
  Campbell nerve root
  Canny Ryall
  carotid
  Carroll-Bennett
  Carroll hand
  centrum
  cerebellar
  cervical disk
  Chandler knee
  Charnley
  Charnley horizontal
  Charnley initial incision
  Charnley knee
  Charnley pin
  Charnley retractor
  Charnley self-retaining
  Charnley vertical
  Cherry brain
  Cherry laminectomy
  Christie gallbladder
  Cloward blade
  Cloward brain
  Cloward cervical
  Cloward-Cushing vein
  Cloward dural
  Cloward-Hoen hemilaminectomy
  Cloward-Hoen laminectomy
  Cloward lumbar lamina
  Cloward nerve root
  Cloward skin
  Cloward small cervical
  Cloward tissue
  cobra

retractor *(cont.)*
  Collin abdominal
  Collis-Taylor
  cone
  cone laminectomy
  cone scalp
  Contour scalp
  Cooley atrial
  Cooley rib
  Coryllos
  Cottle
  Crawford aortic
  Crego
  Crile
  Crile thyroid
  Crotti-Kocher thyroid
  Crotti thyroid
  Cuda
  curved
  Cushing
  Czerny rectal
  David Baker bleph
  Davidson scapula
  Davis
  Davis brain
  Davis ribbon
  Deaver
  DeBakey-Cooley
  decompression
  Delaginiere abdominal
  Denis Browne abdominal
  Desmarres lid
  Doane knee
  Dohn-Carton brain
  Dott
  double-ended right-angle
  double-hook Lovejoy
  Downey hemilaminectomy
  Downing
  Doyen abdominal
  dural
  Durham
  D'Errico
  D'Errico-Adson

retractor *(cont.)*
    East-West
    Eccentric "Y"
    Echols
    Elite Farley
    endaural
    EndoRetract
    Endotrac
    Enker brain
    eXpose
    Fahey
    fan
    Farabeuf
    Farr spring-wire
    Farr wire
    fat pad
    Favaloro sternal
    Fine cross action
    finger
    Finochietto
    Fisch
    flexible
    FlexPosure endoscopic
    Foerster abdominal ring
    Foss bifid gallbladder
    Foss biliary duct
    Franz abdominal
    Frazier laminectomy
    Frazier lighted brain
    Friedman perineal
    Fritsch abdominal
    Fujita snake
    Fujita suction
    Fukushima
    gallows-type
    Garrett
    GasFree Omni-Lift
    Gazayerli endoscopic
    Gelpi
    Gelpi pediatric
    Gelpi perineal
    Gelpi self-retaining
    Genz-Arm pneumatic
    Gibson-Balfour abdominal

retractor *(cont.)*
    Gifford mastoid
    Gilvernet
    Glaser automatic laminectomy
    Goelet
    goiter
    Goligher
    Gosset appendectomy
    Goulet
    Grant gallbladder
    Green
    Greenberg Universal
    Green thyroid
    Haight-Finochietto rib
    hand
    handheld
    Hands Free
    Hardy spinal
    Harrington
    Harrington splanchnic
    Hartzler rib
    Haverfield-Scoville hemilaminec-
        tomy
    Haynes
    Hays hand
    Heaney
    Heaney hysterectomy
    heavy-duty two-tooth
    Hedblom rib
    Heiss soft tissue
    hemilaminectomy
    Henley carotid
    Henner T-model endaural
    Henning
    Hertzler rib
    Hibbs
    Hill rectal
    Hill-Ferguson rectal
    Himmelstein sternal
    Hoen
    Hohmann
    Holscher
    Holzheimer
    horizontal

retractor *(cont.)*
   House-Fisch dura
   humeral head
   humpback Weitlaner
   Hupp trachea
   Hurd tonsil dissector and pillar
   IMA (inferior mesenteric artery)
   Inge laminectomy
   initial incision
   insulated Foman ball
   Israel
   Jackson
   Jannetta posterior fossa
   Jansen
   Jansen-Wagner
   Jarit P.E.E.R.
   Joe's hoe
   Johns Hopkins gallbladder
   Johnson
   Joll thyroid
   Jordan-Bookwalter
   Kartush insulated
   Kasdan
   Kelly
   Kelly abdominal
   Kennerdell-Maroon orbital
   Kilner
   Kilner catspaw
   Kilner cheek
   Kilner insulated
   Kirklin atrial
   Kirschner abdominal
   Kleinert-Ragdell
   Klemme
   Knighton
   Kocher
   Koerte rake
   Kuz-Medics total knee
   Lahey thyroid
   Lahey tissue
   lamina
   laminectomy
   Landon
   Lange-Hohmann bone

retractor *(cont.)*
   Langenbeck
   Langenbeck-Kocher
   LaparoLift Airlift balloon
   laparoscopic
   laser ball
   lateral collateral ligament
   leaflet
   Leyla
   LIMAvator chest wall
   Little
   Lloyd Davies pelvic
   Lone Star
   Love
   Love nerve
   Lowman hand
   Luer
   Luer trachea
   Lukens trachea
   lumbar lamina
   Luongo
   Magrina-Bookwalter
   Maison
   Malcolm-Lynn C-RXF cervical
      retractor frame
   Malcolm-Rand
   Malis brain
   malleable
   malleable ribbon
   Marberger hilar
   Markham-Meyerding
   Mark II
   Mark II Chandler
   Martin nerve root
   Mason-Judd suprapubic
   mastoid
   Mathieu
   Mayo abdominal
   Mayo-Adams abdominal
   Mayo-Adams appendectomy
   Mayo-Collins
   Mediflex-Gazayerli
   meniscus
   metacarpal

retractor *(cont.)*
 Meyerding finger
 Meyerding laminectomy
 Meyerding self-retaining
 Micro-Retractor
 microretractor
 Middeldorpf
 Mikulicz abdominal
 Mikulicz fiberoptic
 Millan retropubic
 Miller-Senn
 mini Hohmann podiatric
 mini Metzenbaum
 mini Roux
 Miskimon
 Mollison
 Moon rectal
 Morris
 Murphy
 Murphy gallbladder
 Myers knee
 narrow blade
 narrow neck mini-Hohmann
 Navratil
 Nelson rib
 nerve root
 Nevyas drape
 Norfolk-Norwich
 North-South
 Oberhill laminectomy
 Ochsner ribbon
 Oettingen abdominal
 Oldberg brain
 Olivier
 Ollier rake
 Omni
 Omni-Lift
 Omni-Tract adjustable wishbone
 ophthalmic
 optical
 orbital
 O'Sullivan-O'Connor abdominal
 Paparella
 Parker

retractor *(cont.)*
 Parks anal
 Parks sphincterotomy
 Paulson knee
 pediatric ribbon
 pediatric Deaver
 Penfield
 Percy amputation
 Percy-Wolfson gallbladder
 Perkins
 Perkins left
 Perkins otologic
 Perkins right
 pin
 pitchfork
 Pitie-Salpetriere saphenous vein
  hook
 Pittman IMA
 Plester self-retaining
 Polytrac Gomez
 Poppen-Gelpi laminectomy
 posterior fossa
 Pratt bivalve
 Protractor wound
 Quervain abdominal
 Ragnell-Davis
 Ragnell handheld
 rake
 RC Mini-Open lighted
 Rehne abdominal
 retropubic
 rib
 ribbon
 Richards abdominal
 Richardson abdominal
 Richardson appendectomy
 Richardson-Eastman
 Rigby appendectomy
 right-angle
 ring abdominal
 R-Med mini retractor
 Robin-Masse abdominal
 Robotrac passive retraction system
 Rochard abdominal

retractor *(cont.)*
>   Rollet
>   Roos brachial plexus root
>   Rosenberg
>   Rosenkranz pediatric
>   Rosenkranz pediatric sternal
>   Rosenkranz universal malleable
>   Roux
>   Roux-Magnus
>   Rowe capsular
>   Rowe humeral head
>   S
>   Sachs vein
>   SaphLITE, SaphLITE II
>   Sauerbruch
>   Sawyer rectal
>   scalp
>   Schink
>   Schoenborn trachea
>   Schwartz laminectomy
>   Scoville
>   Scoville-Haverfield
>   Scoville-Richter
>   Seletz-Gelpi
>   self-retaining
>   Semb lung
>   Senn double-end
>   Senn-Green
>   Senn-Kanavel
>   Senn-Miller catspaw
>   Sewell
>   sharp
>   Sheldon hemilaminectomy
>   Sherwin knee
>   Simon abdominal
>   Sims
>   single-hook auto
>   SJM Rosenkranz pediatric
>   skid humeral head
>   skin (trachea)
>   small rake
>   Smillie knee
>   Smillie meniscus hook
>   Smith anal

retractor *(cont.)*
>   Smith-Buie rectal
>   Smith nerve root suction
>   Smith rectal
>   snake
>   Snitman endaural
>   Sofield
>   Space-OR flexible internal
>   Spacekeeper
>   splanchnic
>   spoon
>   spring-wire
>   Spurling nerve root
>   S-shaped
>   St. Mark's deep pelvic
>   Stack hand
>   staple-shaped
>   sternal
>   stiff ribbon
>   Stiwer
>   straight
>   Stryker illuminated
>   Stuck
>   suction
>   "sweetheart" (Harrington)
>   Sydney Hospital
>   Taylor self-retaining
>   Teflon-coated brain
>   Temple-Fay
>   tibial
>   Tiemann shoulder
>   toothed
>   tracheal
>   Travers
>   trigeminal nerve
>   Tuffier abdominal
>   Tuffier-Raney
>   Tupper
>   two-prong rake
>   U.S.
>   U.S.A.
>   U.S. Army
>   universal
>   University of Minnesota

retroperitoneal injury
retroperitoneal mass lesion
retroperitoneal organ
retroperitoneal region
retroperitoneal sarcoma
retroperitoneal space
retroperitoneal varices
retroperitoneal veins
retroperitoneally
retroperitoneoscopy
retroperitoneum
retropharyngeal approach
retropharyngeal position
retropubic prostatectomy
retropubic retractor
retrorectal abscess
retrosternal chest pain
retrovascular goiter
retrovirus, human mammary tumor
Retter aneurysm needle
Retter knot tier and ligature carrier
return of bowel sounds
Retzius
    space of
    system of
    vein of
REU (rectal endoscopic ultra-
    sonography)
reusable cannula
reusable grasper
ReVele imaging agent
Reverdin abdominal spatula
Reverdin epidermal free graft
Reverdin suture needle
reverse cutting suture
reversed Mercedes Benz sign
reversed peristalsis
reverse sphincterotome
reverse T3 or rT3
reverse-transcriptase polymerase chain
    reaction (RT-PCR) analysis
reverse Trendelenburg position
Revised Trauma Score
RevitaLase erbium cosmetic laser

Rexam Medical Packaging
Rex-Cantli-Serege line
Reye syndrome
Reynold pentad (Charcot triad plus
    altered mental status and shock)
Reynolds dissecting scissors
Reynolds vascular clamp
Rezipas (aminosalicylic acid)
Rezulin (troglitazone)
Rezyme
RFLP (restriction fragment length
    polymorphism)
R.F. tissue ablation device
RGEA (right gastroepiploic artery)
rhabdoid suture
rhabdomyolysis
rhabdomyoma
rhabdomyosarcoma
rhabdovirus
Rheaban (activated attapulgite)
Rheinstadter curette
Rheomacrodex (dextran 40) plasma
    volume expander
rhesus rotavirus-tetravalent vaccine
    (RRV-TV)
rheumatic lesion
rheumatoid panel
rheumatology panel
Rhinelander pin
Rhinoline endoscopic system
RhoC gene
RhoC GTPase gene
rhodanine stain
Rhode Island dissector sponge
Rhodes Inventory of Nausea and
    Vomiting
Rhoton ball dissector
Rhoton bayonet scissors
Rhoton bipolar forceps
Rhoton cup forceps
Rhoton curet
Rhoton-Cushing forceps
Rhoton dissecting forceps
Rhoton elevator

Rhoton enucleator
Rhoton forceps
Rhoton fork
Rhoton hook
Rhoton loop curet
Rhoton-Merz suction tube
Rhoton micro curet
Rhoton micro dissector
Rhoton needle
Rhoton needle holder
Rhoton osteotome
Rhoton pituitary curet
Rhoton punch
Rhoton scissors
Rhoton sellar punch
Rhoton spatula dissector
Rhoton spoon curet
Rhoton suction tip
Rhoton-Tew bipolar forceps
rhTSH (recombinant human thyroid-
    stimulating hormone)
RHV (right hepatic vein)
RIA (radioimmunoassay)
rib contractor
rib elevator
rib forceps
rib hook
rib rasp
rib retractor
rib shears (see shears)
Riba 3.0 SIA reagent kit for hepatitis C
RIBA (recombinant immunoblot assay)
RIBA HCV 3.0 SIA (strip immunoblot
    assay)
ribavirin and interferon alfa-2b
Ribble bandage
ribbon, iridium
ribbon retractor
ribbon stools
ribonuclease
ribovirus
rice-flour breath test
rice-fruit diet
rice-water stool

Richard Allen clip applier
Richards abdominal retractor
Richards angle guide
Richards mallet
Richards reamer
Richards reconstruction nail
Richards side plate
Richards-Hirschhorn plate
Richardson abdominal retractor
Richardson appendectomy retractor
Richardson-Eastman retractor
Richardson retractor
Richardson rod
Richard Wolf instruments and devices
Riches artery forceps
Riches diathermy artery forceps
Richet bandage
Richet fascia umbilicus
Richmar external ultrasound unit
Richter-Heath clip-removing forceps
Richter hernia
Richter laminectomy punch forceps
Richter-Monroe line
rickets, celiac
rickettsial infection
Ricord rectal speculum
ridge extension
ridge, pectineal
Ridlon plaster knife
Riechmann rod
Riedel lobe
Riedel struma
Riedel thyroiditis
Riepe-Bard gastric balloon
Riester economy otoscope
rifaximin
Rift Valley fever virus
Rigby appendectomy retractor
Riger, classic triad of
right adrenalectomy
right and left lateral coronary ligament
right and left lobes of the liver
right-angle chest tube
right-angle clamp

ring *(cont.)*
   internal
   internal abdominal
   internal inguinal
   intrahaustral contraction
   Kayser-Fleischer
   Ochsner
   pyloric
   Schatzki
   Silastic
   silicone elastomer
   sphincter contraction
   superficial inguinal
ring abdominal retractor
ring abscess
Ring catheter
ring-cutter blade
ring cutter, finger
Ringer lactate
ring forceps
ring insertion tool
ringlike contractions
Ring–McLean sump tube
ring of esophagus, A or B
ring retractor
ring-shaped cluster
ring-wall lesion
Riopan (magaldrate)
Riopan Plus 2
Riordan pin
Ripstein anterior sling rectopexy
Rish periosteal elevator
rising hematocrit
rising intracranial pressure
risk factor
risk marker
risk of perforation
Ritebite biopsy forceps
Ritter SpeedClave
Ritter UltraClave
Rivas vascular catheter
Riwolith Impalso Pressure Generator
Riza-Ribe grasper needle
RLP (rectal linitis plastica)

RLQ (right lower quadrant)
RLT (reduced liver transplant)
R-Med mini retractor
R-Med plug
RNA molecule
RNA polymerase, virally encoded
RNA tumor virus
RNA virus (ribovirus)
Ro-Bile
Robbers forceps
Robengatope radioactive agent
Robert Jones bulky soft dressing with
   Hemovac drainage
Robert Jones dressing
Robert Shaw bronchus tube
Roberts artery forceps
Roberts-Gill periosteal elevator
Robertson sign
Robertson suture
Roberts rib shears
Robin-Masse abdominal retractor
Robinson catheter, red rubber
Robinson-Kepler-Power water test
Robinul, Robinul Forte (glycopyrrolate)
robin's egg–blue gallbladder
robot
   AESOP 2000 and 3000
   ZEUS robotic system
robot-assisted procedure
robot neurosurgical microscope
robotic surgery device, AESOP
   (Automated Endoscopic System
   for Optimal Positioning)
robotics, SurgiScope
Robotrac passive retraction system
Robotrac retractor
Robson point
Robson position
ROC EZ anchor
ROC EZ suture anchor
ROC suture fastener
ROC XS suture anchor
ROC XS suture fastener
Rocaltrol (calcitriol)

ROCAP syringe
Rochard abdominal retractor
Rochester-Carmalt forceps
Rochester gallstone forceps
Rochester lamina elevator
Rochester-Mixter forceps
Rochester-Ochsner forceps
Rochester-Péan clamps
Rochester-Péan forceps
Rochester-Péan hemostats
Rochester spinal elevator
Rockey-Davis incision
rod
  absorbable
  acetabular cup detaching
  acetabular cup push (pushing)
  Acufex TAG
  alignment
  Alta tibial/humeral
  Amset R-F
  auto-reinforced polyglycolide
  bendable metallic
  Bickel intramedullary
  Biethium ostomy
  biodegradable
  C-D or CD (Cotrel-Dubousset)
  colostomy
  compression
  Dacron-impregnated silicone
  degradable polyglycolide
  distraction
  Edwards-Levine
  Edwards reverse ratchet
  Ender
  Fixateur Interne
  fluted medullary
  gram-negative
  grooved titanium
  Hall
  Harrington compression
  Harrington distraction
  Harris condylocephalic
  Hartshill rectangle
  hinge

rod *(cont.)*
  humeral
  Hunter Silastic
  Hunter tendon
  Ilizarov telescoping
  impactor
  Isola
  Jacobs distraction
  Kaneda
  Knodt compression
  knurled
  Kostuik
  Küntscher (Kuentscher) condylo-
    cephalic
  Luque
  Meckel
  Moe distraction
  Moe-modified Harrington
  Moss
  Mouradian
  Olerud PSF
  partially threaded
  pedicular
  PMMA (polymethylmethacrylate)
  polyglactin
  polyglycolide, self-reinforced
  PWB (Puno-Winter-Byrd)
  rectangular
  Reichmann
  resorbable
  Richardson
  Rogozinski spinal
  Rush
  Russell-Taylor reconstruction
  Sage
  Schanz
  Schmidt
  Schneider
  Seidel humeral
  Seidel intramedullary
  Selby I and II
  Serrato forearm
  Silastic
  silicone flexor

rongeur *(cont.)*
   Cloward intervertebral disk
   Cloward pituitary
   Codman-Kerrison laminectomy
   Codman-Leksell laminectomy
   Codman-Schlesinger cervical
     laminectomy
   Cohen
   Colclough-Scheicher laminectomy
   Corbett bone
   Cottle-Kazanjiann
   cranial
   curved bone
   Cushing
   Cushing cranial
   Cushing intervertebral disk
   Cushing pituitary
   Dahlgren cranial
   Dale first rib
   Dean bone
   Decker microsurgical
   Decker pituitary
   Defourmentel bone
   DeVilbiss cranial
   disk
   double-action
   down-biting
   duckbill
   Echlin bone
   Echlin duckbill
   Echlin laminectomy
   Echlin-Luer
   Ferris Smith intervertebral disk
   Ferris Smith-Kerrison laminectomy
   Ferris Smith laminectomy
   Ferris Smith pituitary jaw
   Ferris Smith-Spurling disk
   Fine-Kerrison cervical
   first rib
   Fisch bone
   FlexTip
   FlexTip intervertebral
   Friedman bone
   Frykholm bone

rongeur *(cont.)*
   Fulton laminectomy
   Geiger
   Giertz
   gooseneck
   Gruenwald neurosurgical
   Guleke bone
   Hajek antrum
   Hajek-Koffler laminectomy
   Hakansson bone
   Hartmann bone
   Hein
   Hoen intervertebral disk
   Hoen laminectomy
   Horsley bone
   Hudson cranial
   Husk bone
   intervertebral disk
   Jackson intervertebral disk
   Jansen
   Jarit-Kerrison laminectomy
   Jarit-Liston bone
   Jarit-Ruskin bone
   Kerrison
   Kerrison down-biting
   Kerrison laminectomy
   Kleinert-Kutz bone
   Kleinert-Kutz synovectomy
   laminectomy
   Lebsche
   Leksell laminectomy
   Leksell-Stille thoracic
   Lempert bone
   Liston bone
   Liston-Littauer bone
   Littauer-West
   Love-Gruenwald intervertebral disk
   Love-Gruenwald pituitary
   Love-Kerrison cervical
   Love-Kerrison laminectomy
   Luer bone
   Luer-Friedman bone
   Luer-Hartmann
   Malcolm-Lynn

rongeur *(cont.)*
    Markwalder bone
    Marquardt bone
    Mayfield
    McIndoe bone
    Mead
    Mead bone
    Micro-Kerrison
    microlaminectomy
    Midas-Rex
    Miltex-Kerrison cervical
    mini-Ruskin
    monster rongeur
    Montenovesi
    Mount laminectomy
    Müller (Mueller)
    Nicola pituitary
    Oldberg intervertebral disk
    Oldberg pituitary
    Olivecrona
    osteophyte nipper
    peapod intervertebral disk
    Peiper-Beyer laminectomy
    Pilling-Liston
    pituitary
    Poppen intervertebral disk
    Raney laminectomy
    Reiner bone
    Rottgen-Ruskin bone
    Ruskin bone
    Ruskin-Jansen bone
    Ruskin-Jay
    Ruskin-Liston bone
    Ruskin-Rowland bone
    Rust
    Sauerbruch-Coryllos
    Sauerbruch rib
    Sauerbruch-Stille
    Schell bone
    Schlesinger cervical
    Schlesinger intervertebral disk
    Schlesinger laminectomy
    Schlesinger pituitary

rongeur *(cont.)*
    Selverstone intervertebral disk
    Semb
    Semb-Stille bone
    Shearer
    single-action
    Smith-Petersen laminectomy
    Spence intervertebral disk
    Spurling intervertebral disk
    Spurling-Kerrison cervical
    Spurling-Kerrison laminectomy
    Spurling-Kerrison up-biting and
        down-biting
    Spurling pituitary
    Stellbrink synovectomy
    Stille-Horsley bone
    Stille-Leksell
    Stille-Liston bone
    Stille-Luer bone
    Stille-Luer duckbill
    Stille-Luer-Echlin
    Stille-Ruskin bone
    Stookey cranial
    straight bone
    straight pituitary
    Strully-Gigli
    Strully-Kerrison
    synovectomy
    Takahashi
    thoracic
    up-biting
    Urschel first rib
    Walton-Liston bone
    Walton-Ruskin bone
    Watson-Williams intervertebral disk
    Weil-Blakesley intervertebral disk
    Whitcomb-Kerrison laminectomy
    Wilde intervertebral disk
    Yasargil pituitary
    Zaufel-Jansen bone
rongeur forceps
roof of abdomen
roof plate

room
   insufflation tank
   laparoendoscopic
   postanesthesia recovery
room air
Roos brachial plexus root retractor
Roos first rib shears
Roosevelt clamp
root
   anatomical
   brachial plexus
   lung
   nerve
root needle
root of small bowel mesentery
root of sigmoid mesentery
ROPA (Regional Organ Procurement
   Agency)
ropivacaine
ropy bile
Roschke rectal speculum
Rosch-Uchida transjugular liver access
   needle-catheter
rose bengal sodium (^{131}I-labeled)
   hepatic function test
rose bengal test
Rose-Bradford kidney
rosebud sponge
Rosenbach sign
Rosenbach-Gmelin test
Rosenberg retractor
Rosen elevator
Rosen fenestrometer
Rosen incision knife
Rosenkranz deep retractor blade
Rosenkranz pediatric retractor system
Rosenkranz pediatric sternal retractor
Rosenkranz universal clamp
Rosenkranz universal malleable
   retractor
Rosenkranz wire-basket retractor
Rosen needle
Rosen separator
Rosen suction tube

Rosenthal test
Rose position
Rose retractor
rose-thorn ulcer
rosette appearance of anus
rosette Beaver blade
rosette blade
Rosetti stitch
Rosetti technique for Nissen fundoplica-
   tion
Rosidal bandage
rosiglitazone maleate
Rosser crypt hook
Rossetti modification of Nissen fundo-
   plication
rosuvastatin
Rotablator abrasive bur
ROTACS guidewire
Rotalink flexible-shaft reamer
Rotamune vaccine
rotary basket punch
rotary forceps
rotary gamma scalpel
rotary punch
rotary scissors
RotaShield vaccine (rotavirus, live)
rotating lock
rotating sphincterotome
rotating wheel, large
Rotator Cuff Buttress (RCB) plate
rotatory scissors
rotavirus antigen
rotavirus diarrhea
rotavirus DNA virus
rotavirus gastroenteritis, diarrhea
rotavirus in stool specimen
Rotazyme test
Rotex cutting biopsy needle
Rotex II biopsy needle
Roth Grip-Tip suture guide
Roth polyp retrieval net
Roth retrieval net
roticulating endograsper
roticulator, Endo Grasp

roticulator stapler
Rotor syndrome
Rotter lymph node
Rotter node
Rottgen-Ruskin bone rongeur
rotund abdomen
roughage
round cell infiltration
round cell sarcoma
round cup forceps
round ligament (ligamentum teres)
round nose grasper
round stick sponge
round-tapped periosteal elevator
round ulcer
roundworm (nematode)
Rous-associated virus (RAV)
Rous sarcoma virus (RSV)
Rousek extractor
route, enteral administration
route of spread
routine magnification view
Roux-en-Y (also Roux-Y)
Roux-en-Y anastomosis
Roux-en-Y biliary bypass with
    antrectomy
Roux-en-Y chimney surgical technique
Roux-en-Y choledochojejunostomy
Roux-en-Y cystojejunostomy
Roux-en-Y distal jejunoileostomy
Roux-en-Y esophagojejunostomy
    reconstruction
Roux-en-Y gastric bypass
Roux-en-Y gastroenterostomy
Roux-en-Y gastrojejunostomy
Roux-en-Y hepaticojejunostomy
Roux-en-Y jejunoileostomy
Roux-en-Y limb
Roux-en-Y limb to gastric pouch
Roux-en-Y loop
Roux-en-Y pancreaticojejunostomy
Roux-en-Y procedure with vagotomy
Roux limb
Roux-Magnus retractor

Roux retractor
Rovsing sign
Rowasa (mesalamine) enema
Rowe capsular retractor
Rowe disimpaction forceps
Rowe glenoid punch
Rowe glenoid-reaming forceps
Rowe-Harrison bone-holding forceps
Rowe humeral head retractor
Rowe-modified Harrison forceps
roxatidine, roxatidine acetate HCl
Roxicodone (oxycodone)
Roxin (roxatidine acetate HCl)
Roy-Camille cervical plate
Roy-Camille occipitocervical plate
Roy-Camille pedicle plate
Royl-Derm wound cleanser/dressing
rPAF-AH (platelet-activating factor
    acetylhydrolase, recombinant)
RPC (recurrent pyogenic cholangio-
    hepatitis)
RP-HPLC (reverse phase-high perform-
    ance liquid chromatography)
RPR (rapid plasma reagin) test
RPT (rapid pull-through) technique
RQ (respiratory quotient)
RR (respiratory rate)
rRNA ribosomal RNA
RRV-TV (rhesus rotavirus-tetravalent)
    vaccine
RSLT (reduced-size liver transplant)
RSP thermocoupler
RSP thermocouple sensor
rubber band hemorrhoidal ligator
rubber band hemorrhoidectomy
rubber band ligation of hemorrhoid
rubber band ligature
rubber band loader
rubber dam
rubber drain
rubber pickup
rubber seton
rubber-shod clamp
rubber tube

rubbery change
rubbery consistency
rubbery gray mass
rubbery nodule
rubbery texture
rubella virus
Ruben gouge
Rubens flap for breast reconstruction
Rubin rasp
Rubin-Quinton small bowel biopsy tube
Rubinstein-Taybi syndrome
Rubio-TC wire twister
rubitecan
Rubratope-57 radioactive agent
ructus
Rudd-Clinic hemorrhoidal forceps
Rudd-Clinic ligator
Rudd hemorrhoidal ligator
rudimentary lung
Ruel forceps
ruga (pl. rugae)
rugal folds
rugal pattern
rule, Goodsall
rule of nines (9's)
rule of tens (10's)
rule of two (2)
rule of two-thirds (2/3)
rule out sepsis
RuLox (aluminum hydroxide;
    magnesium hydroxide)
rumble (bowel sounds)
rumbling bowel sounds
Rumel artery forceps
Rumel thoracic clamp
Rumel tourniquet flex cannula
rumination
running lock suture
running suture
runny stools
runs (noun) (diarrhea)
runs an oblique course
runting syndrome

rupture
    aneurysm
    appendix
    bladder
    blunt
    complete
    congenital aneurysm
    cystic duct
    delayed splenic
    diaphragmatic
    duodenal
    ERCA-induced
    esophageal
    gastric
    hepatic
    hernia
    intramural esophageal
    intraperitoneal viscus
    large bladder
    Mallory-Weiss mucosal
    membrane
    mesenteric
    peritoneal
    portal vessel
    postemetic esophageal
    splenic
    splenic vessel
    spontaneous
    traumatic
    umbilical hernia
ruptured AAA (abdominal aortic
    aneurysm)
ruptured aneurysm
ruptured aortic atheromatous plaque
ruptured appendix
ruptured disk
ruptured duodenum following blunt
    abdominal trauma
ruptured ectopic pregnancy
ruptured fallopian tube
ruptured follicle
ruptured hernia
ruptured intraperitoneal viscus
ruptured membrane

ruptured perineum
ruptured spleen
RUQ (right upper quadrant)
Ruschelit PVC tracheostomy tube
Rush awl reamer
rushes (bowel sounds), peristaltic
Rush flexible medullary nail
Rush mallet
Rush pin
Rush rod
Ruskin antrum trocar needle
Ruskin bone-cutting forceps
Ruskin bone rongeur
Ruskin bone-splitting forceps
Ruskin-Jansen bone rongeur
Ruskin-Jay rongeur
Ruskin-Liston bone cutter
Ruskin-Liston bone-cutting forceps
Ruskin-Liston bone rongeur
Ruskin rongeur forceps
Ruskin-Rowland bone-cutting forceps
Ruskin-Rowland bone rongeur
Russe bone graft
Russell gastrostomy kit
Russell percutaneous endoscopic
    gastrostomy
Russell-Taylor (R-T) nail
Russell-Taylor interlocking medullary
    nail
Russell-Taylor reconstruction rod
Russian forceps
Russian tissue forceps
Rust amputation saw
rust-colored papule
Rust rongeur
Rutherford-Morrison tissue forceps
Rutkow and Robbins
Rutkow-Robbins-Gilbert classification
    of groin hernias (types 1–7)
Rutkow sutureless plug and patch
Rutzen ileostomy bag
Ruysch disease
RX Herculink 14 biliary stent system
RX Herculink 14 premounted stent
    system
Rydell nail
Ryder micro needle holder
Ryder needle
Ryder needle holder
Ryder-TC needle holder
Ryerson bone graft
Ryle tube

S, s

Saathoff test
Saber BT blunt tip surgical trocar
saber-cut incision
Sable catheter
Sabreloc conventional spatula
Sabreloc spatula
Sabreloc spatula needle
Sabreloc suture
sac
  abdominal
  air
  anal
  aneurysmal
  aortic
  endolymphatic
  enterocele
  fluid-filled
  gestational
  greater peritoneal
  hernia
  indirect hernia
  lesser peritoneal
  pericardial
  peritoneal
  Pleatman
  redundant hernia
  wide-mouth
saccharin
sacciform kidney
saccular colon
sacculation
Sachs brain suction tube
Sachs dural hook
Sachs nerve separator and spatula
Sachs suction tube
Sachs vein retractor
Sacks-Vine feeding gastrostomy tube
Sacks-Vine PEG (percutaneous
    endoscopic gastrostomy) tube
sacral anesthesia
sacral fixation
sacral promontory
sacral regression
sacrifice of facial nerve
sacrifice of lateral cremasteric bundle
sacroabdominoperineal pull-through
sacrococcygeal teratoma
sacrocolposuspension
sacrofixation operation
sacrogenital fold
sacroperineal approach
sacrosidase enzyme replacement
    therapy
saddle anesthesia

saddle block anesthesia
saddle clamp
S-adenosyl-methionine (SAMe)
Sadowsky hook wire
Saf-Clens chronic wound cleanser
SafeTap tapered spinal needle
Safetrak epidural needle
Safety AV fistula needle
safety shield
safety-shielded trocar
Saf-Gel hydrogel dressing
Safil synthetic absorbable surgical
    suture
Saf-T E-Z translucent needle shield
sage-grain stools
Sage rod
SAGES (Society of American
    Gastrointestinal Endoscopic
    Surgeons)
Sage triangular nail
sagittal cranial suture
sagittal plane
sagittal septum of rectus sheath
sagittal surgical saw
sagittal ultrasonography
sago-grain stool
sago liver
Sahli biopsy and aspiration needle
Sahli glutoid test
Sahli-Nencki test
Saint triad
SAL (suction-assisted lipectomy)
SAL (suction-assisted lipoplasty)
salazosulfapyridine
Salem duodenal sump tube
Salenius meniscus knife
Salibi carotid artery clamp
salicylate abuse
salicylate poisoning
salicylazosulfapyridine
saline breast implant
saline cleansing enema
saline continence test
saline drop test

saline flows freely
saline flush
saline infusion
Salinem infection
saline-moistened sponge
saline, normal
saline solution
saline test
Salinetrode electrode
Salisbury common cold virus
saliva aspiration
salivary amylase (S-type)
salivary calculus
salivary gland tumor
salivary gland virus
salivary stone
salivary tumor
Salkowski and Schipper test
Salkowski-Schipper test
salmon-patch hemorrhage
salmon-pink epithelium
Salmonella and *Campylobacter*-specific
    mass spectrometry
Salmonella colitis
Salmonella food poisoning
Salmonella osteomyelitis
salmonellosis
Salofalk (mesalamine)
Salomon test
salt and pepper duodenal erosion
salts, bile
Sal-Tropine (atropine sulfate)
salvage cytology
salvage surgery
SAMBA (simultaneous areolar masto-
    pexy and breast augmentation)
SAMe (S-adenosyl-methionine)
sample, endoscopic tissue
SampleMaster biopsy needle
sampling of lymph node
Sampson medullary nail
Samuels forceps
sandbag
Sand gland

Sandhill P32 pH antimony probe
Sandifer syndrome
Sandimmune (cyclosporine)
Sandostatin
Sandostatin LAR Depot (octreotide
   acetate)
Sandoz suction/feeding tube
sandpaper gallbladder
sandwich radioimmunoassay
sandwiched iliac bone graft
sandy material
SangCya (cyclosporine; alcohol)
Sanger-Brown syndrome
sanguineous fluid
sanguineous infiltration
sanguinopurulent
sanguinoseropurulent
sanguinoserous
Sani-Scope anoscope
Sani-Supp (glycerin)
Santiani-Stone classification of
   pancreatitis
santonin test
Santorini, duct of
SaO$_2$ (oxygen saturation)
saphenofemoral junction
saphenous varix
saphenous vein extracranial-intracranial
   bypass graft
SaphFinder surgical balloon dissector
SaphLITE/SaphLITE II retractor
   system
SAPHtrak balloon dissector
Sapimed anoscope
Sapimed rectoscope
saponification of fat
Saratoga (zinc oxide; boric acid;
   eucalyptol)
sarcoepiplocele
sarcoid of Boeck
sarcoidosis, hepatic
sarcoma
   Abernethy
   alveolar soft-part

sarcoma *(cont.)*
   ameloblastic
   angiolithic
   botryoid
   endometrial stromal
   Ewing
   fascicular
   gastric Kaposi
   giant cell
   giant cell monstrocellular
   granulocytic
   hemangioendothelial
   immunoblastic
   intracolonic Kaposi
   Ito cell
   Jensen
   juxtacortical osteogenic
   Kaposi
   Kupffer cell
   leukocytic
   lipoblastic
   lymphatic
   medullary
   mixed cell
   multiple idiopathic hemorrhagic
   myelogenic
   myeloid
   neurogenic
   osteogenic
   periosteal
   reticulum cell
   retroperitoneal
   round cell
   Rous
   soft tissue
   spindle cell
   synovial
   telangiectatic osteogenic
   vasoablative endothelial (VABES)
sarcoma of retroperitoneal
sarcomatoid degeneration
sarcoplasmic material
sarcoplasmic reticulum
sargramostim

Sarmiento nail
Sarns electric saw
Sarns intracardiac suction tube
Sarot artery forceps
Sarot bronchus clamp
Sarot needle
Sarot needle holder
Sarot-TC needle holder
SART (standard acid reflux test)
satchel drape
satellite lesion
satellite metastasis
satellite nodule
satellite phenomenon
satellite structure
satellite virus
Satietrol Complete
satiety, early
SatinCrescent knife
SatinShortcut knife
Satinsky aortic clamp
Satinsky scissors
Satinsky vascular clamp
Satinsky vena cava clamp
Satin-Slip stylet
Satric-500
Satterlee amputating saw
Satterlee bone saw
satumomab pendetide
satumomab pendetide monoclonal
    antibody
saturated blood
saturation index (SI) of bile
saturation, oxygen
saturnine colic
saucerize
saucer-shaped excavation
Sauerbruch-Britsch rib shears
Sauerbruch-Coryllos rongeur
Sauerbruch-Frey bone punch
Sauerbruch-Frey rib shears
Sauerbruch retractor
Sauerbruch rib elevator
Sauerbruch rib forceps

Sauerbruch rib shears
Sauerbruch rongeur
Sauerbruch-Stille rongeur
Saundby test for blood in stool
Saunders disease
Saunders-Paparella stapes hook
Saunders-Paparella straight needle
Saunders-Paparella window rasp
Sauvage graft
Savage suture
Savary bougie
Savary-Gilliard dilator
Savary-Miller grading scale
Savary tapered thermoplastic dilator
saw
    Accutom low-speed diamond
    Adams
    Adson wire
    Aesculap
    air-powered
    amputating
    Bailey-Gigli
    Bailey wire
    bayonet
    Beaver
    Bier amputation
    Bishop
    bone
    bow-type
    Brun metacarpal
    cast
    Charriere amputating
    Charriere bone
    circular
    Cottle
    counter rotating
    craniotomy
    crosscut
    Cushing
    Davis
    Davis guide for Gigli
    DeMartel wire
    electric cast
    end-cutting reciprocating

saw *(cont.)*
  Engel plaster
  fenestration
  Gigli
  Gigli wire
  Hall air-driven oscillating
  Hall Micro E oscillating
  Hall Micro E reciprocating
  Hall Micro E sagittal
  Hall sternal
  Hall Versipower oscillating
  Hall Versipower reciprocating
  Herbert
  Langenbeck metacarpal
  Lebsche wire
  Luck-Bishop bone
  metacarpal
  micro sagittal
  MicroAire oscillating
  micro oscillating
  Midas Rex craniotomy
  Mueller (Müller)
  Olivecrona-Gigli
  Orthair oscillating
  oscillating
  oscillating sternotomy
  Oscillo III plaster
  Percy amputating
  plaster
  Poppen
  power oscillating
  power-driven
  Raney
  reciprocating motor
  reciprocating
  Rust amputation
  sagittal surgical
  Sarns electric
  Satterlee amputating
  single-blade
  Skilsaw
  sternotomy
  straight oscillating
  Strully-Gigli

saw *(cont.)*
  Stryker
  twin-blade oscillating
  Tyler-Gigli
  Weiss amputation
  Wigmore plaster
  wire
  Zimmer oscillating
SAWA shoulder brace
saw blade
sawcut
saw guide
  Adson
  Bailey Gigli
  Blair
  Cushing
  Cushing-Gigli
  Davis
  Gigli
  Lebsche
  Poppen Gigli
  Raney
saw handle, Strully Gigli
Sawtell artery forceps
Sawtell tonsil hemostatic forceps
sawtooth appearance sign
sawtooth configuration
sawtooth irregularity of bowel contour
sawtooth pattern
Sawyer rectal retractor
Sawyer rectal speculum
SAXX renal stent
Sayre bandage
Sayre periosteal elevator
SB, S-B (Sengstaken-Blakemore) tube
SBE (small bowel enteroscopy)
SBGM (self blood glucose monitoring)
SBO (small bowel obstruction)
SBP (spontaneous bacterial peritonitis)
SCA-EX ShortCutter catheter
scab, chronic
scale (see *classification*)
scale, Detecto weight
scale of 1 to 10

Schoemaker anastomosis
Schoemaker gland scissors
Schoenberg intestinal forceps
Schoenborn trachea retractor
Schoenrock inserter
Schrader air
Schrader Endo-Flo
Schroeder tenaculum forceps
Schubert biopsy forceps
Schuchart rib shears
Schuknecht suction tip
Schuknecht wire-cutting scissors
Schüller (Schueller) view
Schumacher biopsy forceps
Schumacher rib shears
Schumacher scissors
Schumaker aortic clamp
Schwachman-Bodian syndrome
Schwachman-Diamond syndrome
Schwann cell lipidosis
Schwann cell tube
schwannoma
Schwartz clamp
Schwartz clip-applying forceps
Schwartz laminectomy retractor
Schwartz micro clip
Schwartz-Pregenzer urethropexy
Schwartz temporary clamp-applying
 forceps
Schwartz temporary intracranial artery
 clamp
Schwartze chisel
Schwarz test
Schweitzer pin
Schweitzer spring plate
sciatic hernia
SCID (severe combined immuno-
 deficiency)
Sci-Med Express Monorail balloon
scintigraphic balloon
scintigraphic study
scintigraphy (see *imaging*)
 hepatobiliary
 quantitative hepatobiliary (QHS)
 radioistope

scintimammography (SMM)
scintiscan (see *imaging*)
 biliary
 gastroesophageal
scirrhous adenocarcinoma
scirrhous cancer
scirrhous carcinoma of breast
scirrhous lesion
scirrhous tumor
scissor dissection
scissor leg
scissors (see also *shears*)
 Abel
 Acme
 Acufex
 Adson ganglion
 Adson-Toennis
 alligator
 arthroscopic
 Aufricht dissecting
 Babcock wire-cutting
 Babcock wire
 baby Metzenbaum dissecting
 baby Reynolds dissecting
 bandage
 bandage and utility
 Bantam wire-cutting
 Barnes perineorrhaphy
 bayonet-shaped
 Beall circumflex artery
 Beebe wire-cutting
 Bellucci alligator
 bipolar cautery
 bladder
 blunt-tipped iris
 Bonn
 bowel
 Bowman
 brain
 Braun episiotomy
 Braun-Stadler
 bronchoesophageal
 Brook stitch
 Buck

scissors *(cont.)*
    Buie rectal
    Busch suture
    Busch umbilical
    cartilage
    Castanares facelift
    Castroviejo
    Church
    circumflex
    coronary artery
    Crafoord thoracic
    crown and collar
    CTS Harvester bipolar
    curved
    curved dissecting
    curved double-action Metzenbaum
    curved Mayo
    curved unipolar
    cuticle
    Dandy neurosurgical
    Dandy trigeminal nerve
    Dean dissecting
    Deaver
    DeBakey dissecting
    DeBakey endarterectomy
    DeBakey valve
    Decker alligator
    Decker micro
    Decker microsurgical
    DeMartel neurosurgical
    DeMartel vascular
    diathermy
    Diethrich coronary
    Diethrich-Hegemann
    Diethrich valve
    Diethrich vascular
    dissecting
    Don Duralap
    Don peritoneal
    Doyen abdominal
    Dubois
    Duffield
    dural
    Duralap Metzenbaum

scissors *(cont.)*
    Electroscope disposable laparo-
      scopic
    embryotomy
    endarterectomy
    Endo Shears
    ENT (ear, nose, and throat)
    enterotomy
    enucleation
    episiotomy
    Esmarch plaster
    Evershears and Evershears II bipolar
    facelift
    Ferguson
    Finochietto-Metzenbaum
    Finochietto thoracic
    Fiskars Softouch
    fistula
    F. L. Fischer microsurgical
      neurectomy bayonet
    Forman rhinoplasty
    Frazier dural
    Friedland
    Fukushima-Giannotta
    Giertz-Stille
    gland
    Glassman dissecting
    Goldman dissecting
    Goligher abdominal
    Gorney
    Gradle
    Haimovici arteriotomy
    Halsey nail
    Harrington
    Harrington-Mayo thoracic
    Harvey suture
    Harvey wire-cutting
    Haynes
    Heath ligature
    Heath suture
    Hercules plaster and bandage
    hook
    hook, single-action
    Howell coronary

scissors *(cont.)*
   iris
   Jacobson microneurosurgical
   Jameson
   Jannetta-Kurze dissecting
   Jorgenson
   Joseph dissecting
   Joseph nasal
   Kahn dissecting
   Kantrowitz vascular
   Karmody venous
   Kaye-TC
   Kelly dissecting
   Kelly fistula
   Kelly-Locklin
   Kilner dissecting
   Kitner dissecting
   Kleencut
   Knapp
   Knowles bandage
   Koenig nail-splitting
   Kreuscher
   Kurze dissecting
   Lahey
   LaparoSonic coagulating
   LaserScissors
   Lawson Tait perineorrhaphy
   ligature
   Lincoln
   Lincoln-Metzenbaum
   Lister
   Lister bandage
   Littauer stitch
   Little dissecting
   Litwak mitral valve
   Lloyd Davies
   Luque rod
   Malis bipolar cautery
   Malis neurological
   Martin
   Martin cartilage
   Martin stitch
   Mayo dissecting
   Mayo dressing

scissors *(cont.)*
   Mayo-Harrington
   Mayo-Lexer
   Mayo-Noble
   Mayo-Stille
   Mayo straight dissecting
   McCain TMJ
   McIndoe
   Medco Lister bandage
   Medi plaster
   meniscectomy
   meniscus
   Metzenbaum dissecting
   Metzenbaum-TC
   micro
   microneurosurgical
   Micro-One
   Micro-Two
   microscopic
   microsurgery or microsurgical
   microvascular
   Miller rectal
   Mills arteriotomy
   Mills vascular
   moleskin
   monopolar
   MPC scissors
   nail
   nail-splitting
   Nelson
   neurological or neurosurgical
   Nicola
   Northbent stitch
   Noyes iris
   Noyes microscopic
   nurses
   Nu-Tip disposable
   O'Brien
   Olivecrona dural
   Olivecrona trigeminal
   operating
   Ormon rectal
   Oxo kitchen
   Panzer gallbladder

scissors *(cont.)*
Peck-Joseph dissecting
Penn umbilical
Penn wire-cutting
pituitary
Pivotal
plaster
Potts-DeMartel vascular
Potts right-angled
Potts 60° angled
Potts-Smith
Potts-Smith vascular
Potts tenotomy
Potts-Yasargil
Pratt rectal
Quimby
Ragnell dissecting
Re-New laparoscopic
Real coronary artery
Rees
Reynolds
Rhoton bayonet
right-angle
Rogers wire-cutting
rotary
rotatory
Satinsky
Schmieden
Schmieden dural
Schoemaker gland
Schuknecht wire-cutting
Schumacher
Seutin plaster
Shea
Shortbent stitch
Siebold abdominal
Sims abdominal
Sistrunk dissecting
Slip-N-Snip
Smillie meniscus
Smith
Smith bandage
Smith wire-cutting
Snowden-Pencer

scissors *(cont.)*
Spay
Spencer
Spencer stitch
spring-handled
Stevens tenotomy
Stille-Mayo
stitch
Stiwer
Storz wire-cutting
strabismus
straight
straight dissecting
straight double-action
straight double-action monopolar
straight micro
Strully dissecting
Strully dural
Strully neurological
Supercut dissecting
surgical
suture
Sweet esophageal
Sweet pituitary
Tagit antibacterial
Take-Apart
Taylor brain
Taylor dural
tenotomy
Tessier undermining
thoracic
Thorek-Feldman gallbladder
Thorek gallbladder
Tindall
Toennis dissecting
trigeminal
Turner Warwick diathermy
Twisk
umbilical cord
valve
Vannas micro
Vantage iris
Vantage Knowles bandage
Vantage Lister bandage

scissors *(cont.)*
    Vantage Metzenbaum
    Vantage operating
    Vantage Spencer stitch
    Vantage strabismus
    Vezien abdominal
    Waldmann
    Walton
    Webster meniscectomy
    Weck microsuture cutting
    Wertheim
    Westcott dissecting
    Westscott
    Wiet otologic
    Willauer abdominal
    Willauer thoracic
    Wilmer dissecting
    wire
    wire-cutting
    Yankauer
    Yasargil bayonet
    Yasargil micro
    Z-Scissors
scissors dissection
scissors-excision hemorrhoidectomy
scissors sharpener, Miltex
Scivoletto test
SCLC (small cell lung carcinoma)
sclera (pl. sclerae)
    anicteric
    icteric
    nonicteric
scleral icterus
scleroderma bowel disease
scleroderma-like esophagus
scleroderma of esophagus
scleroderma, systemic
ScleroLaser laser
Scleromate sclerosant
ScleroPlus HP laser
sclerosant
    absolute alcohol
    bucrylate
    ethanolamine oleate

sclerosant *(cont.)*
    morrhuate
    polidocanol
    Scleromate
    sodium tetradecyl sulfate
    Sotradecol
    thrombin-Keflin-sotredochal
sclerosing adenosis of breast
sclerosing agent
sclerosing cholangitis
sclerosing encapsulating peritonitis
sclerosing hemangioma
sclerosing hepatic carcinoma (SHC)
sclerosing inflammation
sclerosing solution
sclerosing therapy
sclerosing well-differentiated carcinoma
sclerosis
    central hyaline
    endoscopic injection
    esophageal variceal
    gastric
    hepatic
    hepatoportal
    laser
    variceal
Sclerosol intrapleural aerosol
sclerotherapist
sclerotherapy
    emergent endoscopic
    endoscopic
    esophageal variceal
    fiberoptic injection (FIS)
    hemorrhoidal
    injection
    intravariceal
    paravariceal
sclerotherapy needle
sclerotic kidney
sclerotic stomach
SCNB (stereotactic core needle biopsy)
scolex (pl. scoleces)
scoliocide

scoop
    abdominal
    common duct
    Desjardins gall stone
    Desjardins gallbladder
    Ferguson gallstone
    gallbladder
    Klebanoff gallstone
    Luer-Koerte gallstone
    malleable
    Mayo common duct
    Mayo gallstone
    Moore gallstone
    Moynihan gallstone
    rigid
    Volkman
SCOOP 1 catheter
SCOOP 2 catheter
scope (see *endoscope*)
ScopeSeal endoscope patch
Scopinaro pancreaticobiliary bypass
score (also see *classification*)
    Beppu
    "bother"
    Braden
    Champion Trauma Score (CTS)
    Colon Injury (CIS)
    Demeester
    fecal incontinence
    Gleason
    Injury Severity
    KESS constipation
    Knodell periportal inflammation
    Revised Trauma
scoring incision in surgery
scorpion bite
Scotchcast 2 casting tape
Scott attic cannula
Scott jejunoileal bypass
Scott-McCracken periosteal elevator
Scott nasal suction tube
Scott silicone ventricular catheter
Scott ventricular cannula
scout film

Scoville blade
Scoville brain clip-applying forceps
Scoville brain spatula forceps
Scoville cervical disk retractor
Scoville-Haverfield hemilaminectomy
    retractor
Scoville hemilaminectomy retractor
Scoville nerve root hook
Scoville nerve root retractor
Scoville retractor
Scoville-Richter laminectomy retractor
Scoville ventricular needle
screw
    Barouk micro
    Doyen myoma
    Guardsman femoral
    Herbert bone
    Herbert-Whipple bone
    Howmedica Universal compression
    In-Fast bone
    Jeter lag
    KLS Centre-Drive
    lag
    Lindorf lag
    Magerl
    Propel cannulated interference
    Reddick-Saye
screw-holding forceps
scrotal ecchymosis
scrotal hernia
scrotum
Scudder forceps
Scudder intestinal clamp
Scudder intestinal forceps
scultetus bandage
scultetus binder
scybalous stools
SDI (Surgical Dynamics, Inc)
S*D*sorb meniscal stapler
sea anemone ulcer
sea-blue histiocyte syndrome
Seabrook pump
seabuckthorn seed oil
Sea-Clens wound cleanser

seal
   AccuPort
   Karaya 5
   optimal tracheal
   orbital reducer
sealant (see also *adhesive*)
   CoSeal surgical sealant
   CoStasis
   fibrin
   FloSeal matrix hemostatic
   FocalSeal
   FocalSeal-L
   FocalSeal-S
   Hemaseel APR fibrin
   Hemaseel HMN biological tissue
      glue
   HemaSyst
   Peri-Strips Dry
   Peri-Strips wound
   Proceed hemostatic
   Tisseel fibrin
   TraumaSeal
   VITEX fibrin
Seal-Up II reducer
seasick
seasickness
SeaSorb alginate wound dressing
seatbelt neck injury
seating chisel
Seawell rasp
sebaceous carcinoma
sebaceous cyst
Sebileau periosteal elevator
seborrheic keratosis
sebum
secondary adhesion
secondary adrenocortical insufficiency
secondary bacterial infection
secondary biliary cirrhosis
secondary biliary fibrosis
secondary biseptal cirrhosis
secondary cholangitis
secondary closure
secondary contraction

secondary hepatic cancer
secondary hyperaldosteronism
secondary hyperparathyroidism
secondary hypersplenism
secondary hypothyroidism
secondary infection
secondary jejunal ulcer
secondary lesion
secondary local ischemia
secondary malabsorption
secondary nontropical sprue
secondary peristaltic wave
secondary suture
secondary thyroid hyperplasia
second cyst recurrence
second degree hemorrhoid
second-look laparotomy
second-look operation
Secretin Ferring (secretin)
secretin-pancreozymin test
secretin provocation testing for
   gastrinoma
secretin-stimulated MRCP
secretin stimulation test
secretion
   basal acid
   exocrine
   gastric
   gastric acid
   ileal
   massive acid
   pituitary
   serous
   thin
   thyrocalcitonin
   watery
secretory diarrhea
section
   abdominal
   cross-
   deep
   fresh frozen
   frozen
   permanent

selective cytokine inhibitory drug
(SelCID)
selective mesenteric angiography
selective proximal vagotomy (SPV)
selective sampling
selective serotonin 5-HT (hydroxytrypt-
amine) blocker
selective serotonin reuptake inhibitor
(SSRI)
selective splenic arteriogram
selective vagotomy
selective venous sampling for gastrin
selective visceral hypersensitivity
Selector ultrasonic aspirator
selenium-75 (^{75}Se) radioisotope
selenomethionine (^{75}Se) pancreatic
function test
selenomethionine radioactive agent
(^{75}Se)
Seletz-Gelpi laminectomy retractor
Seletz nonrigid ventricular catheter
self-adhering bandage
self-aspirating cut-biopsy needle
self blood glucose monitoring (SBGM)
self-broaching nail
self-broaching pin
self-centering bone-holding forceps
self-centering reamer
self-esteem disturbance
self-examination
self-expanding metallic wall stent
self-expanding metal stent
self-induced vomiting
self-limited
self-locking nail
self-positioning balloon
self-retaining clamp
self-retaining laryngoscope
self-retaining retractor
self-retaining table-mounted retractor
system
self-splint when coughing
sella punch forceps
Sellheim elevating spoon

Sellors rib contractor
Selman clamp
Selman vessel forceps
Selverstone carotid artery clamp
Selverstone cordotomy hook
Selverstone intervertebral disk rongeur
Selverstone rongeur forceps
semantic conditioning
Semb bone forceps
Semb ligature carrier
Semb lung retractor
Semb rib forceps
Semb rib rasp
Semb rib shears
Semb rongeur
Semb-Stille bone rongeur
semiclosed anesthesia
semielemental diet
semiflexible endoscope
semiformed stools
semi-Fowler position
semifundoplication (Toupet)
semi-invasive portal decompression
semilunar cartilage knife
semilunar fold
semilunar hiatus
semilunar incision
semilunar line
semilunar-shaped fold
seminal fluid
semiopen anesthesia
semirigid endoscope
semirigid sigmoidoscope
semisitting position
semisolid material
semisolid sebaceous debris
semisolid stools
semitendinosus graft
semitubular compression plate
Semken bipolar forceps
Semken delicate forceps
Semken tissue forceps
Semliki Forest virus
Semm biopsy suction curette

Semm rigid laparoscope
Semm-Wisap laparoscope
SEMS (self-expanding microporous
    stent [aneurysm])
Sendai virus
Senexon (senna concentrate)
Sengstaken balloon esophageal
    dilatation
Sengstaken-Blakemore (S-B) tamponade
    balloon
Sengstaken-Blakemore (S-B) tube
Senn double-end retractor
Senn-Green retractor
Senn-Kanavel retractor
Senn-Miller catspaw retractor
Senn plate
Senn retractor
senna concentrate
Senna-Gen (senoside)
Senning bulldog clamp
Senographe 2000D digital
    mammography imaging system
Senokot (senna concentrate)
SenoScan mammography
senosides
Sensability breast examination sheet
Sensability lubricated plastic sheet for
    breast self-examination
sensation
    burning
    foreign body
    globus
    phantom breast
sensation deficit
sensor
    anal EMG PerryMeter
    BIS Sensor
    BreastAlert differential temperature
        (DTS)
    gastrotonometer electronic
    globus
    Mon-a-therm skin temperature
    Optical
    Oxygen

sensor *(cont.)*
    PerryMeter anal EMG
    RSP thermocouple
    side-hole
    sleeve
    snaptrace silver chloride
    TAB thermocouple
    temperature
    thermistor
    Vasotrax blood pressure/heart rate
Sensorcaine MPF (bupivacaine)
sensorium change
sensory innervation
Sensory Threshold Tester
Sensostrip
sentinel blood clot
sentinel fold
sentinel gland
sentinel loop of small bowel
sentinel lymph node (SLN)
sentinel node
sentinel pile (hemorrhoid)
sentinel skin paddle graft
sentinel tag
Sepacell RZ-2000 leukoreduction
    device
separator, Benson pylorus
Sepracoat coating solution
Seprafilm bioresorbable membrane
Seprafilm tissue barrier
Sepragel bioresorbable gel
Sepramesh biosurgical composite mesh
    graft
Sepramesh prosthetic surgical mesh
Sepramesh suture
SEPS (subfascial endoscopic perforator
    surgery)
sepsis
    catheter
    gram-negative
    incarcerated
    intestinal
    intra-abdominal (IAS)
    intravenous line

sepsis *(cont.)*
  oral
  overwhelming postsplenectomy
    (OPSS)
  postsplenectomy
  puerperal
  Staphylococcus
sepsis syndrome
septal cirrhosis, diffuse
septal elevator
septal forceps
septal mucosa
septal panniculitis
septal tissue
septal wall
septectomy, transampullary
septic cholangitis
septicemia, transient
septic necrosis
septicopyemia
  cryptogenic
  metastatic
  spontaneous
septic shock
septic syndrome
septic wound
Septopal beads
septum, interhaustral
sequela (pl. sequelae)
sequence technique
sequential clamp and suture technique
sequential clamp, cut, and tie technique
sequestered foreign material
sequestrant, bile acid
sequestration, fluid
sequestration of circulating red cells
sequestration of medications
sequestration of platelets
sequestration, splenic
sequestrectomy
sequestrum forceps
Sequoia ultrasound system
Seracult Plus test
Seracult test

serendipity view
SergiScope (robotic microscope)
serial cardiac isoenzymes
serial cardiograms
serial cholangiograms
serial CK enzyme study (also CPK)
serial dilutions
serial hemoglobins
serial insulin measurements
serial lesions
serial liver biopsies
serial observations
serial sections
serially clamped, cut, and ligated
serially sectioned
series, gastrointestinal
sermorelin acetate
seroculture
serocystic
serofibrinous inflammation
serofibrinous pleurisy
serological muscle enzymes
serologic cross-reactivity
serologic markers for hepatitis
serologic testing
Seroma-Cath catheter
Seroma-Cath wound drainage system
seroma, postoperative
seromuscular intestinal patch graft
seromuscular layer
seromuscular stitch
seromuscular suture
seromuscular-to-edge suture
seroprevalence
serosa of GI tract
serosal involvement
serosal patch repair
serosal section
serosal surface
serosal tear
serosal transducers and manometry
serosanguineous discharge
serosanguineous fluid
serosanguinopurulent

serositis
serotinin degradation
serotonergic drug
serotonin antagonist
serous abscess
serous adenocarcinoma
serous atrophy
serous cystadenocarcinoma
serous cystadenoma
serous cystoma
serous diarrhea
serous effusion
serous exudate
serous fluid
serous gland of tongue
serous infiltration
serous inflammation
serous membrane
serous secretion
serpentine appendix
serpentine incision
serpentine plate
serpiginous ulcer
serpiginous ulceration
serrated forceps
serrated jaws
serrated suture
Serratia liquefaciens
Serratia marcescens
Serrato forearm pin
Serrato forearm rod
serratus anterior muscle
serrefine clamp (see *clamp; forceps; hemostat*)
serrefine, Dieffenbach
serum alanine aminotransferase (ALT)
serum ammonia
serum ammonia level
serum amylase
serum aspartate aminotransferase (AST)
serum bile acid
serum bilirubin
serum calcium

serum calcium level
serum carcinoembryonic antigen concentration
serum ceruloplasmin
serum cholesterol
serum complement level
serum concentrations of carbohydrate antigen
serum cortisol
serum creatinine, serum urea, creatinine clearance, urine volume, sodium excretion/UNaV)
serum DHEA level
serum globulin concentration
serum glucose value
serum HCV-specific antibody
serum hepatitis (SH) antigen
serum IgA antiendomysium antibody
serum interleukin
serum iron
serum lactate dehydrogenase (LDH)
serum lactic acid level
serum lipase
serum lipid
serum liver enzyme
serum magnesium
serum marker
serum parathormone level
serum potassium
serum protein
serum PTH
serum sodium
serum thyrocalcitonin level
serum total bilirubin
serum transaminase level
serum triglycerides
Serutan laxative (psyllium)
sessile adenoma
sessile lesion
sessile nodular carcinoma
sessile papule
sessile polyp
sestamibi scan
Sethotope radioactive agent

seton
  anal
  Penrose
  rubber
  silk
seton needle
seton placement
seton suture
seton wound
setophobia
SET three-lumen thrombectomy
  catheter
Seutin plaster scissors
Seutin plaster shears
seven-hole (7-hole) plate
severe acidosis
severe cardiac decompensation
severe hemorrhage
severe hypermetabolic state
severe hypersplenism
severe hypocalcemia
severe pain
severe salt-losing state
severe sunburn
severe thrombocytopenia
Sevrain cranial clamp
Sewall brain clip forceps
Sewall clip-applying forceps
Sewell retractor
sewing machine technique
sex chromatin mass
sex steroid
sexual precosity
sexual transmission
sexually transmitted disease
S-flap incision
Sgambati reaction or test for peritonitis
SGOT (serum glutamic-oxaloacetic
  transaminase) (now *AST*)
SGPT (serum glutamic-pyruvic
  transaminase) (now *ALT*)
shadowing, acoustic
shaking chill
shaking sound

Shaldon catheter
shallow mucosal ulcer
sham feeding test
sham therapy
Shambaugh-Derlacki duckbill elevator
Shambaugh fistula hook
Shambaugh irrigator
Shambaugh microscopic hook
Shambaugh narrow elevator
Shambaugh palpating needle
Shardle towel clip
shark liver oil
sharp and blunt dissection
sharp dissection
sharp hook
sharp knife
sharp retractor
sharp spoon
sharp versus dull
Sharplan SilkTouch flashscan surgical
  laser
Sharplan SilkTouch laser system
shave biopsy
shaver burr and cutter
Shaw aneurysm needle
Shaw catheter
Shaw electrical scalpel
Shaw II Teflon-coated hemostatic
  scalpel
SHC (sclerosing hepatic carcinoma)
Shea alligator forceps
Shea drill
Shea scissors
Shearer rongeur
shears (also see *scissors*)
  Bacon thoracic
  Baer rib
  Bethune-Coryllos rib
  Bethune rib
  biarticular bone
  Boehler plaster
  Brunner rib
  Bruns
  Bruns plaster

shears *(cont.)*
cloth
Collins rib
Cooley rib
Coryllos rib
Endo Shears
Esmarch plaster
first rib
Giertz-shoemaker rib
Gluck rib
Hercules plaster
Horsley-Stille rib
Ice hair trimming
LaparoSonic coagulating
Lefferts rib
Liston-Key-Horsley rib
Lorenz
Mcdicut
plaster
Potts rib
rib
Roberts rib
Roos first rib
Sauerbruch-Britsch rib
Sauerbruch-Frey rib
Sauerbruch rib
Schuchart rib
Schumacher rib
Semb rib
Seutin plaster
Shoemaker rib
Stille-Giertz rib
Stille plaster
Stille rib
subclavian peel-away
utility
Vantage first aid
sheath
anterior rectus
carotid
coaxial
cremasteric
ERA resectoscope
femoral

sheath *(cont.)*
fibrous
Hyfrecator pencil
introducer
Microgyn resectoscope
muscle
musculoaponeurotic
Passager introducing
posterior rectus
rectus
Slide-On EndoSheath
sliding
SLS (Spectranetics laser sheath)
subclavian peel-away
sheath ligament
sheath of muscle
Sheehan chisel
Sheehan gouge
Sheehan syndrome
Sheehy round knife
SheerVision loupe
sheeting, Silastic
Sheffield hand elevator
Sheldon hemilaminectomy retractor
Sheldon-Spatz vertebral arteriogram
needle
shelf
Blumer rectal
intraluminal
mesocolic
rectal
shelled out
shellfish, contaminated
shell out a cyst
shelving edge of Poupart ligament
Sheridan ET A6579CO2 Uncuffed
Sher-I-Temp skin temp sensor (Kendall)
Sherlock threaded suture anchor
Sherman bone plate
Sherpa guiding catheter
Sherwin knee retractor
Sherwood intrascopic suction/irrigation
system (for laparoscopic procedure)

shield
  corneal
  eye
  Fuller rectal
  laparoscope
  laser guard
  safety
  Saf-T E-Z translucent needle
  Slim Stem scleral
  Sutcliffe Boey laser
shifting dullness on percussion
shift of intravascular fluid volume into
  peritoneal space
shift to the left on WBC count
shift to the right on WBC count
Shiley tracheal tube
Shiley tracheotomy tube
Shiner tube
shiny mass
Shirley wound drain
shirt-stud abscess
shock
  anaphylactic
  bacterial
  electrical
  endotoxic
  hemorrhagic
  hypoglycemic
  hypovolemic
  insulin
  septic
  toxic
shock absorption
shock kidney
shock liver
shock lung
shock syndrome, toxic
shock with bleeding
shocks given on lithotripsy
shoe cookie (pad)
shoelace technique for delayed primary
  closure of fasciotomy
shoe of the hook
Shoemaker intestinal clamp

Shoemaker rib shears
Shohl solution
short angled curette
short axis parasternal view
short axis view
Shortbent stitch scissors
short-bowel syndrome
short chain fatty acids (SCFA)
ShortCut knife
shorter halflife
short esophagus
short gastric artery
short gastric vein
short gastric vessel (SGV)
short gastrics from the spleen
short gut syndrome
shorthand vertical mattress stitch
short length hepatic vein stenosis
  (SLHVS)
short limb Roux-en-Y gastroenteros-
  tomy
short loose 360° fundoplication
short right-angle dissector
short-scar procedure in breast reduction
short-scar tumescent reduction
  mammoplasty
short segment Barrett esophagus
  (SSBE)
short spatula electrode
short-term treatment
short vessel graft
shotgun pellet embolism
shotty breast
shotty lymph node
Shouldice herniorrhaphy
Shouldice operation for hernia repair
Shriner pin
shrinking liver volume
shrunken liver
shrunken lung
shunt
  Allen-Brown vascular access
  atriocaval
  barium sulfate impregnated

shunt *(cont.)*
   biliopancreatic
   Cordis-Hakim
   CSF (cerebrospinal fluid)
   cysto-atrial
   cystoperitoneal
   Denver hydrocephalus
   Denver peritoneal venous
   distal splenorenal (DSR)
   Drapanas
   DVP flush
   end-to-side portacaval
   end-to-side splenorenal
   endarterectomy
   endolymphatic
   esophageal
   FloCoil
   gastric venacaval
   Gott
   Hakim-Cortis ventriculoperitoneal
   hermetic external
   Heyer-Schulte neurosurgical
   high-pressure
   Hyde
   infant
   intrahepatic transjugular porto-
      systemic
   intrapulmonary
   Javid
   Kasai peritoneal venous shunt
   LeVeen peritoneal
   Linton
   low pressure
   lumbar arachnoid peritoneal
   lumbar thecoperitoneal
   lumboperitoneal (LP)
   medium pressure
   mesocaval H-graft
   mesocaval interposition
   mesocaval shunt (MCS)
   migration of
   modified Blalock-Taussig (MBTS)
   Ommaya ventriculoperitoneal
   one-piece

shunt *(cont.)*
   peritoneal-atrial
   peritoneal-venous
   peritoneocaval
   peritoneovenous (PVS)
   portacaval
   portal-systemic
   portopulmonary
   portosystemic
   portosystemic shunting
   posterior atrial fossa
   proximal splenorenal
   Pruitt-Inahara
   Pudenz
   side-to-side portacaval
   silicone elastomer
   small bowel
   Spetzler lumboperitoneal
   splenorenal
   subdural-to-peritoneal
   Sundt loop
   surgical
   surgical portosystemic
   thecoperitoneal
   transjugular intrahepatic porto-
      systemic (TIPS or TIPSS)
   T-tube
   UNI-SHUNT hydrocephalus
   ventriculoperitoneal
   ventriculoatrial (VA)
   ventriculojugular (VJ)
   ventriculoperitoneal (VP)
   ventriculosubarachnoid (VS)
   ventriculovenous
   Warren splenorenal
shunt failure, intermittent
shunt fraction
shunt function, cerebrospinal fluid
shunting of cerebrospinal fluid
shunting procedure
shunt malfunction
shunt patency test
shunt-related metastasis
shunt reservoir

shunt reversal
shunt revision
shunt syndrome
shunt tap
shunt tube
shunt valve
Shur-Clens wound cleanser
Shutt Mantis retrograde forceps
Shy-Drager syndrome
SI (International System of Units)
SI (saturation index) of bile
SI (sucrose-isomaltose)
SIA (strip immunoblot assay)
SIADH (syndrome of inappropriate
  antidiuretic hormone)
sialodochoplasty
sialography
sialolithotomy
sialorrhea
SIBS (surgical isolation bubble system)
sibutramine HCl
sickle cell anemia
sickle cell crisis
sickle cell disease
sickle knife
sickle-shape Beaver blade
sickle-shape blade
side-aspirating biopsy needle
side-biting clamp
side cutter
side-cutting spatulated needle
side effects of chemotherapy
side-hole recording site
side-hole sensor
side, ipsilateral
side-lying position
side-opening hook
side plate
sideropenic dysphagia
siderotic splenomegaly
side-to-side anastomosis
side-to-side anastomosis choledocho-
  choledochostomy

side-to-side anastomosis with small
  bowel
side-to-side portacaval shunt
side-viewing endoscope
sidewall of the bowel
sidewall, pelvic
SIDS (sudden infant death syndrome)
Siebold abdominal scissors
Siegel-Cattan-Mamou syndrome
Sieman irrigation injection needle
sieving of solid food
Siewerling-Creutzfeldt disease
SIF10 Olympus enteroscope
Siffert method
sigmaS serum tumor marker for breast
  cancer
sigmoidal artery
sigmoid anastomosis clamp
sigmoid artery
sigmoid carcinoma
sigmoid colectomy
sigmoid colon
sigmoid colon involvement
sigmoid colon reservoir
sigmoid colon twisted in counterclock-
  wise direction (sigmoid volvulus)
sigmoid colon volvulus
sigmoid colostomy
sigmoid curve
sigmoid diverticulitis
sigmoidectomy, hand-assisted
sigmoid-end colostomy
sigmoid flexure
sigmoid fold
sigmoiditis
  allergic
  dietetic
  infectious
sigmoid fossa
sigmoid kidney
sigmoid loop
sigmoid loop rod colostomy
sigmoid mesocolon

sign *(cont.)*
    "double duct"
    Federici
    fifth vital (pain)
    flapping tremor
    Fox
    Gilbert
    Grey Turner
    Grocco
    guarding
    hamburger
    Hamman
    Henning
    Horn
    Howship-Romberg
    iliopsoas
    inverted loop
    inverted V
    Kantor
    Kehr
    Klemm
    Kussmaul
    Lennhoff
    Leser-Trelat
    linguine
    liver flap
    lollipop tree (on x-ray)
    McBurney
    McCort
    meniscus
    moulage
    Murphy
    obturator
    omega
    pathognomonic (of a fistula)
    peritoneal
    pillow
    pruning
    psoas
    puddle
    pyloric string
    rat-tail
    RCS (red color)
    rebound

sign *(cont.)*
    red color (RCS)
    reversed Mercedes Benz
    Rigler
    Robertson
    Rosenbach
    Rovighi
    Rovsing
    sawtooth appearance
    Sister Mary Joseph
    stable vital
    Strauss
    string
    Sumner
    Terry fingernail
    tethered-bowel
    thumbprinting
    Trimadeau
    Troisier node
    Trousseau
    Turner
SignaDress hydrocolloid dressing
    material
Signa Special Procedures (SP) system
signet ring appearance
signet ring carcinoma
signet ring cell
signet ring cell carcinoma
signet ring pattern
signet ring type of gastric carcinoma
significant comorbid disease
significant long-term weight loss
signs and symptoms
signs of infection
signs of serosal involvement
Silace-C (docusate sodium)
Silastic catheter
Silastic collar-reinforced stoma
Silastic drip drain
Silastic ring
Silastic rod
Silastic sheeting
Silastic silo reduction of gastroschisis
Silastic stent

Silastic tape dressing
Silastic tube
Silberg graft passer
S ileal reservoir
S incision
silent abdomen
silent gallstone
silent reflux
silent thyroiditis
Silhouette laser system
silicone breast implant
silicone carving block
silicone catheter
silicone donut prosthesis
silicone elastomer band
silicone elastomer ring
silicone elastomer ring vertical gastro-
    plasty (SRVG)
silicone elastomer shunt
silicone flexor rod
silicone gel implant
silicone implant
silicone ring
silicone rubber Dacron-cuffed catheter
siliconized silk
silicon-velvet composite graft
Silkam suture
silk glove sign
Silk guidewire
Silk Laser aesthetic carbon dioxide
    laser for skin resurfacing
silk ligature
silk mesh gauze dressing
silk pop-off suture
silk seton
silk suture
Silk Touch laser skin resurfacing laser
silk traction suture
silo-filler's lung
Silon tent for gastroschisis
Silon wound dressing
Siltex silicone gel breast implant
Silvadene (silver sulfadiazine)
SilverBullet electrode

silver cell
silver filigree
silver finisher's lung
silver-fork deformity
Silverlon wound packing strips
Silverman-Boeker needle
Silverman needle
silver nitrate
silver probe
silver stools
silver sulfadiazine (SSD, SSD AF)
SIM (small intestine mesentery)
Simaal Gel 2 (aluminum hydroxide;
    magnesium hydroxide; simethicone)
simaldrate
Simeco
simethicone
simethicone-coated cellulose suspension
    (SCCS)
Similac with iron formula
Simmonds disease
Simmons chisel
Simmons plate
Simon abdominal retractor
Simonsen technique for large recto-
    vaginal fistula repair
Simplate bleeding time (BT)
simple cyst
simple goiter
simple liver amebic abscess
simple mastectomy
simple mechanical obstruction
simple obesity
Simple Suction Probe cannula
simple suture
Simplex adhesive
Simpson atherectomy catheter
Simpson forceps
Simpson-Luikart forceps
Simpson peripheral AtheroCath catheter
Simpson-Smith rectal suction tube
Sims abdominal scissors
Sims connector
Sims curette

Sims irrigation nozzle
Sims Portex
Sims position
Sims rectal speculum
Sims retractor
Sims uterine scissors
Sims vaginal speculum
Simulect (basiliximab) monoclonal
    antibody
SIMV (synchronous IMV)
sincalide
single-action jaws
single-action monopolar hook scissors
single-action rongeur
single and rapid polymerase chain
    reaction/restriction fragment length
    polymorphism (PCR/RFLP)
single-armed suture
SingleBAR electrode
single-blade saw
single cannula tracheal tube
single-chain intracellular precursor
single-contrast barium
single clamp
single fiber electromyography electrode
single-hook auto retractor
single-layer continuous closure
single-lumen papillotome
single onlay cortical bone graft
single-patient use (SPU) instrument
single pedicle flap
single pedicle TRAM flap
single photon emission tomography
    (SPECT)
single polyp
single-port, double-puncture
    laparoscopy
single-port laparoscopy
single-post Mayo stand
single-puncture laparoscope
single-stripe colitis (SSC)
single-use cannula
Singley intestinal forceps
Singley-Tuttle tissue forceps

singultus (hiccups)
sinogram
sinus
    anal
    medullary
    perineal
    pilonidal
    piriform
    Rokitansky-Aschoff
    sigmoid
    thyroglossal duct
sinus dressing
sinus tract
sinusitis
sinusoidal congestion
sinusoidal fibrosis
sinusoidal lymphocytes
sinusoidal pressure
sinusoid, hepatic
Sipple syndrome (MEA type II)
Sippy diet
Sippy esophageal dilator
sirolimus
SIRS (systemic inflammatory response
    syndrome)
SIRS/sepsis (systemic inflammatory
    response syndrome)
SIS wound dressing
Sisson fracture reducing elevator
Sister Mary Joseph lymph node
Sister Mary Joseph node
Sister Mary Joseph sign
Sistrunk dissecting scissors
site
    exit
    hormone receptor
    incision
    port
    puncture
    recipient
    side-hole recording
    stoma
    surgical
    trocar

SiteGuard MVP transparent adhesive film dressing
site of phagocytosis
Site ~ Rite 3 ultrasound system
SiteSelect percutaneous breast biopsy system
SITEtrac endoscope
situs inversus
situs inversus viscerum
sitz bath
Sitzmarks radiopaque marker
six-hole (6-hole) plate
six-strand suture
six-wire basket
SJM Rosenkranz pediatric retractor
Sjögren syndrome
skate-flap technique of nipple reconstruction
skeletal hyperostosis
skeletal metastasis
skeletal muscle cell
skeletal traction pin
skeletonize (verb)
skeletonized
Skene tenaculum forceps
skid humeral head retractor
ski-jump view
Skil saw
skin
    anicteric
    Composite Cultured Skin (CCS)
    dimpling of
    dusky
    fair
    hyperpigmentation of
    icteric
    jaundiced
    nonicteric
    pale
    perianal
    peristomal
    scaly
skin adhesive (see *adhesives*)
skin approximation

skin blade
skin blade knife
skin change
skin cleanser (see *cleanser; medications*)
skin clip
skin crease incision
skin defect
skin edema
skin flap
skinfold thickness
skinfold thickness test
skin glue
skin graft (see also *graft*)
    Braun
    Douglas
    Dragstedt
    Esser
    free
    full-thickness
    Krause-Wolfe
    Ollier-Thiersch
    pedicle
    postage-stamp type
    split-thickness
skin graft material
skin hook
skin incision
skin induration
skin infection
skin knife
skin lesion
Skinlight erbium YAG laser
skin line
Skinmarker and Ruler markers
skin markings of lymphedema (peau d'orange)
Skinmate marker
skin necrosis
skin preparation
skin replacement (see *skin substitute*)
skin retraction
skin staple
skin stapling

skin stone
skin striae
skin substitute (also see *graft*)
    Biobrane adhesive
    Biobrane glove
    Biobrane/HF
    Dermagraft-TC
    TransCyte
skin suture
skin tag
skin temperature monitoring probe
skin turgor, decreased
skin ulcer
Skin retractor (trachea)
Skin Skribe skin marker in surgery
skinny Chiba needle
skinny needle
skinny needle technique
Skinny dilatation catheter
Skinscan laser surgery device
SkinTegrity hydrogel dressing
Skinvisible hypoallergenic hand lotion
skip area
skip lesion (of Crohn disease)
ski position
Sklar disposable anoscope
skull bone graft
skull clamp
skull film
skull pin
skull plate
skull punch
skull punch forceps
Skylight system
skyline view
slave balloon
SLE (systemic lupus erythematosus)
SLE-like syndrome
sleep apnea
sleeve
    Dent
    laparoscopic
    laparoscopic trocar
    Pneumo Sleeve
    Williams overtube

sleeve of laparoscope
sleeve sensor
SLHVS (short-length hepatic vein stenosis)
Slick endotracheal styler
Slide-On EndoSheath
slide plate
slide, ThinPrep
sliding barrel hook
sliding clamp
sliding component
sliding esophageal hiatal hernia
sliding hernia
sliding hiatal hernia
sliding inlay graft
sliding sheath
Slim Fit Flex Camp
Slim Stem scleral shield
sling
    fascial
    Hemi Sling
    puborectalis
    SurgiSis sling/mesh
sling and swathe bandage
sling muscle fibers
Slinky catheter
slip joint pliers
slipknot
Slip-N-Snip scissors
slipped Nissen fundoplication
slit/cut mesh graft
slitlike defect
Slocum meniscal clamp
Slocum nail
slotted anoscope
slotted cannula
slotted femur plate
slotted hammer
slotted mallet
slotted needle
slotted speculum
sloughing of mucosa
slough of nipple
slough of skin

slow bleed
slow colonic transit
slow-growing skin mass
slowing of gastric emptying
slow intermittent blood loss
slowly enlarging mass
slow virus
SLP1000 (super long-pulse) diode laser
   system
SLS (Spectranetics laser sheath)
SLS Chromos 694 long-pulse ruby laser
   system
sludge
   bile
   biliary
   blood
   gallbladder
sludged blood
slurry of stool
slush machine
slush machine drape
SMA (smooth muscle antibody)
SMA (superior mesenteric artery)
SMA chemistry panel
SMA formula
SMAC ("smack") panel
small accessory vein
small aperture
small bowel
small bowel congenital abnormality
small bowel contrast study
small bowel enema
small bowel enteroscopy (SBE)
small bowel fistula
small bowel follow-through
small bowel infarct
small bowel injury
small bowel meal
small bowel mesentery
small bowel mucosa
small bowel obstruction (SBO)
small bowel perforation
small bowel plus liver transplantation
small bowel resection

small bowel series
small bowel shunt
small bowel transit time
small bowel transplantation
small bowel tube
small-caliber esophagogastro-
   duodenoscopy
small-caliber stools
small cell anaplastic carcinoma
small cell carcinoma
small cell lung carcinoma (SCLC)
small cell tumor
small-droplet fatty liver
small egress cannula
small fibroadenoma
small granule cell
small hernia defect
small inferior artery to the thyroid
small intestine
small intestine bacterial overgrowth
   (SIBO)
small intestine dysmotility
small intestine endoscopy
small intestine enteroscopy
small intestine gland
small intestine leiomyosarcoma
small intestine malignant lymphoma
small intestine transit time
small lymphocytic lymphoma
small noncleaved cell lymphoma
small of back pain
small rake retractor
small round cell carcinoma
small round cell infiltrate
small-stomach syndrome
small to intermediate lymphoid cells
small vessel to the splenic pulp
small window
S.M.A.R.T. (shape memory alloy
   recoverable technology) biliary stent
SmartDose prefilled infusion system
smart loop coagulator
SmartNail
SmartNeedle

Smart Scalpel
SMAS (superior mesenteric artery
   syndrome)
Smead-Jones closure
smear (see also *stain, test*)
   AFB (acid-fast bacillus)
   air-dried
   alimentary tract
   bacteriologic
   blood
   bronchoscopic
   cul-de-sac
   cytologic
   eosinophil
   fast
   feces
   fungal
   KOH
   lower respiratory tract
   malaria
   nasal
   oral
   Pap (Papanicolaou)
   peripheral
   peripheral blood
   potassium hydroxide (KOH)
   pus
   sputum
   stool
   Tzanck
   urine
   wet
Smedberg hand drill
Smedberg twist drill
SMF (streptozocin, mitomycin C, and
   5-FU) chemotherapy protocol
Smiley-Williams arteriogram needle
smile incision
smiling incision
Smillie-Beaver knife
Smillie cartilage chisel
Smillie cartilage knife
Smillie hook
Smillie knee retractor

Smillie meniscotomy chisel
Smillie meniscus hook retractor
Smillie meniscus knife
Smillie meniscus scissors
Smillie nail
Smillie perforator
Smith & Nephew Richards rod
Smith & Nephew video camera system
Smith anal retractor
Smith automatic perforator drill
Smith bandage scissors
Smith bone clamp
Smith-Buie rectal retractor
Smith-Buie rectal speculum
Smith cartilage knife
Smith cranial drill
Smith nerve root suction retractor
Smith-Petersen chisel
Smith-Petersen curved gouge
Smith-Petersen femoral neck nail
Smith-Petersen gooseneck gouge
Smith-Petersen intertrochanteric plate
Smith-Petersen laminectomy rongeur
Smith-Petersen pin
Smith-Petersen plate
Smith-Petersen reamer
Smith-Petersen straight gouge
Smith-Petersen transarticular nail
Smith rectal retractor
Smith scissors
Smith test
Smith wire-cutting scissors
Smithwick button hook
Smithwick clip-applying forceps
Smithwick hook
Smithwick nerve hook
Smithwick nerve hook and dissector
Smithwick sympathectomy hook
SMM (scintimammography)
SMO (supramalleolar orthosis) plate
smoke eliminator, Core laparoscopic
smoke evacuation unit
smoke plume
smoker's lung

SmokEvac electrosurgical probe
SmokEvac trumpet-valve smoke
  evacuator
smoking
smooth diet
smooth goiter
smooth muscle
smooth muscle antibody (SMA)
smooth muscle motility disorder
smooth Steinmann pin
smooth-tipped jeweler's forceps
smooth tissue forceps
smooth tongue
SMV (superior mesenteric vein)
SMX/TMP (sulfamethoxazole and
  trimethoprim)
snake retractor
Snap Kover
snapper plunger lock
snaptrace silver chloride sensor
snap-twist plunger lock
snare
    Carr-Locke
    diathermy rectal
    Douglas rectal
    electrosurgical
    endoscopic
    Eve tonsil
    Frankfeldt rectal
    Frankfeldt rectal diathermy
    Krause nasal
    long-nose retriever
    Nakao I and II
    Norwood rectal
    Olympus disposable
    polypectomy
    rectal
    Tydings tonsil-seizing
    Weston rectal
    Wilson-Cook polypectomy
snare cautery
snared
snare loop biopsy
snare resection (band and snare)

snare technique
snare wires
Snitman endaural retractor
Snowden-Pencer forceps
Snowden-Pencer scissors
snuffbox, anatomical
Snugs bandage
Snugs dressing
Soaker Catheter
soapsuds enema (SSE)
Soave abdominal pull-through operation
Soave endorectal pull-through operation
social drinker
Society of American Gastrointestinal
  Endoscopic Surgeons (SAGES)
Society of Laparoendoscopic Surgeons
socket pin
SOD (sebaceous cysts, osteomas,
  desmoid tumors)
SOD (sphincter of Oddi dysfunction)
sodium (Na)
sodium amidotrizoate
sodium bicarbonate
sodium citrate
sodium diatrizoate with Menoquinon
sodium/H_2O retention
sodium iodine (^{131}I)
sodium iodine (^{123}I) thyroid function
  test
sodium iodine (^{125}I) thyroid function
  test
sodium iodipamide
sodium iopamide contrast medium
sodium iopodate
sodium iothalamate
sodium ioxaglate
sodium ipodate
sodium lactate, compound solution of
sodium loading
sodium metrizoate
sodium morrhuate
sodium nitroprusside (SNP)
sodium oxybate
sodium perborate

sodium phosphate
sodium restriction
sodium stibogluconate
sodium tetradecyl (STD) sulfate
sodium tetradecyl sulfate sclerosant
sodium tyropanoate
Soehendra dilator
Soehendra stent retriever
Sof-Band bulky bandage dressing
Sofield pin
Sofield retractor
Sof-Kling dressing
Sofpulse pulsed magnetic energy device
Sofrature gauze
Sof-Rol dressing
Sofsilk braided silk suture
Sofsilk nonabsorbable silk suture
SofSilk suture
SofSorb absorptive dressing
soft abdomen
Sof-Tact glucose monitor
soft bland diet
soft bulky dressing
Softcat chromic suture
Softcat plain suture
SoftCloth absorptive dressing
SoftFlex computer glove
soft food dysphagia
soft goiter
Soft Guard XL Skin Barrier for ostomy
    skin
Softgut surgical chromic suture
soft laser
SoftLight laser
Soft N Dry Merocel sponge
soft palate
soft papilloma
Softscan laser mammography system
Softscan laser scanner
soft spleen
soft stool
Soft Thoracoport obturator
soft tissue
soft tissue abscess

soft tissue mass
soft tissue necrosis
soft tissue sarcoma
soft tissue shaving cannula (liposhaver)
soft tissue stranding
Soft Torque uterine catheter
Soft-Vu Omni flush catheter
Sof-Wick drain sponge
Sof-Wick dressing
Sof-Wick lap pad
Sof-Wick sponge dressing
solid bolus challenge
solid crystals
solid food dysphagia
Solidifier fluid solidification system,
    The
solid mass
solid organ transplant
solid organ transplantation
solid sphere test
solid state esophageal manometry
    catheter
solitary adenoma
solitary benign adenoma
solitary gland of large intestine
solitary lactiferous duct
solitary lesion
solitary lymph node
solitary myeloma
solitary nodule
solitary rectal ulcer syndrome (SRUS)
solitary thyroid nodule
solitary tumor
solitary ulcer syndrome
Solo catheter with Pro/Pel coating
    catheter
SoloPass catheter
SoloPass stent/catheter
Solo-Prep topical scrub
Solos cystoscope
Solos endoscope
SoloSite hydrogel dressing
SoloSite wound gel
Solos rigid laparoscope

Spacemaker VBD-300 dissector
space-occupying disease
space-occupying lesion
space of Bogros
space of Retzius
Space-OR flexible internal retractor
SpaceSEAL cannula
Spachmann tube
span
   digit
   levator
   liver
Spand-Gel dressing
Sparkles (sodium bicarbonate; citric
   acid; simethicone)
spasm
   anal
   bladder
   diffuse esophageal (DES)
   esophageal
spasmodic colic
spasmodic stricture
Spasmolin (atropine sulfate; scopol-
   amine hydrobromide; hyoscyamine
   hydrobromide; phenobarbital)
Spasmophen
spastic colon
spastic constipation
spastic esophagus
spastic ileus
Spastosed (calcium carbonate;
   magnesium carbonate)
spatula
   bladder
   bow-shaped
   Davis
   distal
   Haberer abdominal
   Kocher bladder
   micropoint
   Reverdin abdominal
   Sabreloc conventional
   Sachs nerve
   spoon-shaped

spatula *(cont.)*
   Tuffier abdominal
   Ultima
spatula electroprobe
spatula electrode
spatula forceps
spatula One-Piece cannula
spatula-tip Toomey syringe cannula
Spay scissors
Speare dural hook
specialized columnar cells
specialized intestinal metaplasia
specialized tissue-aspirating resecto-
   scope (STAR)
specific gravity
specific, layered infiltration
specimen knife
specimen retrieval bag
   Endo Catch
   Endobag laparoscopic
   EndoMate endoscopic
specimen, yarn-collected
speckled appearance
speckled pattern
SPECT (single photon emission
   computerized tomography) scan
Spectranetics laser sheath (SLS) laser
SpectraScience biopsy forceps
SpectraScience Optical Biopsy system
SpectraScience reusable biopsy forceps
spectrometry, *Salmonella* and
   Campylobacter-specific mass
spectroscopy
   fluorescence
   light-scattering
   reflectance
Spectrum adjustable breast implant
speculum
   Alan-Parks rectal
   Auvard
   Barr rectal
   Barr-Shuford rectal
   Beckman nasal
   Bensaude rectal

speculum *(cont.)*
  beveled
  Bodenhammer rectal
  Brewer
  Brinkerhoff rectal
  Chelsea Eaton anal
  Cook rectal
  Cusco vaginal
  Cusco "Swiss pattern" vaginal
  Czerny rectal
  David rectal
  Fansler
  Ferguson-Moon
  Fergusson
  Gabriel rectal
  Graves
  Graves vaginal
  Halle infant
  Hartmann nasal
  Hinkle-James rectal
  Hirschman
  House stapes
  Kelly rectal
  Killian rectal
  Killian septum
  KleenSpec disposable
  Kogan
  Kogan-Burke
  Kristeller
  Martin-Davis rectal
  Mathews rectal
  Mathier trivalve rectal
  Mathieu rectal
  Miltex
  Naunton Morgan rectal
  Parks rectal
  Pederson
  Pennington rectal
  Pratt rectal
  rectal
  Ricord rectal
  Roschke rectal
  Sawyer rectal

speculum *(cont.)*
  Sims rectal
  slotted
  Smith-Buie rectal
  SRT (smoke-retrieval tube) vaginal
  vantage Graves vaginal
  Vernon-David rectal
  Vienna nasal
Speedy balloon catheter
Spence intervertebral disk rongeur
Spence rongeur forceps
Spence, tail of
Spencer disease
Spencer scissors
Spencer stitch scissors
Spencer Wells artery forceps
Spenco breast prosthesis
Sperma-Tex preshaped mesh graft
spermatic cord
spermatic vessel
Spetzler lumboperitoneal shunt
Spexil (trospectomycin)
sphenoethmoidal suture
spheno-occipital suture
spheno-orbital suture
sphenoparietal suture
sphenopetrosal suture
sphenosquamous suture
sphenotemporal suture
sphenovomerine suture
spherical lesion
spherical neoplasm
spherical reamer
spherocytosis
spheroplast, mycobacterial
sphincter
  anal
  anorectal
  antral
  artificial
  basal
  bicanalicular
  biliary
  Boyden

sphincter *(cont.)*
  canalicular
  cardiac (stomach)
  cardioesophageal
  choledochal
  colic
  cricopharyngeal
  duodenal
  duodenojejunal
  esophageal
  external anal
  external rectal
  extrinsic
  first duodenal
  gastroesophageal
  Giordano
  hyperactive
  hypertensive lower esophageal
  Hyrtl
  incompetent
  inferior esophageal
  inguinal
  internal anal (IAS)
  internal rectal
  lower esophageal (LES)
  Lütkens (Luetkens)
  mechanically defective
  Nélaton
  Oddi
  O'Beirne
  pancreatic duct
  pancreaticobiliary
  pharyngoesophageal
  prepyloric
  pyloric
  rectal
  upper esophageal (UES)
sphincteral achalasia
sphincter atony
sphincter contraction ring
sphincter dysfunction
sphincterectomy
sphincteric mechanism
sphincter of anal canal, involuntary

sphincter of bile duct
sphincter of hepatopancreatic ampulla
sphincter of Oddi dysfunction (SOD)
sphincter of Oddi manometry
sphincter of Oddi pressure measure-
  ment
sphincter of Oddi spasm
sphincteroplasty
  anal
  transduodenal
sphincteroscope
sphincterotome
  balloon
  basket
  Demling-Classen
  hybrid
  needle knife
  Olympus
  precut
  reverse
  rotating
  Wilson-Cook (modified) wire-
    guided
sphincterotomy (see also *operations*)
  biliary
  Doubilet
  endoscopic (ES)
  internal
  lateral internal
  Mulholland
  Parks
  Parks partial
  precut
  retrograde
  transduodenal
  "zipper"
sphincterotomy basket
sphincterotomy of papilla
sphincterotomy with stone extraction
sphincter-saving operation
sphincter tone
sphincter urethral muscle
sphingomyelin accumulation in liver
  and spleen

sphygmomanometer
  analog
  Diagnostix
  digital
  Multikuf
  Prosphyg
  Tycos aneroid
SPI-Argent II peritoneal dialysis
  catheter
spica bandage
spiculated mass
spiculations on colon
spicule in profile
spicy food
spider angioma (pl. angiomata;
  angiomas)
spider nevus (pl. nevi)
spider telangiectasia
spider-web clot
Spiess 25 4 mm rigid laparoscope
Spiess endoscope
spigelian fascia
spigelian hernia
spigelian hernia belt
Spigelian line
spike a fever
spike-burst electrical activity
spike burst on electromyogram of colon
spike, fever
spiking fever
spillage of tumor cells
spilled gallstones
spinach stool
spinal afferent
spinal anesthesia
spinal cord injury, concomitant
spinal cord removal instrument
spinal drain
spinal elevator
spinal epidural abscess (SEA)
spinal fluid
spinal fusion gouge
spinal fusion position
spinal headache

spinal immobilization
spinal medulla
spinal needle
spinal perforating forceps
spinal retractor blade
spinal rod
spinal stenosis
spindle cell carcinoma
spindle cell sarcoma
spindle cell thymoma
spindle colonic groove
spindle-shaped incision
spine, anterior superior iliac
SpineCATH intradiscal catheter
Spinelli biopsy needle
SpineScope percutaneous endoscope
spinocan spinal needle
spiral bandage
spiral basket forceps
spiral computed tomography
spiral cortical reamer
spiral CT
spiral drill
spiral fold
spiraling of rectal mucosa
spiral-shaped bacteria
spiral trochanteric reamer
spiral valve of Heister
SpiraStent ureteral stent
spirit lamp
spirochetal jaundice
spirochetosis, Lancereaux-Mathieu-
  Weil
SpiroFlo bioabsorbable prostate stent
spirometry, incentive
spironolactone
Spiros inhaler
Spivack valve
splanchnic anesthesia
splanchnic AV fistula
splanchnic nerve
splanchnic pressure
splanchnic retractor
splanchnic vasoconstriction

splenium
splenobronchial fistula
splenocolic ligament
splenogastric omentum
splenoid gland
splenomegalic cirrhosis
splenomegaly
   chronic congestive
   congenital
   congestive
   Egyptian
   fibrocongestive
   Gaucher
   hemolytic
   infectious
   infective
   myelophthisic
   siderotic
   spodogenous
splenoportal hypertension
splenoportography, magnetic resonance
splenoptosis
splenorenal anastomosis
splenorenal angle
splenorenal ligament
splenorenal recess
splenorenal shunt
splenorenal vein anastomosis
splenorenal venous operation
splenorrhaphy
splenosis, thoracic
splinter forceps
splinting of abdomen
splinting of incision with pillow
split calvarial bone graft
split ileostomy
split incision
split overtube
split-sheath catheter
split-thickness skin graft
SPN (support parenteral nutrition)
spodogenous splenomegaly
SpO$_2$ finger probe for pulse oximetry

sponge
   absorbable
   absorbable collagen
   absorbable gelatin
   Actifoam
   autocount
   Avitene Ultrafoam collagen
      hemostatic
   bronchial
   butterfly
   cherry
   cherry dissector
   cherry endosponge
   cherry-pit
   Col-R-Sponge
   corneal shield
   cylindrical
   Delicot
   diamond knife
   dissecting
   dissector
   ear packing
   ear wick
   Eder rectal
   eye spear
   eye wick
   fibrin
   flat stick
   4 x 4
   gauze
   gelatin
   Helistat absorbable collagen
      hemostatic
   impregnated
   Incert
   Incert bioabsorbable implantable
   instrument wipe
   Ivalon
   K-dissector
   Kerlix disposable laparotomy
   Kittner
   Kling
   Krimpt
   K-Sponge

spot film
spot view
S pouch, ileal
spout, ileal
Sprague Rappaport stethoscope
Spratt curet
SprayGel Adhesion Barrier System
spreader
    Benson pylorus
    bladder neck
    cast
    Finochietto rib
    Hennig cast
    Mayo-Adams
    Millin bladder neck
    pyloric
    rib
    Tuffier rib
spreader graft
spreading forceps
spread suture
Spring Clip surgical stapler
Spring Grip surgical stapler
spring-handled scissors
spring hook
spring-loaded nail
spring-loaded, retractable blunt inner
    protective tube
spring-wire retractor
Sprinz-Dubin syndrome
Sprinz-Nelson syndrome
Sprotte needle
sprue
    celiac
    collagenous
    nontropical
    secondary nontropical
    tropical
S/P (status post) surgical blade
SPT (station pull-through) technique
S-P-T (thyroid, desiccated porcine)
SP-303, SP-501 Sonoprobe endoscopy
    system
SPTL-1b vascular lesion laser

SPU (single-patient use) instrument
spud and needle
spud dissector
spur-crushing clamp
Spurling intervertebral disk rongeur
Spurling-Kerrison cervical rongeur
Spurling-Kerrison laminectomy rongeur
Spurling-Kerrison rongeur forceps
Spurling-Kerrison up-biting and down-
    biting rongeur
Spurling nerve root retractor
Spurling pituitary rongeur
spurting blood
sputum smear
SPV (selective proximal vagotomy)
Spyglass angiography catheter
Spyrogel hydrogel wound and burn
    dressing
SQS-20 subcuticular skin stapler
squamocolumnar junction
squamocolumnar mucosal junction
squamosomastoid suture
squamosoparietal suture
squamososphenoid suture
squamous anal intraepithelial lesion
squamous carcinoma
squamous carcinoma in situ
squamous cell carcinoma (SCC)
squamous cell carcinoma antigen
squamous cell carcinoma of the
    esophagus
squamous intraepithelial lesion
squamous island
squamous lining
squamous metaplasia
squamous papilloma
squamous suture
square hollow chisel
square knot
square-L electrode
square reamer
square-shaped awl
squeeze pressure profile of anal
    sphincter

squeeze, sphincteric
Squirt wound irrigator
S retractor
SRH (stigmata of recent hemorrhage)
SRMD (stress-related mucosal disease)
S-ROM total hip system
SRT (smoke removal tube) vaginal
    speculum
SRUS (solitary rectal ulcer syndrome)
SRVG (silicone elastomer ring vertical
    gastroplasty)
SS (somatostatin)
Ssabanejew-Frank gastrostomy
SSBE (short segment Barrett
    esophagus)
SSC (single-stripe colitis)
SSD, SSD AF (silver sulfadiazine)
SSE (soapsuds enema)
S-shaped brain retractor
S-shaped ileal pouch
S-shaped incision
S-shaped reservoir
S660 small vessel stent
SSRI (selective serotonin reuptake
    inhibitor)
stabilization plate
stabilizer, Octopus tissue
stabilizing staple
stable diabetes mellitus
stable vital signs
stab incision
stab wound
stab wound incision
Stack autoperfusion balloon
Stack hand retractor
Stader pin
stage A Hodgkin disease
stage B Hodgkin disease
stage, Hinchey diverticulitis
stage I or II medullary carcinoma
staghorn calculus
staghorn stone
staging (see *classification*)

staging and defining arterial and venous
    involvement
staging celiotomy
staging laparotomy
staging neoplasm
staging of cancer, surgical
staging of cervical carcinoma
staging of malignancy
staging of malignant melanoma
staging operation
stagnant bile
stagnant loop syndrome
stagnation of blood
Stahl clip applier
stain (see also *dye*)
    anti-Schiff
    esterase
    Gram
    hematoxylin and eosin (H&E)
    indigo carmine
    Lugol solution
    methylene blue
    oil-red-O
    PAS
    peroxidase
    rhodanine
    Sudan
    toluidine blue
    Wright
    Ziehl-Neelsen
stainless steel clamp
stainless steel mesh
stainless steel plate
stainless steel preformed skull plate
stainless steel staple
stainless steel surgical blade
stainless steel suture
stainless steel wire
stainless steel wire suture
stairstep air-fluid levels
stale fish syndrome
stalk of polyp
Stamey-Malecot catheter

stapler *(cont.)*
 circular
 Cobe
 curved circular
 DePalma
 double-headed PI90
 EEA (end-to-end anastomosis)
 EEA Auto Suture
 Endoclip II surgical
 Endo Close surgical
 Endo GIA surgical
 Endo GIA II
 Endo Hernia
 Endo Hernia surgical
 Endo Hernia Universal
 Endopath EMS hernia
 Endopath ES reusable endoscopic
 Endopath EZ45 No Knife endo-
  scopic linear
 Endopath linear cutter
 Endopath multifeed
 Endopath no-knife
 Endo Stitch
 endoscopic articulating (EAS)
 endoscopic multifeed (EMS) TA-90
 GIA (gastrointestinal anastomosis)
  surgical
 hemoclip
 ILS (intraluminal stapler) surgical
 In-Tac bone anchor
 LDS surgical
 linear
 Multifire Endo GIA
 Multifire Endo Hernia
 Multifire GIA surgical
 Multifire TA surgical
 Multifire VersaTack
 No Knife
 Origin Tacker
 PI surgical
 PolyGIA
 Premium CEEA circular
 Premium Plus CEEA disposable
  stapler

stapler *(cont.)*
 ProTack
 Proximate flexible linear
 Proximate ILS curved intraluminal
 Proximate linear cutter
 Roticulator
 S*D* sorb
 Spring Clip
 Spring Grip surgical
 SQS-20 subcuticular skin
 stainless steel
 Surgeons Choice
 Surgigrip
 Surgineedle surgical
 TA-30 Auto Suture
 TA-55 Auto Suture
 TA90-BN
 3M
 TL-90
 VCS Clip adapter
 VersaTack
 Visistat
stapler-facilitated rectal eversion
staple-shaped retractor
staple the mesoappendix
staple the overlying peritoneum shut
stapling device
stapling esophagodiverticulostomy by
 endoscopy
stapling, gastric
stapling off of small gastric pouch
STAR (specialized tissue-aspirating
 resectoscope)
STAR (study of tamoxifen and
 raloxifene)
StarBAR electrode
STAR excimer laser system
starch bandage
starch blocker
starch peritonitis
Starck dilator
Starion thermal cautery hook
Starline select instruments
Starlix (nateglinide)

Stellbrink synovectomy rongeur
stem base plate
stem cell autograft
stenosis
   ampullary
   anal
   antral
   aortic valve
   arterial
   benign papillary
   bowel
   bronchial
   cardiac valvular
   cervical
   choledochoduodenal junctional
   congenital hypertrophic pyloric
   congenital pyloric
   discrete
   esophageal
   hiatal
   hypertrophic pyloric
   inflamed (of sigmoid colon)
   intestinal
   left-sided segmental portal
   mitral
   papillary
   pulmonary
   pyloric
   rectal
   short length hepatic vein (SLHVS)
   spinal
   stomal
stenosis of anastomosis
stenosis of breast duct
stenosis of esophageal hiatus
stenosis of pouch
stenosis of renal artery
stenotic lesion
stenotic segment
Stenotrophomonas maltophilia
stent
   Acculink self-expanding
   ACS Multi-Link OTW Duet
   ACS RX Multi-Link

stent *(cont.)*
   Amsterdam
   Anaconda
   Anastaflo
   AneuRX
   AngioStent balloon-expandable
   autologous vein-covered
   balloon-expandable
   Bard Memotherm colorectal
   Bard XT bifurcated
   beStent
   beStent Rival
   biliary
   BioSorb resorbable urology
   Biostent
   Bx Velocity
   Bx Velocity coronary artery
   Bx Velocity sirolimus-coated
   carboplatin-coated plastic biliary
   Champion nitinol
   choledochal
   colorectal
   Cook Oasis biliary
   coronary
   CrossFlex LC
   CrossFlex TMLC coronary
   crutched stick-type biliary duct
   Czaja-McCaffrey rigid
   double pigtail
   DoubleStent biliary endoprosthesis
   Dynalink self-expanding biliary
   EES (expandable esophageal)
   endobiliary
   ENDOcare nitinol
   EndoCoil biliary
   EndoCoil esophageal
   endoscopic biliary
   endovascular
   Enforcer SDS
   EsophaCoil self-expanding
     esophageal
   esophageal
   esophageal Z-Stent with Dua
     antireflux valve

stent *(cont.)*
    expandable metal
    Firlit drip
    flexible
    Flexima biliary
    French
    GFX 2
    Gianturco expandable (self-expanding) metallic biliary
    Gianturco-Rösch Z-stent
    Gianturco-Roubin flexible coil
    GR II
    Harrell Y
    Hemobahn
    Hepamed-coated Wiktor
    Herculink 14 biliary
    HIPS (heparin infusion prior to stenting)
    Hood stoma
    Horizon
    INR neurological
    InStent self-expanding
    IntraStent DoubleStrut biliary endoprosthesis
    IntraStent DoubleStrut XS
    IntraStent LP biliary
    intravascular
    INX stainless steel
    iridium-192-loaded
    IRIS coronary
    IsoStent radioisotope
    Lubri-Flex
    Megalink biliary
    Memotherm biliary
    Memotherm colorectal
    Memotherm Flexx biliary
    Memotherm nitinol
    Memotherm nitinol self-expanding
    Merogel
    Microvasive Rapid Exchange biliary system
    Mini Crown
    MPD (main pancreatic duct)
    Multi-Flex

stent *(cont.)*
    Multi-Link Tetra
    neurovascular
    NexStent carotid
    NIR ON Ranger
    NIR Primo Monorail
    Niroyal Elite Monorail
    Niroyal Monorail
    nitinol
    Olympus biliary
    OmniStent
    ostiomeatal
    Palmaz
    Palmaz balloon-expandable
    Palmaz Corinthian
    Palmaz Corinthian transhepatic biliary
    Palmaz-Schatz
    Palmaz-Schatz balloon-expandable
    Palmaz-Schatz Crown
    Palmaz-Schatz Crown balloon-expandable
    Palmaz-Schatz Mini Crown
    Palmaz-Schatz (PSS)
    Palmaz vascular
    pancreatic
    pancreatic duct
    Paragon Champion
    Paragon coronary
    Percuflex Plus
    percutaneous
    Perflex
    Perflex stainless steel
    pigtail
    Pilling Weck Y-stent forceps
    pliable
    PowerGrip
    preoperative endoscopic biliary
    ProstaCoil self-expanding
    radioisotope
    Radius
    RX Herculink
    RX Herculink 14 biliary
    RX Herculink 14 pre-mounted

stent *(cont.)*
    S.M.A.R.T. (shape memory alloy recoverable technology) biliary
    S660 small vessel
    SAXX renal
    self-expanding metal
    self-expanding metallic wall
    self-expanding microporous (SEMS)
    SEMS (self-expanding microporous)
    Silastic
    SMART biliary
    SoloPass
    SpiraStent ureteral
    SpiroFlo bioabsorbable prostate
    splenic vein
    straight
    Strecker
    Supra G
    Symphony
    Symphony nitinol
    Talent LPS
    transhepatic biliary
    T-tube
    T–Y
    Ultraflex Diamond biliary
    Ultraflex
    Uni-trac
    UroCoil self-expanding
    UroLume
    U-tube
    Vistaflex biliary
    Wallstent
    Wiktor
    Wiktor GX Hepamed
    Wilson-Cook French
    X-Trode
    XT
    Z
stent-assisted angioplasty
stent dressing
stenting, endobiliary
stent placement
stent remover, Carr-Locke
stent retriever, Soehendra

Stenver view
Stenzel rod
step-cut reamer
step-down effect
step drill
Step minimally invasive surgical access device
step-on can
step section
stercolith, appendiceal
stercoraceous vomiting
stercoral appendicitis
stercoral diarrhea
stercoral ulcer
stercoral ulceration
StereoEndoscope
StereoGuide stereotactic needle core biopsy
StereoScope camera head
stereotactic aspiration biopsy
stereotactic biopsy needle
stereotactic brain biopsy
stereotactic breast biopsy
stereotactic core needle biopsy (SCNB)
stereotactic laser microsurgery
stereotactic (or stereotaxic) operating microscope
stereotactic transsphenoidal hypophysectomy
stereotaxic endoscope
stereotaxically guided interstitial laser therapy
Stericare glycerine hydrogel dressing
Steri-Drape plastic incise drape
sterile drape
sterile dressing
sterilely prepared and draped
sterilely prepped and draped
sterile necrotizing pancreatitis
sterile pancreatic necrosis
sterile paper drape
steri-stripped incision
Steri-Strips dressing
Steri-Strips suture

sternal pleural reflection
sternal retractor
sternal split approach
sternal-splitting incision
sternal wire suture
Sternberg-Reed cell
sternocleidomastoid muscle or forearm
    autograft of parathyroid gland
sternocostal hiatus
sternotomy incision
sternotomy saw
steroid
    contraceptive
    nonabsorbable
steroid-dependent patient
steroid foam enema
steroid synthesis inhibition
steroid taper
Sterrad sterilization system
Stethodop, Adscope
stethoscope
    Bowles
    DeLee-Hillis
    Littmann Cardiology III
    Littmann Classic II S.E.
    Littmann Master Cardiology
    Littmann Master Classic II
    Littre hernia
    Mon-a-therm esophageal
    Sprague Rappaport
Stetten intestinal clamp
Stevens-Johnson syndrome
Stevenson alligator forceps
Stevenson grasping forceps
Stevens tenotomy scissors
Stewart crypt hook
St. George hemorrhoid-seizing forceps
stick sponge
stick-tie
Stieglitz splinter forceps
Stifcore aspiration needle
stiff ribbon retractor
stigmata of recent hemorrhage (SRH)
Stiles seizing forceps

Stiles tissue-grasping forceps
still camera
Stille-Barraya intestinal forceps
Stille bone chisel
Stille bone drill
Stille bone gouge
Stille cranial drill
Stille-Crawford clamp
Stille elevator
Stille gallstone forceps
Stille-Giertz rib shears
Stille hand drill
Stille-Horsley bone forceps
Stille-Horsley bone rongeur
Stille-Leksell rongeur
Stille-Liston bone cutter
Stille-Liston bone rongeur
Stille-Liston bone-cutting forceps
Stille-Luer bone rongeur
Stille-Luer duckbill rongeur
Stille-Luer-Echlin rongeur
Stille-Luer rongeur
Stille-Luer rongeur forceps
Stille-Mayo scissors
Stille plaster shears
Stille rib shears
Stille-Ruskin bone rongeur
Stille-Sherman bone drill
Stille vessel clamp
Stimson dressing
stimulant laxative
stimulated gastric secretion test
stimulation (also see *test*)
    cholecystokinin
    endogenous
    excess TSH
    faucial thermal-tactile
    gastrin
    LARSI
    long-acting thyroid (LAT)
    nerve
    nerve root
    pentagastrin
    repetitive nerve

stool *(cont.)*
  occult blood in
  oily
  pale
  pea soup
  pelleted
  pencil-like
  pipestem
  progressive thinning of
  rabbit
  reducing substance in
  residual
  retention of
  ribbon
  rice-water
  runny
  sago-grain
  scybalous
  semiformed
  semisolid
  silver
  slurry of
  soft
  spinach
  tarry black
  undigested food in
  unformed
  watery
  white fatty
  Wright stain of
stool color
stool consistency
stool culture
stool cytoxin test
stool electrolyte test
stool for occult blood
stool for ova and parasites (O&P)
stool guaiac
stool guaiac negative
stool guaiac positive
stool incontinence
stooling
stool osmotic gap test
stool smear

stool softener
stool specimen
stool urobilinogen
Stoppa posterior approach
Stoppa-Rives giant prosthetic repair
  of the visceral sac
storage disease
store (pl. stores)
  glycogen
  hepatic glycogen
  hepatic iron
  iron
  liver iron
storm
  thyroid
  thyrotoxic
Storz 26033 AP 0° 10 mm rigid
  laparoscope
Storz 26033 BP 0° 10 mm rigid
  laparoscope
Storz 9050B AutoexposureColor
  endoscopic camera
Storz AP 26003 0° 10 mm rigid
  laparoscope
Storz bronchoscope
Storz camera
Storz cholangiograsper
Storz cystoscope
Storz dolphin-nose grasper
Storz endoscope
Storz esophagoscope
Storz high-flow insufflator pump
Storz high insufflator
Storz high-speed insufflator
Storz Hopkins laparoscope
Storz hysteroscope
Storz KSA-2S SuperCam endoscopic
  camera
Storz laparoscope
Storz laparoscopic telescope
Storz laparoscopic video camera
Storz LaproFlator
Storz Microsystems cranial fixation
  plate

Storz Microsystems microplate
Storz Microsystems plate-holding
  forceps
Storz Microsystems pliers
Storz minilaparoscope
Storz OR1 electronic endoscopy system
Storz printer
Storz proctoscope
Storz resectoscope
Storz rigid laparoscope
Storz videoscope
Storz wire-cutting scissors
Storz 0° 10 mm telescope
Stovkis test
strabismus scissors
straight biopsy cup forceps
straight bone rongeur
straight chain fatty acid
straight chest tube
straight chisel
straight clamp
straight Crile forceps
straight cutting needle
straight dissecting scissors
straight dissector
straight double-action monopolar
  scissors
straight dura hook
straight-end cup forceps
straight forceps
straight gouge
straight incision
straight Kelly forceps
straight knife
straight micro grasper
straight micro scissors
straight oscillating saw
straight periosteal elevator
straight pituitary rongeur
straight reamer
straight retractor
straight scissors
straight stent
straight taper point
straight threaded rod

strain-gauge manometry
straining at defecation
straining at stool
stranding
  fascial
  mesenteric
  mesenteric fat (on CT scan)
  soft tissue
strangulated bowel
strangulated bowel obstruction
strangulated hemorrhoid
strangulated hernia
strangulated paraesophageal hernia
strangulated viscus
strangulation, intestinal
strangulation necrosis
strangulation obstruction
strangulation of hernia
strangulation of inguinal hernia
strap muscles
Strassburg test
StrataSorb composite wound dressing
stratified clot
Stratis II MRI system
Stratte needle
Stratte-TC needle holder
Strauss rectoscope
Strauss sign
strawberry gallbladder
strawberry hemangioma
strawberry nevus
straw-colored ascites
straw-colored fluid
streaking
Strecker stent
Street medullary pin
Street nail
Strelinger colon clamp
strep (streptococcus)
  anhemolytic
  beta hemolytic
  group B (GBS)
  hemolytic
  nonhemolytic

streptavidin-polyperoxidase
Streptococcus viridans
streptozocin, mitomycin C, and 5-FU
  (SMF) chemotherapy protocol
streptozotocin
stress Broden view
stress eversion view
stress film
stress gastritis
stress incontinence
stress-induced gastritis
stress-induced organ dysfunction
stress, intra-abdominal sheer
stress inversion view
stress reduction with regional anesthesia
stress-related mucosal disease (SRMD)
Stresstein (multiple branched-chain
  amino acids)
Stresstein liquid feeding
stress tolerant position
stress ulcer
stress ulceration
stress view
Stretta device for delivery of radio-
  frequency energy
stria (pl. striae)
striae distensae
striated muscle
Strickland suture
Strickland suture technique
stricture
  anal
  annular esophageal
  antral
  benign biliary
  bile duct
  biliary
  chronic (of the small bowel)
  cicatricial
  contractile
  cricopharyngeal
  division of
  esophageal
  gastric outlet

stricture *(cont.)*
  hilar
  intrahepatic
  irritable
  longitudinal esophageal
  peptic
  pharyngeal
  postsurgical
  pyloric
  rectal
  recurrent
  spasmodic
  ureteral
strictured segment
stricture formation
stricturoplasty
stridor
strike-through
string cell carcinoma
string guideline
string-of-beads appearance
string sign in terminal ileum
string test
strip
  bovine pericardium
  Chin-Up Strip
  glucose monitoring test
  Gore-Tex
  Oxycel
  reagent
  Steri-Strips
  tricortical iliac
strip biopsy
strip biopsy method
stripe, properitoneal flank
strip immunoblot assay (SIA)
stripper
  Matson rib
  Mayo external vein
  Meyer vein
  Nabatoff vein
strobe flash endoscopic light source
stroke
Stromagen

stromal fibrosis
stromal hemorrhage
stromal necrosis
Stromectol (ivermectin)
Strong Iodine (iodine; potassium
    iodide)
strongyloidiasis
structural aberration
structural homology
structural lesion
Strully dissecting scissors
Strully dural
Strully dural hook
Strully-Gigli rongeur
Strully-Gigli saw
Strully-Kerrison rongeur
Strully neurological scissors
Strully scissors
struma fibrosa
struma lymphomatosis
struma nodosa
strut bone graft
strut template
strut-type pin
struvite stone
StrykeFlow electrocautery probe
StrykeFlow suction irrigator
Stryker cartilage knife
Stryker endoscopy video camera system
Stryker illuminated retractor
Stryker laparoscope
Stryker microdebrider
Stryker microsurgery drill
Stryker notch view
Stryker saw
Stryker stent
Stryker 380-10, 0° 10 mm rigid
    laparoscope
Stryker 380-11, 0° 10 mm rigid
    laparoscope
Stryker 380-12, 30° 10 mm rigid
    laparoscope
Stryker 590 color endoscopic camera
Stryker trumpet valve

Stryker wedge suture anchor
ST segment
STSG (split-thickness skin graft)
Stuck laminectomy retractor
Stucker bile duct dilator
studding
    omental
    peritoneal
study (see also *test*)
    APC (adenoma prevention with
        celecoxib) study
    coagulation
    colonic transit
    contrast
    Early Treatment Diabetic
        Retinopathy Study
    enema contrast
    esophageal motility
    fecal fat
    gastric motility
    gastrografin contrast
    HALT-C (hepatitis C antiviral
        long-term treatment to prevent
        cirrhosis)
    kinetic gallbladder
    manometric
    marker transit
    mecholyl
    noninvasive localization
    nuclear technetium-99
    nuclear-tagged red blood cell
        bleeding
    pelvic floor function
    serial CK enzyme
    small bowel contrast study
    upper GI contrast
    videoendoscopic swallowing (VESS)
stump
    appendiceal
    blind
    cervical
    distal cremasteric
    distal artery
    duodenal

stump *(cont.)*
   gastric
   limb
   rectal
stump ligation
St. Vincent tube occluding clamp
stylet
   intubation
   malleable aluminum
   pediatric video optical intubation
   plastic-sheathed malleable
     aluminum
   Satin-slip
   TFX Medical catheter
   video optical intubation
Stylet internal esophageal MRI coil
S-type amylase (salivary)
Stypven time test
subacute appendicitis
subacute granulomatous thyroiditis
subacute hepatic necrosis
subacute hepatitis
subacute inflammation
subacute necrosis
subacute necrotizing encephalo-
   myopathy
subacute nodular migratory panniculitis
subacute nonspecific peritonitis
subacute obstruction
subacute pancreatitis
subacute perforation
subacute thyroiditis
subannular mattress suture
subaponeurotic abscess
subarachnoid anesthesia
subarachnoid block
subarachnoid catheter
subarachnoid hemorrhage
subareolar duct, dilation of the
subcapsular hematoma
subcarinal node
subcecal appendix
subcholangiopancreatoscope
subchondral bone plate

subchondral drill
subclavian catheter
subclavian-external carotid artery graft
subclinical hepatitis
subclinical infection
subclavian line
subclavian peel-away sheath
subclavian vein
subcostal incision
subcostal margin
subcostal plane
subcu (subcutaneous)
subcutaneous breast implant
subcutaneous catheter tunnel
subcutaneous emphysema
subcutaneous fat
subcutaneous fat necrosis
subcutaneous gas
subcutaneous inflammation
subcutaneous injection artifact
subcutaneous layer
subcutaneous mastectomy
subcutaneous nodule
subcutaneous pannus
subcutaneous structure
subcutaneous suture
subcutaneous tissue
subcutaneous tissue flap
subcutaneous tunnel
subcutaneous ulcer
subcutaneous ventricular reservoir
   catheter
subcutaneous wound
subcuticular layer
subcuticular suture
subdiaphragmatic abscess
subdiaphragmatic diverticulum
subdiaphragmatic perirenal region
subdural abscess
subdural drainage catheter
subdural effusion
subdural hematoma
subdural hemorrhage
subdural-to-peritoneal shunt

subendoscope
subfascial bleeder
subfascial endoscopic perforator surgery (SEPS)
subfascial hematoma
subgaleal abscess
subglandular augmentation mammoplasty
subglottic airway
subhepatic abscess
subhepatic area
subhepatic cecum
subhepatic phlegmon
subhepatic space
subhepatic space fluid
subjective dysphagia
submandibular space
submassive hepatic necrosis
submassive necrosis
submental space
submental vertex view
Sub-Microinfusion catheter
submucosa
submucosal abscess
submucosal carcinoma of the thoracic esophagus
submucosal development
submucosal dissection
submucosal esophageal venous plexus
submucosal fluctuance
submucosal hematoma
submucosal hemorrhage
submucosal saline injection technique
submucosal thickening
submucosal tumor
submucosal tunnel technique
submucosal venous plexus
submuscular breast implant
subnormal serum calcium concentration
suboptimal film
suboptimal thyroid hormone production
subperiosteal abscess
subperiosteal bone resorption
subperitoneal appendicitis

subperitoneal space
subphrenic abscess
Subramanian clamp
subsequent hernia formation
subsequent reanastomosis
subsequent T-tube track ductal dilatation and postoperative choledochoscopy
subserosal hemorrhage
subserosal layer
subserosal needle catheter jejunostomy
subserosal tumor
subsigmoid fossa
substernal extension from an enlarged thyroid
substernal gland
substernal goiter
substernal pain
substernal thyroid gland
substituted benzimidazole
subtotal colectomy
subtotal gastrectomy
subtotal lesion
subtotal pancreatectomy
subtotal parathyroidectomy
subtotal thyroidectomy
subtraction film
subumbilical incision
subumbilical space
subungual abscess
subungual melanoma
subvesical duct
subxiphoid trocar
subxiphoid view
subxiphoid window
succinylacetone
succussion sound
succussion splash (over the stomach)
sucker, sump
sucking chest wound
sucralfate
sucrose intolerance, congenital
sucrose-isomaltose (SI) deficiency

sucrose-isomaltose malabsorption,
   congenital
suction (see also *tube*)
   bulb
   closed
   continuous NG
   DeLee
   Endo-AID suction irrigation
   flexible dental
   FlowGun
   Gomco
   lavage and
   low intermittent
   mucosal resection
   nasogastric (NG)
   nasogastric tube (NTS)
   pinpoint
   Poole
   Res-Q-Vac hand-powered
   suctioned
   Wangensteen
suction-assisted lipoplasty (SAL)
suction biopsy
Suction Buster catheter
suction cannula
suction cap method of endoscopic
suction-coagulator, Cameron-Miller
suction-coagulator with valves
suction cup, endoscopic
suction drain
suction handle
   Medi-Vac Flexi-Clear
   Medi-Vac Yankauer
suction irrigation electrode (SIE)
suction irrigation probe
suction/irrigation system, Sherwood
   intrascopic
suction-irrigator, House-Radpour
suction-ligator
suction liner
   Medi-Vac CRD
   Medi-Vac Flex Advantage
suction lipectomy
suction port

suction retractor
suction tip
suction tube
Sudan stain
sudden cardiac death
sudden infant death syndrome (SIDS)
sudden onset of pain
Sudeck point
suffocative goiter
sugar-icing liver
Sugita right-angle aneurysm clamp
Sugiura esophageal variceal transection
sulciolar gastric mucosa
sulcus, inframammary
Sulfalax Calcium (docusate sodium)
Sulfamylon (mafenide acetate)
sulfasalazine
sulfasalazine enema
sulfasalidine (Azulfidine; Azulfidine
   EN-tabs)
sulfate ($SO_4{}^{2-}$)
sulfobromophthalein sodium test
sulfonamide
sulfonylurea
sulfur colloid liver scan
Sumner sign
sump (see *drain; tube*)
sump drain
sump nasogastric tube
sump sucker
sump syndrome
sun exposure
Sunday staphylorrhaphy elevator
Sundt loop shunt
sunrise view
sunset view
SuperAnchor suture anchor
Superblade blade
SuperChar
Supercut dissecting scissors
superficial abscess
superficial basal epithelial membrane
   (SBEM)
superficial circumflex iliac artery

suppressor T cell
suppuration
suppurative appendicitis
suppurative appendix
suppurative cholangitis
suppurative cholecystitis
suppurative choledochitis
suppurative infection
suppurative pancreatitis
suppurative peritonitis
suppurative thyroiditis
supraceliac aorta
supraceliac aortic cross-clamp
supraclavicular block anesthesia
supraclavicular lymphadenopathy
supraclavicular lymph node
supracolic compartment
supracondylar plate
supracrestal plane
supraduodenal approach
Supra G coronary stent
suprahepatic abscess
suprahepatic caval cuff
suprahepatic space
suprahepatic vena cava
suprahyoid neck dissection
supralevator abscess
supralevator space
Supramid Extra suture material
supramylohyoid
supranuclear lesion
suprapatellar cannula
suprapubic pain
suprapubic region
suprapubic trocar
suprarenal aortic cross-clamp
suprarenal impression
suprasphincteric fistula
suprasternal notch view
supraumbilical DPL
supravaterian duodenum
Supreme electrophysiology catheter
Supreme II blood glucose meter
sural nerve biopsy

suramin sodium
SureBite biopsy forceps
Sure-Closure skin-stretching system
graft
SureCuff catheter
SureCuff tissue in-growth cuff
SureFit electrosurgical grounding pad
Sure-Flex dilatation catheter
SureLac (lactose enzyme)
SurePress compression dressing
Sureshot metal sheathed injection
needle
SureSite transparent adhesive film
dressing
SureStep glucose monitor
SureStep Pro blood glucose monitor
Suretac suture
surface (see *facies*)
surface electrode
surface elevation
surface epithelium
surface of gland
surface of liver bed
surface umbilical pyloromyotomy
Surfak (docusate calcium)
Surfit adhesive
Sur-Fit AutoLock ostomy device
Sur-Fit Mini Pouch (ostomy)
Sur-Fit Natura ostomy device
Sur-Fit Pouch Cover
Sur-Fit Stoma Cap
Surgalloy needle
Surgenomic endoscope
surgeon square knot
Surgeons Choice stapler
surgeon's knot
surgery (see *operation*)
antireflux
bariatric
complication of
debulking
definitive
emergent
exploratory

surgery *(cont.)*
  flexible endoscopic
  HALS (hand-assisted laparoscopic
    surgery)
  keyhole
  laparoscopic
  minimally invasive
  salvage
Surgiblade sterile scalpel blade
surgical abdomen
surgical airway
surgical anesthesia
surgical approach for drainage
surgical catgut
surgical clipper
surgical complication
surgical cricothyroidotomy
surgical debridement
surgical decompression
surgical drainage
Surgical Dynamics aspiration probe
surgical emphysema
surgical excision
surgical exploration
surgical field
surgical gut
surgical gut suture
  chromic
  plain
surgical herniorrhaphy
surgical intervention
surgical isolation bubble system (SIBS)
surgical laparoscopy
surgically bypassed from fecal stream
surgically correctable hypertension
surgically implanted hemodialysis
  catheter (SIHC)
surgical margins
surgical mesh
surgical microinstruments
Surgical No Bounce mallet
surgical palliation
surgical portosystemic shunting

surgical reinforcement material,
  Enteryx biopolymer
surgical resection with wide margins
surgical scar
surgical scissors with TC blades
surgical scrub (see *cleanser*)
surgical sealant (see *adhesive; glue;
  hemostat; medications*)
surgical shunt
Surgical Simplex P adhesive
surgical site infection
surgical solution
surgical splenectomy
surgical staging of cancer
surgical stainless steel suture
surgical stapling
surgical steel skin clip
surgical therapy
surgical treatment of morbid obesity
surgical ulcer
surgical vagotomy
surgical wrap
Surgicel fibrillar absorbable hemostat
Surgicel gauze
Surgicel Nu-Knit absorbable hemostat
Surgicel Nu-Knit hemostatic agent
Surgicel pads (cellulose, oxidized)
Surgicel strips
Surgiclip
Surgidac braided coated polyester
  Dacron suture
Surgidac braided polyester suture
Surgidac suture material
Surgidyne
Surgiflex Wave suction/irrigation system
Surgifoam absorbable gelatin sponge
Surgigrip stapler
Surgigut chromic suture
Surgigut plain suture
Surgi-Kleen skin cleanser
Surgilase CO_2 laser
Surgilase Nd:YAG laser
Surgilase 150 laser
SurgiLav irrigation instrument

suture *(cont.)*

approximation
ArthroSew
atraumatic
atraumatic chromic
Auto Suture
Auto Suture ABBI system
Auto Suture One-Shot anastomotic
  device
Auto Suture Soft Thoracoport
Auto Suture SurgiStitch
Auto Suture universal retractor base
Bard endoscopic suturing
baseball stitch
basilar
basting
Becker
Bell
bioabsorbable
BioSorb
Biosyn monofilament synthetic
  absorbable
Biosyn synthetic monofilament
biparietal
black
blue and white
blunt-point
bolster
Bondek absorbable
Bone Bullet
braided
braided Ethibond
braided Mersilene
braided Nurolon
braided silk
Bralon braided nylon
bregmatomastoid
bridging
bridle
bunching
bundle
Bunnell crisscross
Bunnell wire pullout
buried

suture *(cont.)*

buried interrupted
buried-knot
Capio CL suture-capturing device
cardinal
cardiovascular silk
catgut
cerclage
chain
chromic
chromic catgut
chromic gut
chromic interrupted
circular
circular wire
circumferential
Closer
clove-hitch
coapting
coated
coated Vicryl
coated Vicryl Rapide
collagen
colposuspension
compression stay
Connell
continuous
continuous running
convertible slip knot
Corkscrew suture anchor
coronal
cosmetic conventional cutting
cosmetic reverse cutting
cotton
coupled
cranial
crisscross
crossed-swords technique
cruciate four-strand
Cushing
Cutalon nylon polyamide surgical
Czerny
Czerny-Lembert
Dacron

suture *(cont.)*

Dacron-bolstered
Dafilon surgical
Dagrofil
deep
deep retention
Deklene II
Deknatel
delayed closure of
dentate
Dermabond
dermal
Dermalene
Dermalon
Dexon
Dexon Plus
Dexon II
DG Softgut
diastasis of
Donati
double-armed (DAS)
doubly ligated
dural tack-up
dural tenting
dural traction
Endoknot
Endoloop
Endo Stitch
Endosuture
end-to-end
end-to-side
EPTFE (expanded polytetra-
    fluoroethylene) vascular
Ethibond
Ethibond Excel polyester
Ethicon
Ethicon Excel
Ethiflex
Ethilon
Ethilon monofilament nylon
Ethilon nylon
ethmoidolacrimal
ethmoidomaxillary
everting

suture *(cont.)*

everting mattress
Excel polyester
extracorporeal knot
fascial
fast absorbing surgical gut (plain)
FASTak suture anchor
figure-of-8
fine
fisherman's knot
fishmouth
flat
Flexon steel
four-strand
four-strand Savage
Frater
frontal
frontolacrimal
frontomaxillary
frontonasal
frontoparietal
frontosphenoid
frontozygomatic
funicular
furrier
Gambee
Gely
GI (gastrointestinal)
Giampapa
gift wrap technique
Gillies
Gillies horizontal dermal
granny knot
grasping loop
Gregory stay
Gruber
Gussenbauer
gut
Halsted
Harpoon suture anchor
Hawkeye
heavy monofilament
heavy silk
heavy wire

suture *(cont.)*

nonmutagenic surgical
Novafil
Nurolon
Nurolon braided nylon
nylon
occipital
occipitomastoid
occipitoparietal
occipitosphenoid
orienting
out-in-out technique
over-and-over
over-and-over whip
overlapping
Owen silk
Pagedas self-locking
Panacryl
Panacryl absorbable
parietal
parietomastoid
parieto-occipital
patch-reinforced mattress
PDS (polydioxanone suture) II
    Endoloop suture
PDS II (polydioxanone)
PDS Vicryl
pericostal
Perma-Hand braided silk
Perma-Hand silk
PermaMesh
petrobasilar
petrosphenobasilar
petrospheno-occipital
petrosquamous
PGA synthetic absorbable
Pilot
plain
plain catgut
plain gut
plastic
pledgeted
pledgeted Ethibond
pledgeted mattress

suture *(cont.)*

plication
poliglacaprone absorbable
polybutester
Polydek
polydioxanone (PDS)
polyester
polyglacine
polyglactin 370 absorbable
polyglactin 910 absorbable
polyglycolic acid
polyglyconate absorbable
PolySorb
pop-off
Potts tie
PRE 2
prematurely closed
Premilene
premium point reverse cutting
premium point spatula
preplaced
primary
Prolene
Prolene polypropylene
Pronova
Pronova nonabsorbable
Pronova Poly
Protector meniscus
P-3
pullout
pullout wire
Pulver-Taft fishmouth
pursestring or purse-string
pyroglycolic acid
quilted
radiopaque
Rapide
reabsorbable
Reddick-Saye
reinforcing
relaxation
retention
retraction
reverse cutting

suture *(cont.)*
    rhabdoid
    Richardson angle
    Robertson
    Roth Grip-Tip suture guide
    running
    running interlocking
    running lock
    running locking
    Sabreloc (spatula needle)
    Safil synthetic absorbable surgical
    sagittal cranial
    Savage
    secondary
    Sepramesh
    seromuscular
    seromuscular-to edge
    serrated
    seton
    shorthand vertical mattress stitch
    silk
    Silkam
    silk pop-off
    silk traction
    simple
    single-armed
    six-strand
    skin
    slipknot
    Sofsilk braided silk
    Sofsilk nonabsorbable silk
    Softcat chromic
    Softcat plain
    Softgut surgical chromic suture
    sphenoethmoidal
    spheno-occipital
    spheno-orbital
    sphenoparietal
    sphenopetrosal
    sphenosquamous
    sphenotemporal
    sphenovomerine
    splayed cranial
    spread

suture *(cont.)*
    squamosomastoid
    squamosoparietal
    squamososphenoid
    squamous
    stainless steel wire
    staple
    Statak
    stay
    Steelex
    Steri-Strips
    sternal wire
    stick-tie (suture ligature or
        transfixion suture)
    stitch
    Strickland
    subannular mattress
    subcutaneous
    subcuticular
    superior rectus
    SuperStitch
    Supramid
    Supramid Extra
    Suretac
    surgical catgut
    surgical gut
    surgical linen
    surgical silk
    surgical stainless steel
    Surgidac braided coated polyester
        Dacron
    Surgigut chromic
    Surgigut plain
    Surgilene
    Surgilon
    Surgipro mesh
    Surgipro monofilament polypropy-
        lene
    Surgitie ligating loop
    Sutralon
    SutraSilk
    Suturamid
    Suture Clinch
    Sutured-Clip

suture *(cont.)*
 Suture Lok
 Sutureloop
 Sutureloop colposuspension
 swaged-on
 synthetic
 Synthofil
 tack
 taper point
 tapercutting
 Teflon
 Teflon-coated Dacron
 Teflon-pledgeted
 Teflon-pledgeted mattress
 temporal
 tenting
 Tevdek
 The Closer
 Thiersch
 three-strand
 through-and-through
 through-and-through continuous
 through-the-wall mattress
 Ti-Cron (also Tycron)
 tight
 Tom Jones closure suture
 traction
 transfixion
 transition
 transosseous
 transverse
 Trumbull
 twisted
 two-strand
 Tycron (also Ti-Cron)
 U double-barrel
 umbilical tape
 undyed
 undyed braided polyglycolic acid
 undyed Vicryl
 Vascufil
 vertical
 vertical mattress
 Vicryl

suture *(cont.)*
 Vicryl Rapide synthetic absorbable
 whipstitch
 white
 white silk
 wing
 wire
 wire pullout
 X-PRESS
 Z
 Zimmer Statak
suture abscess
suture anchor (see *anchor*)
Suture Assistant endoscopic suturing
 device
Suture Assistant knot-tying device
suture bite
suture bridge fixation
suture button
Suture Clinch fastener
Suture Clinch suture
suturectomy
Sutured-Clip clip
Sutured-Clip suture
suture displacement
suture "ears"
suture fastener
 ROC
 ROC XS
 Suture Clinch
suture forceps
suture grasper
suture guide
 Investa
 Pilot
suture hook
suture isometry
suture joint
sutureless closure
sutureless electrode lead
sutureless myocardial electrode
suture ligated
suture ligature
suture limb

Swiss celia and suture forceps
Swiss jewelers forceps
Swiss lithoclast
Swiss lithoclast lithotriptor
Swiss-pattern blade breaker
swivel clamp
swivel knife
SYBIOL (synthetic bio-liver) device
Sydney Hospital retractor
Syllact (psyllium seed husks)
Syme aneurysm needle
Symlin (pramlintide acetate)
symmetric chest expansion
symmetrical breast prosthesis
sympathectomy hook
sympathetic ganglion
sympathetic nervous system
sympathetic nervous system symptom
sympathetics
sympathomimetic drug
Symphony nitinol stent (extremities/
　biliary)
symptom
　compressive
　dyspeptic
　obstructive
　postcibal
　pressure
　prodromal
　relief of
　sympathetic nervous system
symptomatic attack
symptomatic esophagitis
symptomatic gallstone
symptomatic hyperglycemia
symptomatic hyperparathyroidism
symptomatic hypocalcemia
symptomatology
Symptom Distress Scale
symptoms of sympathetic discharge
synchronized videofluoroscopy and
　manometry
syncopal episode
syncope
syncytial knot formation

syndromatic hepatic ductular hypoplasia
syndrome (see also *disease*)
　Aagenaes (cholestasis-lymphedema)
　Aarskog
　abdominal muscle deficiency
　ablepharon-macrostomia
　absent abdominal muscle
　Achard-Thiers
　acquired immunodeficiency (AIDS)
　ACTH deficiency
　adrenogenital
　afferent loop
　AIDS (acquired immunodeficiency)
　Alagille
　albatross
　Albright
　Algid malaria
　alpha chain
　Alstrom
　anorexia-cachexia
　anterior abdominal wall
　APECED (autoimmune polyendo-
　　crinopathy; candidiasis; ecto-
　　dermal dysplasia)
　apple-peel syndrome
　Arias
　Armenian
　Asherson
　asplenia
　bacterial overgrowth
　Banti
　Barrett
　Bartter
　basal cell nevus
　Bassen-Kornzweig
　Bearn-Kunkel-Slater
　Beckwith
　Beckwith-Wiedemann
　Bedford
　Behçet
　Bernard-Sergent
　Bessauds-Hilmand-Augier
　Biörck
　blind (stagnant) loop

syndrome *(cont.)*
  Bloodgood
  Bloom
  blue diaper
  blue rubber bleb nevus
  Boerhaave
  Bouveret
  Bowen
  Brachmann-de Lange
  Brandt
  Brennemann
  Budd
  Budd-Chiari
  buried bumper
  Burnett
  burning vulvar syndrome
  café coronary
  Canada-Cronkhitc
  carbohydrate-deficient glycoprotein,
    type 1a
  carcinoid
  carnitine-deficiency
  Caroli
  Carpenter
  Carter-Horsley-Hughes
  cast
  cat-eye
  caudal regression
  celiac artery compression
  cerebrohepatorenal
  CHARGE (coloboma, heart, atresia
    of the choanae, retardation of
    growth and development, genital
    and urinary anomalies, and ear
    anomalies [also tracheoesopha-
    geal fistula])
  Chiari-Budd
  Chilaiditi
  cholestasis-lymphedema
  cholestatic
  chronic fatigue and immune
    dysfunction (CFIDS)
  chronic intestinal pseudo-obstruction
  Clarke-Hadefield

syndrome *(cont.)*
  Cohen
  colonic solitary ulcer
  complex regional pain (CRPS)
  Conn
  Cornelia de Lange
  Courvoisier-Terrier
  couvade
  CREST
  Crigler-Najjar
  Cronkhite-Canada
  CRPS (complex regional pain)
  Cruveilhier-Baumgarten
  Cushing
  cyclic vomiting
  Danbolt-Closs
  Dejerine-Sottas
  descending perineum
  diencephalic
  DiGeorge
  DIMOAD (diabetes insipidus,
    diabetes mellitus, optic atrophy
    and deafness)
  Down
  Drummond
  Dubin-Johnson
  Dubin-Sprinz
  dumping
  Eagle-Barrett
  ectopic ACTH
  Ehlers-Danlos
  eosinophilic gastroenteritis
  euthyroid sick (ESS)
  exomphalos-macroglossia-gigantism
  familial polyposis
  Felty
  fibrocystic breast
  fish-odor
  Fitz-Hugh–Curtis (perihepatitis)
  Flood
  flulike
  Forbes-Albright
  Fröhlich (Froehlich)
  full-blown

syndrome *(cont.)*
    functional bowel
    gallstone ileus
    Gardner
    gas-bloat
    gastrocardiac
    gastroesophageal laceration-
        hemorrhage
    gastrointestinal dysmotility
    gastrojejunal loop obstruction
    gay bowel
    Gee-Herter-Heubner
    Gianotti-Crosti
    Gilbert
    glucagonoma
    Goldberg-Maxwell
    Gopalan
    gourmand
    Guillain-Barré
    Hadefield-Clarke
    Hanot-Chauffard
    Heerferdt-Waldenstrom
    HELLP (hemolysis with a micro-
        angiopathic blood smear, elevated
        liver enzymes, and low platelet
        count)
    hemolytic-uremic (HUS)
    hepatopulmonary
    hepatorenal (HRS)
    hereditary MEA
    Hermansky-Pudlak
    Howel-Evans
    Hutchinson-Weber-Peutz
    hypoglycosylation, type 1a
    impaired regeneration (IRS)
    inhibitory
    inspissated bile
    inspissated sump
    insulin-resistance
    intestinal polyposis-cutaneous
        pigmentation
    irritable bowel (IBS)
    Ivemark
    Jegher

syndrome *(cont.)*
    jejunal
    Kelly-Paterson
    Kimmelstiel-Wilson
    kinky hair
    Klinefelter
    Koenig (König)
    Kunkel
    Ladd
    Laubry-Soulle
    Laurence-Moon-Bardet-Biedl
    leaky gut
    lentigo-polypose-digestive
    levator ani
    Lloyd
    locker room
    Lofgren
    loin pain hematuria (LPHS)
    Lucey-Driscoll
    lupus-like
    Lyell
    lymphadenopathy (LAS)
    lymphoproliferative
    Lynch I
    Lynch II
    malabsorption
    malignant B cell
    Mallory-Weiss
    MEA (multiple endocrine adeno-
        matosis)
    meconium plug
    Meigs
    MEN I (multiple endocrine
        neoplasia I)
    mesenteric artery
    milk-alkali
    Mirizzi
    Mosse
    mucosal neuroma (MEA type III)
    multiorgan dysfunction syndrome
        (MODS)
    multiple endocrine deficiency,
        type II
    multiple hamartoma

syndrome *(cont.)*
    Munchausen
    non-Lynch
    obesity hypoventilation (OHS)
    Obinsky
    Ogilvie
    Oldfield
    Osler-Weber-Rendu
    overlap (connective tissue disease)
    pancreatic cholera
    pancreaticohepatic
    paraneoplastic
    Paterson-Brown-Kelly
    Paterson-Kelly
    pericolic membrane
    perihepatitis
    periodic peritonitis
    Peutz-Jeghers (PJS)
    Peutz-Jeghers familial gastro-
        intestinal polyposis
    Peutz-Touraine
    pharyngeal pouch
    pituitary Cushing
    pituitary tumor
    Plummer-Vinson
    Polhemus-Schafer-Ivemark
    polyglandular autoimmune (PGA II)
    polyglandular deficiency, type II
    polyps and spots
    polysplenia
    postcholecystectomy (PCS)
    postcolonoscopy distention
    postfundoplication
    postgastrectomy
    postgastric surgery
    postpolio
    postpolypectomy coagulation
    postsurgical nonabsorption
    postvagotomy
    Potter
    Prader-Willi
    prune-belly
    pseudo-obstructive
    Purtilo

syndrome *(cont.)*
    Reichmann
    Reimann
    reperfusion
    respiratory distress
    retained antrum
    Reye
    Riley-Day (familial dysautonomia)
    Roger
    Rotor
    Rubinstein-Taybi
    runting
    Sandifer
    Sanger-Brown
    Schmid-Fraccaro
    Schmidt
    Schwachman
    Schwachman-Bodian
    Schwachman-Diamond
    sea-blue histiocyte
    sepsis
    Sheehan
    short-bowel
    short-gut
    Shy-Drager
    Siegel-Cattan, Mamou
    Sipple (MEA type II)
    Sjögren (Sjoegren)
    SLE-like
    small stomach
    solitary rectal ulcer (SRUS)
    solitary ulcer
    somatostatinoma
    splenic agenesis
    splenic flexure
    Sprinz-Dubin
    Sprinz-Nelson
    stagnant loop
    stale fish
    steakhouse
    Stein-Leventhal
    Stevens-Johnson
    sump
    superior mesenteric artery (SMAS)

syndrome *(cont.)*
  systemic inflammatory response (SIRS)
  Takahara
  terminal reservoir
  TORCH (toxoplasmosis; other agents; rubella; cytomegalovirus; herpes simplex)
  Torres
  Townes Brooks
  toxic shock (TSS)
  Turcot
  Turner
  type I hepatorenal
  type II hepatorenal
  VACTERL (vertebral anomalies; anal atresia; congenital cardiac disease; tracheoesophageal fistula; renal anomalies; radial dysplasia; and other limb defects) syndrome
  Verner-Morrison
  Vinson
  vulvar vestibulitis
  Waldenstrom macroglobulinemia
  wasting
  Waterhouse-Friderichsen
  watery diarrhea
  Watson-Alagille
  WDHA (watery diarrhea, hypokalemia, achlorhydria)
  Weil
  Welt
  Wermer (MEA type I)
  Werner
  Wernicke-Korsakoff
  Wiedemann-Beckwith
  Wiscott-Aldrich
  Wolfram
  X-linked lymphoproliferative (XLP)
  ZE
  Zellweger
  Zieve
  Zollinger-Ellison (ZES)

syndrome of inappropriate antidiuretic hormone (SIADH)
syndrome of inappropriate secretion of antidiuretic hormone [ADH]
Synercid (quinupristin/dalfopristin)
Synergraft
Synergy ultrasound system
syngeneic transplant
Synovator arthroscopic blade
synovectomy blade
synovectomy rongeur
synovial biopsy
synovial fluid
Synsorb Cd
Synsorb-PK (8-methoxycarbonyloctyl oligosaccharides)
Syntel latex-free embolectomy catheter
Synthaderm dressing
Synthaderm occlusive wound dressing
Synthamin amino acid solution
Synthes cervical plate
Synthes dorsal distal radius plate
Synthes drill
Synthes Microsystems cranial fixation plate
Synthes Microsystems microplate
Synthes Microsystems pliers
Synthes Microsystems plate-holding forceps
Synthes mini L-plate
Synthes rod
Synthes transbuccal trocar
Synthes wire guide
synthesis, impaired lecithin
synthetic ^{13}C-urea lyophilized powder
synthetic cortisol
synthetic mesh
synthetic mesocaval H-graft
synthetic suture
Synthofil suture
Synthroid (levothyroxine sodium)
syphilis
syphilitic cirrhosis
syphilitic necrosis

syphilitic peritonitis
Syracuse I plate
syringe
   Asepto irrigation
   aspiration
   Autoblock safety
   CoverTip safety
   Daxor quantitative injection syringe
     kit
   EasySafe disposable
   ENSI syringe
   Humalog Pen
   Humulin Pen
   Inject-Ease 100
   Lewy Teflon glycerine mixture
   Luer-Lok
   Medex Protégé 3010 infusion pump
   monojet Toomey
   Omnican Piston
   Pritchard
   Pritchard lipiodol
   ROCAP
   Schimmelbusch bladder
   Ultraject prefilled
   Uni-Matic infiltration
Syringe Avitene dressing
Syringe Avitene endoscopic delivery
   system
system (see also *device*)
   Aastrom CPS (cell-production)
   ABBI (advanced breast biopsy
     instrumentation)
   Ablatherm HIFU (high-intensity
     focused ultrasound)
   ADICOL insulin delivery
   AeroView optical intubation
   AERx diabetes management
   AERx pain management
   AESOP (Automated Endoscopic
     System for Optimal Positioning)
   AESOP 2000; 3000 endoscope
   Airis II open MRI
   Alexa 1000 noninvasive breast lesion
     diagnostic

system *(cont.)*
   AlgoMed drug infusion
   alimentary
   Allon
   Anaconda device and delivery
   AngioStent balloon-expandable stent
     and delivery
   Aspen ultrasound
   Atlas 2.0 diagnostic ultrasound
   AU5 system, ultrasound
   Aurora diode laser
   Aurora MR breast imaging
   AutoSonix
   Auto Suture ABBI
   autotransfusion
   Autovac autotransfusion
   Autovac LF autotransfusion
   Bard Composix mesh graft material
   Bard endoscopic suturing
   BAT (B-mode acquisition and
     targeting)
   Beacon Technology (BTS)
   Beamer injection stent
   BiCAP hemostatic
   Biofield diagnostic
   BioLogic-DT (now Liver Dialysis
     Unit)
   BioLogic-HT (now ThermoChem-
     HT)
   BiPAP S/T-D 30 ventilatory support
   BI-RADS (Breast Imaging Reporting
     and Data System)
   B-mode acquisition and targeting
     (BAT)
   BSD-2000
   CathTrack catheter locator
   CDIS (controlled distention irriga-
     tion system)
   CDI 2000 blood gas monitoring
   Cell Recovery (CRS)
   Cell Saver Haemolite autotrans-
     fusion
   Cenflex central monitoring
   Centauri Er:YAG laser

system *(cont.)*
  CFC BioScanner
  closed
  closed drainage
  Coaguloop
  CollectFirst autotransfusion
  Colormate TLc BiliTest
  Computerized Thermal Imaging
  Core Entree Plus laparoscopic trocar
    and cannula
  CRYOcare
  CRYOguide
  CSM Stretta
  CycloTech cyclosporine delivery
  da Vinci surgical
  DBx diagnostic
  DermaLase Er,Cr:YSGG laser
  DermaScan
  Dialock hemodialysis access
  DOBI (Dynamic Optical Breast
    Imaging)
  EDC endoscopic imaging
  800 series KTP/YAG surgical laser
  EndoALPHA integrated endosur-
    gical
  EndoCinch suturing
  EndoMed laparoscopic
  E-Z Tac soft tissue reattachment
  F.A.S.T. 1 (First Access for Shock
    and Trauma)
  FemRx Soprano cryotherapy
  Flo-Stat fluid management
  Fluid Alarm System (FAS) glove
    integrity
  FluoroNav virtual fluoroscopy
  GE Senographe 2001 digital
    mammography
  GITS (gastrointestinal therapeutic)
  Given Diagnostic Imaging
  GliaSite implantable radiation
    therapy
  Guidant Origin
  GVHD (graft-versus-host disease)
    grading

system *(cont.)*
  HDI 3000 ultrasound
  Hemasure r/LS red blood cell
    filtration
  Hemopure
  Hercules Nd:YAG laser
  Hinchey diverticulitis grading/
    staging
  Illumina PROSeries laparoscopy
  Intercept Platelet
  intermittent open
  Intuitive
  IRMA blood analysis
  Irrijet DS debridement and irrigation
  Isolex 300i stem cell selection
  IsoMed constant-flow infusion
  IVAC SmartSite needleless
  Kaplan PenduLaser 115 surgical
    laser
  KOH colpotomizer
  KTP/YAG surgical laser
  LAGB gastric banding
  Laparolife gasless laparoscopy
  Lap-Band adjustable gastric banding
    (LAGB)
  LifeShirt monitoring
  Liver Dialysis Unit
  LORAD StereoGuide stereotactic
    breast biopsy
  LSTAT (life support trauma and
    transport)
  Luxtec fiberoptic
  lyophilized liposomal delivery
  Lyra laser
  Mammex TR mammography
  Mammotest breast biopsy
  Mammotest Plus breast biopsy
  MCAS (modular clip application)
  medicated urethral system for
    erection (MUSE)
  Medstone STS-T transportable
    lithotripsy
  MIBB breast biopsy
  Multitak suture

system *(cont.)*
  Navion BioNavigation
  Navitrack
  NeoCure cryoablation
  Octopus2 tissue-stabilization
  Olympus CV-1 endoscopic
  Olympus CV-100 endoscopic
  On-Q pain management
  Opdima digital mammography
  Optical Biopsy
  Optical Tracking System (OTS)
  Optistar MR contrast delivery
  ORI electronic endoscopy
  Origin distention balloon
  Palpagraph breast examination
  PDB laparoscopic balloon
  Photon radiosurgery
  Photon Radiosurgery System (PRS)
  portal venous
  POSICAM
  PowerCut gold surgical
  PowerCut pneumatic power
  PowerSculpt cosmetic surgery
  pressurized pulsatile irrigation
  Profore four-layer bandaging
  ProLease drug delivery
  Protectiv I.V. catheter safety
  PRS (Photon Radiosurgery System)
  PSA 4000 anesthesia monitoring
  Pulsavac III wound debridement
  Repose surgical
  Retzius
  Romano surgical curved drilling
  Senographe 2000D digital
    mammography imaging
  Sherwood intrascopic suction/
    irrigation system for laparoscopic
    procedures
  SiteSelect breast biopsy
  SJM Rosenkranz pediatric retractor
  SmartDose prefilled infusion
  Softscan laser mammography
  Sonoprobe SP-501 system for
    endoscopic procedures

system *(cont.)*
  Soprano cryoablation
  SpectraScience Optical Biopsy
  Squirt wound irrigation
  Storz OR1 electronic endoscopy
  Sure-Closure skin-stretching
  surgical isolation bubble (SIBS)
  SurgiLav Plus hydrodebridement
  Ternamian EndoTIP
  ThermoChem-HT (formerly
    BioLogic-HT system)
  Thermo-STAT
  Thora-Klex chest drainage
  3DC endoscopic imaging
  TLc.BiliTest
  TraumaJet wound debridement
  videoendoscopc
  Xillix LIFE-GI fluorescence
    endoscopy
  Xillix LIFE-Lung GI fluorescence
    endoscopy
  XPS Sculpture System
  Zone Specific II meniscal repair
systemic carnitine deficiency
systemic circulation
systemic effects carcinoma
systemic fungal infection
systemic glucocorticosteroids (GCS)
systemic infection
systemic inflammation
systemic inflammatory response
  syndrome (SIRS)
systemic lesion
systemic disseminated lupus
  erythematosus
systemic lupus erythematosus (SLE)
  diffuse
  focal
systemic mast cell disease
systemic mastocytosis
systemic mercury intoxication
systemic necrotizing arteritis
systemic pressure
systemic scleroderma

systemic therapy
system of Retzius
systolic blood pressure
systolic pressure gradient

systolic spleen
Szabo-Berci needle driver
Szabo test

T, t

TAB (tumescent absorbent bandage)
Tabb double-ended flap knife
Tabb elevator
Tabb myringoplasty knife
Tabb pick knife
TAB thermocouple sensor
Tabb 3 mm ruler
TAB wound dressing
table
   Maquet endoscopy
   sigmoidoscopy
tabletop Stone staple
TAC (total abdominal colectomy)
TACE (transcatheter arterial chemo-
   embolization)
tachyarrhythmias
tachycardia
tachygastria
Tacit threaded anchor
tack
tacked behind the uterus
tacked down
tacker, Origin
tack suture
tack-up
tacrolimus
Tactilaze angioplasty laser catheter
tactile anesthesia

tactile probe
TAE (total abdominal evisceration)
taenia (also tenia) strip of soft tissue
Taenia (genus of tapeworm)
Taenia saginata
Taenia solium
taeniacide
tag
   edematous
   external skin
   hemorrhoidal
   perianal skin
   sentinel
   tonsil
Tagamet HB (cimetidine)
tagged ligament
tagged RBC study
tagged red blood cell bleeding scan
TAG suture anchor
tail, axillary
tail of breast
tail of breast tissue
tail of pancreas
tail of Spence
Tait graft
Takahara syndrome
Takahashi forceps
Takahashi rongeur

TAPP (transabdominal preperitoneal)
hernia repair
TAPP (transabdominal preperitoneal)
laparoscopic hernioplasty
tar cancer
tardive dyskinesia
target cell
targeted brain biopsy
targeted cryoablation device
Targeted Ablation Therapy
target lesion
target organ complications of type 1
diabetes
target organ deterioration of diabetes
Targis microwave catheter-based system
tarry black stools
tarsal plate
taurolidine
Taut cystic duct catheter
taxanes, taxoids
Taxol (paclitaxel)
Taxotere (docetaxel)
Taylor brain scissors
Taylor delicate forceps
Taylor dressing forceps
Taylor dural scissors
Taylor gastric balloon
Taylor percussion hammer
Taylor scissors
Taylor self-retaining spinal retractor
Taylor spinal retractor blade
Tazocin
tazofelone
TBZ (thiabendazole)
^{99m}Tc (see *technetium*)
T cell
T cell lymphoma
TCA (trihydrocoprostanic acid)
TCD/CBDE (transcystic duct/common
bile duct exploration)
TcHIDA scan
TC (tungsten carbide) needle holder
TCR (T cell receptor)
TD glucose monitoring system

TDMS (Trex digital mammography
system)
TDT (transmission disequilibrium test)
Teale forceps
tear (rupture)
capsular
diastatic serosal
esophageal
flap
gastric
liver
Mallory-Weiss
Mallory-Weiss mucosal
mesenteric
micro
post-emesis longitudinal
post-retching longitudinal
serosal
teardrop breast prosthesis
teardrop radiographic appearance of
cecal bascule
tearing pain
tear of liver and capsule
tear stone
tear-tip cover
teasing needle
Tebamide (trimethobenzamide HCl)
technetium-99m (^{99m}Tc)
^{99m}Tc albumin colloid
^{99m}Tc albumin microspheres
^{99m}Tc arcitumomab
^{99m}Tc DISIDA
^{99m}Tc disofenin
^{99m}Tc DMSA
^{99m}Tc DTPA aerosol
^{99m}Tc GHP
^{99m}Tc HDP
^{99m}Tc HIDA
^{99m}Tc IDA scan
^{99m}Tc lidofenin
^{99m}Tc MAA (macroaggregated
albumin)
^{99m}Tc MDP
^{99m}Tc medronate

technetium-99m *(cont.)*
    ^{99m}Tc murine MAb to human alfa-
        fetoprotein (AFP)
    ^{99m}Tc pentetic acid
    ^{99m}Tc pertechnetate
    ^{99m}Tc PIPIDA
    ^{99m}Tc polyphosphate
    ^{99m}Tc PYP (pyrophosphate)
    ^{99m}Tc SC (sulfur colloid)
    ^{99m}Tc sestamibi
    ^{99m}Tc sodium pertechnetate
    ^{99m}Tc solesomab monoclonal
        antibody
    ^{99m}Tc SPP (stannous pyrophosphate)
technetium-labeled autologous red
    blood cell scan
technetium-labeled red blood cell scan
technetium-labeled stannous methylene
    disphosphonate
Techni-Care surgical scrub
technique (see also *method*; *operation*)
    autosuture
    bipolar surgical
    Burhenne
    clamp, cut, and tie
    continuous pull-through
    cross-sectional imaging
    EMR (endoscopic mucosal resec-
        tion) suction cap method
    endoscopic reversal
    endoscopic sewing machine
    extraction balloon
    finger-fracture
    Giampap suture
    Hofmeister
    J needle
    Karydakis
    microsurgical
    modified Delphi
    modified tumescent
    PhotoPoint light-activated
    Polya
    polyp snare

technique *(cont.)*
    preperitoneal patch and plug hernia
        repair
    rapid pull-through esophageal
        manometry
    Rosetti
    RPT (rapid pull-through)
    sequential clamp and suture
    Simonsen
    snare
    SPT (station pull-through)
    station pull-through esophageal
        manometry
    Thermal Quenching cooling
    three-trocar cholecystectomy
    tip deflection
    transabdominal preperitoneal
        approach
    transanal double-stapling
    transduodenal drainage
    transgastric drainage
    transpapillary drainage
    Traverso-Longmire
    tumescent
    Turnbull
    Vayre suturing
    vertical pedicle in breast reduction
technology
    antisense
    Beacon
    Coblation
    FACT (Focal Angioplasty Catheter)
    islet separation
    LAST (large-area sensing)
    Masimo SET (signal extraction)
    MCAT (modular coded aperture)
    SET (signal extraction)
    S.M.A.R.T. (shape memory alloy
        recoverable)
    USS-Trex Universal advanced
        radiology
    XenoMouse
Technomed Sonolith 3000 lithotriptor

Technos ultrasound system
Tee connector
TEF (tracheoesophageal fistula)
TefGen-guided tissue membrane
Teflon-coated brain retractor
Teflon-coated Dacron suture
Teflon-coated driver
Teflon-coated guidewire
Teflon-coated hollow-bore needle
Teflon drain, nasobiliary
Teflon ERCP catheter
Teflon insulated coating
Teflon nasobiliary tube
Teflon-pledgeted mattress suture
Teflon sling rectopexy
Teflon sling repair
Teflon suture
Teflon tube
Tegaderm HP transparent dressing
Tegaderm transparent dressing
Tegagel hydrogel dressing and sheet
Tegagen HG alginate wound dressing
Tegagen HI alginate wound dressing
Tegapore contact-layer wound dressing
tegaserod
Tegasorb hydrocolloid dressing
Tegtmeier elevator
telangiectasia
    blanching spider
    gastrointestinal
    hereditary hemorrhagic (HHT)
    Osler-Weber-Rendu
    spider
telangiectatic angioma
telangiectatic lesion
telangiectatic osteogenic sarcoma
telangiectatic vessel
Telecam DX
Telecam SL
TeleMed reusable biopsy forceps
telemetry, multiple parameter (MPT)
Telepaque (topanoic acid)
Telepaque contrast medium

telescope (also see *endoscope; laparoscope*)
    Hopkins II
    Hopkins II forward oblique
    Storz laparoscopic
    Storz 0° 10 mm
    Wolff
telescope bridge
telescopic rod
telescopic wire guide
telescoping medullary rod
telescoping nail
Teletrast absorbable surgical gauze
television monitor
Telfa gauze dressing
Telfa gel
telithromycin
telomerase transcription
telomere-specific probe
TEM (transanal endoscopic microsurgery)
Temnolaparoscopy device
temperature sensor
Temperlite saw blade
Temple-Fay laminectomy retractor
Temple University nail
Temple University plate
Tempo (aluminum hydroxide; magnesium hydroxide; calcium carbonate; simethicone)
temporal artery biopsy
temporal fascia graft
temporal suture
temporary colostomy
temporary end colostomy
temporary enteroscope
temporary fecal diversion
temporary hypoparathyroidism
temporary loop ileostomy
temporary ostomy
temporary pacing wire
TEMPprobes
tenaculum (see *forceps*)
tenaculum-reducing forceps

tertiary hyperparathyroidism
Terumo guidewire
Tesamone (testosterone)
Teslac (testolactone)
Teslascan (mangafodipir trisodium)
Tessier undermining scissors
test (see also *assay*)
    acid clearance (ACT)
    acid perfusion
    acid reflux
    acidification of stool
    ACS:180 BR breast cancer
      screening
    Actalyke activated clotting time
      (ACT)
    Adenovirus EIA
    alanine aminotransaminase (ALT)
      (formerly SGPT) liver function
    AlaSTAT latex allergy
    Alatest Latex-specific IgE allergen
    Alexagram breast lesion diagnostic
    alpha-2 antiplasmin functional assay
    ALT (alanine aminotransferase)
      (newer name for SGPT)
    aminopyrine breath
    ammonia N 13
    antiendomysial antibody
    Anti-Pr-3 ELISA autoimmune
    arclofenin (hepatic function)
    argentaffin reaction
    AST (serum aspartate amino-
      transferase) (formerly SGOT)
    ASTRA profile
    Bactigen Salmonella-Shigella
    Baermann
    balloon expulsion
    Bard BTA
    basal secretory flow rate (BSFR)
    B-D Easy A1c
    bentiromide
    bentonite flocculation
    Bernstein esophageal acid infusion
    betazole stimulation
    BTA stat (bladder tumor assay)

test *(cont.)*
    BTA TRAK bladder tumor
    bile acid breath
    bile acid tolerance
    bile solubility
    BiliChek bilirubin
    binder
    Bioclot protein S assay
    Bio-Enzabead
    Biofield diagnostic system
    Biosafe PSA4
    BladderScan
    bladder tumor assay (BTA)
    blood urea level
    Boas gastric ulcer
    bolus challenge
    Bonney stress incontinence
    Bourne
    Bozicevich
    BRACAnalysis genetic susceptibility
    breath hydrogen
    BSP (bromosulfophthalein)
    BTA stat urine
    "cake mix" kit for hematopoietic
      progenitor assay
    cancelling A's (mental test for
      hepatic encephalopathy)
    C&S (culture and sensitivity)
    CA 19-9 (carbohydrate antigen)
    Captopril
    carcinoembryonic antigen (CEA)
    CARDS O.S. mono
    Casoni skin
    C-cholyl-glycine breath excretion
    CEA (carcinoembryonic antigen
    cephalin-cholesterol flocculation
    C-glycocholic acid breath
    chew-and-spit
    cholecystokinin
    Cholestech L.D.X.
    CholesTrak
    Cholestron, Cholestron PRO
    Chymex (bentiromide)
    C lactose

test *(cont.)*
    Clinitest stool
    CLOtest
    coagulation study
    Colaris
    ColoCare
    colonic transit
    Colopath
    Colormate TLc BiliTest
    ColoScreen Self-Test
    ColoScreen Slide
    copper-binding protein
    cornflake esophageal motility
    CSF glutamine
    culture and sensitivity (C&S)
    ^{14}C urea
    D-xylose absorption
    deferoxamine mesylate infusion
    dexamethasone suppression
    Diagnex Blue gastric acid
    DNA flow cytometry
    drop
    duodenal string
    Easy A1C
    E-cadherin expression test for classi-
        fication of breast carcinoma
    edrophonium
    EIA-2 (enzyme-linked immuno-
        assay)
    Einhorn string
    ELISA titer
    ELISA-3 titer
    Elucigene
    Emit 2000 cyclosporine specific
        assay
    EndoCab ELISA
    endogenous TSH stimulation
    Entero-Test
    Entero-Test Pediatric
    Escherichia coli O157:H7 assay
    esophageal acid infusion
    esophageal function
    esophageal manometry
    esophageal motility study

test *(cont.)*
    esophageal pH
    EZ Detect colorectal screening
    Ez-HBT
    fasting gastric bile acid
    FastPack system
    FDL (fluorescein dilaurate)
    fecal alpha$_1$-antitrypsin
    fecal fat study
    fecal leukocyte count
    fecal occult blood (FEOT)
    Fisher exact
    Fishman-Doubilet
    5-HT (5-hydroxytryptamine)
    FlexPack HP
    FLU OIA assay
    flutamine
    Fouchet
    Francis
    free thyroxine (FT$_4$)
    free thyroxine index (FT$_4$I)
    FTI (free thyroxine index)
    gastric acid
    gastric analysis
    gastric bile acid
    gastric content
    gastric emptying
    gastric function
    gastric motility study
    gastric secretion rate
    gastrin
    gastrin-secretin stimulation
    gastrin stimulation
    Gastroccult
    Gastro-Test
    GGT (gamma-glutamyl transferase)
    Gluco-Protein
    Gluco-Protein OTC self-test
    glucose tolerance
    Gluzinski
    Glycacor
    Glycosal diabetes
    glycyltryptophan
    Gmelin

test *(cont.)*
  graded esophageal balloon distention
  Graham
  Gram stain of stool
  Grassi
  Great Smokies intestinal
    permeability
  Gross
  guaiac
  guaiac occult blood
  Guenzberg
  Hamel
  Hanger
  Harrison spot
  hatching
  Hay
  H_2 breath
  Helicobacter pylori breath
  Helisal rapid blood
  Hema-Check
  Hematest
  HemDetect three-field occult blood
  HemeSelect reagent and collection
    kit
  Hemoccult
  Hemoccult SENSA
  Hemoccult II
  Hemochron high-dose thrombin
    time (HiTT)
  HemoQuant fecal occult blood
  Heprofile ELISA (enzyme-linked
    immunosorbent assay)
  HercepTest
  Herp-Check
  Herzberg
  high-dose dexamethasone
    suppression
  Histalog stimulation
  histamine
  Hollander
  Home Access Hepatitis C Check
  Horizons C-13 urea breath for
    H. pylori

test *(cont.)*
  hot-shot PCR (polymerase chain
    reaction)
  Huppert
  Hybrid Capture CMV DNA
  Hybrid Capture cytomegalovirus
    DNA
  Hybrid Capture HPV DNA
  Hybritech Tandem PSA ratio
    (free PSA/total PSA)
    (PSA, prostate-specific antigen)
  hydrochloric acid
  hydrogen breath
  ^{131}I uptake (thyroid function)
  iliopsoas
  IMAGN 2000 cellular analysis
  ImmunoCard STAT! Rotavirus
  indium-labeled (^{111}In) autologous
    leukocyte
  indocyanine green
  INFORM HER-2/neu breast cancer
  Innofluor FPIA (fluorescence-
    polarization immunoassay) assay
  insulin tolerance
  !nSure fecal occult blood
  intraductal secretin (IDST)
  intraesophageal acid
  intraesophageal pH
  intragraft polymerase chain reaction
    (PCR) assay
  intraluminal pH electrode
  intraoperative endoscopic Congo red
    (IECRT)
  IOS immunoassay system
  iprofenin
  IRMA blood analysis system
  IRMA-M
  IRMA SL
  Isletest and Isletest-ICA
  Isletest-GAD
  Jacoby
  Javorski
  Jolles
  Kapsinow

test *(cont.)*
   Kashiwado
   Kato
   Kelling
   Kinberg
   Kleihauer-Betke
   Kleihauer-Betke acid elution
   Krokiewicz
   lactose breath
   lactose breath hydrogen
   lactulose-mannitol
   LAP (leucine aminopeptidase)
   latex fixation
   LDH (serum lactate dehydrogenase)
   Leo
   leuvine aminopeptidase
   levulose
   LFTs (liver function tests)
   LHMT (low-range heparin management)
   Ligat
   lipase
   lipid profile
   litmus milk
   liver function (LFT)
   long-acting thyroid-stimulating hormone (LATS)
   low-dose dexamethasone suppression
   low-range heparin management test (LHMT)
   Lundh
   Lüttke (Luettke)
   Machado-Guerreiro
   MacLean
   magnetic susceptibility
   Maly
   Mann-Whitney U (data analysis)
   manometric
   Marechal-Rosen
   marker transit study
   Masset test for bile pigments in urine

test *(cont.)*
   Matritech NMP22
   MATRIX assay
   McNemar ascites
   McNemar test for ascites
   measurement
   mebrofenin hepatobiliary function
   mecholyl
   methyl red
   Mitscherlich
   Mohr
   Moynihan
   Myers and Fine
   Mylius
   N High Sensitivity CRP (C-reactive protein)
   Nakayama
   NAP hepatitis B virus (HBV) quantitative panel
   Nardi test (morphine-prostigmine)
   NBT-PABA
   Neomark-BU (broxuridine)
   NeoTect
   Neukomm
   nitrogen partition
   NuMA
   O&P (ova and parasites)
   OncoChek immunoassay
   OnCyte assay
   optimized serum pancreolauryl test
   overnight dexamethasone suppression
   PABA (p-aminobenzoic acid)
   palmitin
   Pap (Papanicolaou)
   parathyroid hormone (PTH)
   PAS (periodic acid-Schiff)
   PathVysion HER-2 DNA probe kit
   peak secretory flow rate (PSFR)
   pentagastrin
   pentagastrin gastric secretory
   pentagastrin infusion
   pentagastrin provocative
   pentagastrin stimulated analysis

test *(cont.)*
    Seracult Plus
    serum amylase
    serum complement level
    serum DHEA level
    serum glucose value
    serum iron
    serum protein
    serum transaminase level
    72-hour fecal fat
    Sgambati reaction for peritonitis
    SGOT (now *AST*)
    SGPT (now *ALT*)
    sham feeding
    shunt patency
    SIA (strip immunoblot assay)
    Smith
    sodium iodide (^{123}I or ^{125}I) thyroid
       function
    solid sphere
    squeeze pressure profile of anal
       sphincter
    standard acid reflux (SART)
    Stat*Simple
    stimulated gastric secretion
    Stokvis
    Stoll
    stool cytotoxin
    stool electrolyte
    stool osmolality
    stool osmotic gap
    Strassburg
    string
    strip immunoblot assay (SIA)
    Stypven time
    sulfobromophthalein sodium
    Super Seracult
    Szabo
    Tensilon
    thallium treadmill exercise
    thyroid antibody
    thyroid function (TFT)
    thyroid hemagglutination
    thyroid microsomal antibody

test *(cont.)*
    thyroid-stimulating hormone (TSH)
    thyroid suppression
    thyroid uptake of radioactive iodine
    thyrotropin-releasing hormone
       (TRH) stimulation
    thyroxine ratio, effective (ETR)
    thyroxine/TBG ratio
    thyroxine-binding globulin (TBG)
    TIBC (total iron-binding capacity)
    tilt
    TMT (trail making)
    Topfer
    Torquay
    total fecal weight
    total iron-binding capacity (TIBC)
    total serum T_4 (total serum
       thyroxine)
    total thyroxine
    trail making (TMT)
    transferrin
    transmucosal electrical potential
    Triage *Clostridium difficile* panel
    Triage parasite panel
    triceps skinfold thickness
    Trinity adenovirus EIA
    Trousseau
    Truquant BR radioimmunoassay
       (RIA)
    TSH immunoassay
    24-hour ambulatory pH
    24-hour gastric acidity
    two-stage triolein
    Tyson
    UBT (urea breath test) for
       Helicobacter pylori
    Udranszky
    Uffelmann
    Ultzmann
    Uni-Gold *H. pylori*
    urea breath (UBT)
    urease breath
    URINELISA for *Helicobacter pylori*
    UriSite microalbumin/creatinine
       urine

test *(cont.)*
  Uri-Test
  van den Bergh
  van Jaksch
  Velogene rapid VRE assay
  Virgo antimitochondrial antibody kit
  vitamin B_{12} absorption
  Voges-Proskauer
  V-scan
  Wagner
  water-gurgle
  water recovery
  water-sipping
  water-soluble contrast esophageal
    swallow
  WEST (Weinstein Enhanced
    Sensory Test) for diabetic
    neuropathy
  Whipple triad
  Winckler
  Witz
  Woldman
  Wolff-Junghans
  xylose tolerance
  Zappacosta
  ZstatFlu
  zylose absorption
Tes-Tape reagent strip
test breakfast
test dinner
testicular appendage
testicular artery
testicular atrophy
testicular pain
testicular pampiniform venous plexus
testicular torsion
testicular tumor
testicular vessel
testing fluid
testing hepatitis
testis
  descent of
  free-floating
testis appendix

test meal
testolactone
testosterone
test panel
Testred (methyltestosterone)
tetanus-prone wound
tetany
  hypocalcemic
  parathyroid
  parathyroprival
tethered-bowel sign
tetracaine HCl
tetracycline
tetradecyl sulfate
tetrahydrocannabinol (THC)
tetraiodothyronine (T_4)
tetralogy of Fallot
Tevdek pledgeted suture
Tevdek suture
T-fastener gastropexy
TFE polymer pledget
TFT (thyroid function test)
TFX Medical catheter stylet
Tg bandage
TGF (tissue growth factor)
thalassemia major
Thal esophageal stricture repair
Thal esophagogastrostomy
Thal fundic patch operation
thalidomide
thallium treadmill exercise test
thallium-201 (^{201}Tl)
Thal-Nissen fundoplasty
Thalomid (thalidomide)
Thal repair of esophageal stricture
Thal stricturoplasty
Thatcher forceps
Thatcher nail
THBR (thyroid hormone binding ratio)
THC (tetrahydrocannabinol)
THC (thulium, holmium, chromium):
  YAG laser
THC (transhepatic cholangiography)
THE (transhepatic embolization)

The Bandeau postaugmentation bra
thecal abscess
thecal sac
thecoperitoneal shunt
Theiler virus
thenar space abscess
theophylline level
theophylline olamine enema
theophylline toxicity
The Pinto Cobra
Thera-Boot compression dressing
theraccine, Theratope-STn
Theradigm-HBV (hepatitis B virus)
Theragyn
Theralax
therapeutic anesthesia
therapeutic endoscopy
therapeutic intervention
therapeutic malaria
therapeutic protein
therapeutic transjugular procedure
therapist
   enterostomal
   occupational
   physical
   respiratory
   stoma
therapy
   ablative
   ablative laser
   adjuvant
   adjuvant systemic
   androgen
   anticholinergic
   antigastrin
   antilymphocyte induction
   antimicrobial
   antireflux
   antisecretory drug
   anti-TNF
   antiviral
   beta blockade
   breast-conserving
   CadPlan cancer planning

therapy *(cont.)*
   combined modality
   conservative
   curative
   decompression
   diet
   diuretic
   electrolyte
   electrosurgical
   empirical
   endocrine
   endoscopic injection (EIT)
   enteral nutritional (EN)
   enterostomal
   enzyme replacement
   extracorporeal shock-wave (ESWT)
   gamma brachytherapy
   gene
   Gerson
   Hemopure (hemoglobin glutamer-
     250 [bovine]) oxygen
   herbal
   hormonal
   hormone replacement (HRT)
   highly active antiretroviral (HAART)
   induction
   instillation
   interferon-ribavirin
   intralesional
   intravenous
   lamivudine
   laser
   life-long suppressive
   long-term thyroxine
   low-intensity laser (LILT)
   medical
   mono-
   multiagent
   multimodal
   multipolar electrocoagulation
     (MECT; MPEC)
   neoadjuvant hormonal (NHT)
   nonoperative
   nutritional

therapy *(cont.)*
- palliation
- palliative
- pancreatic enzyme replacement
- parenteral
- pharmacotherapy
- photodynamic (PDT)
- polydrug
- postmastectomy radiation
- Precision Therapy
- Prevacid triple
- pulsed-dye laser
- pump
- radiation
- radioactive
- sclerosing
- sham
- steroid
- suppressive
- surgical
- swallowing
- systemic
- Targeted Ablation Therapy
- TheraSphere radiation
- tumor amplified protein expression (TAPET)
- tumor necrosis (TNT)

TheraSeed palladium-103 implants
TheraSphere radiation therapy
Theratope vaccine
Theratope-STn
Therevac-Plus (docusate sodium; benzocaine)
Therevac-SB (docusate sodium)
Therex (huHMFG1) human monoclonal antibody
Thermacare warm air blower
Thermachoice uterine balloon therapy system
Therma Jaw (or Thermajaw) hot urologic forceps
thermal ablation
thermal anesthesia
thermal necrosis

thermal probe
Thermal Quenching cooling technique for laser treatment
thermal stimulation technique
Thermazene (silver sulfadiazine)
thermistor sensor
ThermoChem-HT lavage system (formerly BioLogic-HT system)
thermodilution
thermodilution catheter
thermometer
- IVAC Core·Check
- IVAC electronic
- talking digital
- Tender Tykes digital

Thermoplas sheet
Thermo-STAT system
TherOx 0.014 infusion guidewire
The Solidifier fluid solidification system
The Viewing Wand (surgical digitizer)
The Wand
thiabendazole (TBZ)
thiazolidinedione
thick adhesion
thick bile
thickened gallbladder wall
thickened material
thickened polypropylene thread
thickened wall
thickening
- asymmetric mural
- breast
- gallbladder wall
- haustral fold
- mediastinal
- mucosal
- multiple inflammatory fibrous
- mural
- submucosal

thickening in breast
thickening of gallbladder wall
thickening of haustral fold
thicker hepatic parenchyma
thickness, skinfold

thick-walled gallbladder
Thiersch anal incontinence operation
Thiersch graft
Thiersch medium split free graft
Thiersch suture
Thiersch thin split free graft
Thiersch wire
thiethylperazine
thin adhesion
THI needle
thin-needle percutaneous cholangio-
  gram
ThinPrep slide
thin secretion
THINSite dressing
THINSite with BioFilm hydrogel
  topical wound dressing
thin-walled gallbladder
Thioplex (thiotepa)
thiosalan
thiotepa
third branchial pouch
third-degree hemorrhoid
third pharyngeal pouch
Third National Health and Nutrition
  Examination Survey (NHANES III)
third space fluid loss
thizide diuretics
THL (Transvaginal Hydro Laparoscopy)
  system
Thomas Allis forceps
Thomas extrapolated bar graft
Thomas walking calipers
thombophilia
thombotic thrombocytopenic purpura
  (TTP)
Thompson carotid artery clamp
Thompson rasp
Thomson Walker clamp
Thomson Walker-TC needle holder
thoracentesis
thoracentesis fluid
thoracentesis needle
thoracic aorta

thoracic arch aortogram
thoracic cavity
thoracic duct
thoracic duct injury
thoracic great vessel injury
thoracic great vessel
thoracic inlet
thoracic kidney
thoracic rongeur
thoracic scissors
thoracic splenosis
thoracic stomach
thoracic wall, abdominal
Thoracic instruments
thoracoabdominal esophagectomy
thoracoabdominal esophagogastrectomy
thoracoabdominal incision
thoracoacromial artery
thoracodorsal nerve
thoracophrenolaparotomy
Thoracoport
thoracoscopic esophagomyotomy
thoracoscopic repair of diaphragmatic
  defect
thoracoscopic surgery
thoracoscopy cannula
thoracoscopy trocar
Thora-Klex chest drainage system
Thora-Klex chest tube
Thoralon biomaterial graft
Thora-Port
thorascopic esophagomyotomy
thorax
Thorek dissecting scissors
Thorek-Feldman gallbladder scissors
Thorek gallbladder forceps
Thorek gallbladder scissors
Thorek-Mixter gallbladder forceps
Thorek scissors
Thornton nail
Thornton nail plate
Thornwald antrum perforator and
  irrigator
Thorotrast contrast exposure

Thorotrast contrast medium
threaded pin
threaded rod
threaded Steinmann pin
threadworm
three-armed basket forceps
three-edge cutting forceps
three-hole (3-hole) plate
three-in-one device
three-loop ileal pouch
three-nail forceps
three-point skull clamp
three-prong fork
three-pronged grasping forceps
three-quadrant hemorrhoidectomy
three-quarters prone position
Three-Spring Reservoir Wound Suction
    Drainage Kit
three-strand semintendinosus tendon
    graft
three-strand suture
three-way stopcock
thresher's lung
Thrombin-JMI (thrombin)
thrombin-Keflin-sotredochal sclerosant
thrombocytopenia associated with drug
    abuse
thrombocytopenia purpura
thrombocytosis
Thrombogen topical thrombin
thrombophlebitis of superficial breast
    vein
thrombophlebitis, portal
thrombosed external hemorrhoid
thrombosis
    arterial
    bland
    deep venous (DVT)
    diffuse microvascular
    extensive portal vein
    hepatic artery (HAT)
    indolent
    mesenteric

thrombosis *(cont.)*
    nonocclusive mesenteric
    portal vein
    splenic vein
    spontaneous
    superior mesenteric artery
    venous
thrombosis of hepatic vein
thrombosis of portal vein
Thrombostat (thrombin)
thrombotic mesenteric infarction
thrombotic occlusion of stent shunt
thrombotic thrombocytopenic purpura
thromboulcerative colitis
thromboxanes
thrombus, residual
through and-through continuous suture
through-and-through incision
through-and-through injury
through-and-through laceration
through-and-through suture
through-the-scope (TTS) dilator
through-the-scope mechanical litho-
    tripsy
through-the-wall mattress suture
thrush, oral
thumb-control suction tube
thumb forceps
thumb handle
thumbprinting of mucosa
thumbprinting sign
thymalfasin
thymectomy
    complete
    partial
    total
thymic anlage
thymic-dependent portion of the
    immune system
thymic hypoplasia (DiGeorge syn-
    drome)
thymic tumor
Thymitaq (nolatrexed dihydrochloride)

thymoma
   epithelial cell
   lymphoid cell
   malignant
   mixed cell
   spindle cell
thymosin alpha 1
thymus-derived (T) lymphocyte
thymus, enlarged
thymus gland
Thypinone (protirelin)
Thyrar (thyroid, desiccated bovine)
Thyrel-TRH (protirelin)
Thyro-Block (potassium iodide)
thyrocalcitonemia
thyrocalcitonin assay
thyrocalcitonin secretion
thyrocervical angiography
thyrocervical trunk
Thyrogen (thyrotropin alfa)
thyroglobulin antibody
thyroglossal cyst
thyroglossal duct
thyroglossal duct cyst
thyroglossal duct sinus
thyroglossal fistula
thyroid
   aberrant
   accessory
   benign inflammatory
   C cells of
   desiccated
   desiccated bovine
   desiccated porcine
   ectopic
   fibrosis of
   glottic
   intrathoracic
   lingual
   long-standing stimulation of
   multicentric
   nodular
   overactive
   retrosternal

thyroid *(cont.)*
   substernal
   suprahyoid
   underactive
thyroid ablation
thyroid adenoma
thyroid antibody
thyroid antibody test
thyroid autoantibody
thyroid-binding globulin
thyroid cancer
   anaplastic carcinoma
   biologically active
   differentiated
   follicular carcinoma
   medullary (MTC)
   papillary carcinoma
thyroid capsulitis
thyroid carcinoma
thyroid "C" cells
thyroid crisis
thyroid cystadenoma
thyroid disease
thyroidectomy
   bilateral
   complete
   endoscopic
   Kocher collar
   near-total
   prophylactic
   subtotal
   total
   unilateral
thyroid function test (TFT)
thyroid gland
thyroid goiter
thyroid hemagglutination test
thyroid hormone (TH)
thyroid hormone binding ratio (THBR)
thyroid hormone replacement
thyroid infarction
thyroid instruments
thyroid irradiation
thyroid isthmus

thyroiditis
    adult pyogenic
    acute suppurative
    atrophic
    autoimmune
    chronic
    chronic fibrous
    chronic lymphocytic
    de Quervain
    fibrous
    giant cell
    granulomatous
    Hashimoto
    iatrogenic
    invasive
    ligneous
    nonsuppurative
    painless
    postpartum
    pyogenic
    radiation
    Riedel
    silent
    subacute
    subacute granulomatous
    suppurative
    viral
    vital
    woody
thyroid lobe appendage
thyroid lobectomy
thyroid mapping
thyroid microsomal antibody (MSA)
thyroid migration
thyroid neoplasm
thyroid nodule
thyroid panel
thyroid parenchyma
thyroid scan
thyroid-stimulating hormone (TSH) test
thyroid storm
Thyroid Strong (thyroid, desiccated)
thyroid suppression test
thyroid tumor

thyroid ultrasonography
thyroid ultrasound
thyroid uptake of radioactive iodine test
Thyrolar (liotrix)
thyromedan HCl
thyrothymic ligament
thyrotoxic crisis
thyrotoxic myopathy
thyrotoxicosis
    factitious
    neonatal
thyrotoxicosis without hyperthyroidism
thyrotoxic storm
thyrotrophic hormone
thyrotrophin
thyrotropic-releasing hormone
thyrotropin alfa
thyrotropin-releasing hormone (TRH)
    stimulation test
thyrotropin, suppressed
thyroxin-binding globulin capacity
thyroxine-binding globulin (TBG) test
thyroxine ^{125}I
thyroxine ^{131}I
thyroxine ratio, effective (ETR) test
thyroxine/TBG ratio test
Thytropar (thyrotropin)
tiabendazole
TIBC (total iron-binding capacity) test
tibial cutter guide
tibial cutting guide
tibial drill guide
tibial drill pin
tibial punch
tibial retractor
tick-borne virus
tickle of pancreas
tickle of spleen
ticklish
Ticlid (ticlopidine)
ticlopidine
Ticon (trimethobenzamide HCl)
Ti-Cron suture (also Tycron)
tidal volume

Tip-Trol handle
tirolimus
Tischler biopsy tip
Tischler cervical biopsy punch forceps
Tischler-Morgan biopsy forceps
Tisseel fibrin sealant
Tisseel "surgical glue"
Tissomat application device
Tissucol fibrin-collagen hemostatic
   material
Tissucol fibrin glue
tissue
   acinar
   adipose
   analogous
   areolar
   autogenous
   bites of
   cicatricial
   connective
   cortical
   dead pancreatic
   debridement
   dense breast
   ectopic pancreatic
   enveloping scar
   extirpation of
   extraperitoneal
   fatty
   fibroadipose
   fibrofatty
   fibroglandular
   fibrous
   fibrous stromal
   fragmented
   friable
   functioning thyroid
   granulation
   gut-associated lymphoid (GALT)
   heterotopic pancreatic
   infected
   lipomatous-like
   morcellation of
   necrosis of

tissue *(cont.)*
   necrotic
   nodal
   nonviable
   parenchymal
   periadrenal
   pericoronal
   peridiverticular
   perinephric
   perirenal
   plug of
   polypoid
   redundant
   resected
   retrocecal
   scar
   septal
   soft
   splenic
   subcutaneous
   surrounding fatty
   suspicious
   tail of breast
   thyroid
   vascularized gastric
tissue adhesive (see *adhesive*)
tissue and cuticle nipper
tissue approximation
tissue catabolism
tissue debridement
   fibrinolysin and desoxyribonuclease
   papain
   sutilains
tissue engineering
tissue equivalent material
tissue extraction
tissue expander
   AccuSpan
   Becker
   Cox-Uphoff International (CUI)
   Heyer-Schulte
   T-Span
tissue-fixed macrophage
tissue forceps

tissue growth factor (TGF)
tissue hypoxia
tissue invasion
tissue irrigation
tissue ischemia
tissue level of porphyrins
TissueLink Monopolar Floating Ball
tissue marker, MicroMark
tissue-mesh interface
tissue occlusion clamp
tissue penetration
tissue perfusion
tissue-selective estrogens
tissue-sparing technique
tissue vascularity
Tis-U-Trap endometrial suction catheter
titanium alloy rod
titanium half pin
titanium microsurgical bipolar forceps
titanium microsurgical needle holder
titanium nail
titanium plate
titanium staple
Titralac (calcium carbonate)
TLc.BiliTest system
TL–90 (Ethicon) stapler
TME (total mesorectal excision)
TMT (trail-making test)
TNB (transthoracic needle biopsy)
TNB (Tru-Cut needle biopsy)
TNF-alpha (tumor necrosis factor-
    alpha) level
TNFa, IL–1b, IL–6, IL–10, KC,
    MCP–1, MIP–2, and RANTES
    (inflammatory cytokines)
TNM classification of carcinoma
TNM classification of malignant tumors
    (T represents size of tumor,
    N clinical status of node, and
    M metastases)
        M0 No distant metastases
        M1 Distant metastases present
        MX Distant metastases not
            assessed

TNM classification *(cont.)*
        N0 Regional lymph node not
            involved
        N1 Regional lymph node
            involved
        NX Regional lymph node not
            assessed
        Stage I, T1–2, N0, M0—No
            extension or node involve-
            ment
        Stage II, T3, N0, M0—Advanced
            extension, unresectable
        Stage III, T1–3, N1, M0—Node
            involvement
        Stage IV, T1–3, N0–1, M1—
            Distant metastases present
        T1 Direct extension of primary
            tumor
        T2 Direct extension of primary
            tumor to specific organs
        T3 Direct advanced extension of
            tumor, unresectable
TNT (tumor necrosis therapy) staging
    system
to-and-fro anesthesia
Todd cirrhosis
Todd-Wells guide
Toennis-Adson dissecting scissors
Toennis dissecting scissors
Toennis dura hook
Toennis dura knife
Toennis tumor forceps
toe plate
toe-to-groin modified Jones dressing
toe ulcer
togavirus
Toggelite
toilet, peritoneal
Toilinox (stainless steel)
tolazamide
tolbutamide-induced cholestasis
tolbutamide sodium
tolbutamide stimulation test
Toldt, white line of

tolerance, activity
tolerance induction to islet allotrans-
 plantation
Tolerex enteral nutritional therapy
Tolinase (tolazamide)
tolrestat
toluidine blue stain
Tom Jones closure suture
Tomac nonconductive breathing
Tomocat (barium sulfate)
tomographic view
tomography (see *imaging*)
Tomudex (raltitrexed)
Tonalin (conjugated linoleic acid)
tongs, Gardner-Wells
tongue
 adder's
 bald
 base of
 beefy
 black hairy
 coated
 cobblestone
 flat
 furry
 raspberry
 smooth
tongue base
tongue blade
tongue pulsive force
tonic contraction
Tonopaque (barium sulfate)
tonsillar crypt
tonsillar forceps
tonsillar pillar
tonsil forceps
tonsil knife
tonsil scissors
tonsil sponge
tonsil sucker
tonsil tag excision
Toomey irrigating syringe
toothed Adson tissue forceps
toothed retractor

toothed tissue forceps
TOPA (topical oropharyngeal
 anesthesia)
topanoic acid (Telepaque)
Topaz CO_2 laser
Topel knot
Töpfer test
topical agent
topical anesthesia (see *anesthesia*)
topical anesthetic
topical bovine thrombin
topical hemostatic agent
topical nitrate
topical pharyngeal anaesthesia
topical podopyllin
topical steroid
top-loading rod
topogram, topography
 balloon
 scintigraphic balloon
toposcopic catheter
Torbot faceplate
TORCH (toxoplasmosis; other agents;
 rubella; cytomegalovirus; herpes
 simplex) syndrome
Torcon NB selective angiographic
 catheter
Torecan
toremifene citrate
Torquay test
torrential bleeding
Torres syndrome
torsion
 biliary tract
 intestinal
 large-bowel
 testicular
 ovarian
torsion forceps
torsion of cyst or fallopian tube
torsion of splenic vein
torso crease
tortuous bile duct
tortuous esophagus

tortuous lesion
Toshiba EccoCee ultrasound system
Toshiba 270 ultrasound system
Toshiba videoendoscope
tositumomab
total abdominal colectomy (TAC)
total abdominal evisceration (TAE)
    organ harvesting technique
total bilateral vagotomy
total bile acid
total bilirubin
total blood loss
total body sodium deficit
total colectomy
total esophagectomy
total fecal weight test
total food intolerance
total fundic wrap (Nissen-Rossetti)
total gastrectomy
total gastric wrap
total gastrin
total hepatectomy
total intravenous anesthesia
total iron-binding capacity (TIBC)
total left lobectomy of liver
total lesion
total lobectomy
total mastectomy
total mesorectal excision (TME)
total necrosis
total pancreatectomy
total pancreatectomy with
    lymphadenectomy
total parathyroidectomy
total parenteral alimentation
total parenteral nutrition (TPN)
total protein
total protocolectomy and ileostomy
total right lobectomy of liver
total sac excision
total serum T_3 (total serum triiodothy-
    ronine) test
total serum T_4 (total serum thyroxine)
    test

total shunt
total spinal anesthesia
total thoracic esophagectomy
total thymectomy
total thyroidectomy
total thyroxine test
total villous atrophy
totally (or total) extraperitoneal laparo-
    scopic hernioplasty
totally intrahepatic gallbladder
Toti trephine drill
Toupet fundoplasty
Toupet fundoplication
Toupet hemifundoplication
Tourguide guiding catheter
Tourni-cot tourniquet
towel clamp
towel clip
Tower sterile packaging
Townes Brooks syndrome
Townley femur calipers
Townley tibial plateau plate
Townsend-Gilfillan plate
Townsend handle
toxemia, hepatic
toxic (diffuse) goiter
toxic atrophy
toxic cirrhosis
toxic colitis
toxic diarrhea
toxic diffuse goiter
toxic dilatation
toxic dilation of colon
toxic drug concentration in blood and
    tissues
toxic gastritis
toxic gastroenteritis
toxic goiter
toxic granulation
toxic granule
toxic hepatitis
toxic inflammation
toxic insult
toxic irrigant

toxicity
  drug
  gastrointestinal
  GI
  hepatic
  oxygen (O_2)
  theophylline
toxic level
toxic megacolon
toxic multinodular goiter
toxic mushroom poisoning
toxic myocarditis
toxic nephrosis
toxic neuritis
toxic nodular goiter
toxic or inflammatory myopathy or
  dysfunctional neuromuscular
  transmission
toxic pneumonia
toxic shock syndrome (TSS)
toxic steatosis
toxic substances test on venous blood
toxic thyroid state
toxic uninodular goiter
toxic vacuolization
toxigenic bacteria
toxin exposure
toxoplasmosis hepatitis
TPN (total parenteral nutrition)
TPN with lipids
TQa (transcutaneous access flow)
  device
trabecula (pl. trabeculae)
trabecular artery
trabecular carcinoma of skin
trabecular cirrhosis
trace edema
trace mineral
trace pedal edema
Tracer blood glucose monitor
Tracer hybrid wire guide for endo-
  scopic surgery
tracheal blade
tracheal hook

tracheal retractor
tracheobronchial mucosal necrosis
tracheoesophageal (TE)
tracheoesophageal fistula (TEF)
tracheoesophageal junction
tracheoesophageal puncture (TEP)
tracheomalacia
tracheostomy tube
Trachlight
Tracker-10 catheter
Tracker-18 Soft Stream catheter
Tracrium (atracurium besylate)
tract
  alimentary
  biliary
  digestive
  fistulous
  gastrointestinal (GI)
  hepatic outflow
  ileal inflow
  iliopubic
  intestinal
  intramural fistulous
  lower gastrointestinal
  mature T-tube
  pancreaticobiliary
  pyramidal
  reproductive
  respiratory
  sinus
  upper gastrointestinal (UGI)
  urinary
traction anchor
traction diverticulum
traction hook
traction pin
traction suture
trail-making test (TMT)
TrakBack ultrasound catheter
TRAM (transverse rectus abdominis
  myocutaneous) flap
Tramex polypropylene mesh
transabdominal preperitoneal laparo-
  scopic hernioplasty

transabdominal repair
transabdominal retroperitoneal node
 dissection
transabdominal sonography
transaminase, hepatic
transampullary septectomy
transanal approach
transanal deflation of sigmoid volvulus
transanal double-stapling technique
transanal endoscopic microsurgery
 (TEM)
transanal pouch advancement
transarterial chemoembolization
 (TACE)
transarticular pin
transaxillary subpectoral mammoplasty
transcatheter arterial chemoemboliza-
 tion (TACE)
transcatheter variceal embolization
transcatheter vessel embolization
transcellular fluid
transcervical route
transcoccygeal approach
transcorpus impalement
transcription factor
transcutaneous electrical nerve
 stimulation
transcystic common bile duct
 exploration
transcystic duct/common bile duct
 exploration (TCD/CBDE)
TransCyte skin substitute graft
transdermal anesthesia
Transderm Scop
transducer
 abdominal
 rectal
 rectal multiplane
 volume displacement
transducer fitting
transduodenal drainage technique
transduodenal endoscopic decompres-
 sion
transduodenal sphincteroplasty

transduodenal sphincterotomy
Transeal transparent adhesive film
 dressing
transect
transected stomach
transected vertical gastric bypass with
 Silastic ring band and gastrostomy
transection
transection of esophagus
transectomy of vagus nerves, truncal
Transelast bandage
transendoscopic catheter placement
transendoscopic electrocoagulation
transendoscopic tube
transesophageal endoscopy
transesophageal ligation of varices
transfemoral liver biopsy
transfer
 free flap
 free jejunum
 microsurgical free tissue
 microvascular flap
 nuclear
transference of muscle and blood
 supply
 latissimus dorsi flap
 rectus abdominis flap
transferrin saturation, percent
transfixing pin
transfixion pin
transfixion suture
transformation, malignant
transfuse
transfusion
 autologous
 donor-specific (DST)
 incompatible blood
 intraoperative autologous (IOT)
 massive blood
 multiple
transfusion hepatitis
transfusion malaria
transfusion of incompatible blood
transfusion of packed cells

transverse hook
transverse incision
transverse-loop rod colostomy
transverse mesocolon
transverse orientation
transverse plane
transverse process hook
transverse rectus abdominis myocuta-
  neous (TRAM) flap for breast
  reconstruction
transverse section
transverse suture
transverse wedge excision
transversostomy
transversotomy
transversus abdominis aponeurosis
transversus abdominis muscle
transversus aponeurosis
transversus arch
trap, DeLee suction
trastuzumab (anti-HER2 humanized
  monoclonal antibody)
Traube neurological percussion hammer
Traube semilunar space
Traum-Aid HBC enteral feeding
trauma
  autoerotic rectal
  blunt
  blunt abdominal
  foreign body
  head
  homosexual rectal
  iatrogenic
  intraoperative
  liver
  massive splenic
  penetrating
  penetrating abdominal
  rectal
  splenic
TraumaCal (multiple branched-chain
  amino acids) enteral nutritional
  therapy

TraumaCal enteral feeding
TraumaJet wound debridement system
TraumaSeal sealant
traumatic anesthesia
traumatic appendicitis
traumatic extraperitoneal perforation of
  duodenal diverticulum
traumatic hernia
traumatic hyphema
traumatic lesion
traumatic placement of nasogastric tube
traumatic rupture
traumatic scar
traumatic tissue grab
traumatopneic wound
trauma zones (I, II, III)
Trautman Locktite prosthetic hook
Trautmann chisel
Travamulsion fat emulsion solution
Travasol in Dextrose
Travasol with electrolytes
Travasorb HN (high nitrogen) powdered
  feeding
Travasorb MCT (medium chain
  triglyceride)
Travasorb MCT enteral nutritional
  therapy
Travasorb MCT food supplement
Travasorb MCT liquid feeding
Travasorb STD enteral nutritional
  therapy
Travasorb STD liquid feeding
traveler's diarrhea
"traveling volvulus"
Travers retractor
traverse, peritoneal
traverse the internal ring
traversing the center
Traverso-Longmire technique
Treace drill
treatment algorithm
treatment modality
treatment protocol

tree
  biliary
  hepatobiliary
trefoil balloon
trefoil deformity
Treitz fossa
Treitz hernia
Treitz, ligament of
Trelex mesh graft
Trelex polypropylene mesh
trematode (fluke)
tremors of the hands and tongue
tremulousness
Trendelenburg position
trephine drill
trephine, Galt cranial
Treponema pallidum
tretromolar trigone
Trex digital mammography system
  (TDMS)
TRH (thyrotropin-releasing hormone)
Triacana (tiratricol; levothyroxine
  sodium)
triad
  Beck
  Charcot
  Dieulafoy
  fragile histidine (FHIT)
  hepatic
  portal
  Rigler
  Saint
  Whipple
triad of liver disease, arterial hypox-
  emia, and intrapulmonary vascular
  dilatation
triad of Rigler
Triage *Clostridium difficile* panel
Triage parasite panel
trial
  Breast Cancer Prevention Trial
  ADOPT (a diabetes outcome
    progression)
  clinical (phases 1–3)

trial *(cont.)*
  DPT–1 (diabetes prevention trial
    type 1)
  randomized (RT)
  randomized double-blind
  6C (cooperative colorectal cancer
    combination chemotherapy
  clinical)
trial base plate
triangle
  Calot
  cardiohepatic
  Charcot
  cystohepatic
  digastric
  gastrinoma
  Grynfeltt
  Henke
  Hesselbach
  iliofemoral
  inferior lumbar
  inguinal
  Keith abdominal
  Labbe
  Lesgaft
  Livingston
  lumbocostoabdominal
  mesenteric
  Petit
  posterior neck
  Scarpa
triangle sponge
triangular bone reamer
triangular ligament of liver
triangular medullary nail
Triban (trimethobenzamide HCl;
  benzocaine)
Tricam SL/IPM
triceps skinfold thickness
trichinosis
trichobezoar
trichocyst
trichomonal colitis
trichomoniasis, intestinal

Trichosporon beigelii
trichosporosis
Trichuris trichiura
Tricodur Epi (elbow) compression
　　support bandage
Tricodur Omos (shoulder) compression
　　support bandage
Tricodur Talus (ankle) compression
　　support bandage
Tricofix bandage
tricortical bone graft
tricortical ilial strip graft
tricuspid orifice
tridihexethyl chloride
Tridrate bowel prep
Tridrate Bowel Evacuant Kit
trifid stomach
triflange nail
triflanged Lottes nail
trigeminal nerve retractor
trigeminal scissors
triglycerides
　　long chain (LCT)
　　medium chain (MCT)
　　serum
triglyceride enzyme deficiency
trihydrocoprostanic acid (TCA)
trilostane
Trilucent breast implant
Trimadeau sign
Trimax fabric
Trimazide (trimethobenzamide HCl)
trimethoprim-sulfamethoxazole
trimethylaminuria (fish-odor syndrome)
trimmer, Little
Trinity adenovirus EIA test kit
Trinkle drill
trioiodothyronine (T_3)
triple antibiotics
triple-lumen catheter
triple-lumen papillotome
triple-lumen Sengstaken-Blakemore
　　tube
triple-lumen tube

Triptone (dimenhydrinate)
triradial resector blade
trisegmentectomy of liver
Tri-State Hospital Supply Corp.
Tritec (ranitidine bismuth citrate)
tri-wing anoscope
Trizivir
Trizyme (amylase; protease; cellulase)
Trocan disposable CO_2 trocar and
　　cannula
trocar
　　abdominal
　　accessory
　　ascites
　　blunt
　　Bluntport
　　Bluntport laparoscopic
　　camera
　　Coakley antrum
　　conical
　　Cooper Surgical
　　Core audible
　　Core Entree Plus
　　Core Entree II
　　Core shielded laparoscopic
　　Davidson thoracic
　　DeRoyal
　　dilating tip
　　Don Congreve
　　Duke
　　Endopath laparoscopic
　　Endopath TriStar
　　Entree Plus
　　Entree II
　　Entree thoracoscopy
　　Ethicon Endo-Surgery
　　Ethicon Surgiport
　　gallbladder
　　Hasson
　　Hunt-Reich
　　Hurwitz thoracic
　　hydrocele
　　Iotec
　　Landau

trocar *(cont.)*
  laparoscopic
  Nelson thoracic
  New Eder Corporation
  Ochsner gallbladder
  Origin
  Patterson
  PediPort
  peritoneal
  pyramidal
  pyramidal tip
  Saber BT blunt-tip surgical
  safety-shielded
  Step minimally invasive surgical
  subxiphoid
  suprapubic
  Surgiport
  Synthes transbuccal
  Ternamian EndoTIP system
  thoracoscopy
  Trocan disposable CO_2
  TroGARD Finesse
  umbilical
  VanAlyea antrum
  VersaPort
  Visiport optical
  Wangsteen
  Wolf
  Yankauer
trocar cannula
trocar hernia
trocar placement
trocar site tumor implant
trocar tent
trocar wound-site complication
trocar and sheath
trochanter, greater
trochanter-holding clamp
trochanter reamer
Troeltsch dressing forceps
TroGARD Finesse dilating trocar
  system
troglitazone
Troisier sign

Trömner (Troemner) percussion
  hammer
Tronolane (pramoxine HCl)
Tronzo elevator
TrophAmine total parenteral nutrition
trophic effect
trophic lesion
tropical sprue
tropical steatorrhea
tropisetron
trospectomycin
Trousseau esophageal bougie
Trousseau sign
Trousseau test
Trousseau trachea dilator
Troutman needle
Troutman rectus forceps
trovafloxacin
Trovan (trovafloxacin)
Trovax
troxacitabine
Tru-Area Determination wound-
  measuring device
Tru-Close wound drainage system
Tru-Cut cutting biopsy needle
Tru-Cut liver biopsy needle
Tru-Cut needle (TCNB) biopsy
true diverticulum (pl. diverticula)
true lateral view
True/Fit femoral intramedullary rod
  system
TruJect auto-injector drug delivery
  system
Trulife silicone breast prosthesis
Trumbull suture
trumpet, Core reposable
Trumpet needle guide
trumpet valve
truncal obesity
truncal vagotomy and gastroenteros-
  tomy
truncal vagotomy and pyloroplasty
trunk, celiac

TruPulse CO_2 laser
Truquant BR radioimmunoassay
Truquant BR RIA test
Tru-Scint AD imaging agent
truss for groin hernia
Tru-Support EW (elastic wrap) bandage
Tru-Support SA (self-adhering) bandage
Trypanosoma cruzi
trypanosomiasis
trypsin, crystallized
tryptophan malabsorption
TSH (thyroid-stimulating hormone)
TSH immunoassay test
TSH-01 transdermal tape
TSH receptor stimulation
TSH secretion
TSH suppression
TSRH (Texas Scottish Rite Hospital)
  hook
TSRH (Texas Scottish Rite Hospital)
  rod
TSS (toxic shock syndrome)
T-tack gastropexy
TTC (T-tube cholangiogram)
TTS (through-the-scope) catheter
TUBA (transumbilical breast augmenta-
  tion)
tube (see also *stent; tubing*)
  Abbott-Miller
  Abbott-Rawson double-lumen
  Activent antimicrobial ventilation
    myringotomy
  Adson brain suction
  Adson suction
  Andrews Pynchon suction
  angled 24F pleural
  angled pleural
  Argyle chest
  Argyle-Salem sump
  Argyle Sentinel Seal chest
  ascites drainage
  Atkinson silicone rubber
  Axiom double sump
  baby Poole suction

tube *(cont.)*
  baby Yankauer suction
  Baker decompression
  Baker intestinal decompression
  Baker jejunostomy
  Baron suction
  Baylor sump
  bent inner
  bilateral pleural
  Biosystems feeding
  Bivona TTS (tight-to-shaft)
    tracheostomy
  Blakemore
  Blakemore-Sengstaken
  blocked shunt
  blue line Murphy tracheal
  Boyce modification of Sengstaken-
    Blakemore
  brain suction
  Brochman suction
  Broncho-Cath endobronchial
  Broncho-Cath endotracheal
  Buie rectal suction
  Buie suction
  calibration
  Caluso PEG (percutaneous endo-
    scopic gastrostomy) tube
  Cantor
  Cattell gallbladder
  Celestin esophageal
  Celestin intraluminal
  Celestin latex rubber
  cement
  chest
  Ciaglia Blue Rhino
  Cole
  colonic
  Combitube
  cone suction
  Cooley graft suction
  Cooley intracardiac suction
  Corflo-Ultra jejunostomy
  Corpak feeding
  Cottle suction

tube *(cont.)*
    crystal tracheostomy
    cuffed endotracheal
    cuffed fenestrated
    Dawson-Yuhl suction
    decompression
    Dennis intestinal
    dePezer gastrostomy
    diathermy suction
    directional endotracheal
    Dobbhoff gastrectomy feeding
    double-lumen
    double-lumen endobronchial
    drainage
    Dreiling
    Dumon-Gilliard prosthesis pushing
    Edlich gastric lavage
    EMT emergency medicine
    endoesophageal
    endotracheal
    Endotrol tracheal
    EntriStar PEG (percutaneous
        endoscopic gastrostomy)
    esophageal
    Ewald
    Ewald evacuator
    Ewald gastric lavage
    Fazier modified suction
    feeding
    feeding gastrostomy
    FELL suction
    fenestrated
    fenestrated tracheostomy
    Ferguson brain suction
    Ferguson-Frazier suction
    Fergusson suction
    fil d'Arion silicone
    filler
    Flexiflo Stomate low-profile
        gastrostomy
    Foley catheter gastrostomy
    four-lumen
    Frazier Britetrac suction
    Frazier-Paparella suction

tube *(cont.)*
    front lifting hood rectoscope
    gastric aspiration
    gastric calibration
    gastric lavage
    gastrointestinal
    gastrostomy
    germination
    Glasser gastrostomy
    Gomco suction
    Gott
    grafting suction
    Guibor Silastic
    guide
    Guilford-Wright suction
    Haldane-Priestley
    Hardy suction
    Harris
    Hemo-Drain wound
    Hi-Lo Evac endotracheal
    Hi-Lo Jet tracheal
    Hi-Lo tracheal
    Hodge intestinal decompression
    Holinger open-end aspirating
    Hollister gastrostomy
    Holter
    House suction-irrigation
    Immergut suction coagulation
    insulated outer
    intermediate Hi-Lo tracheal
    Inverta-PEG
    J
    Jackson laryngectomy
    Jackson Open-End aspirating
    Jackson trachea
    Jackson Velvet eye aspirating
    Jako laryngeal suction
    jejunal feeding
    jejunostomy
    Jergesen
    Jesberg aspirating
    J-shaped
    Kahn-Frazier suction
    Kam Vac suction

tube *(cont.)*
  Kaslow intestinal
  Keofeed feeding
  Killian suction
  K-Tube
  Lanz low-pressure cuff endotracheal
  large-bore gastric lavage
  large-caliber
  laryngoflex laryngectomy
  laser laryngeal suction
  Laser-Flex tracheal
  Lepley-Ernst
  Levin
  Lewis laryngeal
  LGT laryngectomy
  ligament sizing
  Lindholm tracheal
  Linton-Nachlas
  Lo-Contour
  Lo-Pro tracheal
  long intestinal
  Magill insulated suction
  Malecot gastrostomy
  Malis
  Mallinckrodt Laser-Flex tube
  Mallinckrodt Medical tracheal
  Mark IV
  Martin laryngectomy
  Mason suction
  maxillofacial
  McCulloch suction
  Medi-Vac bulk tubing
  Medoc-Celestin pulsion
  mercury-weighted
  metal-weighted Silastic feeding
  MIC gastroenteric
  MIC jejunostomy
  MIC-Key G gastrostomy
  MIC-Key J gastrostomy
  MIC-TJ (transgastric jejunal)
  micro irrigation suction
  Micron bobbin ventilation
  Mik (Mikulicz) gastrostomy
  Miller-Abbott

tube *(cont.)*
  Miller-Abbott intestinal
  Miller-Abbott long gastrointestinal
  Minnesota
  modified Minnesota
  Molteno seton
  Montgomery Safe-T-Tube
  Mosher life-saving
  Moss G-tube PEG kit
  Moss gastrostomy
  Moss nasal
  Moss Suction Buster
  Mousseaux-Barbin intraluminal
  Mousseaux-Barbin prosthetic
  mushroom gastrostomy
  Nasal RAE uncuffed
  nasobiliary
  nasobiliary drainage
  nasoduodenal feeding
  nasogastric (NG) feeding
  nasojejunal (NJ) feeding
  nasopancreatic drainage
  nasotracheal
  Neo tracheal
  neural
  New York Glass suction
  NEW Speaking Tube
  Newvicon vacuum chamber pickup
  NG (nasogastric) feeding
  Nuport PEG
  Nyhus-Nelson gastric decompres-
    sion and jejunal feeding
  obstructed shunt
  Olympus One-Step Button gastros-
    tomy
  oral gastric (OGT)
  oral gastric calibration
  Oral RAE uncuffed
  oroendotracheal
  orogastric
  Ossoff-Karlan microlaryngeal
    suction
  ostiomeatal stent
  Pacifico-type suction

tube *(cont.)*
    Paul-Mixter
    Pedi PEG
    pediatric feeding
    pediatric nasogastric
    pediatric Y
    PEG (percutaneous endoscopic
        gastrostomy)
    percutaneous gastrostomy
    percutaneous jejunostomy
    Pitt talking tracheostomy
    Plester suction
    Pleur-evac suction
    pleural
    polyethylene
    Poole
    Poole abdominal suction
    Precut intermediate Hi-Lo tracheal
    pressure-sensitive valve in shunt
    Pribham suction
    Procter-Livingston
    PTCS
    Pynchon suction
    Quinton
    Radius enteral feeding
    RAE endotracheal
    rectal
    Rehfuss
    reinforced trachea
    Replogle
    Reuter bobbin
    Rhoton-Merz suction
    right-angle chest
    Ring–McLean sump
    Robert Shaw bronchus
    Rosen suction
    rubber
    Rubin-Quinton small bowel biopsy
    Ruschelit PVC tracheostomy
    Ryle
    Sachs brain suction
    Sacks-Vine feeding gastrostomy
    Sacks-Vine PEG (percutaneous
        endoscopic gastrostomy)

tube *(cont.)*
    Salem duodenal sump
    Sandoz suction/feeding
    Sarns intracardiac suction
    Saticon vacuum chamber pickup
    S-B (Sengstaken-Blakemore)
    Schwann cell
    Scott nasal suction
    Sengstaken-Blakemore (S-B)
    Shah permanent
    Shiley tracheal
    Shiley tracheotomy
    Shiner
    shunt
    Silastic
    Simpson-Smith rectal suction
    single-cannula tracheal
    small bowel
    Souttar
    Spachmann
    spring-loaded, retractable blunt
        inner protective
    Stamm
    standard with flex
    stomach
    straight chest
    suction
    Suh ventilation
    sump nasogastric
    Super PEG
    T
    tampon
    Teflon
    Thora-Klex chest
    thumb-control suction
    Tinckler rectal suction
    tracheostomy
    transendoscopic
    transhepatic
    transpyloric
    triple-lumen Sengstaken-Blakemore
    Tru-Arc
    T-shaped silicone shunt
    U

tube *(cont.)*
 uncuffed Magill endo
 Vacutainer
 Value-Line Poole abdominal suction
 Versatome laser fiber
 Vidicon vacuum chamber pickup
 Vivonex Moss
 V. Mueller-Poole suction
 Wagener-Mosher
 Walton-Poole suction
 Walton-Yankauer suction
 Wangensteen suction
 water-seal chest
 Wilson-Cook
 Wookey skin
 Wurbs-type nasobiliary
 Yankauer suction
 Yasargil suction
tube anode
tube cecostomy
tube check
tube clip
tube decompression
tube drainage
tube duodenostomy with feeding
 jejunostomy
tube enteroscope
tube-fed patient
tube feeding
tube flap graft
tube graft (see *graft*)
tube guide
tube-occluding clamp
tubercle of Zuckerkandl
tubercle, pubic
tuberculosis lesion
tuberculosis, peritoneal
tuberculous Addison disease
tuberculous colitis
tuberculous peritonitis
tube thoracostomy
Tubex gauze dressing
Tubigrip bandage
Tubigrip dressing

Tubigrip glove
tubing (see also *tube*)
 CO_2
 corrugated
 HI VAC
 irrigation
 Lamis
 Lamis Y
 large-bore Tygon
 Lysonics handle
 Medi-Vac bulk
 mentor
 nonconducting
 Orthotec handpiece and
 Pennsylvania Hospital
 PSI-TEC
 Tygon venovenous bypass
 Universal female DISS
tubing clamp
tubing connector
Tubinger gastric reconstruction
tubing forceps
tubocurarine chloride
tubogram
tubo-ovarian abscess
tubular adenocarcinoma
tubular adenoma
tubular cancer
tubular carcinoma
tubular elastic bandage
tubular esophagus
tubular lesion
tubular narrowing
tubular necrosis, acute
tubular plate
tubular polyp
tubular punch
tubular stockinette bandage
tubular vertical gastroplasty
tubulovillous adenoma
tubulovillous polyp
tubus digestorius
Tucker spindle-shaped dilator
Tucks Pads

Tudor-Edwards bone-cutting forceps
Tuffier abdominal retractor
Tuffier abdominal spatula
Tuffier laminectomy retractor
Tuffier-Raney retractor
Tuffier rib spreader
tuft, vascular
tuftsin and properdin (opsins)
tulip probe
TULIP (transurethral laser-induced
  prostatectomy device)
tumbler graft
tumbling obstruction
tumescent liposuction technique
tumescent technique of breast reduction
tummy tuck flap
tumor (see also *neoplasm*)
  Abrikosov
  adrenal
  AML (angiomyolipoma) solid renal
  ampullary
  anaplastic
  aneuploid
  Askin
  benign
  benign bile duct
  benign epidermal
  benign liver
  benign primary
  benign vascular (of the liver)
  beta cell (of the pancreas)
  bifurcation
  bladder
  bone
  breast
  Brenner
  brown
  bulky
  carcinoid
  CNS (central nervous system)
  colon
  cortisol secreting
  cutaneous
  D-cell

tumor *(cont.)*
  desmoid
  discrete
  ectopic cortisol-producing
  embryonal
  endocardial
  endocrine (of the pancreas)
  esophageal
  estrogen-receptor-negative (ER–)
  estrogen-receptor-positive (ER+)
  Ewing
  excision of primary
  extraluminal retrorectal
  extraparathyroid
  feminizing (of the adrenal cortex)
  fibrous
  focal
  functioning adrenocortical
  gastrin-producing
  gastrin-secreting non-beta islet cell
  gastrointestinal
  giant cell
  globular
  glucagon-producing
  glucagon-secreting
  grading
  granular cell
  granulosa cell
  gray
  GRFoma pancreatic endocrine
  gritty
  gross
  gynecologic
  highly vascular
  Hürthle (Huerthle) cell
  ileal primary
  insulin-producing
  insulin-secreting
  intracranial
  invasive
  invasive ductal
  invasive lobular
  islet cell
  kidney

twist drill
twist drill catheter
twist hook
twisted plate
twisted suture
twister, Rubio-TC wire
twisting of the colon on itself about
 its mesentery
TwoCal HN enteral nutritional therapy
two-channel duodenoscope
two-channel endoscope
two-hole (2-hole) plate
two-inch gauze bandage
two-layer anastomosis
two-layer closure
two-layer latex and Marlex closure
 technique
two loop J-shaped ileal pouch
two-lumen catheterization
two-lumen papillotome
two-piece ostomy pouch
two-plane view
two-prong rake retractor
two-quadrant hemorrhoidectomy
two-stage triolein test
two-staged operation
two-strand suture
two-thirds rule
two-tube cuff
two-valved anoscope
two-way laparoscopic port
Tycos aneroid sphygmomanometer
Tycron suture (also Ti-Cron)
Tydings tonsil seizing/snare
Tygon venovenous bypass tubing
tying forceps
Tylenol No. 3 (or #3)
Tyler-Gigli saw

tympanites
tympanitic abdomen
tympanitic dullness
tympany, abdominal
type A, B, or C lesion
type A gastritis
type and cross blood
type and crossmatch
type B chronic gastritis
type B gastritis
type I hepatorenal syndrome
type I hiatal hernia
type 1 plasminogen activator inhibitor
 (PAI-1)
type II hepatorenal syndrome
type II hiatal hernia
typhlitis (appendicitis)
typhloenteritis
typhlomegaly
typhlonous debris
typhlorrhaphy
typhlostenosis
typhlostomy
typhoidal cholangiolitis
typhoidal cholecystitis
Typhoon microdebrider blade
typing and crossmatching of blood
typing system (see *classification*)
Tyrell hook
Tyrex-2 enteral nutritional therapy
tyropanoate contrast medium
tyropanoate sodium
tyrosine
tyrosinemia, hereditary
tyrosyluria
Tyson test
T–Y stent
Tzanck smear

U, u

UA (urinalysis)
UBT (urea breath test) for *Helicobacter pylori* (*H. pylori*)
UC (ulcerative colitis)
UCB (unconjugated hyperbilirubi-nemia)
UCLA pouch
UCP compression plate
UD-BMT (unrelated donor, bone marrow transplantation)
UDCA (ursodeoxycholic acid)
U double-barrel suture
Udranszky test
U-drape
U echovirus
UES (upper esophageal sphincter)
Uffelmann test
UFT (uracil plus tegafur)
UGI (upper gastrointestinal) tract
UGI (upper gastrointestinal) with small bowel follow-through
UGI (upper gastrointestinal) bleeding
UGI contrast study
UICC TNM staging classification
UItrasil material

ulcer (see also *ulceration*)
  acid peptic
  active duodenal
  acute peptic
  amebic
  anastomotic
  anterior wall antral
  antral
  aphthoid
  aphthous
  atheromatous
  atrophic-hyperplastic
  Barrett
  bear claw
  benign
  benign gastric
  buccal
  bulbar peptic
  cervical
  chiclero
  chronic
  chronic peptic
  collar button-like
  corneal
  craterlike (with jagged edges)

umbilicus
  everted
  inverted
  Richet fascia
UMI needle
unattended death
unbanded gastroplasty
uncinate process of pancreas
uncompensated acidosis
uncomplicated acute cholecystitis
unconjugated bilirubin
unconjugated hyperbilirubinemia
uncuffed Magill endotracheal tube
uncuffed tube
underlying hematologic disorder
underlying motor neuron disease
underlying structure
undermine
undermining of muscle
undermining of skin edges
undermining of tissue
undernourished
undernutrition
underperfusion
Undies (trademark)
undifferentiated adenocarcinoma
undifferentiated adenoma
undifferentiated carcinoma
undifferentiated carcinoma of thyroid
  gland
undifferentiated cell
undifferentiated pattern
undifferentiated squamous cell
  carcinoma
undigested food in stool
undigested lactose
undyed braided polyglycolic acid suture
undyed suture
undyed Vicryl suture
unenhanced scan
unexplained abdominal pain
unexplained diarrhea
unformed stool
unguided bougie

unguided sound
Unica CO_2 laser
unicellular organism
Uniflex intramedullary nail
Uniflex polyurethane adhesive surgical
  dressing
uniform uptake throughout
Uni-Gold test for *H. pylori*
Unigraft bone graft material
Unilab Surgibone graft
unilateral adrenalectomy
unilateral anesthesia
unilateral breath sounds
unilateral groin dissection
unilateral hernia
unilateral hyperplasia
unilateral injury
unilateral pleural effusion
unilateral renal parenchymal disease
Unilax (phenolphthalein; docusate
  sodium)
unilobar location
unilobular cirrhosis
Unimar J-Needle
Uni-Matic infiltration syringe
uninodular goiter
uniplane
Uniqcot sponge
UNI-SHUNT hydrocephalus shunt
Uni-Site breathable transparent dressing
UniSpec disposable anoscope
unit (see *device*)
United Bongort Lifestyle pouch
United Max-E drainable pouch
United Network for Organ Sharing
  (UNOS)
United Ostomy Association (UOA)
United Ostomy irrigation set
United Skin Barrier XL Soft-Guard
United States Public Health Service
  (USPHS)
United States Surgical Corporation
  (USSC) devices (see *USSC*)
United Surgical Bongort Lifestyle
  pouch

United Surgical Convex Insert
United Surgical Featherlite ileostomy
  pouch
United Surgical Hypalon faceplate
United Surgical Seal Tite Gasket
United Surgical Shear Plus drainable
  pouch
United Surgical Soft and Secure pouch
United XL 14 Skin Barrier
Unithroid (levothyroxine sodium)
Uni-trac biliary stent
universal colitis
universal critical measurement unit
universal donor cells
Universal female DISS tubing
Universal Plus multi-function
  laparoscopic handpiece
universal retractor
universal ulcerative colitis
University of Minnesota retractor
University of Wisconsin (UW) solution
  for donor organ preservation
unmitigated
Unna boot
Unna-Flex (compressive Unna boot)
  dressing
Unna-Pak compression dressing and
  wrap
unopposed PTH secretion
UNOS (United Network for Organ
  Sharing)
UNOS Liver and Intestinal Organ
  Transplantation Committee
unrelenting diarrhea
unrelenting pain
unrelenting right upper quadrant pain
  or tenderness
unrelieved pain
unremitting pain
unresectable malignancy
unresolving pancreatitis
unroofing of cyst
unsaturated blood
unstable lesion

unstable patient
unsuspected cause of death
Untied Skin Prep for ostomy skin
UOA (United Ostomy Association)
UOS tonic pressure
up-biting biopsy cup forceps
up-biting cup forceps
up-biting rongeur
upper endoscopy
upper esophageal sphincter (UES)
upper gastrointestinal (UGI)
upper gastrointestinal bleeding (UGIB)
upper gastrointestinal endoscopy
upper gastrointestinal tract
upper GI atresia
upper GI bleed
upper GI endoscopy
upper GI with small bowel follow-
  through
upper-hand retractor
Upper Hands self-retaining retractor
  used in liver transplantation
upper inner quadrant
upper motor neuron lesion
upper outer quadrant
upper panendoscopy
upper respiratory infection (URI)
  infection
upper respiratory tract infection (URTI)
UPPP (uvulopalatopharyngoplasty)
upright abdominal film
upright chest x-ray
upright film
upright view
upset stomach
upside-down stomach
uracil plus tegafur (UFT)
Urban operation
urea breath test (UBT)
urea, hepatic
Ureaplasma urealyticum
urease breath test
urease-producing organism
Ureflex catheter

uremia
Uresil laparoscopic cholangiography
    catheter
ureteral or ureteric orifice
ureteral reimplantation
ureteric stone
ureteroileocutaneous anastomosis
ureteroileostomy, Bricker
ureteroscope, flexible
urethral injury
urethral meatus
urethral orifice
urethral papilla
urethropexy, Schwartz-Pregenzer
urethrovaginal fistula
URF-P2 choledochoscope
urgent splenectomy
urge to defecate
uric acid level
uridine diphosphate glucuronosyltrans-
    ferase deficiency
urinalysis (UA)
urinary aldosterone
urinary amylase
urinary calcium excretion
urinary electrolytes
urinary free cortisol
urinary metanephrine
urinary mucosa
urinary potassium
urinary 17-hydroxycorticosteroid
urinary stone
urinary 3-methylhistidine
urinary tract infection (UTI)
urinary tumor
urinary ulcer
urinary VMA
urine 5-HIAA
urine bilirubin
urine cortisol
URINELISA for *Helicobacter pylori*
urine output variations
urine potassium
urine smear

urine urobilinogen
urine vanillylmandelic acid and
    catecholamine excretion
urine-free cortisol
UriSite microalbumin/creatinine urine
    test
Uri-Test
urobilinogen
    fecal
    urine
UroCoil self-expanding stent
UROD (uroporphyrinogen decarboxy-
    lase)
urogenital region
Urografin 290 contrast medium
Urolase fiber laser
UroLume stent
UroMax II catheter
urosepsis
urp (to retch; vomit)
urpiness
urpy
Urschel first rib rongeur
Urso (ursodiol)
ursodeoxycholic acid
ursodiol
urticaria pigmentosa with systemic
    mastocytosis
USA pattern chisel
USA pattern gouge
USA retractor
U.S. Army bone chisel
U.S. Army gouge
U.S. Army pattern bone chisel
U.S. Army retractor
USCI cannula
U.S. Food and Drug Administration
    (FDA)
U-shaped incision
U-shaped retractor
U-sheet
U.S. retractor
U.S. Surgical GIA-30 stapler
Uslenghi plate

USSC (United States Surgical Corporation) devices, including:
ABBI system
CEEA stapler (21, 25, 28, 31)
Endo Babcock clamp
Endo Catch
Endo Close Stapler
Endo Cinch stapler
Endo Dissect
Endo GIA 60 stapler
Endo GIA II stapler
Endo Grasp
Endo Lung
Endo Stitch
Endo Suture
Ento Retract
Endo Universal
MiniSite laparoscope system
Multifire Endo Hernia
Premium CEEA stapler
Premium Plus CEEA stapler
Protack
Purstring (no *e*) device
Surgiview multiple-use disposable laparoscope

USSC *(cont.)*
USSC suture
VCS clip applier
Versaport trocar
USS-Trex Universal advanced radiology technology
uterine cannulas and forceps
uterine cervix carcinoma
uterine corpus carcinoma
uterine forceps
uterine polyp
uterine tumor
uterovesical pouch
uterus, enlarged
utility and sterilizer forceps
utility shears
U tube
U-tube hepaticoenterostomy
U-tube stent
uveal melanoma
uvulectomy
uvulopalatopharyngoplasty (UPPP)
uvulopharyngoplasty
U wave
UW (University of Wisconsin) solution

V, v

vaccine *(cont.)*
   Theratope
   Theratope-STn
   Trovax
   Twinrix (hepatitis A inactivated and hepatitis B [recombinant] vaccine)
   Vaqta (hepatitis A, inactivated)
vaccinia virus
V.A.C. Plus pump
Vac-Rite suction canister
VAC smoke evacuation unit
VACTERL (vertebral anomalies; anal atresia; congenital cardiac disease; tracheoesophageal fistula; renal anomalies; radial dysplasia; and other limb defects) syndrome
Vaculance
Vacutainer tube
vacuum manifold
vagal afferent
vagal efferent tonic response
vagal fibers
vagal innervation
vagal input
vagal stimulation
vagal stimulation of stomach
vagal trunk
vagina
vaginal enterocele
vaginal lengthening
vaginal mucosa
vaginal orifice
vaginal pessary
vagotomy
   bilateral
   highly selective
   medical
   parietal cell (PCV)
   proximal gastric (PGV)
   selective proximal (SPV)
   superselective
   surgical
   total bilateral
   truncal

vagotomy and antrectomy
vagotomy and antrectomy with gastro-duodenostomy
vagotomy and pyloroplasty
vague gastrointestinal dysfunction
vagus nerve
vagus nerve stimulation (VNS)
Valeo lifting glove
Valin hemilaminectomy retractor
valinemia
vallecula (pl. valleculae)
vallecular dysphagia
vallecular pooling
Valleix probe
Valleylab electrocautery
Valleylab electrocautery interchangeable hook
Valleylab SSE-2 cautery unit
Valleylab trigger instrument
Valpin 50
valproic acid
Valsalva maneuver
valsavagenic COPD
Value-Line Poole abdominal suction tube
value, serum glucose
valve
   anal
   antireflux
   aortic
   Bard-Davol trumpet
   Bauhin
   bicuspid
   blunting of
   bulb and air-flow control
   Cabot trumpet
   competent
   competent ileocecal
   CPAP
   failed nipple
   Heister valve
   Holter
   Houston
   ileocecal
   incompetent

valve *(cont.)*
  Kerckring
  LeVeen
  lipomatous ileocecal
  mitral
  nipple
  popoff
  pig
  porcine heart
  pressure-sensitive
  rectal
  shunt
  spiral
  Spivack
  Stryker trumpet
  tricuspid
  Tuohy-Borst
valve hook
valve of Bauhin
valve of Houston
valve of Kerckring
valve scissors
valvular heart disease
valvular regurgitant lesion
Vamin amino acid solution
VanAlyea antrum trocar and wash tube
Van Andel catheter
Van Bogaert disease
Van Buren catheter guide
Van Buren sequestrum forceps
Van Buren urethral bougie
Van Buren urethral sound
vancomycin-resistant enterococci (VRE)
vancomycin-resistant *Enterococcus faecium* (VREF) infection
van den Bergh test
Van Doren biopsy forceps
Vanguard splinter probe
van Heuven anatomic classification of diabetic retinopathy
van Sonnenberg sump drain
vanillylmandelic acid (VMA)
vanishing lung
Vannas micro scissors

Vansil (oxamniquinel)
vanSonnenberg sump
vanSonnenberg-Wittich catheter
Vantage first aid shears
Vantage Graves vaginal speculum
Vantage iris scissors
Vantage Knowles bandage scissors
Vantage Lister bandage scissors
Vantage Metzenbaum scissors
Vantage needle holder
Vantage operating scissors
Vantage Spencer stitch scissors
Vantage strabismus scissors
Vantex central venous catheter
VaporTrode
vapreotide
Vaqta (hepatitis A vaccine, inactivated)
Varco gallbladder forceps
variable-dose patient-controlled anesthesia
variable in location
variable stiffness endoscope
variable stiffness colonoscope
Vari-angle clip applier
variceal bleeding, gastroesophageal
variceal column
variceal decompression
variceal hemorrhage
variceal sclerosis
variceal sclerotherapy in esophagus
variceal wall
varicella-zoster virus (VZV)
varices (pl. of varix) (also varicosity, varicosities)
  actively bleeding
  alcoholic
  bleeding esophageal
  bleeding esophagogastric
  bleeding from esophageal
  bleeding gastric
  colonic
  downhill esophageal
  esophageal
  esophagogastric

varices *(cont.)*
  fundal
  gastric
  ileal
  isolated gastric
  paraesophageal
  radius of
  rectal
  transesophageal ligation of
varices on varices
varicocele
varicose ulcer
varicose vein
varicosity (pl. varicosities) (see *varices*)
variegated uptake of radioiodine
Vari/Moist wound dressing
varioliform gastritis
varix (see *varices*)
Varney pin
Vas-Cath catheter
Vascoray (iothalamate meglumine; iothalamate sodium)
Vascu-Guard bovine pericardial surgical patch graft
Vascufil suture
vascular anastomosis
vascular anomaly
vascular apron
vascular autoregulation
vascular bruit
vascular bundle
vascular cirrhosis
vascular clamp
vascular collapse
vascular compromise
vascular congestion
vascular cutaneous and hepatic tumor
vascular ectasia
vascular encasement
vascular endothelial cell
vascular endothelium
vascular forceps
vascular goiter
vascular hemangioma

vascular injury
vascularized bed
vascularized fibula graft
vascularized gastric tissue
vascular lesion
vascular load
vascular mediator
vascular pedicle
vascular polyp
vascular proliferation
vascular tape
vascular tuft
vasculature of the thyroid gland
vasculitic lesion
vasculitis
  hepatic capsular
  necrotizing bowel
Vascutek graft
vas deferens
Vaseline gauze
Vaseline gauze dressing
Vaseline petrolatum gauze dressing
vasoablative endothelial sarcoma (VABES)
vasoactive intestinal peptide (VIP)
vasoactive intestinal polypeptide (VIP)
vasoactive peptide
vasoconstriction of the mesenteric vessel
vasoconstriction, splanchnic
vasodilation of skeletal and mesenteric vascular beds
vasomotor instability
vasopermeation enhancement (VE)
vasopressin
vasopressin analog
vasopressin deficiency
vasopressin with nitroglycerin
Vasotrax blood pressure/heart rate sensor
vasovagal episode
vasovagal reflex
vasovagal response
VasoView balloon dissection system

Vater
  ampulla of
  papilla of
vaterian segment
VATER (vertebral and/or vascular
  defects; anorectal malformation;
  transesophageal fistula; radial, ray,
  or renal anomaly) syndrome
vault
  rectal
  vaginal
Vayre suturing technique
Vbeam laser
VBG (vertical-banded gastroplasty)
V blade plate
VCARE vaginal-cervical Ahluwalia
  retractor-elevator
VCS clip adapter
VCS clip applier
VDS (ventral derotating spinal)
  compression rod
VE (vasopermeation enhancement)
Vector and VectorX large-lumen
  guiding catheter
vector-borne infection
Vectra VAG (vascular access graft)
vecuronium bromide
vegetarian diet
vegetative lesion
VEGF (vascular endothelial growth
  factor)
vein (see Table of Veins in Appendix)
Veingard transparent dressing
vein graft
vein of Retzius
vein of Sappey
vein retractor
vein stone
vein stripper
Velban (vinblastine sulfate)
Velogene rapid VRE assay
velopharyngeal closure
Velosulin Human BR (insulin)
Velpeau bandage

Velpeau dressing
vena cava compression
vena cava sampling
Venable plate
Venable-Stuck nail
Venable-Stuck pin
venacavography
Venaflow vascular graft
venereal proctocolitis
venereal ulcer
venereal wart
Veni-Gard I.V. stabilization dressing
venocavography, inferior
venodilation
venogram, hepatic
venography (see *imaging*)
veno-occlusive disease (VOD)
veno-occlusive liver disease
venous blood
venous blood gas
venous catheterization
venous drainage
venous hum
venous oozing
venous patency
venous pattern
venous phase of selective splenic
  arteriography
venous plexus
venous return
venous sampling for PTH
venous stasis ulcer
venous supply
venous web disease
venovenous bypass
Ventex wound dressing
ventilated patient
ventilation
  decreased alveolar
  excessive mechanical
  mechanical
  minute
  positive pressure
ventilation-perfusion mismatch

ventilator mode
ventilator settings (mode, tidal volume, ventilator rate, FiO$_2$, PEEP)
venting aortic Bengash-type needle
vent settings
vent the bowel
Ventra catheter
ventral hernia
ventral herniorrhaphy
ventral pancreas
ventral surface
ventricle of larynx appendix
ventricular cannula
ventricular catheter
ventricular needle
ventricular septal defect
ventriculoatrial (VA) shunt
ventriculojugular (VJ) shunt
ventriculoperitoneal (VP)
ventriculoperitoneal drain
ventriculoperitoneal shunt (VPS)
ventriculostomy drain
ventriculostomy needle
ventriculosubarachnoid (VS) shunt
ventriculovenous shunt
ventrolateral hernia
ventroptosis
Ventureyra ventricular catheter
Verbatim balloon catheter
Verbatim balloon probe
Verbrugge bone clamp
Verbrugge bone-holding forceps
Verbrugge clamp
Verbrugge-Hohmann bone retractor
Verbrugge needle
Veress (*not* Verres) needle
Veress cannula
Veress needle
verge, anal
Veridien clamp
Veripath peripheral guiding catheter
Verluma (nofetumobab)
vermicide
vermicular colic

vermiform appendix
vermiform body
vermifuge
vermilionectomy
Vermox (mebendazole)
Verner-Morrison syndrome
vernier calipers
Vernon-David rectal speculum
VerreScope microlaparoscopic entry
verrucous carcinoma
Versabran
Versadopp 10 Doppler ultrasound probe
VersaLight laser
Versalon dressing
Versaport obturator
Versaport Plus reducer
VersaPort trocar
VersaPulse holmium laser
VersaPulse Select holmium laser
Versatack surgical stapler
VersaTack stapler
Versatome laser
Versatrac lumbar retractor
Versed (midazolam HCl)
vertebral body biopsy
vertebral body plate
vertebral body retractor
vertebral pleural reflection
vertical-banded gastroplasty (VBG)
vertical bipedicle flap technique reduction
vertical incision
vertical mattress suture
vertical midline incision
vertical pedicle technique in breast reduction mammoplasty
vertical reduction mammoplasty
vertical retractor
vertical ring gastroplasty (VRG)
vertical Silastic ring gastroplasty
vertical stapled small gastric pouch
vertical suture
very low-calorie diet (VLCD)
very low-density lipoprotein (VLDL)

Vesely-Street split nail
vesical fistula
vesicle, herpetic
vesicoenteric fistula
vesicoureteral reflux
vesicoureterine pouch
vesicouterine fistula
vesicovaginal fistula
vesicular appendix
vesicular pattern
vesiculocolic perforation
VESS (videoendoscopic swallowing
  study)
vessel
  aberrant
  abnormal feeding blood
  afferent
  atypical
  blood
  chyliferous
  cremasteric
  deep epigastric
  epigastric
  gastroepiploic
  great
  hemorrhoidal
  hypogastric
  ileocolic
  iliac
  inferior epigastric
  intercostal
  lacteal
  lymph
  mesocolonic
  perforating
  portal
  short gastric (SGV)
  splenic
  spermatic
  telangiectatic
  testicular
  thoracic
  thoracic great
vessel constriction

vessel hook
vessel knife
vessel loop
vessel retractor
vessel-sizing catheter
vessel transection
vessels were clamped, divided, and
  ligated
vessels were skeletonized
vest-over-pants hernia repair
vestibule of mouth
vestibuloplasty, anterior or posterior
vestigial fold
V-excision
Vezien abdominal scissors
viable omentum
vial decanter
Vianain (ananain; comosain;
  bromelains)
Viasorb wound dressing
Vibra-Surge ultrasonic instrument
Vibrio cholerae
Vibrio jejuni
Vibrio parahaemolyticus
Vickers needle holder
Vickers ring tip forceps
Vicryl knitted mesh
Vicryl Rapide suture
Vicryl Rapide synthetic absorbable
  suture
Vicryl suture
Vicryl woven mesh
vide supra (L. "see above")
video-assisted thoracic surgery (VATS)
video barium swallow
video camera
videoendoscope
videoendoscope-assisted microsurgery
videoendoscopic augmentation
  mammoplasty
videoendoscopic surgical equipment
videoendoscopic swallowing study
  (VESS)

videofluoroscopic swallowing
   evaluation
VideoHydro laparoscope
video image
videolaparoscopic cardiomyotomy
videolaparoscopy
videolaseroscopy
video optical intubation stylet
videorectoscope
videoresectoscope
videoscope (see *endoscope*)
videoscopic fundoplication
video signal enhancer
videothoracoscopy
Vidicon vacuum chamber pickup tube
Vi-Drape
Vienna nasal speculum
view (see also *position, projection*)
   abdominal
   anterior
   AP (anteroposterior)
   AP supine
   apical
   apical lordotic
   axial sesamoid
   axillary
   baseline
   Beath
   Boehler (Böhler) calcaneal
   Boehler lumbosacral
   Breuerton
   Broden x-ray
   brow-down skull
   brow-up skull
   Bucky
   carpal tunnel
   Carter-Rowe
   cine
   clenched fist
   close-up
   coalition
   cone
   coned-down
   cranial angled

view *(cont.)*
   craniocaudad
   craniocaudal
   cross-table
   CTLV (cross-table lateral view)
   decubitus
   dens (cervical spine)
   dorsiflexion
   dorsoplantar
   Dunlop-Shands
   dynamic stress x-ray
   erect
   FCS (full cervical spine)
   Ferguson
   flexion
   fluoroscopic stress x-ray
   frog-leg
   frog-leg lateral
   frontal
   full length
   Harris
   Harris-Beath axial hindfoot
   hemiaxial
   hepatoclavicular
   hip-to-ankle
   Hobb
   Hughston
   infrapatellar view of knee
   intraoperative
   inversion ankle stress
   Jones
   Judet radius
   Knuttsen bending
   LAO (left anterior oblique)
   lateral
   lateral anterior drawer stress
   lateral bending
   lateral decubitus
   lateral oblique
   lateral tilt stress ankle
   limited
   long axial oblique
   long axis
   long-axis parasternal

view *(cont.)*

    lordotic
    mediolateral
    mediolateral oblique
    Merchant
    mortise
    mucosal
    multiplanar fluoroscopic stress
    navicular
    Neer lateral
    Neer transscapular
    no-angulation
    nonstanding lateral oblique
    nonweightbearing
    notch
    oblique
    occipital
    odontoid
    open-mouth odontoid
    orthogonal
    outlet
    overhead
    overhead oblique
    PA (posteroanterior)
    parasternal long-axis
    parasternal short-axis
    patellar skyline
    plain
    planar
    plantar axial
    plantar flexion
    plantar flexion stress
    portable
    postevacuation
    postoperative
    preliminary
    preoperative
    prereduction
    prone
    prone lateral
    Puddu
    push-pull ankle stress
    push-pull hip
    RAO (right anterior oblique)

view *(cont.)*

    recumbent
    right lateral decubitus
    routine magnification
    Schüller (Schueller)
    serendipity
    short-axis
    short-axis parasternal
    ski-jump
    skyline
    spot
    standing dorsoplantar
    standing lateral
    standing weightbearing
    steep LAO (left anterior oblique)
    Stenver
    stress
    stress Broden
    stress eversion
    stress inversion
    Stryker notch
    submental vertex
    submentovertex
    subxiphoid
    sunrise
    sunset
    supine
    supine full
    suprasternal notch
    swimmer's
    tangential
    tangential scapular
    tomographic
    true lateral
    tunnel
    two-plane
    upright
    von Rosen
    Waters
    weightbearing
    weightbearing dorsoplantar
    West Point
    White leg-length
    x-ray

virus *(cont.)*
  epidemic gastroenteritis
  Epstein-Barr (EBV)
  fecal-oral route of transmission
  gastroenteritis virus type A, type B
  HAV (hepatitis A)
  HBV (hepatitis B)
  HBV (hepatitis B)
  HDV (hepatitis D)
  hematogenous dissemination of
  hepadna (hepatitis B-like DNA)
  hepatitis A
  hepatitis B (HBV)
  hepatitis C (HCV) (formerly non-A,
    non-B)
  hepatitis D
  hepatitis E (HEV)
  herpes simplex virus (HSV)
  herpes zoster virus (HZV)
  H5N1
  HGV (hepatitis G)
  HHV-8 (human herpesvirus-8)
  HIV (human immunodeficiency)
  HMTV (human mammary tumor)
  human herpesvirus 6 (HHV-6)
  human mammary tumor (HMTV)
  Juquitiba
  KSHV (Kaposi sarcoma-associated
    virus)
  Laguna Negra
  lymphocytic choriomeningitis
    (LCMV)
  Marburg
  MCV (molluscum contagiosum)
  mutant
  Nipah
  nonsyncytium-inducing (NSI) variant
    of AIDS virus
  Norwalk
  respiratory syncytial (RSV)
  RNA
  rotavirus
  Rous sarcoma
  Sin Nombre (SNV)

virus *(cont.)*
  Theradigm-HBV (hepatitis B)
  varicella zoster (VZV)
  West Nile
  wild-type hepatitis
virus-host interaction
virus-like infectious agent (VLIA)
virus-like particle (VLP) of non-A,
  non-B hepatitis
Visa II PTCA catheter
viscera (see *viscus*)
visceral anesthesia
visceral edema
visceral neuropathy
visceral pain
visceral peritoneum
visceral surface of liver
visceromegaly
visceroptosis
viscid bile
viscous (adj.)
viscous bile
viscous fluid
viscous lidocaine
viscous Xylocaine gargle
viscus (pl. viscera)
  abdominal
  abdominopelvic
  hollow
  intra-abdominal
  intraperitoneal
  perforated
  strangulated
Visi-Black surgical needle
visible peristalsis
visibly and palpably normal
Visicath endoscopic instrument
Visick grading system for dysphagia
Visick grading system for postgastrec-
  tomy carcinoma recurrence
Visicol (sodium phosphate) bowel prep
Visidex II blood glucose testing strips
Visilex polypropylene mesh
Vision PTCA catheter

Visipaque (iodixanol)
Visistat stapler
Visitec circular knife
Visitec crescent knife
Visitec EdgeAhead knife
Visitec stiletto knife
Vistaflex biliary stent
Vistaril
Vistec x-ray detectable sponge
visualization
    direct
    excellent
    good
    inadequate
    poor
Visulas Nd:YAG laser
VISX excimer laser
VISX Star S2 excimer laser
VitaClip clip applier
Vitacuff dressing
Vital Cooley microvascular needle
    holder
Vital-Duval forceps
Vital forceps
Vital High Nitrogen enteral nutritional
    therapy
Vital Ryder microvascular needle
    holder
Vital stapler
Vitallium Küntscher (Kuentscher) nail
Vitallium plate
Vitallium staple
vitamin, ADEKs
vitamin B_{12} absorption test
vitamin, fat-soluble
vitamin K
vitamin, water-soluble
Vita-PMS Plus
vitelline duct
vitelline fistula
vitellointestinal cyst
vitellointestinal duct
Vitesse Cos laser catheter
Vitesse E-II catheter

Vitex tissue adhesive
VITEX fibrin sealant
vivax malaria
Vivonex elemental powdered feeding
Vivonex HN (high-nitrogen) powdered
    feeding
Vivonex jejunostomy catheter
Vivonex Moss tube
Vivonex T.E.N.
V-Lax (psyllium hydrophilic mucilloid)
VLCD (very low calorie diet)
VLDL (very low density lipoprotein)
VLDL cholesterol
V + Loop electrode
VLP (virus-like particle)
V-medullary nail
V. Mueller bulldog clamp
V. Mueller laparoscope
V. Mueller-Poole suction tube
V. Mueller rigid laparoscope
V nail plate
VNS (vagus nerve stimulation)
VNUS Restore catheter
VOD (veno-occlusive disease)
Voges-Proskauer test
volar incision
volar plate
Volkmann bone hook
Volkmann curette
Volkmann hook
Volkmann pancreatic calculus spoon
Volkmann rake retractor
Volkmann retractor
Volkmann spoon for pancreatic calculus
volume
    blood
    circulating blood
    colonic balloon
    end-diastolic
    excess fluid
    fluid
    increased tidal
    intravascular
    mean corpuscular (MCV)

volume *(cont.)*
   shrinking liver
   stroke (SV)
   tidal
volume acquisition (MRI)
volume analysis (MRI)
volume displacement transducer
volume rendering of helical CT data
volume replacement
voluming artifact (MRI)
voluntarily stopping eating and drinking
   (VSED)
voluntary guarding
volvulated Meckel diverticulum
volvulus
   bascule
   cecal
   colonic
   compound
   decompression of
   gastric
   gastric dilatation
   large-bowel
   midgut
   Onchocerca
   recurrent
   sigmoid
   splenic flexure
   transverse colon
   "traveling"
volvulus of splenic flexure
volvulus of transverse colon
Vom Saal pin
vomiting (also emesis)
   bile-stained
   bilious
   bloody
   bright red
   chemotherapy-induced
   coffee-grounds
   concealed
   cyclic
   dry
   epidemic

vomiting *(cont.)*
   episodic
   erotic
   fecal
   feculent
   hysterical
   intractable
   ipecac-induced
   nausea and (N&V)
   nervous
   nonbilious
   periodic
   perioperative
   pernicious
   postoperative
   postprandial
   post-tussive
   profuse
   projectile
   prolonged
   psychogenic
   recurrent bouts of
   self-induced
   stercoraceous
   surreptitious
   vomitus (also emesis)
   winter
vomiting center
vomitus (see *vomiting*)
Von Andel catheter
Von Gierke disease
Von Haberer-Finney anastomosis
Von Haberer gastroenterostomy
von Hippel-Lindau disease
von Jaksch test
von Kupffer test
von Langenbeck periosteal elevator
von Meyenburg complex
Von Petz suturing apparatus
von Recklinghausen disease
von Rokitansky disease
von Rosen view
voodoo death

Vorse-Webster clamp
Vozzle Vacu-Irrigator
VPI ileostomy system
VPI nonadhesive open-end pouch
VPI nonadhesive pouch
VRE (vancomycin-resistant
 enterococcus)
VRG (vertical ring gastroplasty)
V-scan test kit
VSED (voluntarily stopping eating and
 drinking)
VSF (Vermont spinal fixator) clamp
VSF (Vermont spinal fixator) rod
V-shaped incision
V-shaped laceration
V-shaped ulcer
VSP (variable screw placement) plate
V-to-Y closure
vulnerary (agent that promotes wound
 healing)
vulvar lesion
vulvar vestibulitis syndrome
VX-497
Vygon Nutricath S catheter
V-Y plasty

W, w

Wagener-Mosher tube
Wagner acetabular reamer
Wagner closed pin
Wagner retractor
Wagner skin incision
Wagner test
Wainwright plate
Waldenstrom macroglobulinemia
Waldeyer fascia
Waldeyer fossa
Waldmann disease
Waldmann scissors
Walker gallbladder retractor
wall
    abdominal
    anorectal
    anterior abdominal
    axial
    body
    bowel
    carotid
    cavity
    cell
    chest
    entire bowel
    gallbladder
    intra-abdominal
    midabdominal

wall *(cont.)*
    posterior abdominal
    thickened gallbladder
    thoracic
    variceal
wall akinesis
Wallstent
Wallstent biliary endoprosthesis
Wallstent enteral endoprosthesis
Walter-Carmalt splinter forceps
Walter-Liston forceps
Walton biopsy forceps
Walton cartilage clamp
Walton-Liston bone rongeur
Walton meniscus clamp
Walton-Poole suction tube
Walton ribbon retractor
Walton-Ruskin bone rongeur
Walton-Ruskin forceps
Walton scissors
Walton wire-pulling forceps
Walton-Yankauer suction tube
wand
    AccESS
    CLO (Cool Laser Optics)
    CollagENT
    collection
    flexible

wand *(cont.)*
 Hummingbird
 image-guided
 irrigation
 Kaye Lap-Wand
 Lap-Wand with Kittner tip
 laser
 Microblater ArthroWand
 ReFlex
 stereotactic
 surgical
 The Wand
 Viewing Wand
wandering gallbladder
wandering goiter
wandering kidney
wandering liver
wandering spleen
Wangensteen anastomosis clamp
Wangensteen drain
Wangensteen forceps
Wangensteen needle
Wangensteen needle holder
Wangensteen patent ductus clamp
Wangensteen suction
Wangensteen suction tube
Wangensteen tissue forceps
Wangensteen trocar
Wangensteen tube
Ward approximating forceps
Ward needle holder
Ward periosteal elevator
warfarin potassium
warfarin sodium
warm saline solution
Warren splenorenal shunt
wart
 intra-anal
 perianal
 venereal
Warthin (adenolymphoma) tumor
warty papilloma
Was-Cath catheter
washed clot

washing catheter
washing
 bronchial
 gastric
 peritoneal
washings and brushings
Wassmund retractor
wasting, muscle
wasting syndrome
watchful waiting (monitoring tumor
 growth while deferring treatment)
water-borne gastroenteritis
water-borne infection
water brash
waterfall stomach
Waterfield needle
water-filled pouch
water-gurgle test
Waterhouse-Friderichsen syndrome
water-infusion esophageal manometry
 catheter
watermelon stomach
Water Pik, endoscopic
water probe
water recovery test
water retention
water-seal chest tube
watershed area
water-sipping test
water-soluble bilirubin
water-soluble contrast enema
water-soluble contrast esophageal
 swallow
water-soluble vitamins
Waterston's stratification for tracheo-
 esophageal fistula
Waters view
water swallows
water-trap stomach
watery diarrhea
watery diarrhea syndrome
watery secretion
watery stools
Watson-Alagille syndrome

Watson-Cheyne dissector
Watson-Cheyne probe
Watson-Jones bone gouge
Watson-Jones incision
Watson-Jones nail
Watson knife
Watson-Williams intervertebral disk
   rongeur
wattage
Waugh-Clagett pancreaticoduodenos-
   tomy
Waugh diathermy forceps
Waugh dissecting forceps
wave
   abdominal fluid
   flattened T
   fluid
   gastric slow
   inverted T
   peaked T
   peristaltic
   primary peristaltic
   secondary peristaltic
   tetrahertz
   U
WaveWire guidewire
wax pattern
waxy kidney
waxy liver
WBC (white blood cell) count
   bands
   basos (basophils)
   blasts
   differential
   eos (eosinophils)
   immature forms
   leukocytes
   lymphs (lymphocytes)
   monos (monocytes)
   neutrophils
   polys or PMN (polymorphonuclear
      leukocytes)
   segs (segmented neutrophils)
   stabs

WBC, elevated
WBCs (white blood cells)
WDE (wound dressing emulsion)
WDHA (watery diarrhea, hypokalemia,
   achlorhydria) syndrome
weaning, immunosuppressive steroid
Weary cordotomy knife
Weary nerve hook
Weary nerve root retractor
Weaveknit vascular graft
web
   duodenal
   esophageal
   hepatic
   intestinal
   postcricoid
   venous
Webb-Balfour abdominal retractor
Webb-Balfour self-retaining retractor
Weber aortic clamp
Weber-Christian disease
Weber-Christian panniculitis
Weber gland
Weber rectal catheter
Webb nail
Webril bandage
Webril dressing
web space incision
Webster abdominal retractor
Webster meniscectomy scissors
Webster needle
Webster needle holder
Webster-TC needle holder
Weck-Baggish rigid laparoscope
Weck-cel sponge dressing
Weck clamp
Weck clip and applicator
Weck knife
Weck laparotomy pad
Weck microsuture cutting scissors
Weck operating laparoscope
Weck 110405 0° 5 mm rigid
   laparoscope
Weck 110800 rigid laparoscope

wedge biopsy of liver
wedged hepatic venous pressure
    (WHVP)
wedge hepatic biopsy
wedge liver biopsy
wedge resection
weekend drinker
weeping willow appearance
    on venogram
Weibel-Palade granule
weightbearing dorsoplantar view
weightbearing view
weighing, underwater
weight gain
weight, ideal body (IBW)
weight loss, significant long-term
weight loss with hyperphagia
weight-reduction operation
weight-relieving calipers
weights, daily
Weil-Blakesley intervertebral disk
    rongeur
Weil disease
Weil syndrome
Weinberg modification of pyloroplasty
Weinberg pyloroplasty
Weinberg vagotomy retractor
Weiss amputation saw
Weitlaner-Beckman retractor
Weitlaner retractor
Welch Allyn anoscope
Welch Allyn flexible sigmoidoscope
Welch Allyn KleenSpec sigmoidoscope
Welch Allyn upper GI videoendoscope
Welchol (formerly Cholestagel)
welder's lung
welding of suture
well-circumscribed neoplasm
well-differentiated adenoma
well-differentiated carcinoma
Weller cartilage forceps
Weller cartilage scissors
Wellferon (interferon alfa-n1)
Wells posterior rectopexy

Welt syndrome
Wenger plate
Wermer syndrome
Wernicke encephalopathy
Wernicke-Korsakoff syndrome
Wernicke syndrome
Wertheim clamp
Wertheim-Cullen clamp
Wertheim retractor
Wertheim scissors
Wesolowski vascular graft
Wesselsbron virus
Wesson perineal retractor
West bone chisel
West bone gouge
Westcott cutting biopsy needle
Westcott dissecting scissors
Westerman-Jensen needle
WEST (Weinstein Enhanced Sensory
    Test) for diabetic neuropathy
West gouge
West Nile virus
Weston rectal snare
Westphal forceps
Westphal gall duct forceps
Westphal-Strümpell (Struempell) disease
West Point view
West retractor
Westscott scissors
wet colostomy
wet-field cautery
wet lung
wet smear
wet swallow (on esophageal
    manometry)
wet-technique reduction mammoplasty
wetting agent
wet-to-dry dressing
Wharton (cystadenoma) tumor
wheat gliadin
Wheeless surgical construction of J
    rectal pouch
whiplash technique for repositioning
    a catheter

Whipple disease
Whipple pancreatectomy
Whipple pancreaticoduodenectomy
Whipple pancreaticoduodenostomy
Whipple test
Whipple triad
Whipple triad test
whipstitch suture
whipworm
whistle-tip ureteral catheter
Whitacre spinal needle
Whitcomb-Kerrison laminectomy
    rongeur
white bile
white blood cells (WBCs)
White classification for diabetes
    mellitus
white cotton umbilical tape
white fatty stool
White leg-length view
white line of Toldt
white lung
white patch
white phenolphthalein
white pulp of spleen
white silk suture
white suture
Whitehead deformity
Whitehead hemorrhoidectomy
Whitman plate
Whitmore bag
WHO (World Health Organization)
    classification of gastric carcinoma
whole blood
whole transplantation
whorled appearance
WHVP (wedged hepatic venous
    pressure)
Wiberg periosteal elevator
wide excision
wide glucose excursions
wide-mesh petroleum gauze dressing
wide-mouth sac
wide periosteal elevator

widespread bleeding
width of tumor invasion
Wiedemann-Beckwith syndrome
Wiet cup forceps
Wiet otologic scissors
Wigmore plaster saw
Wikstroem artery forceps
Wiktor GX Hepamed coated
Wiktor Prime
Wiktor stent
Wilberg bone staple
wild daisy
Wilde dressing forceps
Wilde ethmoid forceps
wild-type hepatitis virus
Wilde forceps
Wilde incision
Wilde intervertebral disk rongeur
Wilde rongeur forceps
Wilfred Adams diathermy artery
    forceps
Wilkinson abdominal retractor
Wilkinson-Deaver retractor
Willauer abdominal scissors
Willauer-Gibbon periosteal elevator
Willauer thoracic scissors
Williams intestinal forceps
Williams overtube sleeve
Williger bone mallet
Williger curette
Williger periosteal elevator
Willis pancreas
Willis pouch
Willy Meyer incision for mastectomy
Wilmer dissecting scissors
Wilmer scissors
Wilms tumor
Wilson bone graft
Wilson-Cook endoprosthesis
Wilson-Cook esophageal balloon dilator
Wilson-Cook forceps
Wilson-Cook French stent
Wilson-Cook mechanical lithotriptor
Wilson-Cook prosthesis introducer

Wissinger rod
Wister vascular clamp
within normal limits (WNL)
without harm (commensally)
Wittner biopsy forceps
Witz test
Witzel duodenostomy
Witzel enterostomy catheter
Witzel feeding jejunostomy tunnel
Witzel gastrostomy
Witzel jejunostomy
Witzel tunnel for feeding jejunostomy
Wizard balloon replacement device
WNL (within normal limits)
Woelfler gland
Woldman test
Wolf 10/5 (L-angle) operative
    laparoscope
Wolf 170 12 mm rigid laparoscope
Wolf 7732 rigid laparoscope
Wolf 8934.40 rigid laparoscope
Wolf 8937.31 0° 10 mm rigid laparo-
    scope
Wolfe-Boehler mallet
Wolfe full-thickness free graft
Wolfe hand surgery graft
Wolfe-Kawamoto bone graft
Wolff-Junghans test
Wolff telescope
Wolf Lumina rigid laparoscope
Wolfram syndrome
Wolf rigid laparoscope
Wolfson gallbladder retractor
Wolfson intestinal clamp
Wolf trocar
Wolf videoresectoscope
Wolman disease
Wolman xanthomatosis
Wolson gallbladder retractor
Womack procedure
womb stone
Wood lamp
Woodson elevator
Woodward esophagogastrostomy

Woodward hemostat
Wookey skin tube
Workhorse percutaneous transluminal
    angioplasty balloon catheter
working diagnosis
working in a clockwise direction
World Health Organization (WHO)
    classification of gastric carcinoma
worm
    roundworm (nematode)
    tapeworm (cestode)
wound
    abraded
    abscess
    aseptic
    avulsed
    ballistic
    blowing
    burn
    clean
    closed
    contaminated
    contused
    craniocerebral penetrating
    crease
    cross-irrigation of
    cutaneous
    depth of
    exit
    gaping
    glancing
    gunshot (GSW)
    gutter
    high-energy gunshot
    high-velocity gunshot
    incised
    lacerated
    nonpenetrating
    open
    parasternal gunshot
    parasternal stab
    penetrating
    perforating
    plantar puncture

X, x

Xanar 20 Ambulase CO$_2$ laser
xanthelasma
xanthogranulomatous cholecystitis
xanthography
xanthoma cell
xanthoma
   gastric
   skin
xanthomatosis
   biliary hypercholesterolemia
   cerebrotendinous
   Wolman
xanthomatous biliary cirrhosis
Xcytrin (motexafin gadolinium)
XeCl (xenon-chloride) laser
Xeloda (capecitabine)
Xenical (orlistat) capsules
XenoDerm graft
xenograft
XenoMouse Technology
xenon endoscopic light source
xenon flash endoscopic light source
xenon light source
xenon 127 (^{127}Xe)
xenon 133 (^{133}Xe)
xenotransplant with genetically engi-
   neered pig organ
xenotransplantation

Xeroflo dressing
Xeroform dressing
Xeroform gauze
Xeroform gauze dressing
Xillix LIFE-GI fluorescence
   endoscopy system
Xillix LIFE-Lung GI fluorescence
   endoscopy system
xiphoid appendix
xiphoid-to-umbilicus incision
XL-11 catheter
X-linked infantile agammaglobulinemia
   (Bruton-type)
X-linked lymphoproliferative (XLP)
   syndrome
XLP (X-linked lymphoproliferative)
   syndrome
XMB tibial reaming guide
XMG (x-ray mammogram)
Xomed drill
Xomed Kartush insulated retractor
Xpeedior catheter
Xplorer 1000 digital x-ray imaging
   system
Xplorer imaging system
X-Prep (senna extract; alcohol)
X-Prep bowel prep
X-PRESS vascular closure system

XPS Sculpture System
XPS Straightshot
XQ230 Olympus gastroscope
x-ray view
X-shaped micro plate
X-shaped plate
XT coronary stent (radiopaque)

X-trode electrode catheter
X-trode stent
Xylocaine (lidocaine)
Xylo-Pfan (xylose)
xylose absorption test
xylose tolerance test

Y, y

YAG (yttrium-aluminum-garnet) laser
YagLAZR or YagLazr laser
Yale SK poliovirus
Yamada myelotomy knife
Yankauer periosteal elevator
Yankauer punch
Yankauer suction tube
Yasargil arachnoid knife
Yasargil artery forceps
Yasargil bayonet scissors
Yasargil carotid clamp
Yasargil clip-applying forceps
Yasargil elevator
Yasargil hypophyseal forceps
Yasargil knotting forceps
Yasargil ligature guide
Yasargil micro forceps
Yasargil micro rasp
Yasargil micro scissors
Yasargil microvascular knife
Yasargil pituitary rongeur
Yasargil spring hook
Yasargil suction tube
Yasargil tumor forceps
Y bone plate
year, quality-adjusted life (QALY)
yellow atrophy

yellow fever
yellow fever hepatitis
yellow fever virus
yellow jaundice
yellow phenolphthalein
Yeoman biopsy forceps
Yeoman rectal biopsy forceps
Yeoman-Turrell rectal biopsy forceps
Yeoman-Wittner rectal forceps
Yersinia enterocolitica colitis
Yersinia pseudotuberculosis
yersiniasis
YETSS (yuppie executive tight
    sphincter syndrome)
Y incision
yolk sac carcinoma
Yorke-Mason incision
Young forceps
Young intestinal forceps
Young-Millin boomerang needle holder
Yours Truly breast prosthesis
yo-yo dieting
yo-yo weight fluctuation phenomenon
Y-shaped graft
Y-shaped incision
Y-shaped microplate
Y-shaped plate

yttrium-aluminum-garnet (YAG) laser
yuppie executive tight sphincter
    syndrome (YETSS)

Yu pyloroplasty
Y-V anoplasty
Y-V plasty

Z, z

Zachary Cope-DeMartel clamp
zacopride
Zacutex (lexipafant)
Zadaxin (thymosin alpha-1)
zamifenacin
Zanosar (streptozocin)
Zantac 75 (ranitidine)
Zappacosta test
Zaufel-Jansen bone rongeur
Z clamp
Z-clamp forceps
Zebra exchange guidewire
Zeffix (lamivudine)
Zeiss Endolive endoscope
Zeiss operating microscope
Zeiss OPMI surgical microscope
Zeiss Visulas 690s laser
Zellweger cerebrohepatorenal syndrome
Zelmac (tegaserod)
Zemplar (paricalcitol)
Zenapax (daclizumab)
Zenith AAA (abdominal aortic
    aneurysm) endovascular graft
Zenker artery forceps
Zenker diverticulum
Zenker fluid
Zenker necrosis
Zenker pouch
Zenker retractor
Zenotech graft
Zephiran Chloride (benzalkonium
    chloride)
Zeppelin clamp
zero-degree (0°) forward optic laparo-
    scope
ZES (Zollinger-Ellison syndrome)
ZEUS robotic system
Z fixation nail
Zickel intramedullary nail
Zickel rod
Zickel subtrochanteric nail
Zickel supracondylar medullary nail
Ziegler head mirror
Ziehl-Neelsen stain
Zielke gouge
Zielke hook
Zielke rod
Zieve syndrome
zigzag finger incision
zigzag incision
Zika virus
Zimaloy staple
Zimmer caudal hook
Zimmer femoral condyle blade plate
Zimmer gouge
Zimmer hand drill

Zimmer low-viscosity adhesive
Zimmer micro saw
Zimmer oscillating saw
Zimmer pin
Zimmer rigid laparoscope
Zimmer side plate
Zimmer Statak suture/suturing device
Zimmer Y plate
Zimmon papillotome
zinc acetate
Zinca-Pak (zinc sulfate) intravenous
    nutritional therapy
Zinnanti Z-clamp
Zinn retractor
zipper scar
zipper sphincterotomy
zipper stitch
Zipzoc stocking compression dressing
Zipzoc stocking compression wrap
Zixoryn (flumecinol)
Z line
Z-Med catheter
Zoellner rasp
Zofran ODT (ondansetron)
Zoladex (goserelin acetate)
zoledronic acid
Zollinger classification of groin hernias
Zollinger-Ellison syndrome (ZES)
Zometa (zoledronic acid)
zona (pl. zonae)
zonal gastritis
zonal necrosis
zone
    abdominal
    anal transitional (ATZ)
    arcuate
    barrier
    basement membrane
    bloodless, of necrosis

zone *(cont.)*
    calcification
    cloacogenic
    echo
    entry
    hemorrhoidal
    high-pressure (HPZ)
    marginal, of spleen
    medullary
    mucosal
    "no-trocar"
    pectinate
    portal
    proliferation
    transformation
    vascular
Zone Specific II meniscal repair system
zopolrestat
Zosyn (piperacillin sodium; tazobactam
    sodium)
Z-plasty incision
Z-plasty local flap graft
Z-Scissors
Z-shaped plate
ZstatFlu test
Z stent for bile duct and esophageal
    stenosis
Z-stitch suture
Z suture
Zuelzer awl
Zuelzer hook
Zuelzer hook plate
Zuma guiding catheter
Zydone (hydrocodone bitartrate/
    acetaminophen)
zygomycetous fungus
zymogenic cell
Zyoptix laser
Zyvox (linezolid)

Appendix

Table of Arteries

artery	arteria (pl. arteriae)
Abbott's artery	
abdominal aorta artery	arteria aorta abdominalis
aberrant artery	
aberrant obturator artery	
accessory meningeal artery	arteria meningea accessoria
accessory obturator artery	arteria obturatoria accessoria
accessory pudendal artery	arteria pudenda accessoria
accompanying artery of ischiadic nerve	arteria comitans nervi ischiadici
accompanying artery of median nerve	arteria comitans nervi mediani
acetabular artery	ramus acetabularis arteriae circumflexae femoris medialis
acromial artery	
acromiothoracic artery	
Adamkiewicz, artery of	arteria radicularis magna
adipose arteries of kidney	rami capsulares arteriae renis
adrenal artery, middle	arteria suprarenalis media
afferent artery of glomerulus	vas afferens glomeruli
alar artery of nose	
alveolar artery, inferior	arteria alveolaris inferior
alveolar arteries, superior, anterior	arteriae alveolares superiores anteriores
alveolar artery, superior, posterior	arteria alveolaris superior posterior
anastomotic atrial artery	ramus atrialis anastomoticus arteriae coronariae sinistrae
angular artery	arteria angularis
angular gyrus artery	arteria gyri angularis
anonymous artery	
anterior auricular artery	arteria auricularis anterior
anterior cecal artery	arteria cecalis anterior
anterior cerebellar artery	arteria cerebelli anterior
anterior cerebral artery	arteria cerebri anterior
anterior choroidal artery	arteria choroidea anterior
anterior ciliary artery	arteria ciliaris anterior

artery	arteria (pl. arteriae)
anterior circumflex humeral artery	arteria circumflexa humeri anterior
anterior communicating artery	arteria communicans anterior
anterior conjunctival artery	arteria conjunctivalis anterior
anterior descending artery	
anterior ethmoidal artery	arteria ethmoidalis anterior
anterior humeral circumflex artery	
anterior inferior cerebellar artery	arteria cerebelli inferior anterior
anterior inferior segmental artery of kidney	arteria segmenti anterioris inferioris renis
anterior intercostal arteries	rami intercostales anteriores
anterior interosseous artery	arteria interossea anterior
anterior interventricular artery	ramus interventricularis anterior arteriae coronariae sinistrae
anterior labial arteries	arteriae labiales anteriores
anterior lateral malleolar artery	arteria malleolaris anterior lateralis
anterior medial malleolar artery	arteria malleolaris anterior medialis
anterior mediastinal arteries	rami mediastinales arteriae thoracicae internae
anterior meningeal artery	arteria meningea anterior
anterior parietal artery	arteria parietales anterior
anterior peroneal artery	ramus arteriae fibularis anterior
anterior radial carpal artery	arteria radialis carpalis
anterior spinal artery	arteria spinalis anterior
anterior superior alveolar arteries	arteriae alveolares superiores anteriores
anterior superior dental artery	arteria alveolaris anterior superior
anterior superior segmental artery of kidney	arteria segmenti anterioris superioris renis
anterior temporal artery	arteria temporalis anterior
anterior tibial artery	arteria tibialis anterior
anterior tibial recurrent artery	arteria recurrens tibialis anterior
anterior tympanic artery	arteria tympanica anterior
anterolateral central arteries	arteriae centrales anterolaterales
anterolateral striate arteries	arteriae centrales anterolaterales
anterolateral thalamostriate arteries	arteriae centrales anterolaterales
apicoposterior artery	
appendicular artery	arteria appendicularis
arch of aorta	arteria arcus aortae

artery	arteria (pl. arteriae)
arciform arteries	arteriae arcuatae renis
arcuate artery of foot	arteria arcuata pedis
arcuate arteries of kidney	arteriae arcuatae renis
articular artery, proper, of little head of fibula	ramus circumflexus fibulae arteriae tibialis posterioris
ascending artery	arteria ascendens
ascending aorta	arteria aorta ascendens
ascending cervical artery	arteria cervicalis ascendens
ascending palatine artery	arteria palatina ascendens
ascending pharyngeal artery	arteria pharyngea ascendens
atrial anastomotic artery	ramus atrialis anastomoticus arteriae coronariae sinistrae
atrial arteries	arteriae atriales
atrioventricular node, artery to	ramus nodi atrioventricularis
atrioventricular nodal artery	ramus nodi atrioventricularis arteriae coronariae dextrae
auditory artery, internal	arteria labyrinthina
auricular arteries, anterior	rami auriculares anteriores arteriae temporalis superficialis
auricular artery	arteria auricularis
axillary artery	arteria axillaris
axis thoracic artery	arteria thoracica axillaris
azygos arteries of vagina	vaginales arteriae uterinae
basilar artery	arteria basilaris
brachial artery	arteria brachialis
brachiocephalic artery	truncus brachiocephalicus
bronchial arteries	rami bronchiales
buccal artery, buccinator artery	arteria buccalis
bulbourethral artery	arteria bulbi urethrae
bulb of penis, artery of	arteria bulbi penis
bulb of vestibule of vagina, artery of	arteria bulbi vestibuli vaginae
calcaneal arteries	rami calcanei
calcarine artery	
calf, artery of	arteria sural
callosomarginal artery	arteria callosomarginalis
capsular artery	arteria suprarenalis
caroticotympanic arteries	arteriae caroticotympanicae
carotid artery	
caudal artery	arteria sacralis mediana

artery	arteria (pl. arteriae)
caudate lobe, artery of	arteria lobi caudati
cavernous artery	
cecal artery	arteria caecalis
celiac artery	
central arteries	arteriae centrales
central artery of retina, Zinn's artery	arteria centralis retinae
central sulcus artery	arteria sulci centralis
cephalic artery	arteria carotis communis
cerebellar artery	arteria cerebelli
cerebral artery, cerebral arteries	arteria cerebri, arteriae cerebrales
cervical artery	arteria cervicalis
cervicovaginal artery	arteria cervicovaginalis
Charcot's artery	
chief artery of thumb	arteria princeps pollicis
choroid artery, anterior	arteria choroidea anterior
ciliary arteries	arteriae cilliares
circle of Willis	
circumflex artery	ramus circumflexus arteriae coronariae sinistrae
circumflex artery, deep, internal	ramus profundus arteriae circumflexae femoris medialis
circumflex femoral artery, lateral	arteria circumflexa femoris lateralis
circumflex femoral artery, medial	arteria circumflexa femoris medialis
circumflex humeral artery, anterior	arteria circumflexa anterior humeri
circumflex humeral artery, posterior	arteria circumflexa posterior humeri
circumflex iliac artery, deep	arteria circumflexa iliaca profunda
circumflex iliac artery, superficial	arteria circumflexa iliaca superficialis
circumflex scapular artery	arteria circumflexa scapulae
clavicular artery	
clitoris, artery of, deep	arteria profunda clitoridis
clitoris, artery of, dorsal	arteria dorsalis clitoridis
coccygeal artery	arteria sacralis mediana
cochlear artery	ramus cochlearis arteriae labyrinthi
Cohnheim's artery	arteria terminalis
coiled artery	
colic artery	arteria colica
collateral artery	arteria collateralis
common carotid artery	arteria carotis communis
common hepatic artery	arteria hepatica communis

artery	arteria (pl. arteriae)
common iliac artery	arteria iliaca communis
common interosseous artery	arteria interossea communis
common palmar digital artery	arteria digitalis palmaris communis
common plantar digital artery	arteria digitalis plantaris communis
communicating artery of cerebrum	arteria communicans cerebri
companion artery	
conducting artery	
conjunctival artery	arteria conjunctivalis
conus artery	ramus coni arteriosi arteriae coronariae
copper-wire artery	
corkscrew artery	
coronary artery of heart	arteria coronaria
coronary artery of stomach	arteria gastrica
corpus cavernosum	
cortical artery	
costocervical trunk artery	
cremasteric artery	arteria cremasterica
cricothyroid artery	ramus cricothyroideus
crural artery	
cystic artery	arteria cystica
deep artery of clitoris	arteria profunda clitoridis
deep artery of penis	arteria profunda penis
deep artery of thigh	arteria profunda femoris
deep auricular artery	arteria auricularis profunda
deep brachial artery	arteria profunda brachii
deep cervical artery	arteria cervicalis profunda
deep circumflex iliac artery	arteria circumflexa iliaca profunda
deep epigastric artery	arteria epigastrica profunda
deep external pudendal artery	arteria pudenda profunda externa
deep femoral artery	arteria femoralis profunda
deep iliac circumflex artery	arteria circumflexa iliaca superficialis
deep lingual artery	arteria profunda linguae
deep palmar arch	arcus palmaris profundus
deep penis artery	arteria profunda penis
deep plantar artery	ramus plantaris profundus
deep temporal artery	arteria temporalis profunda
deep volar branch of ulnar artery	arteria ulnaris
deferential artery	arteria ductus deferentis
deltoid artery	ramus deltoideus arteriae profundae brachii

artery	arteria (pl. arteriae)
dental artery	arteria alveolaris
descending branch of occipital artery	arteria occipitalis descendens
descending genicular artery	arteria anastomotica magna
descending palatine artery	arteria palatina descendens
descending scapular artery	arteria scapularis descendens
diaphragmatic arteries	arteriae phrenicae inferiores
digital arteries	arteriae digitales
digital collateral artery	arteria digitalis palmaris propria
distributing artery	
dorsal artery of clitoris	arteria dorsalis clitoridis
dorsal artery of foot	arteria dorsalis pedis
dorsal artery of great toe	arteria dorsalis hallucis
dorsal artery of nose	arteria dorsalis nasi
dorsal artery of penis	arteria dorsalis penis
dorsal carpal artery	arteria dorsalis carpal
dorsal digital artery	arteria digitalis dorsalis
dorsal interosseous artery	arteria interossea dorsalis
dorsal metacarpal artery	arteria metacarpalis dorsalis
dorsal nasal artery	arteria dorsalis nasi
dorsalis pedis artery	arteria dorsalis pedis
dorsalis penis artery	arteria dorsalis penis
dorsal metacarpal artery	arteria metacarpea dorsalis
dorsal metatarsal artery	arteria metatarsea dorsalis
dorsal nasal artery	arteria nasi externa
dorsal pancreatic artery	arteria pancreatica dorsalis
dorsal scapular artery	arteria dorsalis scapulae
Drummond, artery of (marginal artery of colon)	
ductus deferens, artery of	arteria ductus deferentis
duodenal arteries	arteriae pancreaticoduodenales inferiores
efferent artery of glomerulus	vas efferens glomeruli
elastic artery	
emulgent artery	arteria renalis
end artery (terminal artery)	
epigastric artery	arteria circumflexa iliaca
epiphyseal artery	
episcleral arteries	arteriae episclerales
esophageal arteries	rami esophagei arteriae gastricae

artery	arteria (pl. arteriae)
ethmoidal artery	arteria ethmoidalis
external carotid artery	arteria carotis externa
external iliac artery	arteria iliaca externa
external mammary artery (lateral thoracic artery)	arteria thoracica lateralis
external maxillary artery (facial artery)	arteria maxillaris externa
external pudendal arteries	arteriae pudendae externae
external spermatic artery (cremasteric artery)	
facial artery	arteria facialis
fallopian artery	areria uterina
femoral artery	arteria femoralis
fibular artery (peroneal artery)	arteria fibularis
foot, artery of, dorsal	arteria dorsalis pedis
frontal artery (supratrochlear artery)	arteria supratrochlearis
frontobasal artery, lateral	arteria frontobasalis lateralis
funicular artery	arteria testicularis
gastric artery	arteria gastrica
gastroduodenal artery	arteria gastroduodenalis
gastroepiploic artery	arteria gastro-omentalis
gastro-omental artery	arteria gastro-omentalis
genicular artery	arteria genicularis
glaserian artery (anterior tympanic)	arteria tympanica anterior
glomerular artery	
gluteal artery	arteria glutealis
great anastomotic artery	arteria radicularis magna
greater palatine artery	arteria palatina major
great pancreatic artery	arteria pancreatica magna
great radicular artery	arteria radicularis magna
great superior pancreatic artery (dorsal)	arteria pancreatica magna superior
helicine arteries of penis	arteriae helicinae penis
hemorrhoidal artery	arteria rectalis
hepatic artery	arteria hepatica
Heubner, artery of (medial striate artery)	
highest intercostal artery (superior)	rami intercostales superiores
highest thoracic artery (superor)	arteria thoracica superior
humeral artery (brachial artery)	arteria humeri
hyaloid artery	arteria hyaloidea
hyoid artery	ramus suprahyoideus arteriae lingualis

artery	arteria (pl. arteriae)
hypogastric artery (internal iliac artery)	arteria iliaca interna
hypophysial artery	arteria hypophysialis
ileal arteries	arteriae ileales
ileocolic artery	arteria ileocolica
iliac artery	arteria iliaca
iliolumbar artery	arteria iliolumbalis
inferior alveolar artery	arteria alveolaris inferior
inferior cerebellar artery	arteria cerebelli inferior
inferior dental artery	arteria alveolaris inferior
inferior epigastric artery	arteria epigastrica inferior
inferior gastroduodenal artery	arteria gastroduodenalis inferior
inferior genicular artery	arteria genicularis inferior
inferior gluteal artery	arteria glutea inferior
inferior hemorrhoidal artery	arteria rectalis inferior
inferior hypophysial artery	arteria hypophysialis inferior
inferior labial artery	arteria labialis inferior
inferior laryngeal artery	arteria laryngea inferior
inferior lateral genicular artery	arteria genus inferior lateralis
inferior medial genicular artery	arteria genus inferior medialis
inferior mesenteric artery	arteria mesenterica inferior
inferior pancreatic artery	arteria pancreatica inferior
inferior pancreaticoduodenal artery	arteria pancreaticoduodenalis inferior
inferior phrenic artery	arteria phrenica inferior
inferior profunda artery	arteria profunda inferior
inferior rectal artery	arteria rectalis inferior
inferior segmental artery of kidney	arteria segmenti inferioris renis
inferior suprarenal artery	arteria suprarenalis inferior
inferior thyroid artery	arteria thyroidea inferior
inferior tympanic artery	arteria tympanica inferior
inferior ulnar collateral artery	arteria collateralis ulnaris inferior
inferior vesical artery	arteria vesicalis inferior
infracostal artery	ramus costalis lateralis arteriae thoracicae internae
infrahyoid artery	arteria infrahyoideus
infraorbital artery	arteria infraorbitalis
infrascapular artery	arteria infrascapularis
innominate artery	truncus brachiocephalicus
inguinal arteries	rami inguinales arteriae femoralis
innominate artery	truncus brachiocephalicus

artery	arteria (pl. arteriae)
insular arteries	arteriae insulares
intercostal arteries	rami intercostales arteriae thoracicae
interlobar arteries of kidney	arteriae interlobares renis
interlobular arteries of kidney	arteriae interlobulares renis
interlobular arteries of liver	arteriae interlobulares hepatis
intermediate atrial artery	ramus atrialis intermedius
intermediate temporal artery	arteria temporalis intermedia
intermetacarpal arteries	arteriae metacarpales palmares
internal auditory artery (labyrinthine)	arteria labyrinthi
internal carotid artery	arteria carotis interna
internal iliac artery	arteria iliaca interna
internal malleolar artery	arteria malleolaris interna
internal mammary artery (thoracic)	arteria thoracica interna
internal maxillary artery	arteria maxillaris interna
internal palpebral artery	arteria palpebralis interna
internal plantar artery	arteria plantaris interna
internal pubic artery	arteria pubicus interna
internal pudendal artery	arteria pudenda interna
internal spermatic artery (testicular)	arteria testicularis interna
internal thoracic artery	arteria thoracica interna
interosseous artery	arteria interossea
interosseous palmar artery	arteria palmaris interossea
intersegmental artery	
interventricular artery	ramus interventricularis
intestinal arteries (ileal or jejunal)	arteriae intestinales
jejunal arteries	arteriae jejunales
kidney, arteries of (segmental arteries of kidney)	arteriae renis
Kugel's anastomotic artery	arteria anastomotica auricularis magna
labial arteries of vulva	rami labiales arteriae femoralis
labyrinthine artery	arteria labyrinthi
lacrimal artery	arteria lacrimalis
laryngeal artery	arteria laryngea
lateral calcaneal artery	arteria calcanei lateralis
lateral circumflex femoral artery	arteria circumflexa femoris lateralis
lateral circumflex artery of thigh	arteria circumflexa femoris lateralis
lateral costal artery	
lateral frontobasal artery	arteria frontobasalis lateralis
lateral inferior genicular artery	arteria genicularis lateralis inferior

artery	arteria (pl. arteriae)
lateral malleolar arteries	rami malleolares laterales
lateral nasal artery	arteria nasi lateralis
lateral occipital artery	arteria occipitalis lateralis
lateral palpebral artery	arteria palpebralis lateralis
lateral plantar artery	arteria plantaris lateralis
lateral sacral artery	arteria sacralis lateralis
lateral striate arteries	arteriae centrales anterolaterales
lateral tarsal artery	arteria tarsea lateralis
lateral thoracic artery	arteria thoracica lateralis
left anterior descending coronary artery	ramus interventricularis anterior arteriae coronariae sinistrae
left colic artery	arteria colica sinistra
left coronary artery	arteria coronaria sinistra
left gastric artery	arteria gastrica sinistra
left gastroepiploic artery	arteria gastro-omentalis sinistra
left gastro-omental artery (left gastroepiploic artery)	
left hepatic artery	ramus sinister arteriae hepaticae propriae
left pulmonary artery	arteria pulmonalis sinistra
lenticulostriate arteries (Charcot's artery) (lateral striate arteries)	
lesser palatine artery	arteria palatina minor
lienal artery (splenic artery)	
lingual artery	arteria lingualis
lingual artery, dorsal	arteria lingualis dorsalis
lobar artery	
long central artery (medial striate artery)	
long ciliary artery	arteria ciliaris longa
long posterior ciliary artery	arteria ciliaris posterior longa
long thoracic artery (lateral)	arteria thoracica lateralis
lowest lumbar arteries	arteriae lumbales imae
lowest thyroid artery	arteria thyroidea ima
lumbar artery	arteria lumbalis
macular arteries	
malleolar artery	arteria malleolaris
mammary artery	arteria thoracica
mandibular artery	arteria alveolaris inferior
marginal artery	ramus marginalis

artery	arteria (pl. arteriae)
marginal artery of colon (artery of Drummond, Riolan's arc)	arteria marginalis coli
masseteric artery	arteria masseterica
mastoid artery	rami mastoidei arteriae auricularis posterioris
maxillary artery	arteria maxillaris
medial artery of foot, superficial	ramus superior arteriae plantaris medialis
medial circumflex femoral artery	arteria circumflexa femoris medialis
medial frontobasal artery	arteria frontobasalis medialis
medial malleolar arteries	arteriae malleolares posteriores mediales
medial palpebral artery	
medial striate artery	
medial tarsal artery	
median artery	arteria comitans nervi mediani
median sacral artery	arteria sacralis mediana
mediastinal arteries, anterior	rami mediastinales arteriae thoracicae internae
mediastinal arteries, posterior	rami mediastinales aortae thoracicae
medullary artery	arteria nutriens
meningeal artery, accessory	ramus meningeus accessorius arteriae meningeae mediae
meningeal artery, anterior	ramus meningeus anterior arteriae ethmoidalis anterioris
meningeal artery, middle	arteria meningea media
meningeal artery, posterior	arteria meningea posterior
mental artery	arteria mentalis
mesencephalic arteries	arteriae mesencephalicae
mesenteric artery	arteria mesenterica
metacarpal arteries	arteriae metacarpales
metaphyseal artery	
metatarsal artery	arteria metatarsae
middle capsular artery	arteria suprarenalis media
middle cerebral artery	arteria cerebri media
middle colic artery	arteria colica media
middle collateral artery	arteria collateralis media
middle genicular artry	arteria articularis azygos
middle hemorrhoidal artery	

artery	arteria (pl. arteriae)
middle meningeal artery	arteria meningea media
middle rectal artery	arteria rectalis media
middle sacral artery	arteria sacralis media
middle suprarenal artery	arteria suprarenalis media
middle temporal artery	arteria temporalis media
middle vesical artery	arteria vesicalis media
Mueller, arteries of	arteriae helicinae penis
musculophrenic artery	arteria musculophrenica
mylohyoid artery	ramus mylohyoideus arteriae alveolaris inferioris
myomastoid artery	ramus occipitalis arteriae auricularis posterioris
nasal artery, dorsal	arteria dorsalis nasi
nasopalatine artery	arteria sphenopalatina
Neubauer's artery	arteria thyroidea ima
nodal artery	
nose, dorsal artery of	arteria dorsalis nasi
nutrient artery	arteria nutricia
obliterated hypogastric artery	
obliterated umbilical artery	
obturator artery	arteria obturatoria
occipital artery	arteria occipitalis
omental artery	
omphalomesenteric artery	
ophthalmic artery	arteria ophthalmica
orbital artery	
orbitofrontal artery (lateral frontobasal)	
ovarian artery	arteria ovarica
palatine artery	arteria palatina
palmar metacarpal artery	arteria metacarpea palmaris
palpebral arteries	arteriae palpebrales
pancreatic artery	arteria pancreatica
pancreaticoduodenal artery	arteria pancreaticoduodenalis
paracentral artery	arteria paracentralis
parietal arteries, anterior and posterior	arteriae parietales anterior et posterior
parieto-occipital artery	arteria parieto-occipitalis
parieto-temporal artery	
pectoral artery	
pelvic artery, posterior	arteria iliaca interna

artery	arteria (pl. arteriae)
penis, deep artery of	arteria profunda penis
penis, dorsal artery of	arteria dorsalis penis
perforating arteries	arteriae perforantes
pericallosal artery	arteria pericallosa
pericardiac arteries, posterior	rami pericardiaci aortae thoracicae
pericardiacophrenic artery	arteria pericardiacophrenica
perineal artery	arteria perinealis
periosteal artery	
peroneal artery, fibular artery	arteria peronea, arteria fibularis
pharyngeal artery, ascending	arteria pharyngea ascendens
phrenic arteries	arteriae phrenicae
plantar artery	arteria plantaris
plantar metatarsal artery	arteria metatarsea plantaris
pontine arteries	arteriae pontis
popliteal artery	arteria poplitea
postcentral sulcal artery	arteria sulci postcentralis
posterior alveolar artery	arteria alveolaris posterior
posterior auricular artery	arteria auricularis posterior
posterior cecal artery	arteria cecalis posterior
posterior cerebral artery	arteria cerebri posterior
posterior choroidal artery	arteria choroidea posterior
posterior circumflex humeral artery	arteria circumflexa humeri posterior
posterior communicating artery	
posterior descending coronary artery	ramus interventricularis posterior arteriae coronariae dextrae
posterior humeral circumflex	artria circumflexa humeri posterior
posterior inferior cerebellar artery	arteria cerebelli posterior inferior
posterior intercostal artery	
posterior interosseous artery	arteria interossea posterior
posterior pancreaticoduodenal artery	arteria pancreaticoduodenalis posterior
posterior scapular artery	arteria scapulae posterior
posterior scrotal artery	arteria scrotalis posterior
posterior septal artery of nose	arteria nasalis posterior septi
posterior spinal artery	arteria spinalis posterior
posterior superior alveolar artery	arteria alveolaris superior posterior
posterior temporal artery	arteria temporalis posterior
posterior tibial artery	arteria tibialis posterior
posterior tibial recurrent artery	arteria recurrens tibialis posterior
posterior tympanic artery	arteria tympanica posterior

artery	arteria (pl. arteriae)
posterolateral central artery	arteriae centrales posterolaterales
posteromedial central arteries	arteriae centrales posteromediales
precentral sulcal artery	arteria sulci precentralis
princeps pollicis artery	arteria princeps pollicis
precuneal artery	arteria precunealis
prepancreatic artery	arteria prepancreatica
presegmental artery	arteria presegmenti
prevertebral artery	arteria prevertebralis
principal artery of thumb	arteria princeps pollicis
profunda brachii artery	arteria profunda brachii
profunda femoris artery	arteria profunda femoris
proper hepatic artery	arteria hepatica propria
proper palmar digital artery	arteria digitalis palmaris propria
proper plantar digital artery	arteria digitalis plantaris propria
pterygoid arteries	rami pterygoidei
pterygoid canal, artery of	arteria canalis pterygoidei
pubic artery	ramus pubicus arteriae epigastricae inferioris
pudendal arteries	arteriae pudendae externae
pulmonary artery	truncus pulmonalis
pyloric artery	arteria gastrica dextra
quadriceps artery of femur	ramus descendens arteriae circumflexae femoris lateralis
radial artery	arteria radialis
radial artery of index finger	arteria volaris radialis indicis
radial carpal artery	
radial collateral artery	arteria collateralis radialis
radial recurrent artery	arteria recurrens radialis
radiate arteries of kidney	arteriae interlobulares renis
radicular arteries	rami spinales arteriae vertebralis
ranine artery	arteria profunda linguae
rectal artery	arteria rectalis
recurrent artery	arteria centralis longa
recurrent artery, radial	arteria recurrens radialis
recurrent artery, tibial, anterior	arteria recurrens tibialis anterior
recurrent artery, tibial, posterior	arteria recurrens tibialis posterior
recurrent artery, ulnar	arteria recurrens ulnaris
recurrent interosseous artery	arteria interossea recurrens
recurrent radial artery	arteria recurrens radialis

artery	arteria (pl. arteriae)
recurrent ulnar artery	arteria recurrens ulnaris
renal artery, renal arteries	arteria renalis, arteriae renales
retinal artery	
retrocostal artery	ramus costalis lateralis arteriae thoracicae internae
retroduodenal artery	arteria retroduodenalis
retroesophageal subclavian artery	artery subclavia retroesophagei
revehent artery	vas efferens glomeruli
right colic artery	arteria colica dextra
right coronary artery	arteria coronaria dextra
right gastric artery	arteria gastrica dextra
right gastroepiploic artery	arteria gastro-omentalis dextra
right hepatic artery	ramus dexter arteriae hepaticae propriae
right pulmonary artery	arteria pulmonalis dextra
round ligament of uterus, artery of	arteria ligamenti teretis uteri
sacral arteries	arteriae sacrales
sacrococcygeal artery	arteria sacralis mediana
saphenous artery	
scapular artery	arteria scapulare
sciatic artery	arteria comitans nervi ischiadici
scrotal arteries, anterior	rami scrotales anteriores arteriae femoralis
scrotal arteries, posterior	rami scrotales posteriores arteriae pudendae internae
segmental artery	arteria segmenti
semilunar ganglion artery	
septal arteries, anterior	rami interventriculares septales
septal arteries, posterior	rami interventricularis posterioris
short central artery	arteria centralis brevis
short ciliary artery	arteria ciliaris brevis
short gastric artery	arteriae gastricae breves
short posterior ciliary artery	arteria ciliaris posterior brevis
sigmoid arteries	arteriae sigmoideae
sinoatrial nodal artery, sinuatrial (S-A) node artery	ramus nodi sinuatrialis arteriae coronaria dextra
somatic artery	
spermatic artery, external	arteria cremasterica
spermatic artery, internal	arteria testicularis
sphenopalatine artery	arteria sphenopalatina

artery	arteria (pl. arteriae)
spinal arteries	rami spinales arteriae vertebralis
spiral artery	
splanchnic artery	
splenic artery	arteria splenica
stapedial artery	
sternal arteries, posterior	rami sternales arteriae thoracicae internae
sternocleidomastoid artery, superior	ramus sternocleidomastoideus arteriae thyroideae superioris
straight arteries of kidney	arteriolae rectae renis
striate arteries	arteriae centrales anterolaterales
stylomastoid artery	arteria stylomastoidea
subclavian artery	arteria subclavia
subcostal artery	arteria subcostalis
sublingual artery	arteria sublingualis
submaxillary glandular artery	
submental artery	arteria submentalis
subscapular artery	arteria subscapularis
sulcal artery	
superficial brachial artery	arteria brachialis superficialis
superficial cervical artery	arteria cervicalis superficialis
superficial circumflex iliac artery	arteria circumflexa iliaca superficialis
superficial epigastric artery	arteria epigastrica superficialis
superficial external pudendal artery	arteria pudenda superficialis externa
superficial iliac circumflex artery	arteria circumflexa iliaca superficialis
superficial palmar arch artery	arteria arcus palmaris superficialis
superficial perineal artery	arteria perinealis superficialis
superficial petrosal artery	
superficial temporal artery	arteria temporalis superficialis
superficial volar artery	
superficial volar arch artery	
superior cerebellar artery	arteria cerebelli superior
superior epigastric artery	arteria epigastrica superior
superior gluteal artery	arteria glutea superior
superior hemorrhoidal artery	arteria rectalis superior
superior hypophysial artery	arteria hypophysialis superior
superior intercostal artery	arteria intercostalis suprema
superior labial artery	arteria labialis superior
superior laryngeal artery	arteria laryngea superior
superior lateral genicular artery	arteria genus superior lateralis

artery	arteria (pl. arteriae)
superior medial genicular artery	arteria genus superior medialis
superior mesenteric artery	arteria mesenterica superior
superior pancreaticoduodenal artery	arteria pancreaticoduodenalis superior
superior phrenic artery	arteria phrenica superior
superior profunda artery	arteria profunda superior
superior rectal artery	arteria rectalis superior
superior segmental artery of kidney	arteria segmenti superioris renis
superior suprarenal arteries	arteriae suprarenales superiores
superior thoracic artery	arteria thoracica superior
superior thyroid artery	arteria thyroidea superior
superior tympanic artery	arteria tympanica superior
superior ulnar collateral artery	arteria collateralis ulnaris superior
superior vesical artery	arteria vesicalis superior
supraduodenal artery	arteria supraduodcnalis
suprahyoid artery	arteria superhyoideus
supraorbital artery	arteria supraorbitalis
suprarenal artery, aortic	arteria suprarenalis media
suprascapular artery	arteria suprascapularis
supratrochlear artery	arteria supratrochlearis
sural artery	arteria suralis
sylvian artery	arteria cerebri media
tarsal artery	arteria tarsalis
temporal artery	arteria temporalis
terminal artery (Cohnheim's artery)	
testicular artery	arteria testicularis
thalamostriate arteries, anterolateral	arteriae centrales anterolaterales
thoracic artery	arteria thoracica
thoracicoacromial artery	arteria thoracoacromialis
thoracodorsal artery	arteria thoracodorsalis
thymic arteries	rami thymici arteriae thoracicae internae
thyroid artery	arteria thyroidea
thyroid artery, inferior, of Cruveilhier	ramus cricothyroideus arteriae thyroideae superioris
thyroid ima artery	arteria thyroidea ima
tibial artery	arteria tibialis
tonsillar artery	ramus tonsillaris arteriae facialis
tracheal artery	
transverse artery of neck	arteria transversa cervicis
transverse cervical artery	arteria transversa cervicis

artery	arteria (pl. arteriae)
transverse facial artery	arteria transversa faciei
transverse perineal artery	arteria transversa perinealis
transverse scapular artery	arteria transversa scapulae
trunk artery	
tubo-ovarian artery	arteria ovarica
tympanic artery	arteria tympanica
ulnar artery	arteria ulnaris
ulnar carpal artery	
ulnar collateral artery, inferior	arteria collateralis ulnaris inferior
ulnar collateral artery, superior	arteria collateralis ulnaris superior
umbilical artery	arteria umbilicalis
upper limb, arteries of	arteriae membri superioris
ureteric artery	
urethral artery	arteria urethralis
urethral bulb artery	
uterine artery	arteria uterina
uterine artery, aortic	arteria ovarica
vaginal artery	arteria vaginalis
venous arteries	venae pulmonales
ventricular arteries	arteriae ventriculares
vermiform artery	arteria appendicularis
vertebral artery	arteria vertebralis
vesical artery, inferior	arteria vesicalis inferior
vesical arteries, superior	arteriae vesicales superiores
vestibular arteries	rami vestibulares arteriae labyrinthi
vidian artery	arteria canalis pterygoidei
visceral artery	
vitelline artery	arteria vitellina
volar carpal artery	
volar interosseous artery	arteria interossea volaris
Zinn, artery of	arteria centralis retinae
zygomatic artery	
zygomatico-orbital artery	arteria zygomatico-orbitalis

Table of Muscles

muscle	musculus (pl. musculi)
abdominal muscles	musculi abdominis
abdominal external oblique muscle	musculus obliquus externus abdominis
abdominal internal oblique muscle	musculus obliquus internus abdominis
abductor digiti minimi muscle of foot (abductor muscle of little toe)	musculus abductor digiti minimi pedis
abductor digiti minimi muscle of hand (abductor muscle of little finger)	musculus abductor digiti minimi manus
abductor hallucis muscle (great toe)	musculus abductor hallucis
abductor pollicis brevis muscle (abductor muscle of thumb, short)	musculus abductor pollicis brevis
abductor pollicis longus muscle (abductor muscle of thumb, long)	musculus abductor pollicis longus
accessory flexor muscle of foot (quadratus plantae muscle)	musculus flexor accessorius
adductor muscle, short	musculus adductor brevis
adductor muscle of great toe	musculus adductor hallucis
adductor muscle, long	musculus adductor longus
adductor muscle, great	musculus adductor magnus
adductor minimus muscle (adductor muscle, smallest)	musculus adductor minimus
adductor pollicis muscle (thumb)	musculus adductor pollicis
Aeby's cutaneomucous muscle	
agonistic muscles	
Albinus' muscle	
anconeus muscle	musculus anconeus
antagonistic muscles	
anterior auricular muscle	musculus auricularis anterior
anterior cervical intertransverse muscles	musculi intertransversarii anteriores cervicis
anterior rectus muscle of head	musculus rectus capitis anterior
anterior scalene muscle	musculus scalenus anterior

muscle	musculus (pl. musculi)
anterior serratus muscle	musculus serratus anterior
anterior tibial muscle	musculus tibialis anterior
antigravity muscles	
antitragus muscle	musculus antitragicus
arrector pili muscles	musculi arrectores pilorum
(erector muscles of hairs)	
articular muscle	musculus articularis
articular muscle of elbow	musculus articularis cubiti
articular muscle of knee	musculus articularis genus
articular muscle of knee	articularis genu musculus
aryepiglottic muscle	musculus aryepiglotticus
auditory ossicles, muscles of	musculi ossiculorum auditus
axillary arch muscle	pectorodorsalis musculus
back muscles	musculi dorsi
Bell's muscle (ureteric bridge)	
biceps brachii muscle	musculus biceps brachii
(biceps muscle of arm)	
biceps femoris muscle	musculus biceps femoris
(biceps muscle of thigh)	
bipennate muscle	musculus bipennatus
Bochdalek's muscle	musculus triticeoglossus
Bovero's muscle ("sucking muscle")	musculus cutaneomucosus
Bowman's muscle (ciliary muscle)	musculus ciliaris
brachial muscle (brachialis)	musculus brachialis
brachiocephalic muscle	musculus brachiocephalicus
brachioradial muscle (brachioradialis)	musculus brachioradialis
Braune's muscle	musculus puborectalis
broadest muscle of back	musculus latissimus dorsi
bronchoesophageal muscle	musculus bronchoesophageus
Brücke's muscle (Crampton's muscle)	
buccinator muscle	musculus buccinator
buccopharyngeal muscles	musculi pars buccopharyngea
(also, constrictor muscles	
of pharynx, superior)	
bulbocavernous muscle	musculus bulbospongiosus
canine muscle	musculus levator anguli oris
cardiac muscle	
Casser's perforated muscle	musculus coracobrachialis
(casserian muscle)	(ligamentum mallei anterius)

muscle	musculus (pl. musculi)
ceratocricoid muscle	musculus ceratocricoideus
cervical iliocostal muscle	musculus iliocostalis cervicis
cervical interspinal muscles	musculi interspinalis cervicis
cervical longissimus muscle (neck)	musculus longissimus cervicis
cervical muscles	musculi colli
cervical rotator muscles	musculi rotatores cervicis
Chassaignac's axillary muscle	
chin muscle	musculus mentalis
chondroglossus muscle	musculus chondroglossus
chondropharyngeal muscles	musculi pars chondropharyngea
(constrictor muscle of pharynx, middle)	(constrictor pharyngis medius)
ciliary muscle	muscularis ciliaris
coccygeal (coccygeus) muscle(s)	musculus coccygeus, musculi coccygei
Coiter's muscle	musculus corrugator supercilii
compressor muscle of naris	
congenerous muscles	
constrictor muscle of pharynx, inferior	musculus constrictor pharyngis inferior
constrictor muscle of pharynx, middle	musculus constrictor pharyngis medius
constrictor muscle of pharynx, superior	musculus constrictor pharyngis superior
coracobrachial muscle (coracobrachialis)	musculus coracobrachialis
corrugator muscle	corrugator supercilii musculus
corrugator cutis muscle of anus	musculus corrugator cutis ani
corrugator supercilii muscle	musculus corrugator supercilii
Crampton's muscle (Bruecke's muscle)	
cremaster muscle (Riolan's muscle)	musculus cremaster
cricoarytenoid muscle, lateral	musculus crico-arytenoideus lateralis
cricoarytenoid muscle, posterior	musculus crico-arytenoideus posterior
cricopharyngeal muscle	musculus cricopharyngeus
cricothyroid muscle	musculus cricothyroideus
cruciate muscle	musculus cruciatus
cutaneomucous muscle	musculus cutaneomucosus
(the "sucking muscle," also called Aeby's muscle, Bovero's muscle, Klein's muscle, Krause's muscle, mucocutaneous muscle)	
cutaneous muscle	musculus cutaneus
dartos muscle of scrotum	musculus tunica dartos
deep muscles of back (true back muscles)	musculi dorsi
deep flexor muscle of fingers	musculus flexor digitorum profundus

muscle	musculus (pl. musculi)
deep transverse perineal msucle	musculus transversus perinei profundus
deltoid muscle	musculus deltoideus
depressor muscle of angle of mouth	musculus depressor anguli oris
depressor muscle of epiglottis	musculus thyroepiglottic
depressor muscle of eyebrow	musculus depressor supercilii
depressor muscle of lower lip	musculus depressor labii inferioris
depressor muscle of septum of nose	musculus depressor septi
depressor superciliary muscle	musculus depressor supercilii
detrusor muscle of urinary bladder	musculus detrusor urinae (musculus detrusor vesicae)
diaphragm, diaphragmatic muscle	diaphragma
digastric muscle	musculus digastricus
dilator muscle	musculus dilatator
dilator muscle of ileocecal sphincter	musculus dilator pylori ilealis
dilator muscle of pupil	musculus dilator pupillae
dilator muscle of pylorus	musculus dilator pylori gastro-duodenalis
dorsal interosseous muscles of foot	musculi interossei dorsalis pedis
dorsal interosseous muscles of hand	musculi interossei dorsalis manus
dorsal muscles (muscles of back)	musculi dorsi
dorsal sacrococcygeal muscle	musculus sacrococcygeus dorsalis
Dupré's muscle	musculus articularis genu
Duverney's muscle	musculus orbicularis oculi
elevator muscle of anus	musculus levator ani
elevator muscle of prostate	musculus levator prostatae
elevator muscles of rib	musculi levatores costarum
elevator muscle of scapula	musculus levator scapulae
elevator muscle of soft palate	musculus levator veli palatini
elevator muscle of upper eyelid	musculus levator palpebrae superioris
elevator muscle of upper lip	musculus levator labii superioris
elevator muscle of upper lip and wing of nose	musculus levator labii superioris alaeque nasi
emergency muscles	
epicranial muscle	musculus epicranius
epimeric muscle	
epitrochleoanconeus muscle	musculus epitrochleoanconaeus
erector muscles of hairs (arrector pili)	musculi arrectores pilorum
erector muscle of penis	musculus ischiocavernosus
erector muscle of spine	musculus erector spinae

muscle	musculus (pl. musculi)
eustachian muscle	musculus tensor tympani
expression, muscles of	musculi faciales
extensor muscle of fingers	musculus extensor digitorum
extensor muscle of great toe, long	musculus extensor hallucis longus
extensor muscle of great toe, short	musculus extensor hallucis brevis
extensor muscle of hand, short (Pozzi's muscle)	musculus extensor digitorum brevis manus
extensor muscle of index finger	musculus extensor indicis
extensor muscle of little finger	musculus extensor digiti minimi
extensor muscle of thumb, long	musculus extensor pollicis longus
extensor muscle of thumb, short	musculus extensor pollicis brevis
extensor muscle of toes, long	musculus extensor digitorum longus
extensor muscle of toes, short	musculus extensor digitorum brevis
extensor muscle of wrist, radial, long	musculus extensor carpi radialis longus
extensor muscle of wrist, radial, short	musculus extensor carpi radialis brevis
extensor muscle of wrist, ulnar	musculus extensor carpi ulnaris
external intercostal muscles	musculi intercostales externi
external oblique muscle	musculus obliquus externus abdominis
external obturator muscle	musculus obturator externus
external pterygoid muscle	lateral pterygoid musculus
external sphincter muscle of anus	
extraocular muscles	musculi bulbi
extrinsic muscles	
eyeball muscles (extraocular muscles)	
facial and masticatory muscles	musculi faciales et masticatores
facial expression, muscles of	musculi faciales
facial muscles	musculi faciales
fast muscle (white muscle)	
fauces (the throat), muscles of	musculi palati et faucium
femoral muscle	musculus vastus intermedius
fibular muscle, long	musculus peroneus longus
fibular muscle, short	musculus peroneus brevis
fibular muscle, third	musculus peroneus tertius
fixation muscles, fixator muscles	
fixator muscle of base of stapes	musculus fixator baseos stapedis
flexor muscle of fingers, deep	musculus flexor digitorum profundus
flexor muscle of fingers, superficial	musculus flexor digitorum superficialis
flexor muscle of great toe, long	musculus flexor hallucis longus
flexor muscle of great toe, short	musculus flexor hallucis brevis

muscle	musculus (pl. musculi)
flexor muscle of little finger, short	musculus flexor digiti minimi brevis manus
flexor muscle of little toe, short	musculus flexor digiti minimi brevis pedis
flexor muscle of thumb, short	musculus flexor pollicis brevis
flexor muscle of thumb, long	musculus flexor pollicis longus
flexor muscle of toes, short	musculus flexor digitorum brevis
flexor muscle of toes, long	musculus flexor digitorum longus
flexor muscle of wrist, radial	musculus flexor carpi radialis
flexor muscle of wrist, ulnar	musculus flexor carpi ulnaris
Folius' muscle	ligamentum mallei laterale
fusiform muscle (spindle-shaped muscle)	musculus fusiformis
Gantzer's muscle	
gastrocnemius muscle	musculus gastrocnemius
Gavard's muscle	
gemellus muscle, inferior	musculus gemellus inferior
gemellus muscle, superior	musculus gemellus superior
genioglossal muscle	musculus genioglossus
geniohyoid muscle	musculus geniohyoideus
glossopalatine muscle (palatoglossus)	musculus palatoglossus
glossopharyngeal muscle	pars glossopharyngea musculi constrictoris pharyngis superioris
gluteal muscle, greatest	musculus gluteus maximus
gluteal muscle, least	musculus gluteus minimus
gluteal muscle, middle	musculus gluteus medius
gracilis muscle	musculus gracilis
great adductor muscle	musculus adductor magnus
greater pectoral muscle	musculus pectoralis major
greater posterior rectus muscle of head	musculus rectus capitis posterior major
greater psoas muscle	musculus psoas major
greater rhomboid muscle	musculus rhomboideus major
greater zygomatic muscle	musculus zygomaticus major
Guthrie's muscle	sphincter urethrae
hamstring muscles	
head, muscles of	musculi capitis
Hilton's muscle	musculus aryepiglotticus
Horner's muscle	musculus orbicularis oculi
Houston's muscle	compressor venae dorsalis penis
hyoglossal (hyoglossus) muscle	musculus hyoglossus

muscle	musculus (pl. musculi)
iliac muscle	musculus iliacus
iliacus minor muscle	musculus iliacus minor
iliococcygeal muscle	musculus iliococcygeus
iliocostal muscle	musculus iliocostalis
iliocostal muscle of neck	musculus iliocostalis cervicis
iliocostal muscle of loins	musculus iliocostalis lumborum
iliocostal muscle of thorax	musculus iliocostalis thoracis
iliopsoas muscle	musculus iliopsoas
incisive muscles of inferior lip	musculi incisivi labii inferioris
incisive muscles of lower lip	musculi incisivi labii inferioris
incisive muscles of superior lip	musculi incisivi labii superioris
incisive muscles of upper lip	musculi incisivi labii superioris
index extensor muscle	musculus extensor indicis
inferior constrictor muscle of pharynx	musculus constrictor pharyngis inferior
inferior gemellus muscle	musculus gemellus inferior
inferior longitudinal muscle of tongue	musculus longitudinalis inferior
inferior oblique muscle	musculus obliquus inferior
inferior oblique muscle of head	musculus obliquus capitis inferior
inferior posterior serratus muscle	serratus posterior inferior musculus
inferior rectus muscle	musculus rectus inferior
inferior tarsal muscle	musculus tarsalis inferior
infrahyoid muscles	musculi infrahyoidei
infraspinous muscle	musculus infraspinatus
innermost intercostal muscle	musculus intercostalis intimus
inspiratory muscles	
intercostal muscles	musculi intercostales
interfoveolar muscle	ligamentum interfoveolare
intermediate great muscle	musculus vastus intermedius
internal intercostal muscle	musculus intercostalis internus
internal oblique muscle	musculus obliquus internus abdominis
internal obturator muscle	musculus obturator internus
internal pterygoid muscle	musculus pterygoideus medialis
interosseous muscles	musculi interossei
interspinal muscles	musculi interspinales
intertransverse muscles	musculi intertransversarii
intra-auricular muscles	
intraocular muscles	
intrinsic muscles	
intrinsic muscles of foot	

muscle	musculus (pl. musculi)
involuntary muscles	
iridic muscles	
ischiocavernous muscle	musculus ischiocavernosus
Jarjavay's muscle	
Jung's pyramidal auricular muscle	
Klein's cutaneomucous muscle	
Kohlrausch's muscle	
Koyter's muscle	musculus corrugator supercilii
Krause's cutaneomucous muscle	musculus cutaneomucosus
Landstrom's muscle (umlaut o)	
Langer's axillary arch muscle	
larynx, muscles of	musculi laryngis
lateral cricoarytenoid muscle	musculus cricoarytenoideus lateralis
lateral great muscle	musculus vastus lateralis
lateral lumbar intertransversarii muscles	musculi intertransversarii laterales lumborum
lateral pterygoid muscle	musculus pterygoideus lateralis
lateral rectus muscle	musculus rectus lateralis
lateral rectus muscle of the head	musculus rectus capitis lateralis
lateral vastus muscle	musculus vastus lateralis
latissimus dorsi muscle	musculus latissimus dorsi
lesser rhomboid muscle	musculus rhomboid minor
lesser zygomatic muscle	musculus zygomaticus minor
levator ani muscle	musculus levator ani
levator muscles (see *elevator muscles*)	
lingual muscles	musculi linguae
long abductor muscle of thumb	musculus abductor pollicis longus
long adductor muscle	musculus adductor longus
long extensor muscle of great toe	musculus extensor hallucis longus
long extensor muscle of thumb	musculus extensor pollicis longus
long extensor muscle of toes	musculus extensor digitorum longus
long fibular muscle	musculus peroneus longus
long flexor muscle of great toe	musculus flexor hallucis longus
long flexor muscle of thumb	musculus flexor pollicis longus
long flexor muscle of toes	musculus flexor digitorum longus
long muscle of head	musculus longus capitis
longissimus muscle	musculus longissimus
longissimus muscle of back (thorax)	musculus longissimus thoracis
longissimus muscle of head	musculus longissimus capitis

muscle	musculus (pl. musculi)
longissimus muscle of neck	musculus longissimus cervicis
longitudinal muscle of tongue, inferior	musculus longitudinalis inferior linguae
longitudinal muscle of tongue, superior	musculus longitudinalis superior linguae
long muscle of head	musculus longus capitis
long muscle of neck	musculus longus colli
long palmar muscle	musculus palmaris longus
long peroneal muscle	musculus peroneus longus
long radial extensor muscle of wrist	musculus extensor carpi radialis longus
lumbar iliocostal muscle	musculus interspinalis lumborum
lumbar interspinal muscles	musculus interspinalis lumborum
lumbar quadrate muscle	musculus quadratus lumborum
lumbar rotator muscles	musculi rotatores lumborum
lumbrical muscles of foot	musculi lumbricales pedis
lumbrical muscles of hand	musculi lumbricales manus
Marcacci's muscle	
masseter muscle	musculus masseter
medial great muscle	musculus vastus medialis
medial lumbar intertransverse muscles	musculi intertransversarii mediales lumborum
medial pterygoid muscle	musculus pterygoideus medialis
medial rectus muscle	musculus rectus medialis
medial vastus muscle	musculus vastus medialis
mentalis muscle	musculus mentalis
Merkel's muscle	musculus ceratocricoideus
mesothenar muscle	musculus adductor pollicis
middle constrictor muscle of pharynx	musculus constrictor pharyngis medius
middle scalene muscle	musculus scalenus medius
mucocutaneous muscle	
Mueller's muscle	musculus orbitalis
multifidus muscles (intermediate layer of transversospinalis muscles)	musculi multifidi
multipennate muscle	musculus multipennatus
mylohyoid muscle	musculus mylohyoideus
nasal muscle	musculus nasalis
neck, muscles of	musculi colli
nonstriated muscle (smooth muscle)	
notch of helix, muscles of	musculus incisurae helicis
oblique arytenoid muscle	musculus arytenoideus obliquus
oblique auricular muscle	musculus obliquus auriculae

muscle	musculus (pl. musculi)
oblique muscle of abdomen, external	musculus obliquus externus abdominis
oblique muscle of abdomen, internal	musculus obliquus internus abdominis
oblique muscle of head, inferior	musculus obliquus capitis inferior
oblique muscle of head, superior	musculus obliquus capitis superior
obturator muscle, external	musculus obturator externus
obturator muscle, internal	musculus obturator internus
occipitofrontal muscle	musculus occipitofrontalis
Ochsner's muscles	
ocular muscles	musculi bulbi
Oddi's muscle (sphincter)	
Oehl's muscles	
omohyoid muscle	musculus omohyoideus
opposing muscle of little finger	musculus opponens digiti minimi
opposing muscle of thumb	musculus opponens pollicis
orbicular muscle	musculus orbicularis
orbicular muscle of eye	musculus orbicularis oculi
orbicular muscle of mouth	musculus orbicularis oris
orbital muscle	musculus orbitalis
organic muscle (visceral musscle)	
palate and fauces, muscles	musculi palati et faucium
palatine muscles	musculi palati
palatoglossus muscle	musculus palatoglossus
palatopharyngeal muscle	musculus palatopharyngeus
palmar interosseous muscle	musculus interosseus palmaris
palmar muscle, short	musculus palmaris brevis
palmar muscle, long	musculus palmaris longus
papillary muscle	musculus papillaris
pectinate muscles	musculi pectinati
pectineal muscle	musculus pectineus
pectoral muscle, greater	musculus pectoralis major
pectoral muscle, smaller	musculus pectoralis minor
pectorodorsalis muscle (axillary arch)	
penniform muscle	musculus unipennatus
perineal muscles	musculi perinei
peroneal muscle, long	musculus fibularis longus
peroneal muscle, short	musculus fibularis brevis
peroneal muscle, third	musculus fibularis tertius
pharyngopalatine muscle	musculus palatopharyngeus
Phillips' muscle	

muscle	musculus (pl. musculi)
piriform muscle	musculus piriformis
plantar interosseous muscle	musculus interosseus plantaris
plantar muscle	musculus plantaris
plantar quadrate muscle	musculus quadratus plantae
platysma muscle	musculus platysma
pleuroesophageal muscle	musculus pleuroesophageus
popliteal muscle	musculus popliteus
posterior auricular muscle	musculus retrahens aurem
posterior cervical intertransverse muscles	musculi intertransversarii posteriores cervicis
posterior cricoarytenoid muscle	musculus cricoarytenoideus posterior
posterior scalene muscle	musculus scalenus posterior
posterior tibial muscle	musculus tibialis posterior
Pozzi's muscle (extensor digitorum brevis muscle of hand)	musculus extensor digitorum brevis manus
procerus muscle	musculus procerus
pronator muscle, quadrate	musculus pronator quadratus
pronator muscle, round	musculus pronator teres
psoas muscle, greater	musculus psoas major
psoas muscle, smaller	musculus psoas minor
pterygoid muscle	musculus pterygoideus
pubococcygeal muscle	musculus pubococcygeus
puboprostatic muscle	musculus puboprostaticus
puborectal muscle (Braune's muscle)	musculus puborectalis
pubovaginal muscle	musculus pubovaginalis
pubovesical muscle	musculus pubovesicalis
pyloric sphincter muscle	musculus sphincter pyloricus
pyramidal auricular muscle (Jung's m.)	musculus pyramidalis auriculae
quadrate (four-sided) muscle	musculus quadratus
quadrate muscle of loins	musculus quadratus lumborum
quadrate muscle of lower lip	musculus depressor labii inferioris
quadrate muscle of sole	musculus quadratus plantae
quadrate muscle of thigh	musculus quadratus femoris
quadrate muscle of upper lip	musculus quadratus labii superioris
radial flexor muscle of wrist	musculus flexor carpi radialis
rectococcygeus muscle	musculus rectococcygeus
rectourethral muscle	musculus recto-urethralis
rectouterine muscle	musculus recto-uterinus
rectovesical muscle	musculus rectovesicalis

muscle	musculus (pl. musculi)
rectus abdominis muscle (rectus muscle of abdomen)	musculus rectus abdominis
rectus muscle of head, anterior	musculus rectus capitis anterior
rectus muscle of head, lateral	musculus rectus capitis lateralis
rectus muscle of head, greater posterior	musculus rectus capitis posterior major
rectus muscle of head, smaller posterior	musculus rectus capitis posterior minor
rectus femoris muscle (rectus muscle of thigh)	musculus rectus femoris
red muscle (slow muscle)	
Reisseisen's muscles	
rhomboid muscle, greater	musculus rhomboideus major
rhomboid muscle, lesser	musculus rhomboideus minor
ribbon muscles	musculi infrahyoidei
rider's muscles (adductor muscles of thigh)	
Riolan's muscle (cremaster muscle)	musculus cremaster
risorius muscle (Albinus' muscle, Santorini's muscle)	musculus risorius
rotator muscles	musculi rotatores
rotator muscles of neck	musculi rotatores cervicis
rotator muscles of back	musculi rotatores lumborum
rotator muscles of thorax	musculi rotatores thoracis
Rouget's muscle	
round pronator muscle	musculus pronator teres
Ruysch's muscle	
sacrococcygeal muscle	musculus sacrococcygeus
salpingopharyngeal muscle	musculus salpingopharyngeus
Santorini's muscle	musculus risorius
sartorius muscle (tailor's muscle)	musculus sartorius
scalene muscle, anterior	musculus scalenus anterior
scalene muscle, middle	musculus scalenus medius
scalene muscle, posterior	musculus scalenus posterior
scalene muscle, smallest (Albinus' m., Sibson's m.)	musculus scalenus minimus
scalp muscle (epicranius muscle)	
Sebileau's muscle	
second tibial muscle	musculus tibialis secundus
semimembranous muscle	musculus semimembranosus
semispinal muscle	musculus semispinalis
semispinal muscle of head	musculus semispinalis capitis

muscle	musculus (pl. musculi)
semispinal muscle of neck	musculus semispinalis cervicis
semispinal muscle of thorax	musculus semispinalis thoracis
semitendinous muscle	musculus semitendinosus
serratus anterior muscle	musculus serratus anterior
serratus posterior inferior muscle	musculus serratus posterior inferior
serratus posterior superior muscle	musculus serratus posterior superior
shawl muscle (trapezius muscle)	
short adductor muscle	musculus adductor brevis
short extensor musscle of great toe	musculus extensor hallucis brevis
short extensor muscle of thumb	musculus extensor pollicis brevis
short extensor muscle of toes	musculus extensor digitorum brevis
short fibular muscle	musculus peroneus brevis
short flexor muscle of great toe	musculus flexor hallucis brevis
short flexor muscle of little finger	musculus flexor digiti minimi brevis
short flexor muscle of little toe	musculus flexor digiti minimi brevis
short flexor muscle of thumb	musculus flexor pollicis brevis
short flexor muscle of toes	musculus flexor digitorum brevis
short palmar muscle	musculus palmaris brevis
short peroneal muscle	musculus peroneus brevis
short radial extensor muscle of wrist	musculus extensor carpi radialis brevis
Sibson's muscle	musculus scalenus minimus
skeletal muscles	musculi skeleti
slow muscle (red muscle)	
smaller muscle of helix	musculus helicis minor
smaller pectoral muscle	musculus pectoralis minor
smaller posterior rectus muscle of head	musculus rectus capitis posterior minor
smaller psoas muscle	musculus psoas minor
smallest scalene muscle	musculus scalenus minimus
smooth muscle (unstriated, unstriped, visceral)	
Soemmerring's muscle (levator muscle of thyroid gland)	
soleus muscle	musculus soleus
somatic muscles	musculi skeleti
sphincter muscle of anus	musculus sphincter ani
sphincter muscle of bile duct	musculus sphincter ductus choledochi
sphincter muscle of hepatopancreatic ampulla	musculus sphincter ampullae hepatopancreaticae
sphincter muscle of pupil	musculus sphincter pupillae

muscle	musculus (pl. musculi)
sphincter muscle of pylorus	musculus sphincter pyloricus
sphincter muscle of urethra	musculus sphincter urethrae
sphincter muscle of urinary bladder	musculus sphincter vesicae urinariae
spinal muscle	musculus spinalis
spinal muscle of head	musculus spinalis capitis
spinal muscle of neck	musculus spinalis cervicis
spinal muscle of thorax	musculus spinalis thoracis
spindle-shaped muscle	musculus fisiform
splenius muscle of head	musculus splenius capitis
splenius muscle of neck	musculus splenius cervicis
stapedius muscle	musculus stapedius
sternal muscle	musculus sternalis
sternochondroscapular muscle	musculus sternochondroscapularis
sternoclavicular muscle	musculus sternoclavicularis
sternocleidomastoid muscle	musculus sternocleidomastoideus
sternocostal muscle	musculus transversus thoracis
sternohyoid muscle	musculus sternohyoideus
sternomastoid muscle (sternocleidomastoid)	
sternothyroid muscle	musculus sternothyroideus
strap muscles	
striated muscle	
styloauricular muscle	musculus styloauricularis
styloglossus muscle	musculus styloglossus
stylohyoid muscle	musculus stylohyoideus
stylopharyngeal muscle	musculus stylopharyngeus
subanconeus muscle	musculus articularis cubiti
subclavian muscle	musculus subclavius
subcostal muscle	musculus subcostalis
subcrural muscle	musculus articularis genu
suboccipital muscles	musculi suboccipitales
subquadricipital muscle	musculus articularis genu
subscapular muscle	musculus subscapularis
subvertebral muscles	musculi hypaxial
superficial back muscles	
superficial flexor muscle of fingers	musculus flexor digitorum superficialis
superficial lingual muscle (of tongue)	
superficial transverse perineal muscle (Theile's muscle)	musculus transversus perinei superficialis
superior auricular muscle	musculus auricularis superior

muscle	musculus (pl. musculi)
superior constrictor muscle of pharynx	musculus constrictor pharyngis superior
superior gemellus muscle	musculus gemellus superior
superior longitudinal muscle of tongue	musculus longitudinalis superior
superior oblique muscle	musculus obliquus superior
superior oblique muscle of head	musculus obliquus capitis superior
superior posterior serratus muscle	musculus serratus posterior superior
superior rectus muscle	musculus rectus superior
superior tarsal muscle (Mueller's muscle)	musculus tarsalis superior
supinator muscle	musculus supinator
supraclavicular muscle	musculus supraclavicularis
suprahyoid muscles	musculi suprahyoidei
supraspinalis muscle	musculus supraspinalis
supraspinous muscle	musculus supraspinatus
suspensory muscle of duodenum (Treitz' ligament)	musculus suspensorius duodeni
synergic or synergistic muscles	
tailor's muscle (sartorius muscle)	
temporal muscle	musculus temporalis
temporoparietal muscle	musculus temporoparietalis
tensor muscle of fascia lata	musculus tensor fasciae latae
tensor muscle of soft palate	musculus tensor veli palati
tensor tarsi muscle	musculus orbicularis oculi
tensor muscle of tympanic membrane (Toynbee's muscle)	musculus tensor tympani
teres major muscle	musculus teres major
teres minor muscle	musculus teres minor
Theile's muscle (superficial transverse perineal muscle)	
third peroneal muscle	musculus peroneus tertius
thoracic interspinal muscle	musculi thoracic interspinalis
thoracic intertransverse muscles	musculi intertransversarii thoracis
thoracic longissimus muscle	musculus longissimus thoracis
thoracic rotator muscles	musculi rotatores thoracis
thorax, muscles of	musculi thoracis
thyroarytenoid muscle	musculus thyroarytenoideus
thyroepiglottic muscle (depressor muscle of epiglottis)	musculus thyroepiglotticus
thyrohyoid muscle	musculus thyrohyoideus

muscle	musculus (pl. musculi)
tibial muscle, anterior	musculus tibialis anterior
tibial muscle, posterior	musculus tibialis posterior
Tod's muscle (oblique auricular muscle)	
tongue, muscles of	musculi linguae
Toynbee's muscle	musculus tensor tympani
tracheal muscle	musculus trachealis
tracheloclavicular muscle	musculus tracheloclavicularis
trachelomastoid muscle	musculus longissimus capitis
tragicus muscle	musculus tragicus
(Valsalva's muscle)	
transverse arytenoid muscle	musculus arytenoideus transversus
transverse muscle of abdomen	musculus transversus abdominis
transverse muscle of auricle	musculus transversus auriculae
transverse muscle of chin	musculus transversus menti
transverse muscle of nape	musculus transversus nuchae
transverse muscle of neck	musculus transversus nuchae
transverse muscle of thorax	musculus transversus thoracis
transverse muscle of tongue	musculus transversus linguae
transversospinal muscle	musculus transversospinalis
trapezius muscle	musculus trapezius
Treitz' muscle (suspensory muscle	
of duodenum)	
triangular muscle	musculus triangularis
triceps muscle of arm	musculus triceps brachii
triceps muscle of hip	musculus triceps coxae
triceps muscle of calf	musculus triceps surae
trigonal muscle	
true (deep) muscles of back	musculi dorsi
two-bellied muscle (digastric muscle)	musculus digastricus
ulnar extensor muscle of wrist	musculus extensor carpi ulnaris
ulnar flexor muscle of wrist	musculus flexor carpi ulnaris
unipennate muscle	musculus unipennatus
unstriated muscle, unstriped muscle	
(smooth muscle)	
urogenital diaphragm, muscles of	musculi diaphragmatis urogenitalis
uvula, muscle of	musculus uvulae
Valsalva's muscle	
vastus intermedius muscle	musculus vastus intermedius
(intermediate great muscle)	

muscle	musculus (pl. musculi)
vastus lateralis muscle (lateral great muscle)	musculus vastus lateralis
vastus medialis muscle (medial great muscle)	musculus vastus medialis
ventral sacrococcygeal muscle	musculus sacrococcygeus ventralis
vertical muscle of tongue	musculus verticalis linguae
visceral muscle (smooth)	
vocal muscle	musculus vocalis
voluntary muscle	
white muscle (fast muscle)	
Wilson's muscle (urethral sphincter)	musculus sphincter urethrae
wrinkler muscle of eyebrow	musculus corrugator supercilii
yoked muscles	
zygomatic muscle, greater	musculus zygomaticus major
zygomatic muscle, lesser	musculus zygomaticus minor

Table of Veins

vein	vena (pl. venae)
accessory cephalic vein	vena cephalica accessoria
accessory hemiazygos vein	vena hemiazygos accessoria
accessory saphenous vein	vena saphena accessoria
accessory vertebral vein	vena vertebralis accessoria
accompanying vein	vena comitans
accompanying vein of hypoglossal nerve	vena comitans nervi hypoglossi
adrenal veins	venae suprarenales
afferent veins	
anastomotic vein, inferior	vena anastomotica inferior
anastomotic vein, superior	vena anastomotica superior
angular vein	vena angularis
anonymous veins	venae brachiocephalicae
antebrachial vein, median	vena intermedia antebrachii
anterior auricular vein	vena auricularis anterior
anterior cardiac veins	venae cordis anteriores
anterior cardinal veins	
anterior cerebral vein	vena cerebri anterior
anterior facial vein	
anterior intercostal veins	venae intercostales anteriores
anterior jugular vein	vena jugularis anterior
anterior labial veins	venae labiales anteriores
anterior pontomesencephalic vein	vena pontomesencephalica anterior
anterior scrotal veins	venae scrotales anteriores
anterior vein of septum pellucidum	vena septi pellucidi anterior
anterior veins of heart	venae ventriculi dextri anteriores
anterior veins of right ventricle	venae ventriculi dextri anteriores
anterior tibial veins	venae tibiales anteriores
anterior vertebral vein	vena vertebralis anterior
appendicular vein	vena appendicularis
aqueduct of cochlea, vein of	vena aqueductus cochleae
aqueduct of vestibule, vein of	vena aqueductus vestibuli

vein	vena (pl. venae)

aqueous veins

arciform veins of kidney

arcuate veins of kidney | venae arcuatae renis

arterial vein | vena arteriosa, truncus pulmonalis

arterial vein of Soemmering | vena portae hepatis

articular veins | venae articulares

ascending veins of Rosenthal | venae inferiores cerebri

ascending lumbar vein | vena lumbalis ascendens

atrial veins of heart, left | venae atriales sinistrae

atrial veins of heart, right | venae atriales dextrae

atrial vein, lateral | vena lateralis atrii

atrial vein, medial | vena medialis atrii

atrioventricular veins of heart | venae atrioventriculares cordis

auditory veins, internal | venae labyrinthinae

auricular veins, anterior | venae auriculares anteriores

auricular veins, posterior | vena auricularis posterior

axillary vein | vena axillaris

azygos vein | vena azygos

basal vein, Rosenthal's | vena basalis

basilic vein | vena basilica

basivertebral vein | vena basivertebralis

Baumgarten's veins

Boyd communicating perforation veins

brachial veins | venae brachiales

brachiocephalic veins | venae brachiocephalicae

Breschet's vein | venae diploicae

bronchial veins | venae bronchiales

Browning's vein

bulb of penis, vein of | vena bulbi penis

Burow's vein

canaliculus of cochlea, vein of | vena aqueductus cochleae

capillary vein

cardiac veins | venae cordis

cardiac veins, anterior | venae ventriculi dextri anteriores

cardiac vein, great | vena cardiaca magna

cardiac vein, middle | vena cardiaca media

cardiac vein, small | vena cardiaca parva

cardiac veins, smallest | venae cardiacae minimae

cardinal veins

vein	vena (pl. venae)
carotid vein, external	vena retromandibularis
caudate nucleus, veins of	venae nuclei caudati
cavernous veins of penis	venae cavernosae penis
central veins of liver	venae centrales hepatis
central vein of retina	vena centralis retinae
central vein of suprarenal gland	vena centralis glandulae suprarenalis
cephalic vein	vena cephalica
cerebellar veins	venae cerebelli
cerebral veins	venae cerebri
cervical vein, deep	vena cervicalis profunda
choroid vein	vena choroidea
choroid veins of eye	
ciliary veins	venae ciliares
circumflex veins	venae circumflexae
cochlear aqueduct, vein of	vena aqueductus cochleae
cochlear canaliculus, vein of	vena aqueductus cochleae
Cockett communicating perforating veins	
colic vein, left	vena colica sinistra
colic vein, middle	vena colica media
colic vein, right	vena colica dextra
common basal vein	vena basalis communis
common cardinal veins (ducts of Cuvier)	
common facial vein	vena facialis communis
common iliac vein	vena iliaca communis
communicating veins (perforating veins)	
companion vein, companion veins	vena comitans, venae comitantes
condylar emissary vein	vena emissaria condylaris
conjunctival veins	venae conjunctivales
coronary vein, left	vena coronaria sinistra
coronary vein, right	vena coronaria dextra
corpus callosum, vein of, dorsal	vena dorsalis corporis callosi
corpus callosum, vein of, posterior	vena posterior corporis callosi
corpus striatum, vein of	
costoaxillary veins	venae costoaxillares
cubital vein, median	vena intermedia cubiti
cutaneous vein	vena cutanea
cutaneous vein, ulnar	vena basilica
Cuvier's veins	
cystic vein	vena cystica

vein	vena (pl. venae)
deep cerebral veins	venae cerebri profundae
deep cervical vein	vena cervicalis profunda
deep circumflex iliac vein	vena circumflexa iliaca profunda
deep veins of clitoris	venae profundae clitoridis
deep dorsal vein of clitoris	vena dorsalis clitoridis profunda
deep dorsal vein of penis	vena dorsalis penis profunda
deep epigastric vein	
deep facial vein	vena faciei profunda
deep femoral vein	vena profunda femoris
deep lingual vein	vena profunda linguae
deep middle cerebral vein	vena cerebri media profunda
deep vein of penis	vena profunda penis
deep temporal veins	venae temporales profundae
digital veins	venae digitales
diploic vein	vena diploica
dorsal callosal vein	vena corporis callosi dorsalis
dorsal veins of clitoris	venae dorsales clitoridis
dorsal vein of corpus callosum	vena corporis callosi dorsalis
dorsal digital veins of foot	venae digitales dorsales pedis
dorsal digital veins of toes	
dorsal lingual vein	venae dorsales linguae
dorsal metacarpal veins	venae metacarpeae dorsales
dorsal metatarsal veins	venae metatarseae dorsales
dorsal veins of penis, deep	vena dorsalis profunda penis
dorsal scapular vein	vena scapularis dorsalis
dorsispinal veins	
emissary vein	vena emissaria
emulgent vein	
epigastric veins, superior	venae epigastricae superiores
episcleral veins	venae episclerales
esophageal veins	venae esophageae
ethmoidal veins	venae ethmoidales
external iliac vein	vena iliaca externa
external jugular vein	vena jugularis externa
external nasal veins	venae nasales externae
external pudendal veins	venae pudendae externae
eyelids, veins of	
facial vein	vena facialis
femoral vein	vena femoralis

vein	vena (pl. venae)
fibular veins	venae fibulares
frontal veins	venae frontales
Galen, veins of	venae internae cerebri
gastric veins	venae gastricae
gastroepiploic vein, left	vena gastro-omentalis sinistra
gastroepiploic vein, right	vena gastro-omentalis dextra
gastro-omental vein, left	vena gastro-omentalis sinistra
gastro-omental vein, right	vena gastro-omentalis dextra
genicular veins	venae geniculares
gluteal veins, inferior	venae gluteae inferiores
gluteal veins, superior	venae gluteae superiores
great cardiac vein	vena cordis magna
great cerebral vein	
great cerebral vein of Galen	vena cerebri magna
great vein of Galen	
great saphenous vein	vena saphena magna
hemiazygos vein	vena hemiazygos
hemorrhoidal veins	venae rectales
hepatic veins	venae hepaticae
hepatic portal vein	
highest intercostal vein	vena intercostalis suprema
hypogastric vein	vena iliaca interna
ileal veins	venae ileales
ileocolic vein	vena ileocolica
iliac vein, common	vena iliaca communis
iliac vein, external	vena iliaca externa
iliac vein, internal	vena iliaca interna
iliolumbar vein	vena iliolumbalis
inferior anastomotic vein	vena anastomotica inferior
inferior basal vein	vena basalis inferior
inferior cardiac vein	
inferior veins of cerebellar hemisphere	venae hemispherii cerebelli inferiores
inferior cerebral veins	venae cerebri inferiores
inferior choroid vein	vena choroidea inferior
inferior epigastric vein	vena epigastrica inferior
inferior eyelid veins	
inferior gluteal veins	venae gluteae inferiores
inferior hemorrhoidal veins	
inferior labial vein	vena labialis inferior

vein	vena (pl. venae)
inferior laryngeal vein	vena laryngea inferior
inferior mesenteric vein	vena mesenterica inferior
inferior ophthalmic vein	vena ophthalmica inferior
inferior palpebral veins	venae palpebrales inferiores
inferior phrenic vein	vena phrenica inferior
inferior rectal veins	venae rectales inferiores
inferior thalamostriate veins	venae thalamostriatae inferiores
inferior thyroid vein	vena thyroidea inferior
inferior ventricular vein	vena ventricularis inferior
inferior vein of vermis	vena vermis inferior
innominate veins	venae brachiocephalicae
innominate cardiac veins (Vieussens' veins)	
insular veins	venae insulares
intercapitular veins	venae intercapitales
intercostal veins	venae intercostales
interlobar veins of kidney	venae interlobares renis
interlobular veins of kidney	venae interlobulares renis
interlobular veins of liver	venae interlobulares hepatis
intermediate antebrachial vein	
intermediate basilic vein	vena intermedia basilica
intermediate cephalic vein	vena intermedia cephalica
intermediate colic vein	vena colica media
intermediate cubital vein	
intermediate vein of forearm	
internal auditory veins	
internal cerebral veins	venae cerebri internae
internal iliac vein	vena iliaca interna
internal jugular vein	vena jugularis interna
internal pudendal vein	vena pudenda interna
internal thoracic vein	vena thoracica interna
interosseous veins	venae interosseae
intersegmental veins	pars intersegmentalis
intervertebral vein	vena intervertebralis
intrasegmental veins	pars intrasegmentalis
jejunal and ileal veins	venae jejunales et ilei
jugular veins	venae jejunales
key vein	
kidney, veins of	venae renis
knee, veins of	venae genus

vein	vena (pl. venae)
Krukenberg's veins	venae centrales hepatis
Labbe's vein (acute e)	vena anastomotica inferior
labial veins	venae labiales
labyrinthine veins	venae labyrinthi
lacrimal vein	vena lacrimalis
large vein	vena magna
large saphenous vein	vena saphena magna
laryngeal vein, superior	vena laryngea superior
Latarget's vein	
lateral atrial vein	vena atrii lateralis
lateral circumflex femoral veins	venae circumflexae femoris laterales
lateral direct veins	venae directae laterales
lateral vein of lateral ventricle	vena atrii lateralis
lateral recess of fourth ventricle, vein of	vena recessus lateralis ventriculi quarti
lateral sacral veins	venae sacrales laterales
lateral thoracic vein	vena thoracica lateralis
left colic vein	vena colica sinistra
left coronary vein	vena coronaria sinistra
left gastric vein	vena gastrica sinistra
left gastroepiploic vein	vena gastro-omentalis sinistra
left gastro-omental vein	vena gastro-omentalis sinistra
left hepatic veins	venae hepaticae sinistrae
left inferior pulmonary vein	vena pulmonalis inferior sinistra
left ovarian vein	vena ovarica sinistra
left superior intercostal vein	vena intercostalis superior sinistra
left superior pulmonary vein	vena pulmonalis superior sinistra
left suprarenal vein	vena suprarenalis sinistra
left testicular vein	vena testicularis sinistra
left umbilical vein	vena umbilicalis sinistra
levoatrio-cardinal vein	
lingual vein	vena lingualis
long saphenous vein	vena saphena longus
long thoracic vein	vena thoracica longus
lumbar veins	venae lumbales
Marshall's oblique vein	
masseteric veins	venae massetericae
mastoid emissary vein	vena emissaria mastoidea
maxillary vein	vena maxillaris
Mayo's vein	

vein	vena (pl. venae)
medial atrial vein	vena atrii medialis
medial circumflex femoral veins	venae circumflexae femoris mediales
medial vein of lateral ventricle	vena atrii medialis
median antebrachial vein	vena intermedia antebrachii
median basilic vein	vena intermedia basilic
median cephalic vein	vena intermedia cephalica
median cubital vein	vena intermedia cubiti
median vein of forearm	vena intermedia antebrachii
median vein of neck	vena mediana colli
median sacral vein	vena sacralis mediana
mediastinal veins	venae mediastinales
median vein	vena intermedia
medulla oblongata, veins of	venae medullae oblongatae
meningeal veins	venae meningeae
mesencephalic veins	venae mesencephalicae
mesenteric vein, inferior	vena mesenterica inferior
mesenteric vein, superior	vena mesenterica superior
metacarpal veins	venae metacarpales
middle cardiac vein	vena cordis media
middle colic vein	vena colica media
middle hemorrhoidal veins	venae rectales mediae
middle hepatic veins	venae hepaticae mediae
middle meningeal veins	venae meningeae mediae
middle rectal veins	venae rectales mediae
middle temporal vein	vena temporalis media
middle thyroid vein	vena thyroidea media
musculophrenic veins	venae musculophrenicae
nasofrontal vein	vena nasofrontalis
oblique vein of left atrium	vena obliqua atrii sinistri
obturator vein	vena obturatoria
occipital vein	vena occipitalis
occipital cerebral veins	venae occipitales
occipital emissary vein	vena emissaria occipitalis
olfactory gyrus, vein of	vena gyri olfactorii
ophthalmic vein, inferior	vena ophthalmica inferior
ophthalmic vein, superior	vena ophthalmica superior
ovarian vein, left	vena ovarica sinistra
ovarian vein, right	vena ovarica dextra
palatine vein	vena palatina

vein	vena (pl. venae)
palmar digital veins	venae digitales palmares
palmar metacarpal veins	venae metacarpeae palmares
palpebral veins	venae palpebrales
pancreatic veins	venae pancreaticae
pancreaticoduodenal veins	venae pancreaticoduodenales
paraumbilical veins	venae paraumbilicales
parietal veins	venae parietales
parietal emissary vein	vena emissaria parietalis
parotid veins	venae parotidea
pectoral veins	venae pectorales
peduncular veins	venae pedunculares
perforating veins	venae perforantes
pericardiac veins	venae pericardiales
pericardiacophrenic veins	venae pericardiacophrenicae
pericardial veins	venae pericardiacae
peroneal veins	venae peroneae
petrosal vein	vena petrosa
pharyngeal veins	venae pharyngeae
phrenic veins	venae phrenicae
plantar digital veins	venae digitales plantares
plantar metatarsal veins	venae metatarseae plantares
pontine veins	venae pontis
popliteal vein	vena poplitea
portal vein	vena portae hepatis
posterior anterior jugular vein	vena jugularis posterior anterior
posterior auricular vein	vena auricularis posterior
posterior cardinal veins	
posterior facial vein	vena retromandibularis
posterior horn, vein of	vena cornus posterioris
posterior intercostal veins	venae intercostales posteriores
posterior labial veins	venae labiales posteriores
posterior vein of left ventricle	vena posterior ventriculi sinistri
posterior marginal vein	vena corporis callosi dorsalis
posterior parotid veins	venae parotideae posterioreae
posterior pericallosal vein	vena corporis callosi dorsalis
posterior scrotal veins	venae scrotales posteriores
posterior vein of left ventricle	vena ventriculi sinistri posterior
posterior vein of septum pellucidum	vena septi pellucidi posterior
posterior tibial veins	venae tibiales posteriores

vein	vena (pl. venae)
precardinal veins	
precentral cerebellar vein	vena precentralis cerebelli
prefrontal veins	venae prefrontales
prepyloric vein	vena prepylorica
pterygoid canal, vein of	vena canalis pterygoidei
pudendal veins	venae pudendae
pulmonary veins	venae pulmonales
pyloric vein	vena gastrica dextra
radial veins	venae radiales
ranine vein	vena sublingualis
rectal veins	venae rectales
renal veins	venae renales
retromandibular vein	vena retromandibularis
Retzius' veins	
right colic vein	vena colica dextra
right gastric vein	vena gastrica dextra
right gastroepiploic vein	vena gastro-omentalis dextra
right gastro-omental vein	vena gastro-omentalis dextra
right hepatic veins	venae hepaticae dextrae
right inferior pulmonary vein	vena pulmonalis inferior dextra
right ovarium vein	vena ovarica dextra
right superior intercostal vein	vena intercostalis superior dextra
right superior pulmonary vein	vena pulmonalis superior dextra
right suprarenal vein	vena suprarenalis dextra
right testicular vein	vena testicularis dextra
Rosenthal's vein	
Ruysch's veins	
sacral veins	venae sacrales
Santorini's vein	
saphenous veins	venae saphenae
Sappey's veins	venae paraumbilicales
scleral veins	venae sclerales
scrotal veins	venae scrotales
septum pellucidum, vein of, anterior	vena anterior septi pellucidi
septum pellucidum, vein of, posterior	vena posterior septi pellucidi
short gastric veins	venae gastricae breves
short saphenous vein	vena saphena breve
sigmoid veins	venae sigmoideae
small vein of heart	vena cardiaca parva

vein	vena (pl. venae)
small cardiac vein	vena cordis parva
smallest cardiac veins	venae cordis minimae
small saphenous vein	vena saphena parva
spermatic vein	vena spermatica
spinal veins	venae spinales
spiral vein of modiolus	vena spiralis modioli
splenic vein	vena splenica
stellate veins of kidney	venulae stellatae renis
Stensen's veins	venae vorticosae
sternocleidomastoid vein	vena sternocleidomastoidea
striate veins	venae thalamostriatae inferiores
stylomastoid vein	vena stylomastoidea
subclavian vein	vena subclavia
subcostal vein	vena subcostalis
subcutaneous veins of abdomen	venae subcutaneae abdominis
sublingual vein	vena sublingualis
sublobular veins	
submental vein	vena submentalis
superficial vein	vena superficialis
superficial cerebral veins	venae cerebri superficiales
superficial circumflex iliac ven	vena circumflexa iliaca superficialis
superficial dorsal veins of clitoris	venae dorsales clitoridis superficiales
superficial dorsal veins of penis	venae dorsales penis superficiales
superficial epigastric vein	vena epigastrica superficialis
superficial middle cerebral vein	vena cerebri media superficialis
superficial temporal veins	venae temporales superficiales
superior anastomotic vein	vena anastomotica superior
superior basal vein	vena basalis superior
superior veins of cerebellar hemisphere	venae hemispherii cerebelli superiores
superior cerebral veins	venae cerebri superiores
superior choroid vein	vena choroidea superior
superior epigastric veins	venae epigastricae superiores
superior eyelid, veins of	
superior gluteal veins	venae gluteae superiores
superior hemorrhoidal vein	vena rectales superior
superior intercostal vein	vena intercostalis superior
superior labial vein	vena labialis superior
superior laryngeal vein	vena laryngea superior
superior mesenteric vein	vena mesenterica superior

vein	vena (pl. venae)
superior ophthalmic vein	vena ophthalmica superior
superior palpebral veins	venae palpebrales superiores
superior phrenic veins	venae phrenicae superiores
superior rectal vein	vena rectalis superior
superior thalamostriate vein	vena thalamostriata superior
superior thyroid vein	vena thyroidea superior
superior vein of vermis	vena vermis superior
supraorbital vein	vena supraorbitalis
suprarenal veins	venae suprarenales
suprascapular vein	vena suprascapularis
supratrochlear veins	venae supratrochleares
supreme intercostal vein	vena intercostalis suprema
sural veins	venae surales
surface thalamic veins	venae directae laterales
sylvian vein, vein of sylvian fossa	vena mediae superficiales cerebri
temporal veins	venae temporales
temporomandibular joint, veins of	venae articulares temporomandibulares
temporomaxillary vein	vena temporomaxillaris
terminal vein	vena thalamostriata superior
testicular veins	venae testiculares
thalamostriate veins	venae thalamostriatae
thebesian veins	venae cordis minimae
thoracic veins	venae thoracicae
thoracoacromial vein	vena thoracoacromialis
thoracoepigastric vein	vena thoracoepigastrica
thymic veins	venae thymicae
thyroid veins	venae thyroideae
tibial veins	venae tibiales
trabecular veins	
tracheal veins	venae tracheales
transverse cervical veins	venae transversae colli
transverse facial vein	vena transversa faciei
transverse veins of neck	venae transversae cervicis
transverse vein of scapula	venae transversae scapulae
Trolard's vein	vena anastomotica superior
tympanic veins	venae tympanicae
ulnar veins	venae ulnares
umbilical vein	vena umbilicalis
uncus, vein of	vena unci

vein	vena (pl. venae)
upper limb, veins of	venae membri superioris
uterine veins	venae uterinae
varicose veins	
vena cava, inferior	vena cava inferior
vena cava, superior	vena cava superior
ventricular veins of heart	venae ventriculares cordis
vermis, inferior vein of	vena inferior vermis
vertebral vein	vena vertebralis
vertebral column, veins of	venae columnae vertebralis
vesalian vein	
Vesalius' vein	
vesical veins	venae vesicales
vestibular veins	venae vestibulares
vestibular aqueduct, vein of	vena aqueductus vestibuli
vestibular bulb, vein of	vena bulbi vestibuli
vidian veins	venae canalis pterygoidei
Vieussens' veins	venae cardiacae anteriores
vitelline vein	vena vitellina
vortex veins (vorticose veins)	venae vorticosae